KU-222-805

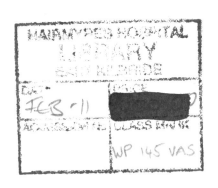

Gynecologic Oncology

Gynecologic Oncology
Evidence-Based Perioperative and Supportive Care

Second Edition

Edited by

Scott E. Lentz, MD
Regional Director of Gynecologic Oncology
Southern California Permanente Medical Group
Los Angeles Medical Center

Allison E. Axtell, MD
Gynecologic Oncology
Southern California Permanente Medical Group
Los Angeles Medical Center

Steven A. Vasilev, MD, MBA
Clinical Professor, Gynecologic Oncology
UCLA-Geffen School of Medicine
Southern California Permanente Medical Group
Los Angeles Medical Center

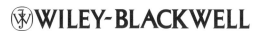

A John Wiley & Sons, Inc., Publication

For general information on our other products and services or for technical support, please contact our
Customer Care Department within the United States at (800) 762-2974, outside the United States at
(317) 572-3993 or fax (317) 572-4002.

Wiley also publishes its books in a variety of electronic formats. Some content that appears in print may
not be available in electronic formats. For more information about Wiley products, visit our web site at
www.wiley.com

Library of Congress Cataloging-in-Publication Data:

Lentz, Scott E.
    Gynecologic oncology : evidence-based perioperative and supportive care /
    Scott E. Lentz, Allison E. Axtell, Steven A. Vasilev. – 2nd ed.
        p. ; cm.
    Rev. ed. of: Perioperative and supportive care in gynecologic oncology:
    evidence-based management / edited by Steven A. Vasilev. c2000.
    Includes bibliographical references.
    ISBN 978-0-470-08340-6 (cloth)
        1. Generative organs, Female–Surgery.   2. Evidence-based medicine.
3. Clinical medicine–Decision making.   I. Axtell, Allison E.   II. Vasilev, Steven A.
III. Perioperative and supportive care in gynecologic oncology.   IV. Title.
        [DNLM: 1. Genital Neoplasms, Female–surgery.   2. Critical Care–methods.
3. Evidence-Based Medicine.   4.Gynecology–methods.
5. Perioperative Care–methods. WP 145]
    RG104.P393 2010
    618.1′059–dc22
                                                                    2010033322
Printed in Singapore

10   9   8   7   6   5   4   3   2   1

This manuscript is humbly offered as an attempt to focus our lives as physicians onto our greatest goal—superior quality care delivered in a compassionate and meaningful way.

The product of this effort would not have been possible without our richest sources of support. For SEL—this is for my children, John, Madison and Timothy, who continually remind me that life is what happens while I'm waiting for the next big thing; and my wife Amelia, a savior in more ways than I can verbalize. For SAV—this is for my mother, Katharina, a lifelong source of support and encouragement; my two sons, Alex and Andrei, sources of emotional inspiration and vibrant reflections of a continuous youthful zeal for learning, and my loving wife Joyce who regularly redirects me towards those people, things and moments that matter most in life.

Most importantly this is for our patients, an endless source of fascination, learning, instruction and inspiration.

Scott E. Lentz, MD
Allison E. Axtell, MD
Steven A. Vasilev, MD, MBA

Contents

Foreword to the Second Edition

The information provided in this edition is much needed in the everyday management of patients with gynecologic cancer. This clinically practical textbook provides guidelines that are critical for excellent preoperative, perioperative, and supportive care of gynecologic oncology patients. Special effort has been made to employ the principles of evidence-based medicine derived from scientific studies, whenever available. A separate discussion on why evidence-based medical treatment is so important is included.

The second edition differs from the first one in several important ways: In this edition, special attention has been paid to evidence-based reviews of each of the major disease sites in gynecologic oncology. Not included in this edition are ancillary topics of the first edition, such as intensive care management, anesthetic issues, and perioperative radiology. These topics, though very important, were felt to distract from the specific goals in the title. A very practical chapter on the prevention and treatment of laparoscopic complications is included. A new, but very useful, section on the management of end-of-life complications (common in patients with advanced gynecologic cancer) such as tumor-related bowel obstruction, persistent ascites, and pleural effusion is also included. In addition, this edition has discussions on the ever-challenging pain management issues faced by the physicians and caregivers at the end of life of the patient. The role of perioperative herbal supplements, along with necessary precautions, is discussed in detail.

Those who perform surgeries for gynecologic cancer as well as those who carry out benign gynecologic procedures will find this edition to be a most helpful guide. Residents and fellows in obstetrics and gynecology will find an abundance of useful information in this text.

LEO D. LAGASSE, MD
Professor Emeritus
Department of Obstetrics and Gynecology
David Geffen School of Medicine at UCLA

Contributors

Denise Aberle, MD, Professor, Department of Radiological Sciences, UCLA School of Medicine, Los Angeles, CA

Malaika E. Amneus, MD, Assistant Professor, Division of Gynecologic Oncology, Olive View-UCLA Medical Center, Sylmar, CA

Allison E. Axtell, MD, Gynecologic Oncologist, Division of Gynecologic Oncology, Southern California Permanente Medical Group, Los Angeles Medical Center, Los Angeles, CA

Margarett C. Ellison, MD, MHA, Gynecologic Oncologist, Piedmont Gynecologic Oncology, Atlanta, GA

Nicole Fleming, MD, Fellow, Division of Gynecologic Oncology, Department of Obstetrics and Gynecology, UCLA Geffen School of Medicine, Los Angeles, CA

Laszlo Z. Galffy, MD, Anesthesia and Pain Management Center of Glendale, CA

Paul Koonings, MD, Director of Gynecologic Oncology, Kaiser Permanente, San Diego, CA

Leo Lagasse, MD, FACS, FACOG, Director of Gynecologic Oncology, Cedars-Sinai Comprehensive Cancer Center, Professor of Gynecology, University of California, Los Angeles, CA

Scott E. Lentz, MD, Regional Director of Gynecologic Oncology Services, Southern California Permanente Medical Group, Kaiser Permanente Los Angeles Medical Center, Los Angeles, CA

Kathryn F. McGonigle, MD, FACS, FACOG, Assistant Professor, UCLA School of Medicine, Division of Gynecologic Oncology, UCLA School of Medicine Los Angeles, CA

Judith McKay, PhD, Psychologist

R. Wendel Naumann, MD, Director Minimally Invasive Surgery in Gynecologic Oncology, Associate Director of Gynecologic Oncology, Blumenthal Cancer Center, Carolinas Medical Center, Charlotte, NC

Matthew Powers, MD, Resident, Department of Surgery, Keck School of Medicine, University of Southern California, Los Angeles, CA

Howard Silberman, MD, FACS, Professor of Surgery, Keck School of Medicine, University of Southern California, Los Angeles, CA

Harriet Smith, MD, Professor, Division of Gynecologic Oncology, Montifiore Medical Center, Bronx, NY

Amy Stenson, MD, Assistant Professor, Department of Obstetrics and Gynecology, UCLA Geffen School of Medicine, Los Angeles, CA

Devansu Tewari, MD, Gynecologic Oncologist, Southern California Permanente Medical Group, Sand Canyon Hospital, Anaheim, CA

Fidel A. Valea, MD, Associate Professor, Division of Gynecology Oncology, Department of Obstetrics and Gynecology, Duke University Health System, Durham, NC

Clayton A. Varga, MD, MHSM, Pasadena Rehabilitation Institute, Pasadena, CA

Alexander Vasilev, BA, AB, Clinical Research Associate, Department of Obstetrics and Gynecology, Kaiser Permanente Los Angeles Medical Center, Los Angeles, CA

Steven A. Vasilev, MD, MBA, FACOG, FACS, Director, Surgical and Radiation Oncology Clinical Trials Director, Gynecologic Oncology Integrative Therapies, Kaiser Permanente Los Angeles Medical Center, Clinical Professor, UCLA David Geffen School of Medicine, Los Angeles, CA

Part One

General Principles

Chapter 1

Introduction

Steven A. Vasilev, MD, MBA and Scott E. Lentz, MD

"Learning without thinking is useless. Thinking without learning is dangerous."

—Confucius

TOWARD EVIDENCE-BASED MEDICAL PRACTICE

The very roots of Osler's apprentice-based medical education and practice, to which we still largely adhere, are being severed. Lest this be interpreted as a call to arms, Osler noted that his textbook of medicine was based on "personal experience correlated with the general experience of others."[1] This is a far cry from practice based on randomized clinical trials or even scientific evidence from observational studies. With all due respect to Osler, it is a fact that his method of practice and learning should have little place in contemporary medicine.

Patients would find it almost laughable that the evolution of current medical care has largely followed a "trial and error" pattern, driven by an educational system that was centered on the apprenticeship model. Our forefathers were educated based on the clinical experience of their mentors, and propagated the perceptions, attitudes, and behaviors with which they were presented. While exceptions to this model clearly existed, it has only been in the very recent past that the medical literature began to demand careful statistical analysis of published conclusions. The era of rigorous review of published material marked the beginning of a sea change in medical thinking.

Information in medicine creates advantage, whether that is due to more rapid diagnosis and treatment or clarity of understanding that opens the doors to discovery and progress. The trouble has been that the discipline of medicine is so broad that no single physician could master every facet and be expected to constantly integrate the rapidly changing landscape of new findings. The effective practice of medicine requires that new information be constantly incorporated, and yet the information

Gynecologic Oncology: Evidence-Based Perioperative and Supportive Care, Second Edition.
Edited by Scott E. Lentz, Allison E. Axtell and Steven A. Vasilev.
© 2011 John Wiley & Sons, Inc. Published 2011 by John Wiley & Sons, Inc.

sources that clinicians typically use fail to provide enough valuable data. To correct this problem, the notion of "evidence-based medicine (EBM)" has grown since its inception in the early 1990s. Evidence-based medicine was so-named as a means of communicating high-quality information to busy clinicians who were overwhelmed by the burgeoning body of literature in their field.

One widely published definition of EBM is "the conscientious, explicit and judicious use of the current best evidence in making decisions about the care of individual patients."[2] This definition highlights a critical piece of the EBM paradigm that is easily overlooked: medical evidence is generated based on evaluations of multiple measurements and yet, this information must be applied in the singular. Phrased another way, if we tell a patient that they have a 35% chance that their cancer will return after treatment, is it unreasonable for them to reply, "Which 35% of my body will the cancer involve?"

> *Evidence-Based Medicine [is] the process of systematically finding, appraising, and using contemporaneous research findings as the basis for clinical decisions. Evidence-based medicine asks (sic) questions, finds and appraises the relevant data, and harnesses that information for everyday clinical practice. Evidence-based medicine follows four steps: formulate a clear clinical question from a patient's problem; search the literature for relevant clinical articles; evaluate (critically appraise) the evidence for its validity and usefulness; implement useful findings in clinical practice.[3]*

Public perception of medical care has evolved over the convoluted history of medicine. Surgeons no longer are double as barbers, and the general distrust of inpatient medicine has been replaced with an apparent reliance on the supremacy of the hospital. The modern era of medicine has heralded a widespread respect and wonder at the seemingly endless series of "miracles" that characterize progress from the days of Lister and childbed fever. In the current market of aggressive competition for faculty and patients, the role of information in medicine has never been more pronounced.

Radical changes are in motion in health-care delivery. So far they have been initiated externally and are often based on business and cost considerations. Much of this has been out of the individual physician's control to say nothing about their understanding. As a result, health care has evolved from a cottage to a mainstream industry and the physician has largely been left out of this evolutionary loop. Is there some fault on the physician's part that has allowed this loss of control? If so, what is it? Is it possible that maximum physician independence, revered above all else and at all costs, has undermined the ability for physicians to regain control of health-care delivery? If physician independence means preserving unexplained practice variance, which is currently out of control, perhaps physicians *are* their own worst enemy.

W. Edwards Deming, a statistician and management leader who taught quality as a system to the Japanese, spoke of variance management as being at the very core of quality improvement.[4] Of course, in contrast to manufacturing, zero tolerance for variance and defects is not often possible in medicine. The focus must instead be on narrowing the range between upper and lower limits of a process. To this end, when a procedure or diagnostic test falls within a reasonable range of indications and evidence, the system process is in control. When procedures performed fall well outside this range, or if the range is exceedingly wide, the system process is out of control. Such is the case with health care, both on a micro- and macroscale. For decades, many studies have documented overuse of specific medical services, which are sometimes solely based on geographic location (e.g., certain cities have higher coronary bypass surgery rates with no local increased epidemiologic risk factors to explain this). Essentially, these practice patterns are "unexplained" by reasonable common causes or indications. In other words, reasonable variation in practice patterns is exceeded too often. One study specifically noted that 10%–27% of hysterectomies among women enrolled in seven health plans were performed for totally inappropriate reasons.[5] Multiple studies performed by the RAND Corporation and others document similar findings and illuminate a quality problem in that patients are being subjected to risk of adverse consequences without documented benefit.[6] It is worth repeating that the goal is not to achieve zero variance, rather merely to reduce practice variance to levels supported by existing evidence of benefit.

Perhaps we are asking the wrong primary questions and setting the wrong goals. For example, a commonly debated question is, "how can we reduce costs?" Should we instead be asking how we could improve the quality of care, minimizing unjustifiable and unexplainable practice variance? Is it possible that costs could be effectively reduced as a byproduct to this alternative and more palatable primary question? If the correct goals were set, could there be an alignment of effort toward true physician driven optimally managed care?

Is practice variance reduction and quality improvement via evidence-based guidelines just another medical "management fad" being foisted upon physicians? After all, there is a veritable alphabet soup proliferation of managed care and business based "buzz" words, reflecting the driving forces in the evolution of health-care delivery, usually not in concert with medical terminology: CQI, TQM, PDCA, EBM, LOS, Juran, Deming, etc. There are also more than 1500 practice guidelines in print and countless critical pathways. Most organizations seemingly have generated a set, but practical impact has been underwhelming. Can these help? How exactly? Are guidelines the same as critical pathways? Are these pathways just a "nursing thing"? How can we expect externally applied forces, embodied by practice guidelines forged by "expert" consensus panels, to be truly incorporated into better practice patterns at the local level? Certainly, unless the very best concepts in guideline development and evidence-based practice are actually implemented, there would be no net effect in patient care and cost efficiencies. Thus far, in fact, there has been no net impact. Perhaps we are not only asking the wrong questions but also taking the wrong approach. Perhaps the best solutions will come from individual physicians self-adjusting practice patterns based on evidence and outcomes rather than directives mandated from externally generated guidelines.

Is there a paradigm among all of the confusion that is workable? Is there a means by which the positive thrust toward value-added (outcomes/cost) care, as opposed to cheapest care, could be directed by physicians? One answer might be to practice the "best medicine" possible. Obviously, this is not a new concept. However, as we generate more and more data and publish it in a forest of journals, the ability to keep up gives way to information overload. Additionally, not all data has the same strength and the quality varies, and thus the *data* may not translate into good practical *information*. Along these lines, the randomized controlled clinical trial has been a gold standard and usually carries more weight than a case report/series or a consensus panel report. However, despite the estimated 250,000 or so randomized clinical trials that have confirmed the relative efficacy of many treatments, there is still a paucity of such studies to guide certain medical practice decisions. Without actually reading every single published journal, often in specialties that do not normally cross our desk, it is simply impossible for the average clinician to keep up with what is proven and what is not, and with what strength of evidence.

Ideally, to optimally obtain and use information, physicians would need electronic databases with continually updated data that is properly analyzed and processed. Most, if not all, practicing physicians either don't have this readily available or are not facile in searching current literature.[7] Problem-based electronic database searches, using tools such as the MEDLINE, to answer specific questions are still infrequently used and may be incomplete since full article text may not be immediately available. In practice, the tendency is to evaluate problems based only on personal and often antiquated experience, or refer to respected authorities.[7] Commonly, we refer to readily available resources such as textbooks to answer specific questions. The challenge inherent to this approach is in maintaining a full and up-to-date library, which is usually impossible.

Printed text, such as this book, will be criticized as being outdated no sooner than its publication. This is a potentially valid criticism. Much of what is summarized in this textbook is in fact not new, and in some areas quite dated but axiomatic. Nevertheless, it represents the best evidence known to the contributors to date. As long as one is aware of this limitation, by the 80/20 rule, it is generally true that 80% of evidence is relatively static and 20% represents new findings. In most cases, it is really the former scenario that is the bigger problem in practice variance minimization. In many instances, the main point is the *lack* of data to support efficacy of generally accepted common interventions. Of greater concern, despite strong data to support one point or another in patient care improvement, is that many physicians continue to practice status quo simply because "that is the way we have always done it." In some cases, the available evidence is rapidly evolving and in other areas good solid evidence in existence for years or even decades has not been incorporated into general practice.

Are we discussing "cookbook medicine" here? Not at all. Medicine is still both an art and science and will continue as such so long as we treat human beings and not machines or biomechanical hybrids. However, we now have the operational tools to maximize the science while still supporting the art of delivering compassionate and effective care. Some of these tools are introduced in this text and the best evidence for perioperative and supportive care issues is presented. Selected chapters contain more axiomatic material than others. We have attempted to highlight controversial areas. However, this is a *synopsis* of evidence regarding general principles of perioperative care. As such, this textbook is not intended to be comprehensive and the reader is referred to the multiple excellent references within each chapter or to other works.

For all of the major technological advances in medicine, it is the struggle between art and science that defines medicine and separates it from aviation or manufacturing "widgets." EBM demands that clinicians integrate the best available information on the behalf of their patients, simultaneously considering the individual patient factors and the best available evidence pertinent to the clinical situation. It is the critical thinking of the physician that allows EBM to thrive and acts as a counterbalance against practice limited by the most proximate clinical experience. Good physicians can integrate individual clinical expertise and the best available evidence because neither alone is enough. The centrality of this concept is summarized expertly by Sackett[2]:

> *Without clinical expertise, a practice risks becoming tyrannised by evidence, for even excellent external evidence may be inapplicable to or inappropriate for an individual patient. Without current best evidence, practice risks becoming rapidly out of date, to the detriment of patients.*

PERIOPERATIVE AND CRITICAL CARE ECONOMICS

At the societal decision-making level, we must ultimately balance the focus on *maximum* acute care with *optimal* care of an aging population. While some chronic and catastrophic diseases, such as cancer, often cannot be cured, patients still need relief from symptoms and minimization of disease-related complications and dysfunction. All of these issues touch upon supply and demand realities and opportunity costs. Maximizing efficiencies and minimizing unexplained practice variance will go a long way toward conservation of scarce resources and improved outcomes, and will contribute to overall cost reduction in health-care delivery services.

If one adopts a classic economic marginal analysis approach toward mortality, morbidity, level and extent of ICU care, complications, and avoidance thereof, one can isolate the incremental impact of each decision on quality and costs. Key questions might be as follows: During preoperative evaluation, prevention of complications is key to decreased morbidity and length of stay. How much more, or perhaps less, is required as a diagnostic input to achieve a given superior quality output? During perioperative care, what incremental opportunities exist for prevention with appropriate surveillance and management that are based on good evidence? In using new technologies, or even older technologies, what is the appropriate incremental use of such resources and what are their limitations toward optimizing outcomes?

EBM exists then as a tool, but not a substitute for the clinician. The proper implementation of EBM has driven the growth of an entire field of medicine, replete with its own experts, critics, proponents, and detractors. The most widely understood conceptual framework of EBM is the idea of the hierarchy of evidence. This is referred to as the first fundamental principle of EBM, and is discussed in more detail in Chapter 2. Even though randomized clinical trials are the gold standard, there absolutely is a place for cohort studies, case–control studies, and other "lesser" evidence. This does not mean that issues that are not defined by randomized trials are incompletely tested. All levels of evidence are worthwhile, and best evidence is exactly that—the best that can be generated for a topic. The second fundamental principle of EBM is the idea that regardless of the level of evidence, value and preference judgments are implicit in every clinical decision.[8]

It is important to recognize that EBM is not without its limitations. As with any effective tool, it is perhaps easier to misuse rather than properly utilize it. Tragedy can result from paying attention to poor quality evidence instead of good quality evidence, and critical appraisal cannot be abandoned for blind acceptance. Many medical schools and training programs, in a form of premature closure, are moving away from teaching the fundamentals of careful evidence appraisal to emphasize the implementation of evidence. The intent of this new focus is to produce high-quality, safe, and low-cost care (i.e., Accreditation Council for Graduate Medical Education competencies of systems-based practice and improvement and practice-based learning). However, abandoning appropriate skepticism regarding the effectiveness of these interventions may lead to large investments in quality improvement, safety, and efficiency activities that fail to yield the expected benefits.

The same can be said for incorrectly applying population-based models to best practices in individual care. Major pronouncements about a particular action or intervention are not served by EBM, and those who try to misuse the literature in this way risk harming the very group that they have sworn to protect. Regardless of one's perspective on EBM, the discipline reflects the desire of all involved in patient care to improve the quality of patient care.

OPERATIONAL TOOLS OVERVIEW

This textbook strives to present the best available evidence for decision making in perioperative and supportive care in the gynecologic oncology patient. It also introduces some operational mindsets and tools. Questions *that this textbooks* addresses include *the following*:

- What is evidence-based medicine? How does one find all the available data? What if there is no good data? How does one evaluate which evidence is best for the given situation?
- What evidence exists toward minimizing unexplained variance and optimizing practice patterns?
- Are there any formal decision analysis methodologies that can help?
- Can these principles translate into practice guidelines that can actually be implemented and contribute to improvement?
- Is this just cookbook medicine? Or, is it a guide toward evolution of best practices specific to each physician's and patient's environment?

This textbook primarily addresses gynecologic oncology care, but can readily apply to complicated gynecologic perioperative care. Key issues are associated with a level of evidence score within the text or in algorithm form. Some chapters also contain more axiomatic information than others, and as such are not always subject to grading. In other subject areas the lack of extensive underlying evidence is striking. Chapter 2 addresses information gathering and interpretation tools. The subsequent clinical chapters present the contributing authors' best efforts to gather and synthesize up-to-date information addressing best approaches to common as well as uncommon problems in perioperative, supportive, and critical care. Some authors found data gathering and grading more second nature than others and so some biases remain. These areas should be apparent and interpreted to mean that the subject area is heavily influenced by level III data. Editing cannot always alleviate this and may confuse the reader if expert opinion meaning is altered.

This second edition is constructed largely as the first. Many of the chapter topics have remained the same, and others have been updated to include major changes in practice since the publication of the first edition. Some chapters have been deleted to narrow the focus on the perioperative nature of the text, and new chapters have been included in herbal and complimentary medicine, end-of-life decision making, and fertility-specific issues pertinent to the gynecologic oncology patient.

In summary, this is an imperfect but focused and genuine effort to present the best available information designed to help decrease practice variance toward predictable improved clinical outcomes. As presented, it is anticipated to be a kernel work in progress, constantly improved through revision, and a guide for reader-directed updating and local adaptation.

REFERENCES

1. OSLER W. The Principles and Practice of Medicine. 8th ed. New York: Appleton and Co.; 1918.
2. SACKETT DL, ROSENBERG WM, GRAY JA, et al. Evidence based medicine: what it is and what it isn't. BMJ 1996;312(7023):71–72.
3. ROSENBERG W, DONALD A. Evidence based medicine: an approach to clinical problem solving. BMJ 1995;310(6987):1122–1126.
4. WALTON M. The Deming Management Method. 1st ed. New York: Putnam Publishing Group; 1986.
5. BERNSTEIN SJ. The appropriateness of hysterectomy: a comparison of care in seven health plans. JAMA 1993;269:2398–2402.
6. CHASSIN MR. Assessing strategies for quality improvement. Health Affairs 1997;16:151–161.
7. OLATUNBOSUN OA, EDOUARD L, PIERSON RA. Physician's attitudes toward evidence based obstetric practice: a questionnaire survey. BMJ 1998;316:365–366.
8. GUYATT GH, HAYNES RB, JAESCHKE RZ, et al.; for Evidence-Based Medicine Working Group. Users' guides to the medical literature: XXV. Evidence-based medicine: principles for applying the Users' Guides to patient care: JAMA. 2000;284(10):1290–1296.

Chapter 2

Evidence-Based Medicine and Decision Support

Steven A. Vasilev, MD, MBA

WHAT IS EVIDENCE-BASED MEDICINE?

Bertrand Russell noted, "The extent to which beliefs are based on evidence is very much less than believers suppose." It is easy to see how this may be directly applicable to medical practice.

Under the protective blanket of the "art" of medical practice, decision making has often been based on anecdotal experience and incomplete utilization of the best available objective data. Physicians tend to practice based more on what their attendings taught them rather than continually researching existing evidence.[1,2] It then becomes a matter of unchanging practice routine to make decisions based mostly on personal experience and intuition. In effect, every physician may be doing what they perceive to be their best, but that is not enough. Data suggest that many decisions are made contrary to available evidence and up to half of decisions are based on weak or no evidence.[2–4] In light of this, it is essential that the medical educational process be carefully scrutinized to see if it requires transformation to optimize decision making and reproducible quality outcomes.[5–7] Largely due to inattention to the above, unexplained practice variance is a significant problem, contributing to runaway costs and a wide range of outcomes.[7–14]

W. Edwards Deming, a leader in cross-industry quality issues, stated that all of his work at the core was based on controlling variance via statistical process control (SPC).[15] What is unexplained or assignable clinical practice variance? In any industry, to maintain the quality of outcomes, operations and processes must be continually inspected and tested to minimize defects. In health care, just as in other industries, there will be variability in outcomes. The goal in health-care services might not be *zero defects* as proposed in some manufacturing scenarios, but rather minimization of variability in outcomes such that the result as a whole is of acceptable quality.

The question then becomes "Is the outcome variability following a given intervention due to chance (random) variation or assignable (nonrandom) unexplained variation?" Chance variation is that which is built into a system, such as the range of normal hemoglobins in the physiologic system of a patient. Assignable variation occurs if some portion of the system is out of control and is amenable to intervention. One of the biggest challenges is to determine if a process or activity is out of control, requiring adjustment, or not.

During the 1920s and 1930s, while at Bell Telephone Laboratories, Walter Shewhart developed *statistical control charts* to help determine when assignable variation has occurred. A repetitive operation, such as caring for a set of patients with a particular problem, will seldom, if ever, produce exactly the same result. However, the outcome variability surrounding a mean value and standard deviation will often produce a normal distribution for the population. As in any other statistical scenario, periodically examining the entire population of interest for variation in the mean is not feasible. Instead, sampling is performed along with selection of an upper control limit (UCL) and a lower control limit (LCL). If the sample mean exceeds control limits, typically set at +/−3 standard deviations in most industries, the possibility that the variation is due to chance is <0.3%. Taken one step further, it is even possible to *predict* assignable variation prior to loss of system control. Also, in some cases, assignable variation can represent improvement in process rather than loss of control and should thus be investigated.

The above brief discussion is meant to introduce the idea that unexplained clinical practice variance should be sought, the reasons identified, and a process improvement implemented. This could be on an individual practice or organizational or even societal level. Details regarding statistical process control are beyond the scope of this textbook, and the interested reader may refer other sources.[16] The key point is that tools are available to assess how unexplained variance can influence outcomes and point to areas requiring attention and correction.

Unexplained variance due to assignable variation has the potential to be significantly influenced by evidence-based medical practice. How scientific can the base for the art of medicine get? During the 1990s, it was estimated that less than 10% of clinical practice was based on solid randomized controlled clinical trial (RCT) data, and more recent reports suggest that many guidelines are still of dubious quality.[3,4,17–19] While this may be a criticism of evidence-based medicine (EBM), it reflects a core misunderstanding of EBM intent.[20,21] In fact, the other 90% of clinical practice should still be based upon the best available level of evidence or at least the understanding that a particular practice pattern or intervention is not well grounded in evidence of any kind.[18,22] This understanding alerts clinicians that their convictions may be on shaky ground and that further evaluation may be required to minimize practice variance.

What is more disturbing is that the 10% of clinical practice that *is* well grounded in solid RCT data is often not incorporated into standard patient care, and unexplained variance is seen in this group of interventions as well. Lag time between publication of compelling data and incorporation can exceed 10 years.[23]

Is EBM a new "managed care" concept? On the contrary, the concept of EBM dates back more than a century.[24,25] Recently, largely due to "managed care" pressures, it has enjoyed a resurgence of interest among divergent groups: clinicians wishing to regain control of medical practice, payors wishing to limit variance and lower costs, health-care purchasers wishing quality initiatives for better value, and the public wishing to understand what the "best" approach really is.[26] Numerous centers and Internet Web sites for evidence-based practice have been established in numerous disciplines. For example, the Cochrane Collaboration, an international multicenter venture with an internet portal (www.cochrane.org), reviews, synthesizes, and distributes data on health-care practices on an ongoing basis.[27,28] A number of EBM journals have also been introduced. Additionally, recommendations for improvement in reporting of clinical trials have been proposed and endorsed by leading journals.[29,30] These recommendations are embodied in CONSORT or Consolidated Standards of Reporting Trials (www.consort-statement.org). Related forms of standardization are proposed, such as STROBE or Strengthening the Reporting of Observational studies in Epidemiology (www.strobe-statement.org), QUOROM or QUality of Reporting of Meta-analyses, and STARD for diagnostic studies (www.stard-statement.org).[31]

This resurgence of interest in EBM has certainly faced significant criticism.[32–35] Some have interpreted it to be a fad, a pure cost cutting device, while others label it "cookbook" medicine, which at its core is an antithesis to the "art" of medicine. Much of this criticism and negative reaction is based upon the misunderstanding of terminology and philosophy. It may also be negatively associated with the decade-long continued backlash against "managed care." However, lost among this is the EBM philosophic thrust toward improvement in the quality of medical practice. Although some believe that quality de facto requires higher costs, the converse is likely true in most cases. There is no question that technology transfer will continue to affect health-care costs. However, the correct application of new and emerging technology and limitation of poor management decisions will serve as a counterbalance. In the optimal scenario, overall quality improvement will decrease costs.[36,37] Additionally, convergence of information technology and computer-assisted decision analysis and support will likely accelerate and contribute to quality improvement and cost control.[38] Thus, it may be axiomatic that true improvements in quality and efficiency will control costs. As long as quality is better defined and becomes the lead issue, and costs are well described and assigned, a relationship between the two will become easier to evaluate and implement process improvement. Currently, neither is the case. Quality is not clearly defined and costs are usually improperly assigned.[39]

Thus, EBM may be poised to utilize the boom in information technology and improve quality through unexplained variance reduction, but it is certainly in a state of evolution. Various interpretations and local adaptations are apparent and will continue while health care is in a state of reorganization. With the above in mind, it may be helpful and illuminating to review what EBM can do and what it will not do.

At its core, EBM may be viewed as a process. This process combines systematically obtaining the best available refined data (i.e., information) on a defined topic with the clinical expertise of the clinician. The resulting knowledge base then is applied to patient care.[5,40] While this may seem like good old-fashioned medical care, the data gathering portion of the process is the first significant challenge. In today's environment of data overload, physicians are challenged to keep up with the myriad of peer-reviewed journal articles, much less assess the adequacy of each study and the strength of evidence presented. A new paradigm and skill set is required, including efficient access to published studies and systematic application of evidence strength analysis.[41]

The second challenge is to continually and systematically incorporate the best evidence into clinical practice. The application of clinical expertise and judgment, heretofore known as the "art" of medicine, is an integral part of compassionate health-care delivery and cannot be summarily replaced by data driven guidelines. Physicians must continue to combine research-based evidence with accumulated clinical expertise.[42–44] The physician is a knowledge worker and the goal should be the development of a learning system within the individual a la a Peter Senge modification of the *learning organization,* which is based upon continually improving systems.[45,46] In a patient-centered environment, hard objective data may point toward one intervention but, based on clinical experience and patient input, the best outcomes may be realized by taking a different path for a given clinical situation. Optimally, both data and expertise should be available, interventions applied and outcomes assessed.

A common misperception is that EBM is equivalent to cookbook medicine. Pat prescriptions for any imaginable condition without regard for individual patient requirements or physician's clinical expertise would fit that definition. However, EBM mandates *integration* of clinical experience and a commitment to using the best available data as a guide to continued improvement and incremental narrowing of practice variance patterns.

EBM cannot and does not have cost reduction as its primary goal. Rather, more effective utilization of diagnostic and treatment resources has as its by-product possible cost reduction. This does not always occur and depends upon how costs are defined and to whom they are assigned.

EBM does not rest entirely upon external research findings with the RCT as the gold standard. While it is true that well-designed and interpreted prospective studies should have a strong influence on shaping practice patterns, they are not the end all. Neither is the compilation of the same via meta-analyses. The process goal is to define the best available external evidence that addresses specific clinical questions. The type of evidence depends on the clinical question at hand. Some questions require a RCT, while others require a cohort study, and still others may merely require an observation of widely disparate efficacy of a given intervention.

Traditional CME has failed to keep physicians abreast of new developments to the extent that these innovations and developments are not readily integrated into practice.[47–49] Worse, the half-life of medical education is getting ever shorter. Without the best current evidence, practice patterns can become dangerous and costly in both an economic and morbidity sense. EBM can help maintain the balance between data-driven guidelines and patient centered "art" of medical practice.[50]

EBM is a philosophic approach to medical practice and education. It is not outcomes research, but can help delineate where evidence is lacking as a basis for future research. It does so by delineating what kind and strength of evidence exists for a particular question and facilitates the gathering and grading of such evidence. As more supporting evidence becomes available, the validation of EBM as a philosophy and generally accepted practice infrastructure appears to be warranted.[51,52]

So how does EBM get incorporated into everyday medical practice? According to Sackett, there are five key steps to incorporating evidence-based practice into day-to-day medical care. First, the clinical problem must be framed into answerable questions. Second, the best available data, which will help answer the question, must be quickly and efficiently tracked down. Third, the evidence must be critically appraised for validity and usefulness as information. Fourth, the appraisal results must be incorporated into daily practice. Fifth, the results of this change in practice patterns must be evaluated for outcomes and other feedback regarding the new practice pattern.[53]

EXTERNAL DATA GATHERING AND RELEVANCE INTERPRETATION TOOLS

As the information age explodes, the total amount of readily available knowledge far exceeds the clinical experience of a single physician or consensus group of experts. Additionally, due to the electronic superhighway and multiple electronic storage media, one no longer needs to read through masses of journals and memorize key references in order to stay current.[54,55]

The following represents a synopsis of helpful sources and strategies for searching the medical literature. For a more comprehensive discussion, refer to the classic Sackett's *Evidence Based Medicine: How to Practice and Teach EBM*.[53]

In general, evidence must be current and credible, applicable to the practitioner's patient population and clinically relevant above and beyond an acceptable p value or confidence interval.

Electronic searches have practically become synonymous with MEDLINE or PubMed searches. As described below, MEDLINE is the largest and most well-known database. However, other sources may be better for focused topic searches. For example, recent research topics and cutting edge information may be best found in Current Contents. On the other hand, for a general review on a particular topic, possibly with CME credit attached to help fulfill licensing requirements, Medscape or other online journal databases should be consulted (Table 2.1). Online structured reviews and guidelines provide an evidence-based synthesis of available literature on a growing number of topics (Table 2.2). The overview given in this chapter is pragmatically structured around latest and most useful Web sites rather than just providing artificial constructs of database vs. search engine classifications

MEDLINE

The most widely available tool to clinicians, and also available directly to the public, is the searchable MEDLINE database through the National Library of Medicine. Most electronic search engines that access this online portion of the National Library of Medicine retrieve references by textwords of medical subject headings (MeSH).

Table 2.1   Evidence-Based E-Journals

Core Evidence	http://www.coremedicalpublishing.com
Anesthesia and Intensive Care	http://www.aaic.net.au/home.html
Anesthesiology	http://www.anesthesiology.org
ACP Journal Club	http://www.acpjc.org
PIER	http://pier.acponline.org/index.html
JAMA	http://www.ama-assn.org/public/journals/jama/ jamahome.htm
New England Journal of Medicine	http://www.nejm.org/
EBM Online	http://ebm.bmj.com
Cochrane Collaboration	http://www.cochrane.org/index.html
UpToDate	http://www.uptodate.com

Searches can be initiated for specific article titles, authors, general subjects, or specific clinical questions.

The most popular and easy to use search engines are PubMed and Ovid via Universities. Abstract availability is free through the NLM (http://ncbi.nlm.nih. gov/PubMed). Abstracts are available for over 75% of the references, comprising 19 million citations from MEDLINE and life science journals indexed from 1966 on.

Basic text keyword searches can certainly provide reams of basic and broad information. Unfortunately, at this point there is so much information published that there is pollution and overload. It is becoming difficult to tell the difference between good and misleading or low quality information. To help address this, search strategies can significantly influence the quantity and quality of data found.[56] First, the MEDLINE database should reflect the available literature for the appropriate time period.[57] Second, *all* evidence for a given topic should be considered, from case series or consensus opinions up to randomized double blind prospective studies. Third, all evidence must describe the specific patient population or clinical problem in reasonable detail. This centers upon entry of the appropriate key words and MeSH headings. Since the early 1990s the MeSH vocabulary has expanded to include specific search string toggles for type of study (e.g., controlled trial vs. cohort) and publication (e.g., meta-analysis).[58] Although validity of studies should be individually appraised, by

Table 2.2   Online Structured Reviews and Guidelines

Society of Critical Care Medicine	http://www.learnicu.org/Quick_Links/Pages/ default.aspx
Evidence-Based Medicine	http://www.acponline.org/clinical_information/ guidelines/current/#acg
JAMA Evidence	http://www.jamaevidence.com
Health Services Technology Assessment Text (HSTAT)	http://text.nlm.nih.gov/
Cochrane Collaborative database	http://www.cochrane.org/index.htm

including these methodology toggles in their search, users of the MEDLINE and other online NLM databases can search by type of studies available. The Health Information Research Unit (HIRU) of McMaster University (http://hiru.mcmaster.ca/hiru/) has suggested strategies for optimal retrieval of relevant citations by methodology based MEDLINE searching.[56] For example, in order to maximize the proportion between relevant and irrelevant citations retrieved, the search strategy (included with other key words or MeSH headings) EXPLODE SENSITIVITY and SPECIFICITY OR PREDICTIVE VALUE (TEXTWORD) can be used. If a personally performed search does not provide appropriate information, librarian consultation should be sought.

Online Journals and Databases

A very brief and incomplete list of available journals most closely pertaining to evidence-based perioperative care is given in Table 2.1. Most of these journals come with an online search engine, many are free or have featured evidence-based article reviews and indexed back to 1995 or earlier.

Textbooks

Textbooks have the distinct advantage of presenting synthesized information on various topics and the information is quickly accessible. The disadvantage lies in the danger of being outdated as of the publication date. Unfortunately, as of a 2005 review of medical library researchers found that physicians still rely primarily on two information resources: colleagues and printed textbooks and journals.[59] This practice has not changed much since 1992, when a similar review was conducted. However, if EBM philosophy is applied and explicit links to evidence are identified, textbooks are still a valuable resource. In particular, there is relative stability of supporting data for 80% of clinical interventions. The other 20% is subject to periodic change, although this ratio may change depending upon how dynamic the given area is. Thus, a textbook synthesis of EBM information can facilitate incorporation into clinical practice those interventions that are clearly well grounded and facilitate removal from clinical practice those interventions that are clearly without basis. In order to capture a current compendium regarding clinical problems and interventions, rapidly updated CD-ROM or online textbooks offer a distinct advantage.

Meta-analysis

A meta-analysis is a secondary systematic review of published primary data, optimally including RCT. Often smaller studies are grouped together in order to apply statistical analysis tools to an increased pooled sample size.[60] While meta-analysis has gained widespread acceptance, the utility of this method has been questioned.[61,62] Standardized approaches have therefore been recommended.[31] Additionally, the results are limited by the quality of the primary data publications. We know that large randomized trials and systematic reviews disagree at a rate greater than chance alone would predict. Therefore, the review must include a description of how the primary data sources were identified, and provide enough information for the reader to be able to assess the possibility of selection and analysis distortion due to various biases. Continuous compilation of clinical trial results and analysis of the results have been suggested and are provided on multiple subject areas by the Cochrane Collaboration.[63] Although not meta-analysis per se, the ACP Journal Club provides online abstracted reviews of primary literature.

EBM Guidelines

Evidence-based guidelines represent an attempt to distill the best available evidence via a structured process for a particular clinical question.[64] Many, if not most, published guidelines, which number in the thousands, do not employ such a rigorous process and should be interpreted accordingly.[65] Guidelines written by external sources also do not enjoy widespread implementation. The GRADE System (Grades of Recommendations Assessment, Development and Evaluation) was introduced in 2004 and endorsed by many organizations, including the Cochrane Collaboration. There is concern that this methodology for rating guidelines is yet to be validated.[66] However, with these caveats in mind, the Society of Critical Care Medicine operates a good online guidelines site pertaining to issues in perioperative and critical care. Additional resources are listed in Table 2.2, including HSTAT (which provides NIH Consensus Statements and AHCPR Evidence Based Guidelines) representing the two extremes of guideline development process.

Grading Published Data

Once a representative data set of published references is obtained, it must be systematically reviewed to determine the quality of data presented. The key question is: "which *data* set translates into the best *information* available for the specific question at hand?" Best may be defined as relevant and with the least methodological flaws. These flaws differ depending upon the type of study design, and are introduced below. Extensive discussion regarding clinical research design is well beyond the scope of this textbook, and there are many excellent textbooks and reviews[67–71] to refer. A particularly comprehensive review series of articles, entitled "User's Guide to the Medical Literature", published by the Evidence-Based Medicine Working Group from McMaster University[72–85] is highly recommended.

The individual studies must then be evaluated for strength of evidence and categorized by evidence-based medicine (EBM) level. This textbook refers to guidelines proposed by the U.S. Preventive Services Task Force (USPSTF).[86,87] Although this system was proposed for the evaluation of clinical preventive services, it is generally applicable to other interventions. These EBM levels may be noted in the text or in the decision algorithm or both, depending upon the chapter and material (e.g., level

I; 3 and Level II-3; 6). When available, the number of "best" studies/reports used to support the evidence are noted after the semicolon.

- **Level I**: Evidence obtained from at least one properly designed and powered RCT; well-conducted systemic review or meta-analysis of homogeneous RCTs.
- **Level II-1**: Evidence obtained from well-designed controlled trials without randomization.
- **Level II-2**: Evidence obtained from well-designed cohort or case–control analytic studies, preferably from more than one center or research group.
- **Level II-3**: Evidence obtained from multiple time series with or without the intervention. Dramatic results in uncontrolled experiments could also be regarded as this type of evidence.
- **Level III**: Opinions of respected authorities, based on clinical experience, descriptive studies, or reports of expert committees.

Other grading systems also exist, such as the Canadian Task Force (www. ctf-phc.org) and the Centre for Evidence Based Medicine (CEBM) at Oxford (www. cebm.net), but are similar in nature.

A letter grade may then be assigned, summarizing the overall strength of evidence. Most grades are specific for the preventive services or screening question at hand. Nonetheless, a general appreciation for the use of levels of evidence as they translate into "grades" is reviewed below. In this textbook, letter grades are not assigned, leaving the reader to make their own assessment based on EBM Level of evidence and applicability to their patient population. The USPSTF made some changes to its grade definitions and introduced a "statement of net benefit" in May 2007. This should be borne in mind when reviewing grades assigned before and after this date. The following represent grades using information from both USPSTF and the CEBM systems.

- **Grade A**: Consistent level I studies (CEBM). The USPSTF recommends this service. There is high certainty that the net benefit is substantial.
- **Grade B**: Consistent level II or III studies or extrapolations from level I studies (CEBM). The USPSTF recommends this service. There is high certainty that the net benefit is moderate or there is moderate certainty that the net benefit is moderate to substantial.
- **Grade C**: Level IV studies or extrapolations from level II and III studies (CEBM). The USPSTF recommends against routinely providing this service to an individual patient. There is at least moderate certainty that the net benefit is small.
- **Grade D**: Level V studies or troublingly inconsistent or inconclusive studies at any level (CEBM). The USPSTF recommends against the service. There is moderate or high certainty that the service has no net benefit or that the harms outweigh the benefits.

- **I Statement** (USPSTF only): The USPSTF concludes that the current evidence is insufficient to assess the balance of benefits and harms of the service. Evidence is lacking, is of poor quality, or is conflicting, and the balance of benefits and harms cannot be determined.

WHAT IS THE "BEST" EVIDENCE?

There is no consensus about which evidence rating system is ideal or which should be universally applied. Additional systems have been proposed, based on the field of medicine or are journal specific. You may find any of these, or a combination hybrid, in use by any given journal.

The "best" source of high quality evidence is generally considered to be the RCT. This study design provides very useful information with the least bias vulnerability, but it is not the appropriate answer to all questions. Many interventions or other clinical questions have not been, nor ever will be, investigated at that level. Or, the clinical question being asked may not be appropriate for evaluation in a randomized controlled fashion. Examples are abundant and include low prevalence conditions, treatment or diagnostic decisions of low impact, low morbidity conditions, and highly complicated very high cost low volume interventions. For example, the Pap smear was never evaluated by RCT. However, enough observational epidemiologic evidence exists and so its role in reducing the incidence of invasive cervical cancer is not generally questioned. Similarly, certain other questions require answers not from RCTs but from observational cohort and case–control studies, outcomes data within a local practice setting, questionnaire or interview-based data, problem modeling data, and other formats.

Intuitively, it is important to consider what type of information an RCT provides. Usually, the RCT compares two or more treatments, which are felt to differ relatively minimally in efficacy, in order to determine which is the better intervention. The true effectiveness of an RCT treatment arm is often inversely proportional to the number of RCTs it has been a part of. Thus, if a significant advance occurs, such as the introduction of the Pap smear or of antibiotics/penicillin, an RCT is not mandated to demonstrate efficacy.

EBM grading schemes *do* place high value on RCTs, but this should not over-shadow the fact that some questions are better answered by alternative study designs. Total homage to and reverence for the "*p* value" is not realistic. Instead, asking the appropriate question usually determines the appropriate study design or data source and is a philosophic underpinning of EBM practice.

EVALUATING PROSPECTIVE RCTs (EBM LEVEL I)

Clinical trials are intervention based on definition, with the subjects prospectively assigned to experimental and control arms. The subjects in both arms should be similar in all or most characteristics, allowing outcomes of a given intervention to be accurately assessed between the arms. While blinded studies are more difficult to design and implement, unblinded studies overestimate benefit by up to 17%.

Major advantages of this study design are as follows. (1) Bias elimination by random assignment of intervention. (2) Facilitates blinding of the investigators as well as participants whenever possible, further reducing bias. 3) Facilitates statistical probability analysis in determining strength of cause–effect relationship.

Study design flaws to watch for may include the following. (1) Invalid methods of randomization. (2) Subjects not matched by key variables. (3) Sample size too small to detect potentially important differences. (4) Compliance problems or loss to follow-up rate affects the outcomes analysis.

EVALUATING CONTROLLED PROSPECTIVE NONRANDOMIZED STUDIES (EBM LEVEL II-1)

Level II-1 studies are also interventional in nature. However, the study and control groups are not prospectively and randomly assigned, introducing biases. When using historical or otherwise unmatched control groups, the reported effects of the intervention being studied are often exaggerated.[88,89]

Study design flaws may include those listed under the Level I category. The main detraction from the highest reliability rating is the nonrandom assignment between the study and control groups. This could unevenly distribute known and unknown variables and factors that can be significant enough to sway the outcome analysis and interpretation.

EVALUATING OBSERVATIONAL STUDIES (EBM LEVELS II-2, II-3, AND III)

These studies represent the bulk of evidence available for the majority of diagnostic and treatment interventions. They include both prospective and retrospective study designs as delineated hereafter.

Level II-2

Case–Control Studies

The design of these studies is generally retrospective. First, the research question is identified and explicitly framed. Then the objective is to identify subjects with and without a disease or condition. A sample population is identified as well as a matched sample population without the condition but with similar demographics. The background of each group is then reviewed in order to find out why the cases developed a given condition whereas the controls did not. The odds that a given intervention or exposure produced the condition in the case group is compared with the control group. As such the output of the study is the *odds ratio*, which approximates the *relative risk* rather well if the prevalence of a condition is not excessively high. The major advantages are as follows. (1) The study can be rapidly performed. (2) It is useful when studying rare conditions.

Major study flaws to watch for include (1) unknown factors that influenced development of a condition inadvertently not taken into consideration, (2) selection bias preferentially included or excluded subjects in either the case or control group, and (3) differential recall bias may affect the ability of either group to remember, admit to, or include certain key exposures being investigated.

Cohort Studies

Cohort studies can be either prospective or retrospective. In each case, a group of subjects is followed through time, usually made up of exposed and unexposed subjects to a given risk factor or intervention. In a *prospective* cohort study, these risk factor exposures have been identified and the incidence of outcomes such as a finding or disease state in both groups is recorded as it occurs. In a *retrospective* cohort study, the risk factor exposure as well as the outcome has already occurred in a well-delineated cohort assembled for another purpose. Most often the control group is internal since comparisons are made between subjects within the single cohort. The outcome is reported as a *relative risk*.

Major study flaws include (1) expensive and inefficient way to study rare diseases or states, (2) confounding variables may exist, which obscure the cause–effect relationship between risk factor and outcome, (3) outcome assessment between groups can be biased, and (4) criteria for risk factor exposure are not accurate.

Level II-3

The following studies fall between classic observational studies (case–control and cohort) and pure descriptive accounts.

Uncontrolled Experiments

Uncontrolled observations of the result of an intervention or exposure that show dramatic outcomes may point to a valid question requiring hypothesis testing. However, since no exact information is provided about exposure and no control groups exist, other methods must be employed to test the hypothesis for a cause–effect relationship. Other factors may have caused the outcome rather than the intervention or exposure being considered.

Cross-Sectional Studies

These observational studies collect data at a single point in time, comparing presence or absence of an exposure or intervention with a given outcome. It is difficult or impossible to assess a temporal relationship, although serial cross-sectional surveys can evaluate general changes over time. This design is hypothesis generating rather than testing and generates prevalence or relative prevalence.

Level III

The least persuasive studies, which offer almost no insight into an exposure to outcome relationship, include (1) pure descriptive studies, (2) case series and reports, and (3) expert opinion or consensus panel reports.

Consensus conferences, which use EBM strategies, provide recommendations based on structured review of available evidence. In this setting, the strength of recommendations is much higher than that coming from a simple round table discussion or expert opinion. In communicating the EBM review results, standards may be set based on Level I data, guidelines introduced at Level II data and options suggested for Level III data.[90]

STATISTICS ISSUES: DESIGN, POWER, SAMPLE SIZE, AND CLINICAL UTILITY

A review of basic statistics, even briefly, is well beyond the scope of this textbook. A brief and very readable synopsis of statistics for the nonstatistician is provided within an excellent review series published recently in the *British Medical Journal*.[91,92]

Without delving into the specifics of statistical analysis tools employed, several key general questions can be asked in assessing the quality of published research. Common errors in study design and reporting surround: (1) inadequate sample size, (2) inadequate power, (3) inadequate follow-up, and (4) statistically significant but clinically irrelevant results.

Sample size should be large enough to provide a high probability of detecting *clinically* relevant effects of a given intervention, if they exist. This is accomplished via published nomograms or computer programs and is determined by the desired power of the study. In other words, what sample size is required to find a true clinical difference between the groups at a moderate, high or very high probability.[71] Too often a power of 80%–90% is not achieved and the given study is prone to a Type II(β) error, meaning the intervention had no effect when if fact it did. Type I(α) errors are less common, defined as reporting a significant difference when in fact no true difference exists.

A study may not be conducted for a sufficiently long period of time or be hampered by subjects who are "lost to follow-up." This results in incomplete detection of late effects and bias within the group not followed to the established endpoint. The latter bias is often in favor of the intervention. Thus, it is the convention to analyze results based on intention to treat rather than actual treatment provided.[93] Additionally, the statistical handling of "outliers" should be specifically addressed in the study methods section.

Regarding significance, the *p* value for an intervention may be statistically significant but the difference fails to approach clinical relevance. Depending on secondary issues such as various assigned costs, the proposed intervention may not be appropriate to recommend. Conversely, a *p* value that is not significant means one of two things: (1) there is no difference or (2) the sample size was too small to demonstrate a difference. Unfortunately, a "nonsignificant" p value does not distinguish between these results. Since the p value is not a measure of association and is an arbitrary construct based on a cutoff point "yes–no" dichotomy, many have questioned its value. Instead, *confidence intervals* (CI) provide a better assessment of evidence strength and definitiveness of the study at hand.[94] A 95% CI implies high probability that the value given is included within the specified range. The larger the clinical trial, the narrower the CI, and thus increasing the likelihood that the result is definitive. If the CI overlaps zero difference (e.g., 95% CI $= -2.0$ to 10) between groups under study, the strength of inference is weaker than a situation with no overlap. Despite the advantages, CI reporting is still not prevalent in the medical literature.

Finally, the ideal clinical interpretation of treatment or diagnostic efficacy will include the likelihood that an effect will be realized if a given intervention is applied. These statements of likelihood are embodied in (1) number needed to treat (NNT), (2) relative and absolute risk reduction in cohort studies, and (3) the odds ratio in case–control studies. These calculations allow comparison of practical clinical applicability between available interventions. In other words, if a given treatment or test is proposed for a patient, what is probability that the intervention will be effective (Table 2.3).

The relative significance of the odds ratio (case control) or relative risk (cohort or RCT) in determining strength of evidence depends upon the clinical scenario. The more the effect carries clinically important consequences, the lower the number that may be considered significant. Also, since a case–control study has greater potential for bias than a cohort study or RCT, a significant odds ratio should exceed 3 or 4. In comparison, a relative risk for a cohort study or RCT may be considered significant at a level of 1 or 2.

However, statements about risk reduction do not always help in making decisions about when to offer a treatment to a particular patient. Thinking about clinical

Table 2.3   Ratios

| Group | Outcome Event | | |
	Yes	No	Total
Control	a	b	a + b
Experimental	c	d	c + d
Number needed to treat (NNT) (in order to achieve a benefit or harm/risk)	$= \dfrac{1}{(a/a + b) - (c/c + d)} = \dfrac{1}{ARR}$		
Relative risk reduction (RRR) (cohort studies)	$= \dfrac{[(a/a + b) - (c/c + d)]}{(c/c + d)} = \dfrac{\text{untreated} - \text{treated}}{\text{trated}}$		
Absolute risk reduction (ARR)(cohort studies)	$= (a/a + b) - (c/c + d) = \text{untreated} - \text{treated}$		
Odds ratio (case–control studies)	$= \dfrac{\text{Odds of outcome in experimental group}}{\text{Odds of outcome in control group}} = \dfrac{c/d}{a/b}$		

Table 2.4 Costs

Cost	A sacrifice of resources, regardless of whether it is accounted for as an asset or expense (NOT = expense per se)
Expense	A cost charged against a revenue in a given accounting period (NOT = cost per se)
Direct medical cost	Costs of medical services provided
Direct nonmedical cost	Costs of additional related services such as transportation and transfer of materials
Indirect cost	Costs indirectly impacting patient care such as administration, housekeeping, engineering
Direct variable cost	Costs that change in direct proportion with changes in volume of service provided
Direct fixed cost	Costs that do not change as volume changes within a relevant range of activity
Semifixed/step cost	Costs that increase in steps with volume or outcome, such as academic salary adjustments
Total cost	Variable costs + fixed costs
Average cost	Total cost divided by the total quantity of output
Marginal cost	Addition to total cost that results from one additional unit of output or benefit
Opportunity cost	A forgone benefit that could have been realized from the best forgone alternative use of a resource: time, money, health benefit, etc.
Intangible cost	Costs of pain and suffering
Morbidity cost	Costs of economic loss due to work missed
Mortality cost	Costs of economic productivity loss due to death

problems using the NNT construct provides the clinician with an idea of how applicable a risk reduction is to a given population or even a particular patient The NNT is calculated by taking the inverse of the ARR (Table 2.4). It tells us how many patients need to be treated with the intervention in question to achieve one additional benefit (i.e., marginal benefit). For example, assume the risk of outcome (O) for new treatment (y) is 40%, and the risk for the same outcome (O) is 65% for control treatment (x). The ARR is: $x - y = 25\%$. Since NNT is the inverse of this number we arrive at $1/0.25 = 4$. In other words, four patients would need to receive treatment y in order to achieve the outcome (O). As the ARR increases, fewer patients need to be treated to achieve the desired outcome. Ideally, the NNT calculation should be bounded by a 95% CI in order to appreciate the precision of the number. The broader the CI, the less convincing the argument is for an intervention or for a statement regarding harm.

Unfortunately, the methodology of NNT reporting is not uniform in the literature and several caveats are critical. First, the NNT can only be calculated from an ARR not a RRR or an OR. The ARR allows the NNT to assess the clinical magnitude of the outcome or treatment effect. The RRR does not discriminate between a 70% reduction of an outcome from 90% to 20% vs. 0.00090% to 0.00020%. In the former situation the NNT is $1/70 = 1.4$ (i.e., less than 2 patients need to be treated), and in the latter it is $1/.00070 = 1429$ (i.e., more than 1400 patients need to be treated).

In case–control studies, OR may be converted to NNT if the particular population patient expected even rate (PEER) is known by the following formula, in which RRR × PEER = ARR[53]:

$$NNT = \frac{1 - [PEER \times (1 - OR)]}{(1 - PEER) \times PEER \times (1 - OR)}$$

The NNT outcome event noted in Table 2.4 can be favorable (benefit) or unfavorable (risk or harm), sometimes denoted as NNH or number needed to harm. It may be desirable to know how many patients would require treatment to yield that one additional (marginal) benefit, harm, or both. Thus an additional modification to the NNT formula, which addresses both the marginal benefit and the marginal harm or risk of a given intervention yields

$$NNT = \frac{1}{(benefit_1 - benefit_2) + (risk_1 - risk_2)}$$

Alternatively, the NNT can be compared to the NNH in order to define the relative benefit associated with providing a treatment. Decision thresholds for the absolute NNT or NNH will depend upon the clinical situation, and the physician's and patient's risk aversion profile. For example, if the adverse outcome is significant or severe enough in terms of harm (i.e., morbidity, mortality, or costs), it may be prudent to increase the threshold for an acceptable NNH before considering the treatment (e.g., NNH = 100 rather than NNH = 5). Of course, all of this depends upon the available alternatives. In- depth consideration of multiple parameters involving risks, benefits, and costs requires formal decision analysis, which is introduced later in this chapter.

Diagnostic Tests Analysis

Evaluation of diagnostic tests is based upon the outcomes possibilities of true positive and negative results versus false positive and negative results. These give rise to the following familiar formulas:

Sensitivity = True positive/(True positive + False negative)

Specificity = True negative/(True negative + False positive)

Most tests have a range that overlaps a diseased versus nondiseased state. Thus, both sensitivity and specificity are influenced by the choice of a test's normal versus abnormal cutoff point within this overlapping range of values. Ideally, the cutoff is set to minimize both false positive and false negative results. The exact point may be influenced by the medical or economic consequences of an excess in sensitivity or specificity. For example, too high of a sensitivity could lead to excess additional testing, resulting in higher cost and possible incremental morbidity.

Assuming an appropriate cutoff point, a negative test result of a highly sensitive test effectively *rules out* a condition. Conversely, a positive result of a highly specific condition *rules in* a diagnosis. As the prevalence of a disease decreases, the more specificity the test must have to be clinically valuable and to minimize false positives. In contradistinction, the more prevalent diseases require very sensitive tests such that the false negative results are minimized.

$$\text{Prevalence} = \frac{\text{Number of persons with disease at a point in time}}{\text{Number of persons at risk}}$$

It is very important to keep in mind that prevalence directly influences the usefulness of the predictive value.

$$\text{Positive predictive value} = \frac{\text{Patients with positive test and disease}}{\text{All patients with positive test}}$$

$$\text{Negative predictive value} = \frac{\text{Patients with negative test and no disease}}{\text{All patients with negative test}}$$

Predictive values are often used to help evaluate diagnostic test usefulness. However, predictive values should only be considered if the ratio of the number of patients in the disease group and the number of patients in the healthy control group is equivalent to the prevalence of the diseases in the studied population. If this is not the case, likelihood ratios are more suited to the task, since they do not depend on prevalence.

$$\text{Positive likelihood ratio} = \frac{\text{Sensitivity}}{(1 - \text{Specificity})}$$

$$\text{Negative likelihood ratio} = \frac{(1 - \text{Sensitivity})}{\text{Specificity}}$$

Further assessment of diagnostic testing modalities includes evaluation of the marginal role of each test toward increasing diagnostic certainty. How much more information does that one additional test provide and at what value cutoff point? None of our testing tools are 100% accurate, so the information obtained from a given test can best be assessed by receiver operating characteristics (ROC) curves. The ROC curve plots sensitivity versus the false positive rate. The inverse relationship between sensitivity and specificity becomes obvious in evaluating a ROC curve, with the perfect test having an area under the curve (AUC) of 1.0, representing sensitivity = 1 and specificity =1. Thus, the most ideal attainable test value approaches the upper left-hand corner of the curve, as depicted in Fig. 2.1.

A poor test has a curve of $45°$ at a diagonal left to right, with an equal loss of specificity for each marginal gain in sensitivity. For most tests, there is a steep ascending portion of the curve that represents excellent gains in sensitivity with minimal loss in specificity. The best cutoff value for a test is the point at which the curve turns the corner and flattens out, representing greater losses of specificity for minimal marginal improvement in sensitivity. In Fig. 2.1, a test value around 55 would be ideal. An attractive feature of ROC curves in diagnostic test selection is that the curves can be compared to determine which test gets closest to the upper left-hand corner and has the largest AUC (i.e., the "best" test).

ROC Curve

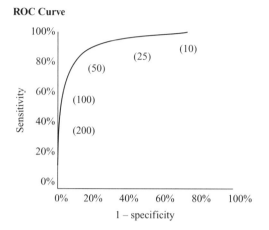

Figure 2.1   **ROC curve.**

A clinically useful way to approach test result analysis is to look at that point/value beyond which the condition or disorder in question becomes highly probable or improbable. This approach moves beyond Gaussian distributions and standard deviations or cutoff points. It minimizes use of redundant testing modalities by introducing an incremental or marginal analysis mind set. In other words, how much more certain am I going to be of the diagnosis after a given test ? Does additional testing beyond this result improve my diagnostic yield by 1% or 20% ?

The first task is to estimate, calculate or use established/published pretest odds that a condition exists. For example, a new 5×6 cm adnexal mass in a 60-year-old patient, with smooth, cystic and mobile characteristics, may represent a 50% chance of malignancy. The 50% odds may have been published in a significant series of adnexal masses or may be calculated if supporting information is provided in the form of a 2×2 table, such as Table 2.4.

$$\text{Prevalence} = (a + c)/(a + b + c + d)$$

$$= \text{outcome present/all patients in sample population}$$

$$\text{Pretest odds} = \text{prevalence}/(1 - \text{prevalence})$$

Can this level of diagnostic certainty be improved such that preoperative planning is optimized? A pelvic ultrasound is quite commonly ordered in these situations. As an illustrative example, a pelvic ultrasound may have a sensitivity of 90% and a specificity of 70% for predicting malignancy findings at surgery. A derivative of these numbers is the likelihood ratio (LR) for a positive or negative test:

$$\text{LR}+ = \text{sensitivity}/(1 - \text{specificity})$$

$$\text{LR}- = (1 - \text{sensitivity})/\text{specificity}$$

Basically, 30% of patients (100% – 70%) with ultrasound characteristics suggestive of malignancy do not turn out to have ovarian cancer. So the LR+ = 90%/30% = 3. Therefore, the pretest odds of malignancy were 50%, or 1:1 by convention. The posttest odds are a product of the LR and the pretest odds. In this case, posttest odds = 3 × 1:1 = 3:1. The posttest probability that the condition exists is 3/3+1 = 75%. The probability of malignancy is now 75%, making this a test that added significant marginal value. Conversely, in order to rule out a cancer, the likelihood ratio of a negative test result (i.e., an ultrasound not suggestive of ovarian cancer) can be calculated in a similar fashion as follows:

$$LR- = 10\%/70\% = 0.14$$

$$\text{Posttest odds} = 1 \times 0.14 = 0.14$$

$$\text{Posttest probability that ovarian cancer exists} = 0.14/1.14 = 12\%$$

The same logic can be applied to determine if CA125, other tumor markers, computerized tomography, or magnetic resonance imaging would provide significant incremental value. Several tests may be equal in incremental value as the primary test, but involve cost considerations. These economic analysis issues are addressed later in this chapter, and the testing sequence may be best determined via formal multifactorial decision analysis.

Diagnostic test results may report multilevel likelihood ratios from a very positive result, through a range of neutral or indeterminate results, to a highly negative result. The pulmonary ventilation-perfusion (V-Q) scan is an example of reporting the probability of pulmonary embolism in this fashion. The V-Q scan results must be correlated with the clinical picture (i.e. pretest odds) in order to make an optimal treatment decision. In general, a highly positive LR (i.e. >10) with pretest probability of >33% will generate posttest probabilities in excess of 83%. On the other hand, with a highly negative LR (i.e. <0.1), pretest probability of <33% translates into a posttest probability of <5%. In the indeterminate LR range, a series of clinical decision sequelae is possible, but depending on the pretest odds, additional testing may be required. Ideally, for any test, the range of LR and pretest probabilities must be correlated in order to determine the posttest probability, the marginal clinical impact and need for further testing. Not doing so, instead relying on the high sensitivity or specificity of a seemingly good test at a given cutoff, may lead to a suboptimal decision. This is because the precise value obtained within the test's range may represent an indeterminate LR approaching 1, reflecting a zero marginal benefit for the test. In other words, the pretest probability equals the posttest probability at best.

For a further in depth discussion of diagnostic test analysis the interested reader is referred to other works.[71,95]

DECISION ANALYSIS PRIMER

Lack of a formal manner by which to approach multifactorial risk decisions is akin to attempting preparation of an annual income tax statement in your head. Some clinical decisions are straight forward, or at least seem to be. However, when multiple diagnostic tests and findings are entertained, a free form decision will fail to take all issues into weighted consideration.

Decision analysis rests upon the concept of *expected value*. Using computer-assisted modeling, such as DATA™ from TreeAge Software Inc.[96] (Williamstown, MA), all uncertainties are put into perspective and analyzed using Markov (recursive) processes.[97] A Markov model is a recursively defined system with a finite number of states. It is used to model changes to an individual or population over time. An influence diagram is usually initially constructed, defining all factors that affect the decision and how they are related. From this, a decision tree is created which includes the following tenets: (1) time flows from left to right and events are placed in proper sequence, (2) all clinically important final outcomes must be represented, (3) nodes are designated as a decision, uncertainty, or an outcome, (4) branches emanating from a decision node represent all available options, (5) branches emanating from a chance node represent all possible clinically important outcomes, and (6) probabilities of events are assigned at each chance node and payoffs are assigned at each terminal outcome node.

In the example above, representing a very rudimentary tree (Fig. 2.2), colorectal cancer screening tests are ordered in several possible combinations. Probabilities, based on best available evidence via EBM approach, are assigned to each chance node. The tree can then be "rolled back" by the computer program in order to determine which path is the most likely to provide the best desired outcome, and at what expected value (i.e., the outcome value that can be expected on average). The utility outcome or payoff measure may be defined as optimal detection, minimal morbidity, optimal cost structure, quality of life, and so on. For any decision or chance node branch, a sensitivity analysis may be performed and a tornado diagram created, visually displaying which decision and chance points have the greatest relative uncertainty effects on the final outcome.

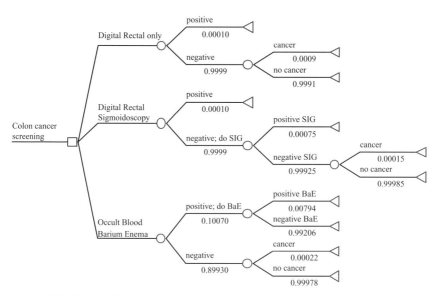

Figure 2.2 Basic decision analysis tree.

Each variable undergoing analysis is represented by a horizontal bar, summarizing the range of possible model outcomes generated by varying the related variable. A wide bar indicates that the associated variable has a large potential effect on the expected value of the model. The graph is called a tornado diagram because the horizontal bars are arranged in order. The widest bar, representing the most critical uncertainty, is displayed at the top. The result is a funnel shaped visual aid displaying a sensitivity analysis comparing key variable impact on the model.

Validity of decision analysis must be iteratively reviewed during model construction as well as at the time of analysis. The following key questions should be kept in mind: (1) Was the appropriate decision model used? (2) Were all appropriate strategies included and in a clinically appropriate sequence? (3) Were all clinically relevant outcomes considered? (4) Was an explicit and appropriate process used to collect and transform the available evidence into the probabilities used within the tree? (5) Were appropriate utilities assigned to the possible outcomes? (6) Were the appropriate sensitivity analyses conducted? The last item is particularly important since the quality of input = quality of output. If the entire result is overly dependent on a chance or decision data point that is not very precise or not well substantiated, the definitiveness of the result is in question.

Serious limitations of decision analysis include (1) availability and quality of data in formulation of chance node probabilities, (2) potential oversimplification of complex medical decisions, and (3) assignment of utilities to the outcomes can be very subjective.

Although decision analysis is a very complex subject, information technology and user friendly inexpensive computer programs are leveling the playing field. Several very useful references can provide enough background to the reader such that basic decision analysis can be readily incorporated into relatively complex clinical decision making.[23,95,98–102]

ECONOMIC ANALYSIS PRIMER

An economic analysis concentrates upon choices and tradeoffs in resource allocation, whether that be established diagnostic testing, treatment intervention or application of emerging technologies. The ultimate economic outcome of interest is usually "cost" in relation to some utilization or outcome parameter. This is problem #1. Costs are exceedingly difficult to correctly define and assign.[103,104] Furthermore, the perspective (e.g., payer vs. provider vs. patient vs. societal) of the analysis determines the types of costs considered. Table 2.4 lists types of costs generally considered in various analyses and their definitions. The list is by no means exhaustive. For example, if a study on cost effectiveness is conducted over a long period of time, issue such as short-term versus long-term costs arise. These two time frames have a different intrinsic distribution of fixed and variable direct costs. Additionally, the economic cost accrued today is not the same as that over a period of time due to inflation and cost of money provided (i.e., interest or hurdle rates), at which point discounting methods need to be employed.[105,106] If the study period exceeds 1 year, a discount rate to adjust for present value should be applied, with published estimates ranging from 3% to 7%.[107]

Because of difficulties in measuring the subjective costs of pain, suffering, morbidity/mortality, and some opportunity costs, most analyses concentrate on the direct costs of providing a medical service. However, this can skew the true clinical meaning and validity of a given study.

The population type also influences the cost issue. For example, older gynecologic cancer patients are often Medicare beneficiaries. Therefore, many economic analyses from the payer perspective have been based upon cost estimates from Medicare data. These are based on diagnostically related groups (DRGs) and are paid by Medicare in a fixed amount per hospitalization. It follows that any additional costs incurred by the provider would not be considered in an analysis based on Medicare DRG cost data, even though it will clearly affect the provider's profit/loss. In general, indirect reference-based measures of cost such as *cost-to-charge ratios* can be very misleading due to charge fluctuations and an inconsistent relationship between true costs for rendering a service and a charge.[108] For this reason, economic analysis validity is enhanced greatly when a direct measurement of cost, such as activity based costing/management, is used.[109]

It should be apparent that even the seemingly simple task of accurately defining and assigning a cost structure is foreboding. However, once that is performed, the next equally challenging step is assigning a value to a given health benefit from an intervention or test. If there is an objective medical measurement such as blood pressure readings, this must be accurately defined and used. In the absence of objective measurements, or as a supplement, quality adjusted life years (QALYs) provide a very common metric for differentiating between interventions that require a patient's subjective preferences as to outcomes.[110–112] An alternative is the health years equivalent (HYE) metric that incorporates the likelihood of deterioration or improvement in condition over time.[113] These metrics have been determined by patient utility preferences as well as community defined preferences, with no consensus as to which is the better metric.[110,114] Unfortunately, there is no good way to assess QALYs and HYEs per intervention when a patient has multiple disabling conditions. Both methods have their critics, but a better alternative is elusive.

Economic analysis studies are often mislabeled. Several different types exist and are dependent upon the goal of the study. First and foremost, prior to any economic analysis, well-documented evidence based data regarding pure clinical effectiveness should be sought. Once clinical effectiveness is established, the goal of economic assessment is defined and questions formulated, yielding the appropriate study design as summarized in Table 2.5.

Cost Minimization Analysis

The simplest analysis determines that is the least costly of clinically equivalent interventions. An example might be comparison of equivalent same generation, same side effects, same coverage spectrum antibiotics from several vendors.

Table 2.5 Economic Analyses

Question	Outcomes Units	Study design
Which of several similar interventions that yield *similar* outcomes should be chosen?	Equal medical outcomes	Cost minimization analysis (CMA)
Which of several interventions that yield clinically *different* outcomes should be chosen?	Medical units,	
	e.g., mm Hg pressure	Cost effectiveness analysis (CEA)
Which of several similar interventions that affect quality of life or patient preferences should be chosen?	QALY or HYE	Cost utility analysis (CUA)
Which of several different interventions with differing outcomes, also expressed in terms of cost, should be chosen?	Monetary	Cost benefit analysis (CBA)

Cost units for *all* study designs is in monetary terms (e.g., dollar).

Cost Effectiveness Analysis

When comparing several interventions with different clinical outcomes, the effectiveness of the intervention is compared using clinical effect on the same medical units (e.g., medication A and B effect on mm Hg reduction in blood pressure). If the outcome units differ, some common denominator must be sought, such as survival. Once a cost and clinical effect for the study interventions are determined, a cost effectiveness ratio (C/E) is reported.[112,115–117]

Although most often an *average* total cost is used in reporting cost effectiveness, the optimal assessment should be based on *marginal* cost versus marginal benefit. In other words, how much more cost is associated with one more unit of benefit or with the next most effective option.[95,118]

An additional requirement of appropriate reporting of C/E studies is presentation of alternative scenario-based sensitivity analyses. This indicates the stability or definitiveness of the reported findings.[116]

Cost Utility Analysis

When utility or preference is the outcome, reported as QALY or HYE, the analysis becomes a specific type of cost effectiveness assessment. It determines the clinical outcome benefits gained in terms of a *time tradeoff* of preference for raw life years gained versus the quality of life in those years. The alternative is a *standard gamble* technique, which asks the patient to rate the utility of a sure outcome (e.g., chronic pain) versus a gamble on a possible alternative outcome with an intervention (e.g., motor nerve damage with surgical intervention).

Cost–Benefit Analysis

This method of analysis is less frequently used because of the difficulty of assigning a monetary amount to an outcome, such as a QALY gained or medical complication avoided. The intervention cost and benefit are both expressed in monetary terms, such that the interventions can be compared for best value for dollar spent in health-care delivery.

Finally, a decision analysis tree can be structured rather than a pure spreadsheet cost model. This offers greater versatility by visually representing the decision and chance issues (nodes) and can calculate effectiveness, cost-effectivness, dollars per QALY (quality adjusted life year) for a given intervention.

TOWARD EFFECTIVE GUIDELINE DEVELOPMENT AND IMPLEMENTATION

Guidelines merely point toward a path of decreasing clinical practice variance. They are NOT standards. This difference is critical to appreciate. A *standard* may be proposed when the outcomes of intervention are known at EBM Level I, and there is unanimous agreement that exceptions are rare. *Guidelines* are recommended when the outcomes are mixed, the evidence is generally EBM Level II, and there is agreement that exceptions are fairly common. Lastly, *options* may be advanced when the outcomes are unknown, or the evidence is generally based on Level III data. The latter may be regarded as pure opinion, although the options are still based upon expert review and are still "guides" in principle when compared to free form intervention decision making.

Currently there are thousands of published guidelines, which in general have failed to reduce clinical practice variance.[119] The most often cited reason is that the guidelines were externally generated, thus failing to achieve a significant local approval. Furthermore, most guidelines are developed without a defined systematic EBM process, instead being generated via consensus approach, which is wide open to bias.[64] Even when the development process is defined, the written guidelines often fail to note which recommendations are based on high level evidence and which are opinions.[120] Beyond this, guidelines will not have an impact unless the outcomes are measurable such that process improvement can be initiated via guideline modification. In other words, guideline implementation should be a dynamic rather than a static process.

Is there a mechanism by which guidelines can be meaningfully generated and implemented? First, one must decide which practice patterns have significant reducible assignable practice variance. Second, one must understand the attributes of good guidelines and what purpose they fulfill (Table 2.6). Third, one must decide if appropriate guidelines already exist for the problem at hand or if new guidelines are required. Fourth, one must design, generate, or modify guidelines. Fifth, one must implement them.[82,121]

Since guideline development is a time and resource intensive process, a more efficient approach at the local practitioner level may be existing guideline assessment

Table 2.6 Guideline Attributes for Development or Assessment

Can provide guidance toward decreasing assignable practice variance

Are systematically developed, evidence based and current

Are clearly defined and optimally categorized by strength of evidence
  • Standards
  • Guidelines
  • Options

Provide flexibility at guideline and option levels, with exceptions noted

The guidelines are implementable

The outcomes are measurable

and/or modification. First it is important to determine who developed the guidelines and whether the guidelines fit the population at hand. Second, the methodology of guidelines development should be determined. The underlying evidence for the guidelines must be substantiated as described in this chapter and explicitly noted. This may require an updated search of primary literature in order to ensure that the recommendations are current. Third, the established measurable outcomes should coincide with the goals for guideline requirement. For example, if a set of guidelines is developed for purposes of improving quality or managing variance, it may not fulfill needs for a cost containment or utilization optimization program. Fourth, the guidelines should be able to close the gap between the current clinical practice outcomes and the outcomes desired. Fifth, the guidelines must be able to be implemented in a cost-efficient and practical fashion. If the effort and use of resources required to implement the guidelines exceed the anticipated benefits, the implementation should be reconsidered.

Implementation is generally regarded as the most difficult phase of the guideline development or incorporation process. Even before development or appropriateness assessment of existing guidelines, the organizational dynamics must be considered. Often, the organization must be prepared for implementation, obtaining buy-in for the process from top to bottom. Additionally, understanding physician behavior modification is a separate skill set that must be sought and developed by the organization.

Table 2.7 represents the relative effectiveness of development, dissemination, and implementation strategies.[122]

Table 2.7 Guideline Strategies

Development Strategy	Dissemination Strategy	Implementation Strategy
Internal	Specific education	Patient specific reminder at time of visit
Intermediate	CME	Patient-specific feedback
External, local	Mailing targeted groups	General feedback
External, national	Journal publications	General reminder

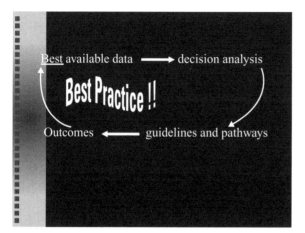

Figure 2.3   Evidence-based continuous feedback loop model.

One of the most important lessons in failed guideline implementation lies in the following. If a set of guidelines fails within an organization, the question should be not what is wrong with the practitioners but rather what is wrong with the guidelines and the implementation process. The guideline process is dynamic and even relative successes should be viewed as works in progress. As new information becomes available, modifications will be required.

BEST PRACTICES LOOP MODEL

Synthesizing all of the above information gathering, evidence grading and analysis tools yields a useful framework toward continually improved best practices. Elements of the cross industry plan-do-check/study-act (PDCA/PDSA) improvement cycle loop are employed.[46] The resulting continuous loop feedback model (Fig. 2.3) promotes the collection, interpretation, and integration into practice of valid, important and relevant patient-reported, clinician-observed, and research-based evidence. The best available evidence, moderated by specific clinical circumstances and judgment, is integrated into evolving practice patterns. The outcomes are continually assessed, which modify the loop along with any newly available and relevant external evidence.

REFERENCES

1. COVELL DG, UMAN GC, MANNING PR. Information needs in office practice: are they being met? Ann Intern Med 1985;103:596–599.
2. OLATUNBOSUN OA, EDOUARD L, PIERSON RA. Physician's attitudes toward evidence based obstetric practice: a questionnaire survey. BMJ 1998;316:365–366.
3. FIELD MJ, LOHR KN. Guidelines for Clinical Practice. Institute of Medicine. Washington, DC:National Academy Press; 1992. p 34.

4. CLANCY CM. Evidence based decision making: global evidence, local decisions. Health Affairs 2005;24(1):151–162.
5. BORDLEY DR, FAGAN M, THEIGE D. Evidence-based medicine: a powerful educational tool for clerkship education. Am J Med 1997;102:427–432.
6. CHASSIN MR, GALVIN RW. The urgent need to improve healthcare quality. JAMA 1998;280:1000–1005.
7. CHASSIN MR, BROOK RH, PARK RE, et al. Variations in the use of medical and surgical services by the medicare population. N Eng J Med 1986;314:285–290.
8. HAMPTON JR. Evidence based medicine, practice variations and clinical freedom. J Eval in Clin Pract 1997;3:123–131.
9. MARWICK C. Proponents gather to discuss practicing evidence based medicine. JAMA 1997;278:531–532.
10. WEINSTEIN MW. Checking medicine's vital signs. New York Times Magazine April 19, 1998: 36–37.
11. WENNBERG DE. Variations in the delivery of health care: the stakes are high. Ann Intern Med 1998;128:866–868.
12. WENNBERG J. Dealing with medical practice variations: a proposal for action. Health Aff Millwood 1984;3(2):6–32.
13. EDDY DM. Clinical Decision Making: From Theory to Practice. A Collection of Essays from JAMA. Boston, MA:Jones and Bartlett Publishers; 1996. p 5.
14. STAFFORD RS, SINGER DE. National patterns of warfarin use in atrial fibrillation. Arch Intern Med 1996;156:2537–2541.
15. WALTON M. The Deming Management Method. New York:Putnam Publishing; 1986.
16. SHAFER SM, MEREDITH JR. Quality control. In:SHAFER SM, MEREDITH JR, editors. Operations Management. New York:John Wiley; 1998. p 741–747.
17. BRASE T. "Evidence based medicine": Rationing care, hurting patients. ALEC The State Factor Dec 2008:1–16.
18. NAYLOR CD. Grey zones of clinical practice: some limits to evidence based medicine. Lancet 1995;345:840–842.
19. RODARTE JR. Evidence based surgery. Mayo Clin Proceed 1998;73:603.
20. SMITH R. Where is the wisdom: the poverty of medical evidence. BMJ 1991;303:798–799.
21. WOOLF SH. Practice guidelines, a new reality in medicine: II. Methods of developing guidelines. Arch Intern Med 1992;152:946–952.
22. SACKETT DL, ROSENBERG WMC, GRAY JAM, et al. Evidence-based medicine: what it is and what it isn't. BMJ 1996;312:71–72.
23. DEEDWANIA PC. Underutilization of evidence based therapy in heart failure. An opportunity to deal a winning hand with an ace up your sleeve. Arch Intern Med 1997;157:2409–2412.
24. KASKA SC, WEINSTEIN JN. Historical perspective. Ernest Amory Codman, 1869–1940. A pioneer of evidence based medicine: the end result idea. Spine 1998;23:629–633.
25. RANGACHARI PK. Evidence based medicine: old French wine with a new Canadian label? J Royal Soc Med 1997;90:280–284.
26. AUPLISH S. Using clinical audit to promote evidence based medicine and clinical effectiveness: an overview of one health authority's experience. J Eval Clin Prac 1997;3:77–82.
27. BERO L, RENNIE D. The Cochrane collaboration: preparing, maintaining and disseminating systematic reviews of the effects of health care. JAMA 1995;274:1935–1938.
28. JADAD AR, HAYNES RB. The Cochrane collaboration: advances and challenges in improving evidence based decision making. Med Decis Making 1998;18:2–9.
29. FREEMANTLE N, MASON JM, HAINES A, ECCLES MP. CONSORT: an important step toward evidence based health care. Consolidated standards of reporting trials. Ann Intern Med 1997;126:81–83.
30. ROSENBERG W, DONALD A. Evidence based medicine: an approach to clinical problem solving. BMJ 1995;310:1122–1126.
31. MOHER D, COOK DJ, EASTWOOD S, et al.. Improving the quality of reports of meta-analyses of randomized controlled trials: the QUOROM statement. Lancet 1999;354:1896–1900.

32. FEINSTEIN AR, HORWITZ RI. Problems in the "evidence" of "evidence based medicine." Am J Med 1997;103:529–535.
33. KERNICK DP. Lies, damned lies, and evidence based medicine. Lancet 1998;351:1824.
34. HORWITZ RI. The dark side of evidence based medicine. Clev Clin J Med 1996;63:320–323.
35. SHAHAR E. A Popperian perspective of the term "evidence based medicine." J Eval Clin Prac 1997;3:109–116.
36. BAIRD MA. Physician-patient-family trust: the bridge to reach evidence based medicine. Fam Med 1996;28:682–683.
37. ELLRODT G, COOK DJ, LEE J, et al. Evidence based disease management. JAMA 1997;278: 1687–1692.
38. COHEN JJ. Higher quality at lower cost: maybe there is a way. Acad Med 1998;73:414–419.
39. CARPENTER CE, BENDER DA, NASH DB, et al. Must we choose between quality and costs? Qual Healthc 1996;5:223–229.
40. Evidence Based Medicine Working Group. Evidence-based medicine: A new approach to teaching the practice of medicine. JAMA 1992;268:2420–2425.
41. RAFUSE J. Evidence based medicine means MDs must develop new skills, attitudes, CMA conference told. CMAJ 1994;150:1479–1481.
42. COOK D. Evidence based critical care medicine: a potential tool for change. New Horiz 1998;6: 20–25.
43. COOK DJ, SIBBALD WJ, VINCENT JL, et al. Evidence based critical care medicine: what is it and what can it do for us? Evidence based medicine in critical care group. Crit Care Med 1996;24: 334–337.
44. VANDERBROUCKE JP. Observational research and evidence based medicine: what should we teach young physicians? J Clin Epidemiol 1998;51:467–472.
45. SENGE PM. The Fifth Discipline: The Art and Practice of the Learning Organization. New York:Bantam Doubleday Dell Publishing; 1990.
46. BERWICK DM. Developing and testing changes in the delivery of care. Ann Intern Med 1998;128:833–838.
47. DAVIS D. The Physician as a Learner. Chicago:AMA Press; 1994.
48. DAVIS DA, THOMSON MA, OXMAN AD, et al. Changing physician performance. A systematic review of the effect of continuing medical education strategies. JAMA 1995;274:700–705.
49. DAVIS DA, THOMSON MA, OXMAN AD, et al. Evidence for the effectiveness of CME: a review of 50 randomized controlled trials. JAMA 1992;268:1111–1117.
50. GREEN ML, ELLIS PJ. Impact of an evidence based medicine curriculum based on adult learning theory. J Gen Intern Med 1997;12:742–750.
51. BENNETT RJ, SACKETT DL, HAYNES RB, et al. A controlled clinical trial of teaching critical appraisal of clinical literature to medical students. JAMA 1987;257:2451–2454.
52. SHIN JH, HAYNES RB, JOHNSTON ME. Effect of problem based, self directed undergraduate education on life-long learning. Can Med Assoc J 1993;148:969–976.
53. SACKETT DL. Evidence Based Medicine: How to Practice and Teach EBM. 2nd ed. London:Churchill Livingstone; 2000.
54. HERSH W. Evidence based medicine and the internet. ACP J Club 1996;125:A14–A16.
55. KILEY R. Evidence based medicine on the Internet. J Royal Soc Med 1998;91:74–75.
56. HAYNES RB, WILCZYNSKI N, MCKIBBON KA, et al. Developing optimal search strategies for detecting clinically sound studies in MEDLINE. J Am Med Infor Assoc 1994;1:447–458.
57. MACPHERSON DW. Evidence based medicine. CMAJ 1995;152:201–204.
58. NWOSU CR, KHAN KS, CHIEN PFW. A two term MEDLINE search strategy for identifying randomized trials in obstetrics and gynecology. Obstet Gynecol 1998;91:618–622.
59. COUMOU HC, MEIJMAN FJ. How do primary care physicians seek answers to clinical questions? A literature review. J Med Libr Assoc 2006;94(1):55–60.
60. THACKER SB, PETERSON HB, STROUP DF. Meta-analysis for the obstetrician gynecologist. Am J Obstet Gynecol 1996;174:1403–1407.
61. OHLSSON A. Systematic reviews – theory and practice. Scan J Clin Lab Invest 1994;54(219):25–32.

62. LELORIER J, GREGOIRE G, BENHADDAD A, et al. Discrepancies between meta-analyses and subsequent large randomized controlled trials. N Engl J Med 1997;337:536–542.

63. LAU J, ANTMAN EM, JIMENIEZ-SILVA J, et al. Cumulative meta-analysis of therapeutic trials for myocardial infarction. N Engl J Med 1992;327:248–254.

64. HEFFNER JE. Does evidence based medicine help the development of clinical practice guidelines? Chest 1998;113:172S-178S.

65. BERG AO. Clinical practice guidelines: believe only some of what you read. Fam Pract Manag 1996;3(4):58–70.

66. KAVANAGH BP. The GRADE system for rating clinical guidelines. PLoS Med 2009;6(9):e1000094. doi: 10.1371/journal.pmed.1000094.

67. BEGG C, CHO M, EASTWOOD S, et al. Improving the quality of reporting of randomized controlled trials: The CONSORT statement. JAMA 1996;276:637–639.

68. CHALMERS TC, SMITH H, BLACKBURN B, et al. A method for assessing the quality of a randomized controlled trial. Control Clin Trial 1981;2:31–49.

69. CHALMERS I, DICKERSON K, CHALMERS TC. Getting to grips with Archie Cochrane's agenda. BMJ 1992;304:786–788.

70. INGELFINGER JA, MOSTELLER F, THIBODEAU LA, et al. Reading a report of a clinical trial. In:Biostatistics in Clinical Medicine. 3rd ed. New York:McGraw Hill; 1994. p 259–279.

71. HULLEY SB, CUMMINGS SR. Designing Clinical Research. Baltimore, MD:William and Wilkins; 1988.

72. OXMAN AD, SACKETT DL, GUYATT GH. User's guide to the medical literature I. How to get started. JAMA 1993;270:2093–2095.

73. GUYATT GH, SACKETT DL, COOK DJ. Evidence-based medicine working group: user's guides to the medical literature II: how to use an article about therapy or prevention A. Are the results of the study valid? JAMA 1993;270(21):2598–2601.

74. GUYATT GH, SACKETT DL, COOK DJ. User's guide to the medical literature II. How to use an article about therapy or prevention B. What were the results and will they help me in caring for my patients? JAMA 1994;271:59–63.

75. JAESCHKE R, GYATT GH, SACKETT DL. User's guide to the medical literature III. How to use an article about a diagnostic test. A. Are the results of the study valid? JAMA 1994;271:389–391, 703–707.

76. JAESCHKE R, GYATT GH, SACKETT DL. User's guide to the medical literature III. How to use an article about a diagnostic test. B.What are the results and will they help me in caring for my patients? JAMA 1994;271:703–707.

77. LEVINE M, WALTER S, LEE H, et al. User's guide to the medical literature. IV. How to use an article about harm. JAMA 1994;271:1615–1619.

78. LAUPACIS A, WELLS G, RICHARDSON S, et al. User's guide to the medical literature. V. How to use an article about prognosis. JAMA 1994;272:234–237.

79. OXMAN AD, COOK DJ, GUYATT GH. User's guide to the medical literature. VI. How to use an overview. JAMA 1994;272:1367–1371.

80. RICHARDSON WS, DETSKY AS. User's guide to the medical literature. VII. How to use a clinical decision analysis. A. Are the results of the study valid? JAMA 1995;273:1292–1295.

81. HAYWARD RSA, WILSON M, TUNIS SR, et al. User's guide to the medical literature. VIII. How to use clinical practice guidelines. A. Are the recommendations valid? JAMA 1995;274:570–574.

82. WILSON M, HAYWARD RSA, TUNIS S, et al. User's guide to the medical literature. VIII. How to use clinical practice guidelines. B. What are the recommendations and will they help you in caring for your patients? JAMA 1995;274:1630–1632.

83. GUYATT GH, SACKETT DL, SINCLAIR JC, et al. User's guide to the medical literature. IX. A method for grading health care recommendations. JAMA 1995;274:1800–1804.

84. NAYLOR CD, GUYATT GH. User's guide to the medical literature. X. How to use an article reporting variations in the outcomes of health services. JAMA 1996;275:554–558.

85. NAYLOR CD, GUYATT GH. User's guide to the medical literature. XI. How to use an article about clinical utilization review. JAMA 1996;275:1435–1439.

86. US Preventive Health Services Task Force. Guide to Clinical Preventive Services. 2nd ed. Baltimore, MD:Williams and Wilkins; 1995.

87. SCHULTZ KF, CHALMERS I, HAYES RJ, et al. Dimensions of methodological quality with estimates of treatment effects in controlled trials. JAMA 1995;273:412–415.

88. COLDITZ GA, MILLER JN, MOSTELLER F. How study design affects outcomes in comparisons of therapy. I: Medical. Stat Med 1989;8:441–454.

89. MILLER JN, COLDITZ GA, MOSTELLER F. How study design affects outcomes in comparisons of therapy. II: Surgical. Stat Med 1989;8:455–466.

90. BULLOCK DR, CHESTNUT R, CLIFTON G, et al. Guidelines for the management of severe head injury. Eur J Emerg Med 1996;3:109–127.

91. GREENHALGH T. Statistics for the non-statistician: I. BMJ 1997;315:364–366.

92. GREENHALGH T. Statistics for the non-statistician. II: "Significant" relations and their pitfalls. BMJ 1997;315:422–425.

93. STEWART LA, PARMAR MKB. Bias in the analysis and reporting of controlled trials. Int J Health Tech Assess 1996;12:264–275.

94. GUYATT G, JAENSCHKE R, HEDDLE N, et al. Basic statistics for clinicians. I. Hypothesis testing. Can Med Assoc J 1995;152:27–32.

95. SOX HC Jr, BLATT MA, HIGGINS MC, et al. Medical Decision Making. Newton, MA:Butterworth-Heimnemann; 1988. p 103–145.

96. DATA™. Decision Analysis Program from TreeAge Software. Williamstown, MA. http://www.treeage.com.

97. SONNENBERG FA, BECK JR. Markov models in decision making: a practical guide. Med Decis Making 1993;13:322–328.

98. DETSKY AS, NAGLIE G, KRAHN MD, et al. Primer on medical decision analysis. Part 1: Getting started. Med Decis Making 1997;17:123–125.

99. DETSKY AS, NAGLIE G, KRAHN MD, et al. Primer of medical decision analysis. Part 2: Building a tree. Med Decis Making 1997;17:126–135.

100. NAGLIE G, MURRAY D, KRAHN MD, et al. Primer on medical decision analysis. Part 3: Estimating probabilities and utilities. Med Decis Making 1997;17:136–141.

101. KRAHN MD, NAGLIE G, NAIMARK D, et al. Primer on medical decision analysis. Part 4: Analyzing the model and interpreting the results. Med Decis Making 1997;17:142–151.

102. NAIMARK D, KRAHN MD, NAGLIE G, et al. Primer on medical decision analysis. Part 5: Working with Markov processes. Med Decis Making 1997;17:152–159.

103. SCHUETTE HL, TUCKER TC, BROWN ML. The costs of cancer care in the United States: implications for action. Oncology 1995;9(11):19–22.

104. DOUBILET PM, WEINSTEIN MC, McNEIL BJ. Use and abuse of the term "cost-effective" in medicine. N Engl J Med 1986;314:253–256.

105. KEELER EB, CRETIN S. Discounting of lifesaving and other monetary benefits. Manag Sci 1983;29:300–306.

106. GOLD MR, SIEGEL JE, RUSSELL LB. Cost-Effectiveness in Health and Medicine. New York:Oxford University Press, 1996.

107. FINKLER SA. The distinction between cost and charges. Ann Intern Med 1982;96:102–109.

108. SAMUELSON WF, MARKS SG. Managerial Economics. 2nd ed. ORLANDO, FL:The Dryden Press/Harcourt Brace; 1995. p 700–715.

109. BOYLE MH, TORRANCE GW, SINCLAIR JC, et al. Economic evaluation of neonatal intensive care very-low-birth-weight infants. N Engl J Med 1983;308:1330–1337.

110. OLDRIDGE N, FURLONG W, FEENY D. Economic evaluation of cardiac rehabilitation soon after myocardial infarction. Am J Cardiol 1993;72:154–161.

111. RUSSELL LB, GOLD MR, SIEGEL JE, DANIELS N, WEINSTEIN MC, Panel on Cost-effectiveness in health and medicine: The role of cost-effectiveness analysis in health and medicine. JAMA 1996;276(14):1172–1177.

112. MEHREZ A, GAFNI A. Quality adjusted life years, utility theory and health year equivalents. Med Decis Making 1989;9:142–149.

113. MAHER M. Cost Accounting. Creating Value for Management. 5th ed. McGraw Hill; 1997. p 231–185

114. NEASE RF Jr, KNEELAND T, O'CONNOR GT. The Ischemic Heart Disease Patient Outcomes Research Team: variation in patient utilities for outcomes of the management of chronic stable angina: implications for clinical practice guidelines. JAMA 1995;273:1185–1190.

115. WEINSTEIN MC, SIEGEL JE, GOLD MR, et al. Panel on Cost effectiveness in Health and Medicine: Recommendations on cost-effectiveness in health and medicine. JAMA 1996;275(15):1253–1258.

116. SIEGEL JE, WEINSTEIN MC, RUSSELL LB, GOLD MR, Panel on Cost-effectiveness in Health and Medicine. Recommendations for reporting cost effectiveness analysis. JAMA 1996;276(16): 1339–1341.

117. SMITH WJ, BLACKMORE CC. Economic analysis in obstetrics and gynecology. Obstet Gynecol 1998;91(3):472–478.

118. WEINSTEIN MC. Principles of cost effective resource allocation in health care organizations. Int J Technol Assess Health Care. 1990;6:93–103.

119. KOSECOFF J, KANOUSE DE, ROGERS WH, et al. Effects of the National Institutes of Health Consensus Development Program on physician practice. JAMA 1987;258(19):2708.

120. WINN RJ, BOTNICK WZ, BROWN NH. The NCCN Guideline Program 1998. Oncology 1998;12:30–34.

121. HUTCHNISON A. The philosophy of clinical practice guidelines: purposes, problems, practicality and implementation. J Qual Clin Pract 1998;18:63–73.

122. GRIMSHAW JM, RUSSELL IT. Effects of clinical guidelines on medical practice: a systematic review of rigorous evaluations. Lancet 1993;342:1317–1322.

Chapter 3

Vascular Access and Other Invasive Procedures

Paul Koonings, MD and Scott E. Lentz, MD

INTRODUCTION

Venous access is an important technique in the care and management of gynecological patients. There are two major types of venous access available—peripheral and central.[1] Peripheral venous access is the preferred method unless there is a contraindication to its use. In general, the closer venous access is toward the heart, the greater the frequency and severity of complications.

VASCULAR ACCESS PROCEDURES

Short-Term Central Venous Catheterization

Central venous catheterization has emerged as an integral part of the management of gynecological oncology patients.[2] Multiple venipunctures and the prolonged administration of intravenous agents lead to venous irritation, as many house officers and patients can attest. The resultant phlebitis produces a gradual sclerosis with subsequent destruction of the peripheral veins.[3] Hyperosmolar solutions, chemotherapeutic agents, and other irritating intravenous agents are particularly destructive. This absence of adequate peripheral veins may not only delay the administration of chemotherapeutic agents but can also result in a higher complication rate secondary to the extravasation of these particularly toxic drugs.

Central venous catheterization has been used in many of these situations to circumvent these problems, allowing for reliable venous catheterization albeit their placement and maintenance is not without risk. Indications for central venous catheterization include the absence of peripheral veins, prolonged intravenous therapy, parenteral hyperalimentation, hemodynamic monitoring, and the administration

Gynecologic Oncology: Evidence-Based Perioperative and Supportive Care, Second Edition.
Edited by Scott E. Lentz, Allison E. Axtell and Steven A. Vasilev.
© 2011 John Wiley & Sons, Inc. Published 2011 by John Wiley & Sons, Inc.

of intensive chemotherapy. Short-term (less than 30 days) catheterization is primarily used in the perioperative or immediate postoperative period. The usual indications for short-term central venous catheterization include infusion of large amounts of intravenous solutions including blood products and the need to monitor central venous pressure or placement of a Swan–Ganz catheter. Short-term parenteral hyperalimentation may also be given through these devices.

Technique

There are two primary approaches to central venous catheterization used in a gynecological patient: the internal jugular approach and the subclavian approach. Familiarity with each method is recommended; however, most institutions use either the internal jugular or the subclavian vein exclusively.[3,4] Needless to say, it is of great importance to understand the anatomy involving each approach. It is precisely because of the anatomy that the right side is preferred for each technique. On the left side, the dome of the lung and the pleura are elevated while the thoracic duct empties nearby, exposing these structures to possible trauma. Moreover, there is a more direct route to the right atrium when using the right internal jugular approach. This approach should be exclusively used on ventilator patients requiring a central venous line since a lung puncture can result in a tension pneumothorax.

General Preparation of the Patient   Once the decision for central venous access has been made, informed consent should be obtained from the patient or guardian. Information involving risks, benefits, and alternatives are included in this discussion. All questions of the patient must be addressed.

Following informed consent, the proposed introduction site is prepared with an antiseptic solution approximately 5–10 cm around it. Hirsute sites should be depilated with electric clippers. Insertion discomfort should be dealt with aggressively. Intravenous medication (e.g., morphine sulfate and Versed) along with a generous amount of local anesthetic will usually suffice. After the local anesthetic is drawn up in a syringe, it is slowly injected subcutaneously using a 25-gauge or smaller needle along the proposed needle tract.

Once the area has been adequately prepped and anesthetized, the clinician should use sterile gloves. If the procedure is nonemergent, the use of sterile drapes, gown, cap, and mask is recommended.

The clinician should be familiar with the prepackaged kits available. A spare kit should be available during insertion in case the original becomes unusable.

Internal Jugular Vein Approach

Anatomy   The internal jugular vein extends from the base of the skull adjacent to the carotid artery entering the chest to join the subclavian vein behind the clavicle. It is initially lateral to the carotid artery and moves anterior to the internal carotid artery at the level of C6. It lies posterior to the sternocleidomastoid muscle.

Insertion Technique[5-7] The following steps should be followed for internal jugular vein insertion.

1. The patient undergoes general preparation.
2. The patient is placed in Trendelenburg position (15–30 degrees).
3. The patient's head is turned contralateral to the insertion site at approximately 45 degrees.
4. The anatomical landmarks are identified. This includes the apex of the triangle formed by the sternocleidomastoid muscle and the base of the trapezius near the clavicle.
5. If the ipsilateral carotid artery can be palpated, it is gently retracted medially.
6. The needle is inserted at the apex of the triangle at a 20- to 30-degree angle to the frontal plane, aiming just lateral to the ipsilateral nipple. It is advanced with continuous gentle negative pressure. The jugular vein is usually entered within 3 cm; if the needle catheter is inserted beyond 5 cm, the risk of pneumothorax or arterial puncture increases.
7. Once the vein has been identified and blood may be easily aspirated, the modified Seldinger technique is used to insert the selected catheter.[8] A J-shaped guidewire is gently passed through the needle. This wire must never be forced as this can result in vessel rupture. Moreover, the wire should never be retracted with the needle in place as this may result in wire shearing. If the guidewire is advanced too far, it may cause premature ventricular beats. In these circumstances, it should be retracted so the ectopic beats abate. The wire should be constantly held through these maneuvers.
8. The needle is now removed and replaced with the vein dilator and the catheter. Occasionally the skin puncture site needs to be enlarged sharply. Once the catheter is in place, the dilator and guidewire are removed. Flow of blood is then confirmed and the catheter connected to the appropriate intravenous solution.
9. The catheter is then anchored to the skin and covered with a gauze dressing.
10. A mandatory end-expiration chest X-ray is checked for proper catheter placement and the presence of a pneumothorax.

Subclavian Vein Insertion

Anatomy The subclavian vein, a continuation of the axillary vein, arches gently across the first rib in front of the anterior scalene muscle and inferior to the clavicle. Its course approximates that of the deeper subclavian artery which can be palpated posterior to the clavicular head of the sternocleidomastoid muscle. The thoracic duct enters at the junction of the left subclavian and internal jugular veins.[9-11]

Insertion Technique The following steps should be followed for subclavian vein insertion.

1. The patient is prepared and positioned similar to that for internal jugular intravenous catheterization except that a small pillow is placed between the scapula to elevate the clavicular heads.

2. The puncture site should be located lateral to the midpoint of the clavicle, approximately 1–2 cm below it.

3. Once inserted it should be parallel to the frontal plane just below the clavicle. It is unnecessary to "walk the needle" under the clavicle as this causes extreme pain and discomfort. The index finger may be placed gently in the suprasternal notch to indicate the target area. Mild constant aspiration is applied during needle advancement. Once the free flow of blood is achieved, the needle is advanced a further 5 mm to confirm intraluminal placement.

4. The needle bevel is then oriented toward the heart.

5. A guidewire is threaded through the needle while the patient performs the Valsalva maneuver to prevent an air embolus.

6. The needle is replaced with a vein dilator followed by the catheter. It is extremely important not to let go of the guidewire during this procedure. Once the catheter is placed, the guidewire is removed. Blood flow is confirmed and the catheter is connected to the appropriate intravenous solutions. The catheter is then anchored and covered. Its position and the absence of a pneumothorax are confirmed by a postprocedure end expiration chest X-ray. The catheter tip should be in the superior vena cava above the pericardial reflection.

Complications

Complications of central venous catheterization may occur as a result of insertion or continued catheter presence. Insertion complications include the inability to cannulize the vein, cardiac arrhythmias, pneumothorax, arterial puncture, and air embolism. It appears that a failed initial insertion is the biggest predictor of other complications. Insertion complications can be avoided as a function of increasing experience and meticulous attention to details. It is the responsibility of the surgeon to not only be able to diagnose these complications but to treat them in a timely manner.

Insertion Complications

Inability to Identify or Cannulize the Central Vein Rarely, one is unable to identify and aspirate the central vein after several attempts. In such incidences, the anatomy should be reviewed to make sure that landmarks are correctly identified. The patient's position is checked to ensure that he or she is in steep Trendelenburg position, with the head turned toward the opposite side. If the patient has a peripheral venous catheter, hydration is useful. If these exercises are unsuccessful, there are two further approaches the physician may use. The first approach is to use ultrasound to identify the intended central vein.[12, 13] A 5- to 7.5-MHz transducer may identify the vein and allow easier targeting. If this does not work, an alternate approach may be used.[14] This should be performed on the ipsilateral side if subclavian vein catheterization was attempted in order to obviate the risk of bilateral pneumothorax or paratracheal hematoma.

Cardiac Arrhythmia   Occasionally, premature ventricular beats are encountered during catheter placement. These ectopic beats are primarily due to ventricular irritation from the guidewire. Withdrawing the guidewire will usually stop these ectopic beats. Rarely are anti-arrhythmia agents required.

Pneumothorax   The risk of pneumothorax appears inversely related to the experience of the physician.[15] It has been estimated that experienced physicians have one-half the complication rate of inexperienced physicians. Therefore, a physician experienced in central line placement should be present during the actual procedure. The risk of pneumothorax is also related to the approach used. The subclavian approach appears to have a higher preponderance of pneumothorax compared to the internal jugular approach.[16] As previously mentioned, left-sided placements have a higher pneumothorax rate. Chest X-ray is the gold standard for diagnosing a pneumothorax. An end expiration film enhances the diagnosis of pneumothorax. After central venous catheterization has been attempted or completed it is prudent to obtain a chest X-ray. Clinically the patient may complain of sudden onset of chest pain with radiation to the neck as well as shortness of breath. Physical findings occasionally reveal absent breath sounds with tactile phemitus. The treatment for pneumothorax is discussed under "Chest Tube Thoracostomy."

Hematoma   The risk of massive hematoma following central venous placement is low.[17] A thorough understanding of the anatomy combined with experience and good technique will reduce this complication. Any history of a bleeding disorder should be evaluated with the appropriate coagulation studies before this procedure is undertaken. Occasionally, internal jugular venous cannulization can result in an inadvertent carotid artery puncture. Palpation and medial retraction of the carotid artery is helpful. If the carotid artery is inadvertently punctured, direct pressure is usually adequate to control bleeding. Subclavian site bleeding is more difficult to control, as direct pressure of the involved vessel is difficult. An expanding hematoma may result in respiratory embarrassment secondary to a paratracheal hematoma. Thoracic surgery consultation should be considered to assist in the management of this complication.

Air Embolism   The deadliest, rarest, and most preventable complication associated with central venous placement is air embolism. Air embolism occurs when there is a break in the circuit allowing atmospheric pressure to push air into the circulation. A fatal dose of air (100 mL) can be delivered in less than 1 second. The primary opportunities for this devastating condition occur during insertion or removal of the catheter and during line breaks when the intravenous components are changed.

Careless technique or equipment failure allows air to enter the venous circulation, which is then pumped into the right ventricle, thereby interrupting blood flow. The patient may complain of chest pain with shortness of breath as well as anxiety. Clinical findings reveal hypotension tachycardia and cogwheel cardiac murmur. The association of air embolism with the site of insertion of central venous catheters was reported in a small retrospective study of 26 patients. The results are notable in that there seemed to be no preponderance of emboli specific to a single insertion site. While the largest number of emboli did occur in patients with subclavian insertions, the authors acknowledge a presumed bias as this method comprised the vast majority of line insertions[18] (**Level II-3**).

Air embolism can be prevented during vein cannulation by placing the vein in a dependent position while the patient exhales.

Once air embolism is diagnosed or suspected the patient should be placed in the left lateral Trendelenburg position (Durant's position) and given 100% oxygen immediately. Some authors suggest that hyperbaric oxygen can accomplish the same effect, but studies have failed to clarify whether hyperbaric oxygen therapy is superior to 100% inspired oxygen.[19] The source of the air leak should be located and closed off. A thoracic surgery consult should be considered as well as direct suction of the heart.

Complications Related to Catheter Presence   Infection, thrombosis, and positional obstruction are the most common problems associated with catheter presence.[20] The physician who places these catheters must know how to recognize and treat these challenges to patient well-being. Long-term complications as a result of prolonged catheter presence are discussed in a separate section.

Infection   Estimates of catheter infection range from 5% to 25%,[21–26] and intravascular devices are the most important cause of iatrogenic blood stream infection.[27–31] The conventional reporting method for catheter-related infections has been to express a rate "per 100 devices," but current recommendations have changed the reporting to rates per 1000 catheter days. This change more accurately reflects the infection rates originating from the catheter's presence.[32–35] The incidence of infection is directly time-related and becomes more common after 72 hours. Diagnosis is made by a physical examination, primarily by checking the patient's temperature and the catheter site as well. Blood and catheter cultures are obtained to confirm the diagnosis. A basic line sepsis algorithm is shown in Fig. 3.1. There appear to be several maneuvers available which decrease the infection rate. Subclavian vein catheterization has a lower infection rate than internal jugular venous catheterization, which is believed to be secondary to the difficulty in keeping the neck area sterile. Therefore, the subclavian approach should be specifically considered in neutropenic patients. Several studies have examined whether changing the catheter site, changing the catheter over a guidewire, or continued use of the same site until clinically indicated is of benefit in decreasing the infection rate.[36–39] Prospective studies revealed no difference between these aforementioned techniques. An arbitrary rule dictating catheter change every 3–7 days appears to be of little, if any, benefit. Therefore, the catheter can be

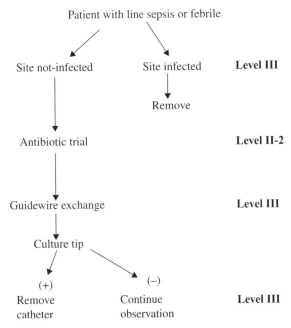

Figure 3.1   Suggested management of central venous line sepsis.

left in place unless there are clinical signs of infection. After the initial enthusiasm for semipermeable dressings for central venous catheterization, recent studies have revealed no advantage over the plain gauze dressing.[40] They may in fact lead to increased infection rate. It is therefore recommended that the catheter exit site be covered with an antibiotic ointment if desired and then covered with a plain gauze dressing. Another issue is whether single, double, or triple lumen catheters have a higher infection rate. In general, the multilumen catheters require more connections, thereby permitting more opportunities for technique breakdown and bacterial contamination. Therefore, as in other situations, the right catheter for the right indication should be selected.

A comprehensive analysis of catheter-related infection events by authors from the University of Wisconsin Medical School attempted to quantify the relative risks particular to each intravascular device[41] (**Level II-2**). Prospective analysis of blood stream infections was the primary inclusion criterion and there were 200 such reports available in the literature for analysis. All commonly used intravascular devices were represented across a wide variety of disease states, including hematology and oncology. These reports are also notable for the fact that the authors calculated infection rates using both methods, i.e., per 100 devices as well as per 1000 catheter days. The distinction in reporting is more than academic. Reporting results per 1000 catheter days is the currently recommended method, as it better reflects blood stream infections directly attributable to the catheter rather than infections coincident with catheter presence.[32–35] The results are dramatically different and instructive in terms

Table 3.1   Rates of Intravascular Device Related Bloodstream Infections[a]

Type of Device	Number of Studies	Pooled Mean (Per 1000 Catheter Days)	95% CI[b]
Peripheral plastic catheter	110	0.5	0.2–0.7
Arterial catheter	14	1.7	1.2–2.3
PICC[b]	15	1.1	0.9–1.3
Central catheter—nontunneled, nonmedicated	79	2.7	2.6–2.9
Central catheter—nontunneled, medicated	18	1.6	1.3–2.0
Cuffed and tunneled central catheter	29	1.6	1.5–1.7
Subcutaneous central venous port	14	0.1	0.0–0.1
Pulmonary artery catheter	13	3.7	2.4–5.0
Hemodialysis catheter, temporary	18	4.8	4.2–5.3
Hemodialysis catheter, long-term	18	1.6	1.5–1.7

[a]Excerpted from Reference 41.
[b]PICC, peripherally inserted central catheter; CI, confidence interval.

of catheter management (Table 3.1). The leading conclusions of the authors are as follows.

- All intravascular catheter devices pose a risk of blood stream infection.
- Arterial catheters pose an infection risk similar to that seen with nontunneled, noncuffed multilumen central catheters (1.7 vs. 2.7 per 1000 catheter days) and deserve further study as a source of catheter-related blood stream infection.
- Peripherally inserted central catheter (PICC) lines are more likely to lead to blood stream infection when compared with cuffed and tunneled central venous catheters (3.5 vs. 1.6 per 1000 catheter days).
- Noncuffed hemodialysis catheters are substantially more likely to lead to blood stream infections than their cuffed counterparts (4.8 vs. 1.6 per 1000 catheter days).
- Surgically implanted central ports are much safer than cuffed and tunneled catheters (0.1 vs. 1.6 per 1000 catheter days), but this advantage may be mitigated if the implanted port is accessed repeatedly or for a prolonged period.
- Tunneling a noncuffed catheter can reduce the catheter-related infection risk by 33% (2.7 vs. 1.7 per 1000 catheter days), but this may be impractical in patients who are anticoagulated or coagulopathic.

Thrombosis Secondary to Catheter Presence   The incidence of catheter-related thrombosis is related to the length of time for which the catheter is left in place, and the combination of catheter presence and coexistent cancer confers a twofold increase in risk (adjusted OR, 43.6; 95% CI, 25.5–74.6).[42,43] Significant thrombosis is unusual in catheters left in place for 2 weeks or less. Inherited mutations in Factor V Leiden and prothrombin G20210A have been shown to increase the overall risk of upper-extremity deep vein thrombosis (DVT) by threefold.[44] It is not clear how many upper-extremity DVT events are caused solely by heritable mutations; published rates range from 10% to 26%. Because of this, routine screening for these mutations is recommended only in cases of unexplained thrombosis[45] (**Level III**).

The clinical signatures of central venous thrombosis are edema, erythema, and pain in either upper extremity. Duplex ultrasound will diagnose venous obstruction while radiographic dye infusion through the catheter will characterize the thrombus. Other clinical clues to the presence of thrombosis include the inability to aspirate and inject through the catheter. As in the lower extremity, contrast venography is the gold standard, but this is not the usual practice standard because of the invasive nature of the test and the potential risks associated with repetitive contrast dosing. Alternatively, ultrasound-based methods have been shown to be the most reliable noninvasive method.[46,47] Once the diagnosis of catheter-related thrombosis is made, treatment is indicated (Fig. 3.2). The patient is heparinized with catheter removal until asymptomatic and then placed on Coumadin for approximately 3 months.[48] If continued catheter use is warranted in the face of thrombosis, urokinase or streptokinase infusion may resolve the thrombosis; however, a bleeding diathesis may be significant. Ultimately, if the catheter is not removed, the thrombosis will recur.

The continued need for venous catheterization in cancer patients means that catheter-related thrombosis presents a real challenge to continuing therapy. The requirement to remove a catheter in order to successfully treat a thrombosis has been questioned in a pilot fashion in a single cohort from multiple institutions. All patients were actively receiving chemotherapy and suffered an upper-extremity thrombosis. Instead of removing the lines, patients were treated with concurrent low molecular weight heparin (5 days) and oral warfarin (3 months). In an intent-to-treat analysis, 100% of patients were able to maintain their catheters without repeat thrombosis. One patient (4% of study population) did suffer a catastrophic hemorrhage which resulted in death, a rate consistent with other published studies in anticoagulant therapy in cancer patients. The authors conclude that cancer patients with indwelling lines can maintain their catheters while receiving anticoagulation for a catheter-induced thrombosis[19,49] (**Level II-3**). Conflicting information concerning the role of prophylactic anticoagulation in upper-extremity venous catheters has failed to define a standard management method in these patients. Notably, studies that have examined the role of prophylactic therapy have failed to include a safety analysis, an important consideration in determining the need for preventive therapy.[44]

Positional Obstruction Positional obstruction can occur with subclavian catheters.[50] It is related to the medial location of the catheter. This allows the catheter to be pinched off between the clavicle and the first rib. This obstruction is usually intermittently relieved when the shoulder is elevated, alleviating rib pinching. If not corrected, this condition may result in catheter fracture with subsequent embolus.

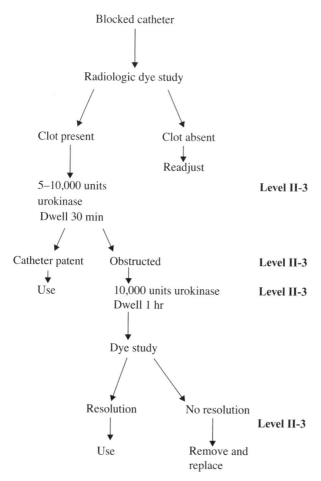

Figure 3.2   Suggested management of central venous line blockage.

This complication can be avoided by using an alternate access site once positional obstruction is recognized. To prevent this complication the venous puncture should be made lateral to the midclavicular line so that the catheter will be inside the lumen of the subclavian vein and therefore protected as it passes over the first rib.

Long-Term Venous Catheterization

Over the past two decades, long-term venous catheterization devices have emerged as the benchmark for reliable venous access in patients requiring lengthy intravenous therapy. The decision of whether to place a long-term central venous catheterization device in the patient is dependent on many factors. These factors include the patient's current condition, availability of effective therapy, and the patient's life expectancy.

Patients with malignancy requiring chemotherapy, administration of blood products, and parenteral nutrition have an improved quality of life with these devices. They may also be used for blood draws. It is estimated that approximately 400,000 long-term intravenous catheterization catheters are implanted yearly in the United States alone.[1]

Once the decision to place the long-term central venous access catheter has been made, a device needs to be selected. Currently, there are two major catheter systems used: those with and without a reservoir. A port-a-cath is an example of the reservoir type. The reservoir system is completely buried underneath the epidermis. The advantages of this system include minimal maintenance, freedom from dressings and activity restrictions, better cosmesis, and minimal maintenance when compared to the nonreservoir system. A special needle (Huber) that displaces rather than punctures the diaphragm is used to access the reservoir. Examples of the nonreservoir type include a Broviac or Hickman catheter. The nonreservoir system usually requires frequent flushing and dressing changes. Moreover, it penetrates the epidermis constantly reminding the patient of her disease and limits physical activities including swimming and showering. The major disadvantage of the reservoir type is the increased time (approximately 15 minutes) required to place the reservoir and technical skill. However, its advantages easily outweigh its disadvantages, leading it to become the device of choice.

Insertion Technique

The insertion technique involves the following steps.

1. Informed consent should be given to the patient.

2. The site of the reservoir or exit site of the nonreservoir system should be identified. It is best to do this while the patient wears her brassiere so the device can be located in such a manner that it will not interfere with or irritate the patient. The reservoir/exit site should not be so far lateral that the patient rubs the device when moving her arm from the device. In patients with large breasts, the port should be located medially so that it can be easily palpated for access.

3. The internal jugular or subclavian vein is located and accessed as previously mentioned, leaving the J-wire *in situ* with a clamp to prevent migration.

4. The proposed reservoir/exit site is infiltrated with marcaine and an incision is made. If a reservoir port is going to be used, the incision should be approximately 4–5 cm long.

5. A 21-gauge spinal needle is then used to infiltrate marcaine along the proposed catheter track.

6. An introducer/dilator is then introduced from the exit of the J-wire to the proposed reservoir/exit side of the catheter.

7. The catheter is then attached to the dilator and tunneled in the subcutaneous tissue to where the J-wire is located. The Dacron cuff is placed well within the tunnel. If a reservoir is used, a small crevice is made for it to prevent

migration. The reservoir must be anchored to the chest fascia using nonabsorbable monofilament sutures.

8. The catheter is then placed on the chest along its proposed course through the vascular system. It is tailored to a length usually 1 or 2 cm below the sternal notch approximating the location of the superior vena cava.

9. A peel-away catheter introducer is then inserted along the J-wire into the venous system.

10. The J-wire is then removed and the catheter is threaded while the patient performs the Valsalva maneuver.

11. The peel-away introducer is then retracted, peeled, and removed. Catheter placement is then confirmed using fluoroscopy. The catheter tip should be in the superior vena cava 1–2 cm from the right atrium. The incision sites are then closed using either steri strips or subcuticular stitches. The reservoir or catheter can be accessed following a chest X-ray to confirm position and to rule out pneumothorax. This should be done only with a Huber needle in the case of the reservoir.

Pulmonary Artery Catheterization

The Swan–Ganz catheter was first developed and described over a quarter century ago.[51] Although proposed indications for its use are myriad, its benefits have not been conclusive.[52] A common recommendation made by most investigators is to use the Swan–Ganz catheter in a judicious manner.[52–54] Like most tools in medicine, if not totally familiar with its use, consultation should be obtained. To quantify this effect, a prospective, randomized controlled trial in ICU patients from the National Health Service in the United Kingdom was performed. Outcome measures included hospital mortality, length of ICU stay, length of in-hospital stay, as well as economic evaluation. No differences were seen in mortality (68.4% vs. 65.7%) or length of hospital stay (in either ICU or other inpatient ward). The adjusted hazard ratio (catheter vs. no catheter) was 1.09[55] (**Level I**). The Swan–Ganz catheter can be inserted via any vein used for central venous catheterization.

Insertion Technique

The insertion technique involves the following steps.

1. Informed consent should be obtained from the patient.

2. The equipment should be checked to make sure that all the necessary parts are present for insertion and use and are in working order. Technical difficulties with the equipment are frustrating and can be easily avoided by examining the equipment prior to use. It is mandatory to examine the catheter balloon for leakage, size, and shape by injecting it with 1.5 mL of air prior to insertion. The expiration date on the catheter should also be checked. Fluid should not

be injected into the balloon port. All ports must be flushed and checked for patency.

3. The internal jugular vein or subclavian vein is accessed with the J-wire as previously mentioned.

4. The skin incision is then enlarged and a vessel dilator with an introducer stealth is advanced along the J-wire into the vein. Do not let go of the J-wire.

5. The J-wire and the dilator are then removed and replaced by the pulmonary artery catheter. The pulmonary artery catheter is gently threaded through the introducer.

6. The tip will approximate the right atrium when it is 10–15 cm from the entrance of either the internal jugular vein or subclavian vein. The balloon is then inflated to 1.5 mL.

7. It is then advanced smoothly and rapidly using continuous electrocardio-graphic and pressure monitoring. The catheter will transverse the tricuspid valve, enter and exit the right ventricle at approximately 35–40 cm, traverse the pulmonary artery, and ultimately wedge at approximately 60 cm. Proper position is identified using the characteristic pressure changes. Congestive heat failure may require fluoroscopic assistance.

Balloon deflation should reveal a pulmonary artery pressure pattern. If the catheter continues to reveal a wedge pressure it should be retracted slowly. Once a correct positioning has been confirmed, using the pressure tracing a postprocedure chest X-ray must be obtained. The catheter can be secured and covered in the usual manner.

Complications of the Swan–Ganz Catheter

Complications associated with cannulizing the appropriate central vein are similar to those previously described for venous catheterization. Placement of the Swan–Ganz catheter itself is associated with its own unique types of complications. Arrhythmias associated with Swan–Ganz insertion placement are common, occurring in up to 50% of insertions.[56] A vast majority of these arrhythmias are not hemodynamically significant and will often disappear after withdrawing the catheter into the superior vena cava and reintroducing it. It is incumbent on the physician to be able to diagnose and manage any arrhythmias that may be encountered. These arrhythmias are primarily of ventricular origin secondary to cardiac muscle irritation. Although anti-arrhythmic drugs are rarely needed, they should be readily available. In general, the only ones requiring intervention are complete heart block (requires transvenous pacer therapy) and persistent ventricular tachycardia (requires pharmacotherapy). Arrhythmias are more common when the patient has underlying cardiac disease or a previous history of arrhythmias.

Thrombosis is also occasionally encountered. Its management is similar to that described for central venous catheterization. Increased thrombosis rates are associated with left-sided central catheterization and prolonged duration of catheterization.

Whether low dose heparin or Coumadin is of benefit in this setting is unknown. Infections complicating Swan–Ganz catheter presence may also occur. The previous discussion is applicable in this situation. Sterile technique is mandatory to help reduce this problem. Unfortunately, even with sterile technique, prolonged catheterization will result in infection. These need to be treated on an individual basis, which may involve removal of the catheter and use of antibiotics. Pulmonary infarction is fortunately rare when the catheter is routinely inspected to ensure proper location. The pressure pattern is "key" in this situation. Prolonged wedging will result in pulmonary infarction. It is mandatory that the monitors be regularly checked to rule out persistent wedging. Balloon malfunction is another complication of Swan–Ganz catheters. Balloon rupture occurs primarily with repeated inflations or excessive inflation volumes. The average balloon capacity is less than 1.5 mL and should not be exceeded. If balloon rupture is encountered, the decision should be made on whether pulmonary artery diastolic pressures are sufficient in lieu of wedge pressures before replacement is contemplated. Less common complications include pulmonary artery rupture, which occasionally occurs in patients who have pulmonary hypertension. It is associated with balloon inflation and excess catheter looping. Therefore, the balloon should be inflated for only short periods of time with the right volume and catheter redundancy should be avoided. Complete heart block is an unusual complication associated with preexisting left bundle branch block. Pacemaker insertion is the treatment of choice in this situation. Cardiac tissue injury usually occurs when the balloon is not deflated and the catheter roughly withdrawn. The catheter may disrupt the cordia in this circumstance. Balloon deflation before catheter withdrawal will avoid this devastating complication. Catheter knotting, a rare but serious complication, is associated with patients with congestive heart failure and cardiomegaly.[57] When this situation is encountered, it is prudent to place the Swan–Ganz catheter with fluoroscopic guidance. If a knot is encountered, it can involve one of the tricuspid cordia. Occasionally it can be loosened with gentle traction. If it is unsuccessful, atriotomy is necessary to release the catheter. Force should never be used, as this may rupture the cordia, resulting in massive heart failure and death.

PLEURAL CAVITY PROCEDURES

Thoracentesis

Thoracentesis is the most common invasive pulmonary procedure performed by gynecologists. There are two major types of thoracentesis: diagnostic and therapeutic.[58] Diagnostic thoracentesis is performed when the pleural effusion is of unknown etiology. Once fluid is obtained it is evaluated for LDH, protein, infection, and malignant cells. This allows one to differentiate transudates from exudates. Transudates are usually related to cardiac, liver, or renal dysfunction. Once the responsible organ dysfunction has been corrected, the effusion will correct. An exudative pleural effusion requires a thorough investigation to determine its origin. The vast majority of exudative pleural effusions encountered in gynecology are associated with ovarian malignancy. These effusions are usually associated with ascites. Occasionally, benign ovarian disease can cause a pleural effusion. Meigs described the classic syndrome of ovarian fibroma, ascites, and pleural effusion. It is important for the physician to determine whether the pleural effusion is malignant or not as this will have an impact on the patient's treatment and survival. A therapeutic thoracentesis is primarily performed to relieve the symptoms of dyspnea. It may be combined with a diagnostic thoracentesis if not previously performed by sending the aspirated fluid for the appropriate laboratory evaluation. A patient who undergoes a therapeutic thoracentesis will accumulate pleural fluid in 3–7 days if the underlying disorder is not corrected. Multiple therapeutic thoracentesis can be performed for continued relief of symptoms. Persistent, recurrent pleural effusions should be treated with a chest tube and pleurodesis as described later.

Procedure

A chest X-ray including a lateral decubitus film should be obtained. Classic findings include a hemithorax opacification which follows the effect of gravity, ruling out loculations. If the fluid layers to less than 1 cm, ultrasound guidance should be used.[59] If the patient has an abnormal bleeding history or is receiving anti-coagulant therapy, coagulation studies should be ordered and acted upon in a judicious manner. Informed consent should be obtained. The patient is placed in a comfortable sitting position with arms supported at shoulder height and the head resting on the pillow. If the patient leans too far forward, the fluid accumulates beyond the reach of the needle. The needle entrance should be placed one to two rib spaces below where the percussion note becomes dull, but not below the ninth rib. It should be inserted superior to the inferior rib to prevent damage to the neurovascular bundle. Numerous thoracentesis kits are available. The physician should be familiar with them and have an extra one on hand. The proposed thoracentesis site is cleansed with antiseptic solution and draped appropriately. A skin wheal is created using marcaine with a 25-gauge needle. This is followed by injection along the proposed needle tract. The thoracentesis needle is then slowly introduced while gently aspirating. Once fluid is withdrawn, the needle is stabilized, asking the patient to expire, and the plastic catheter is advanced into the pleural space. Aspiration is performed with a three-way stopcock and vacuum bottles. Aspirated fluid is processed in the appropriate manner. Once the fluid has been aspirated, the needle should be withdrawn in a quick manner and a Band-Aid applied. A post-thoracentesis expiratory chest X-ray should be obtained to rule out pneumothorax.

Complications

Pneumothorax is the most common complication following thoracentesis.[60,61] Approximately 10% of patients undergoing thoracentesis will develop a pneumothorax. Optimally, only one-fifth of these patients will ultimately require a chest tube. A common cause of pneumothorax during thoracentesis is faulty technique. This is usually due to a break in the system allowing atmospheric pressure to enter into the pleural space. Lung laceration secondary to needle trauma is a rare cause of pneumothorax. Other complications encountered during thoracentesis include cough and vasovagal reaction. Both of these are felt to be secondary to pleural irritation. Removal of the needle will usually result in resolution of the cough. A vasovagal reaction may require the administration of atropine in rare instances. Infrequently, laceration to the abdominal organs may occur. Improper needle placement is the cause in this situation. Failure to produce pleural fluid (dry tap) may be corrected using ultrasound guidance.

The volume of fluid withdrawn can also contribute to postprocedure complications. The concept of "reexpansion pneumonitis" results when the collapsed lung is permitted to expand into the space recently vacated by the effusion. If this happens too rapidly, pulmonary edema can result from a massive rush of pulmonary arterial flow, which overwhelms the venous return. This is generally felt to be unlikely at volumes below 1.5 L, but in chronic effusions some authors advocate a limit of only 1 L[62, 63] (**Level III**).

Chest Tube Thoracostomy

Chest tubes have been used since the dawn of medicine, first described during the time of Hippocrates.[64] Pneumothorax represents one of the most common causes for chest tube insertion in gynecology. In turn, central line placement and mechanical ventilation barotrauma are the usual causes of pneumothorax. Classical teaching recommended chest tube insertion for all pneumothoraces. Recent studies have indicated that a pneumothorax does not automatically require a chest tube insertion.[65] Asymptomatic, nonventilating patients with an iatrogenic pneumothorax of less than 25% can be safely observed in most cases. Approximately 1.5% of the initial volume of the pneumothorax will be absorbed every 24 hours, taking approximately 3 weeks for the pneumothorax to completely resolve. Repeat chest X-ray should be performed 4–6 hours after the initial film to confirm that the pneumothorax is not enlarging. This is repeated in 1–2 days to document absorption. A patient with a symptomatic pneumothorax or one larger than 25% may undergo an aspiration thoracentesis to resolve this condition. If unsuccessful or if chest tube placement is indicated, the tube is left in place for a minimum of 24 hours following lung expansion under water seal and then removed. Suction to evacuate air is unnecessary and can be counterproductive by increasing the probability of persistent bronchopleural leak. All patients on mechanical ventilators developing pneumothoraces should undergo chest tube placement as tension pneumothorax develops rapidly in the setting of positive pressure ventilation. Another indication for chest tube placement is symptomatic recurrent pleural effusions from malignancy. A larger bore tube is placed as a precursor to pleurodesis. Once the chest tube is inserted, the lung is reexpanded for a minimum of 24 hours, and the patient is stable with no evidence of reexpansion pulmonary edema or extensive shunting, pleurodesis may be attempted.

The two most common areas for chest tube insertion are the third intercostal space in the midclavicular line or the fourth/fifth intercostal space in the midaxillary line.

The midaxillary although initially uncomfortable to the patient has better cosmesis. It is important for the physician not to place the tube posterior to the midaxillary line as this will result in the patient being unable to lie comfortably on her back.

Procedure

The patient should be given the rationale for placement of the chest tube and informed consent should be obtained. The proposed location for chest tube placement should be identified and the area fully anesthetized with marcaine as previously mentioned. The pleura should be generously anesthetized where the tube will penetrate. A 3-cm incision can be made parallel to the interspace above the superior edge of the inferior rib. The incision should be taken down to the muscle without cutting it. A hemostat may then be used to dissect the intercostal muscle to the parietal pleural. The chest tube is then grasped with the hemostat and pushed through the parietal pleura into the pleural space. For evacuation of pneumothorax, a smaller bore tube should be used and advanced in an anterior and superior direction, where air will collect with the patient in a supine position. For drainage of effusions, a larger bore tube should be advanced in a posterior direction, with the superior direction adjusted depending on effusion size and patient position. The chest tube should then be anchored and covered with sterile petroleum gauze to ensure an airtight seal. The tube is then connected to a closed three-chamber collecting system.

A three-chamber collecting system consists of a collection chamber, a water seal chamber, and a suction control chamber. The collection chamber collects any fluid from the pleural cavity and allows air to pass through to the water seal chamber without generating back pressure. The water seal chamber has the intake submerged to create a one-way valve, which imposes a back pressure, preventing air at atmospheric pressure to reenter the pleural cavity. If bubbles are noted at the intake of this chamber, then a persistent bronchopleural or system tubing leak is present. The suction control chamber is configured in such a way as to limit the suction imposed on the system to 20 cm H_2O. Bubbling in this chamber simply means that atmospheric air is being entrained via an ambient air intake valve.

A postprocedure chest X-ray is obtained to confirm placement. The decision to remove the chest tube is made once the pneumothorax or drainage from the pleural effusion has resolved with complete lung expansion for a minimum of 24 hours. The tube is quickly removed while the patient performs the Valsalva maneuver and the wound site is covered with petroleum gauze.

Complications

The major complication of chest tube insertion and placement is patient discomfort. Adequate anesthesia during insertion and placement easily relieves such discomfort. If local anesthesia is not effective, a combination of Versed and intravenous morphine sulfate are effective. Ectopic chest tube location is unusual. Once recognized this situation should be corrected by removal and correct insertion. Infectious complications can occur and should be treated with antibiotics and timely removal of the chest tube. Occasionally subcutaneous emphysema may develop. This can occur when not all the catheter perforations are in the pleural space. Careful placement will avoid this problem.

Pleurodesis

Background Indications

Pleurodesis is used primarily for recurrent pneumothoraces and malignant pleural effusions. Chest tube placement is first accomplished and once the lung has reexpanded for a minimum of 24 hours, pleurodesis is considered. Classically, tetracycline has been the pleural irritant used.[66,67] It has recently been removed from the market. Alternative agents commonly used in lieu of tetracycline are bleomycin, minocycline, doxycycline, or talc slurry. Randomized trials comparing pleurodesis agents have not shown a benefit of one agent over another, but talc has emerged as a commonly used substance based on its easy availability and low cost[68–70] (**Level II-2**).

Procedure

First the lung has to be completely reexpanded before an attempt is made to perform pleurodesis. If the lung has not reexpanded pleurodesis is futile and pleurectomy is indicated. Once the lung has reexpanded, lidocaine 3–4 mg/kg is infused into the pleural space through the chest tube. The tube is then clamped and for the next 10 minutes the patient is repositioned so the entire parietal pleura is anesthetized. The patient is given intravenous sedation as well. Sixty units of Bleomycin are then infused into the pleural space. The chest tube is then clamped for 2 hours and the patient repositioned frequently to ensure that this sclerotic agent contacts all pleural surfaces, resulting in pleural space obliteration. Once the tube is released, it is attached to a negative pressure of 20 cm of H_2O for a minimum of 24 hours. Once the pleural drainage is less than 150 mL/day, the chest tube can be removed.

Long-term drainage in recurrent pleural effusions has been managed by subcutaneous implantable ports with periodic access or through a transdermal catheter with a unidirectional valver to prevent only egress of pleural fluid. Initial reports of this method led to the development and approval of a device known as the PleurX catheter. This is a 15.5 French silicone catheter that has been designed for long-term placement into a pleural effusion. Since its introduction, a large body of literature has demonstrated its benefit in terms of patient comfort and cost savings. In addition to drainage of pleural fluid, the PleurX catheter is associated with spontaneous pleurodesis once the entire volume of effusion has been drained. This occurs in rates less than that seen with pleurodesis, but is not associated with the potential side effects that a sclerotic agent may bring. Symptomatic improvement is very high and offers patients an excellent opportunity to avoid repeated procedures and hospital visits. A summary of several recent publications related to the usage of the PleurX catheter in persistent pleural effusions is given in Table 3.2.

Table 3.2 Series Reporting PleurX Tunneled Catheters to Manage Malignant Pleural Effusions[a]

Series	Symptomatic Improvement (%)	Spontaneous Pleurodesis (%)	Significant Recurrent Effusions (%)
Putnam 2000[72]	81	21	8
Pollak 2001[73]	93	42	16
Musani 2004[74]	100	58	8
Tremblay 2006[75]	96	44	8
Pien 2001[76]	91	0	9

Adapted from Reference 71.

Complications

The major complication of pleurodesis is pain, often relieved by intrapleural lidocaine. Occasionally intravenous Versed with morphine sulfate are required. Another complication of pleurodesis is failure. Failure rates are increased if the lung is not expanded or there is a pleural effusion. Adequate chest expansion with drainage prior to pleurodesis is the key to success of this procedure. The reported failure rate for both bleomycin or minoxicycline are approximately 10%–20%. Other adverse effects associated with bleomycin infusion are fever, nausea, alopecia, and skin rash. Fever can be controlled with antipyretic agents.

ABDOMINAL CAVITY PROCEDURES

Paracentesis

Unlike other procedures in gynecology, a nonindication for this procedure is paramount. An undiagnosed abdominal pelvic mass is not an indication for paracentesis. Paracentesis in this picture can change a potentially curable localized neoplasm into an incurable metastatic disease. The extenuating circumstances that justify an exception to this tenet are indeed rare.

The most common gynecologic indication for this procedure is the relief of ascites postoperatively which causes respiratory embarrassment.[77] This is particularly justified if the patient has not yet received chemotherapy. Once chemotherapy is initiated, the ascites will usually resolve. Patients with end-stage malignancy not responding to treatment who develop symptomatic ascites can be temporarily relieved with paracentesis. Unfortunately, the ascites will reaccumulate requiring multiple taps. Prudent use of this technique is required in order to balance immediate patient relief versus future procedures. Recently, considerable discussion with regard to the amount of fluid removed through paracentesis has been devoted to the literature.[78–80] While the majority of this work has been done with patients with liver disease, it does appear to be applicable to ovarian cancer patients. Recent studies have shown that removal of large amounts of fluid (greater than 5 L) is not detrimental to the patient's health. Whether the intravenous fusion of albumin should be done currently is debatable. Each case should be managed on an individual basis.

Procedure

The patient should be informed of the need for paracentesis and informed consent obtained. Ultrasound examination of the abdomen will reveal the deepest fluid pocket and any loculation should be noted. The area through which the needle is to be introduced should be cleansed and a sterile towel should be placed. Prepackaged kits are available and an extra kit should be prepared. Most kits utilize a single-lumen flexible catheter for fluid drainage. Recently, the use of a triple-lumen vascular catheter has been described for use in paracentesis, which is reported to decrease the probability of occlusion of the single-lumen catheter. Additionally, in cases of therapeutic paracentesis, ascites can be withdrawn in higher volumes with the multi-lumen approach[81] (**Level III**). Various local anesthesia should be infused into the skin and along the proposed needle track using a small gauge needle. A Z-track method should be used to prevent postprocedure leakage. A 14- to 16-gauge 3-inch needle with a flexible catheter should be introduced utilizing ultrasound guidance. The fluid should then be removed either manually using a syringe or with the use of vacuum bottles. After the fluid has been removed, the needle can be removed and a Band-Aid applied. Initially, the patient should have an intravenous access available during this procedure.

Complications

The major complication is infection. This can be prevented using the sterile technique. If infection is encountered, it can be treated in the appropriate method after cultures have been obtained. Bowel injury can be avoided by ultrasound guidance. If the bowel is struck by the needle, the needle can be inserted at a different angle to avoid the bowel. Another complication is continued leakage of intraperitoneal fluid. This may be reduced by using the Z-track technique.

Intraperitoneal Catheters

With the cure for ovarian cancer still elusive, different methods of chemotherapy administration have been sought. Among these methods, intraperitoneal chemotherapy has been evaluated in patients with ovarian cancer in an attempt to improve survival.[82, 83] The role of peritoneal chemotherapy was significantly advanced after a 2006 GOG study demonstrated a dramatic difference in overall and progression-free survival in epithelial ovarian cancer patients receiving this treatment. In spite of the dramatic differences in outcomes, the treatment method was also shown to carry considerable toxicity, leading to incomplete treatment in more than half of the patients studied.[84, 85] Theoretically, intraperitoneal chemotherapy administration offers the advantage of increased dose concentration to intraperitoneal tumor compared to systemic administration. Catheter-related complications were among the chief reasons for failure to complete planned intraperitoneal therapy, and various authors have advocated for differing peritoneal catheters in order to reduce complications related to the infusion device itself. These catheters are similar in appearance to catheters used for long-term central venous catheterization therapy; the primary differences between them are based on the catheter structure (fenestrated versus closed), the number of ports (single versus multiple), and the cutaneous interface (transdermal versus subcutaneous). If intraperitoneal chemotherapy is only to be given once as in the administration of P32, a Tenckhoff-type catheter is recommended. These catheters have no subcutaneous port. Alternatively, a Jackson Pratt drain can be utilized for this function. Emerging literature on the different forms of peritoneal catheters has not shown a demonstrable difference between the fenestrated and the closed catheters. No differences were seen in a single institution study of 85 patients receiving peritoneal chemotherapy when compared for number of completed cycles, catheter-related complications, or reasons for discontinuation[86] (**Level III**).

Technique

The rational for placement of the intra-abdominal catheter is given to the patient entrance site and an informed consent is obtained. Local anesthesia is injected at the exit site and along the catheter's tract at the level of the umbilicus just lateral to the intra-abdominal rectus abdominus muscle. The catheter is placed into the abdomen through a small incision. A subcutaneous tunnel is then made on the ipsilateral side to the lower quadrant. The Dakron cuff is placed in subcutaneous tissue 2 cm from the exit site. Implanted subcutaneous ports are placed on the ipsilateral side along the lower rib cage on the midclavicular line. The port is then anchored to the chest wall fascia and closed in the subcuticular manner and steri strips placed.

Complications

Most abdominal access complications are similar to those encountered with central venous access devices. However, bowel perforation is encountered in approximately 3% of patients. Etiology is believed to be catheter erosion. Peritonitis is reported 5%–10% of the time and usually mandates catheter removal.

Subcutaneous infections are unusual. However, if associated with a tunnel infection removal appears indicated. A decision on whether to place an intraperitoneal catheter currently with large bowel surgery has been discussed by several authors. Although there is no definite evidence that a catheter with large bowel surgery will increase the risk of peritonitis, it appears prudent to delay placement. Complications include infusion and aspiration difficulties. A fibrous sheath coating the catheter is usually responsible. If an intraluminal wire placement is unsuccessful in dislodging the obstruction, laparoscopy may be helpful, otherwise catheter replacement is required.

REFERENCES

1. GROEGER J, LUCAS A, et al. Venous access in the cancer patient. Principle Pract Oncol 1991;5(3):2–14.
2. GLEESON N, FIORICA J, et al. Externalized Groshong catheters and Hickman ports for central venous access in gynecologic oncology patients. Gynecol Oncol 1993;51:372–376.
3. KOONINGS P, GIVEN F. Long-term experience with a totally implanted catheter system in gynecologic oncologic patients. J Am Coll Surg 1994;178:164–166.
4. BROTHERS T, VON MOLL L, et al. Experience with subcutaneous infusion ports in three hundred patients. Surg Gynecol Obstet 1988;166:295–301.
5. CIVETTA J, GABLE J, et al. Internal-jugular-vein puncture with a margin of safety. Anesthesiology 1972;36:622–625.
6. VAUGHAN RW, WEYGANDT GR. Reliable percutaneous central venous pressure measurement. Anesth Analg, Curr Res 1973;52:709–712.
7. PRINCE SR, SULLIVAN RL, et al. Percutaneous catheterization of the internal jugular vein in infants and children. Anesthesiology 1976;44:170–174.
8. SELDINGER SI. Catheter replacement of needle in percutaneous arteriography: new technique. Acta Radiol 1953;39(5):368–376.
9. WILSON JN, GROW JB, et al. Central venous pressure in optimal blood volume maintenance. Arch Surg 1962;85:563–578.
10. TOFIELD J. A safer technique of percutaneous catheterization of the subclavian vein. Surg, Gynecol Obstet 1969;128:1069–1071.
11. MOGIL R, DELAURENTIS D, et al. The infraclavicular venipuncture. Arch Surg 1967;95:320–324.
12. SHERER D, ABULAFIA O, et al. Ultrasonographically guided subclavian vein catheterization in critical care obstetrics and gynecologic oncology. Am J Obstet Gynecol 1993;169:1246–1248.
13. MANSFIELD P, HOHN D,et al. Complications and failures of subclavian vein catheterization. N Engl J Med 1994;331:1735–1738.
14. VYSKOCIL J, KRUSE J, et al. Alternative techniques for gaining venous access. J Crit Illn 1993;8(3): 435–442.
15. LAFFER U, DURIG H, et al. Vascular access problems and implantable devices. Recent Results Cancer Res 1991;121:189–197.
16. NELSON B, MAYER A, et al. Experience with the intravenous totally implanted port in patients with gynecologic malignancies. Gynecol Oncol 1994;53:98–102.
17. EASTRIDGE B, LEFOR A, et al. Complications of indwelling venous access devices in cancer patients. J Clin Oncol 1995;13(1):233–238.
18. HECKMANN JG, LANG CJ. Neurologic manifestations of cerebral air embolism as a complication of central venous catheterization. Crit Care Med 2000;28:1621–1625.
19. BROCKMEYER J, SIMON T, et al. Cerebral air embolism following removal of central venous catheter. Mil Med Mil Med 2009;174(8):878–881.
20. RICHARDSON D, BRUSO P. Vascular access devices. J Intraven Nurs 1993;16(1):44–49.
21. KEUNG Y, WATKINS K, et al. Comparative study of infectious complications of different types of chronic central venous access devices. Cancer 1994;73(11):2832–2837.
22. JOHNSON A, OPPENHEIM B. Vascular catheter-related sepsis: diagnosis and prevention. J Hosp Infect 1992;20:67–78.
23. BRINCKER H, SAETER G. Fifty-five patient years' experience with a totally implanted system for intravenous chemotherapy. Cancer 1986;57:1124–1129.
24. SCHWARTZ C, HENRICKSON K, et al. Prevention of bacteremia attributed to luminal colonization of tunneled central venous catheters with vancomycin-susceptible organisms. J Clin Oncol 1990;8(9):1591–1597.
25. LECCIONES J, LEE J, et al. Vascular catheter-associated fungemia in patients with cancer: analysis of 155 episodes. Clin Infect Dis 1992;14:875–883.
26. MUELLER B, SKELTON J, et al. A prospective randomized trial comparing the infectious and noninfectious complications of an externalized catheter versus a subcutaneously implanted device in cancer patients. J Clin Oncol 1992;10:1943–1948.

27. MAKI DG. Nosocomial bacteremia: an epidemiologic overview. Am J Med 1981;70:719–732.
28. BANERJEE SN, EMORI TG, CULVER DH, et al. National Nosocomial Infections Surveillance System. Secular trends in nosocomial primary bloodstream infections in the United States, 1980–1989. Am J Med 1991;91:86S–89S.
29. CRNICH CJ, MAKI DG. The role of intravascular devices in sepsis. Curr Infect Dis Rep 2001;3:496–506.
30. MAKI DG, CRNICH CJ. Line sepsis in the ICU: prevention, diagnosis, and management. Semin Respir Crit Care Med 2003;24:23–36.
31. CRNICH CJ, MAKI DG. Infections caused by intravascular devices: epidemiology, pathogenesis, diagnosis, prevention, and treatment. In: APIC Text of Infection Control and Epidemiology. Vol. 1, 2nd ed. Washington, DC: Association for Professionals in Infection Control and Epidemiology, Inc; 2005. p 24.21–24.26.
32. National Nosocomial Infections Surveillance System. National Nosocomial Infections Surveillance (NNIS) System Report, data summary from January 1992 to June 2002, issued in August 2002. Am J Infect Control 2002;30:458–475.
33. Centers for Disease Control and Prevention (CDC). Monitoring hospital-acquired infections to promote patient safety: United States, 1990–1999. *MMWR Morb Mortal Wkly Rep* 2000;49:149–153 [published correction appears in *MMWR Morb Mortal Wkly Rep* 2000;49:189–190].
34. Joint Commission on the Accreditation of Healthcare Organizations. Accreditation Manual for Hospitals. Chicago, IL: Joint Commission on the Accreditation of Healthcare Organizations; 1994. p 121–140.
35. SAINT S. Prevention of intravascular catheter-associated infections. In: SHOJANIA KG, DUNCAN BW, MCDONALD KM, WACHTER RM, editors. Making Health Care Safer: A Critical Analysis of Patient Safety Practices. Rockville, MD: Agency for Healthcare Research and Quality; 2001. p 163–184.
36. COBB D, HIGH K, et al. A controlled trial of scheduled replacement of central venous and pulmonary catheters. N Engl J Med 1992;327:1062–1068.
37. EYER S, Brummit C, et al. Catheter-related sepsis: prospective, randomized study of three methods of long-term catheter maintenance. Crit Care Med 1990;18:1073–1079.
38. GREGORY J, SCHILLER W. Subclavian catheter changes every third day in high risk patients. Am Surg 1985;51:534–536.
39. CARLISLE E, BLAKE P, et al. Septicemia in long-term jugular hemodialysis catheters: eradicating infection by changing the catheter over a guidewire. Int J Artif Organs 1991;14(3):150–153.
40. WEINER, ES. Catheter sepsis: the central venous line Achilles' heel. Semin Pediatr Surg 1995;4(4):297–314.
41. MAKI DG, KLUGER DM, et al. The risk of bloodstream infection in adults with different intravascular devices: a systematic review of 200 published prospective studies. Mayo Clin Proc 2006;81(9):1159–1171.
42. LOKICH J, BECKER B. Subclavian vein thrombosis in patients treated with infusion chemotherapy for advance malignancy. Cancer 1983;52:1586–1589.
43. BLOM JW, DOGGEN CJM, OSANTO S, et al. Old and new risk factors for upper extremity deep venous thrombosis. J Thromb Haemost 2005;3:2471–2478.
44. BERNARDI E, PESAVENTO R, PRANDONI P. Upper extremity deep venous thrombosis. Semin Thromb Haemost 2006;32:729–736.
45. HENDLER MF, MESCHENGIESER SS, BLANCO AN, et al. Primary upper-extremity deep vein thrombosis: high prevalence of thrombophilic defects. Am J Hematol 2004;76:330–337.
46. KNUDSON GJ, WIEDMEYER DA, ERICKSON SJ, et al. Color Doppler sonographic imaging in the assessment of upper extremity deep venous thrombosis. AJR Am J Roentgenol 1990;154:399–403.
47. BAXTER GM, KINCAID W, JEFFREY RF, et al. Comparison of color Doppler ultrasound with venography in the diagnosis of axillary and subclavian vein thrombosis. Br J Radiol 1991;64:777–781.
48. BERN M, LOKICH J, et al. Very low doses of warfarin can prevent thrombosis in central venous catheters. Ann Intern Med 1990;112:423–428.
49. KOVACS MJ, KAHN SR, et al. A pilot study of central venous catheter survival in cancer patients using low-molecular-weight heparin (dalteparin) and warfarin without catheter removal for the treatment of upper extremity deep vein thrombosis (The Catheter Study). J Thromb Haemost 2007;5:1650–1653.

50. AITKEN D, MINTON J, et al. The "pinch off sign": a warning of impending problems with permanent subclavian catheters. Am J Surg 1984;148:633–636.

51. SWAN H, GANZ W, FORRESTER J, et al. Catheterization of the heart in man with use of a flow-directed balloon-tipped catheter. N Engl J Med 1970;283:447–451.

52. SHOEMAKER W. Use and abuse of the balloon tip pulmonary artery (Swan–Ganz) catheter: are patients getting their money's worth? Crit Care Med 1990;18(11):1294–1296.

53. BERLAUK J, ABRAMS J, et al. Preoperative optimization of cardiovascular hemodynamics improves outcome in peripheral vascular surgery. Ann Surg 1991;214(3):289–299.

54. ROSEN M, BERGER D, et al. Practice guidelines for pulmonary artery catheterization. Anesthesiology 1993;78:380–394.

55. HARVEY S, STEVENS K, et al. An evaluation of the clinical and cost-effectiveness of pulmonary artery catheters in patient management in intensive care: a systematic review and a randomised controlled trial. Health Technol Assess 2006;10(29).

56. BENNETT D, BOLDT J, et al. Expert panel: the use of the pulmonary artery catheter. Intensive Care Med 1991;17:I–VIII.

57. TREMBLAY N, TAILLEFER J, et al. Successful non-surgical extraction of a knotted pulmonary artery catheter trapped in the right ventricle. Can J Anaesth 1992;39(3):293–295.

58. GROGAN D, IRWIN R, et al. Complications associated with thoracentesis. Arch Intern Med 1990;150:873–877.

59. KOHAN J, POE R, et al. Value of chest ultrasonography versus decubitus roentgenography for thoracentesis. Am Rev Respir Dis 1986;133:1124–1126.

60. GROGAN D, IRWIN R, et al. Complications associated with thoracentesis. Arch Intern Med 1990;150:873–877.

61. COLLINS T, SAHN S. Thoracocentesis clinical value, complications, technical problems, and patient experience. Chest 1987;91(6):817–822.

62. TARVER RD, BRODERICK LS, CONCES DJ. Reexpansion pulmonary edema. J Thorac Imaging 1996;11:198–209.

63. MAHFOOD S, HIX WR, AARON BL, et al. Reexpansion pulmonary edema. Ann Thorac Surg 1988;45:340–345.

64. SILVER M, BONE R. Techniques for chest tube insertion and pleurodesis. Crit Procedures 1993;86:631–637.

65. LIGHT R. Iatrogenic pneumothorax. In: Pleural Diseases. 2nd ed. Philadelphia: Lea & Febinger; 1990. p 251–253.

66. LYNCH T. Management of malignant pleural effusions. Chest 1993;103(4):385S–389S.

67. KELLER S. Current and future therapy for malignant pleural effusion. Chest 1993;103(1):63S–67S.

68. TAN C, SEDRAKYAN A, BROWNE J, et al. The evidence on the effectiveness of management for malignant pleural effusion: a systematic review. Eur J Cardiothorac Surg 2006;29:829–838.

69. ZIMMER PW, HILL M, CASEY K, et al. Prospective randomized trial of talc slurry vs bleomycin in pleurodesis for symptomatic malignant pleural effusions. Chest 1997;112:430–434.

70. LYNCH TJ Jr, KALISH L, MENTZER SJ, et al. Optimal therapy of malignant pleural effusions: report of a randomized trial of bleomycin, tetracycline and talc and a meta-analysis. Int J Oncol 1996;8:183–190.

71. SPECTOR M, POLLAK JS. Management of malignant pleural effusions. Semin Respir Crit Care Med 2008;29:405–413.

72. PUTNAM JB Jr, WALSH GL, SWISHER SG, et al. Outpatient management of malignant pleural effusion by a chronic indwelling pleural catheter. Ann Thorac Surg 2000;69:369–375.

73. POLLAK JS, BURDGE CM, ROSENBLATT M, et al. Treatment of malignant pleural effusions with tunneled long-term drainage catheters. J Vasc Interv Radiol 2001;12:201–208.

74. MUSANI AI, HAAS A, SEIJO L, et al. Outpatient management of malignant pleural effusions with a tunneled pleural catheter: pleurodesis without sclerosing agents. Respiration 2004;71:559–566.

75. TREMBLAY A, MICHAUD G. Single-center experience with 250 tunneled pleural catheter insertions for malignant pleural effusion. Chest 2006;129:362–368.

76. PIEN GW, GANT MJ, WASHAM CL, et al. Use of an implantable pleural catheter for trapped lung syndrome in patients with malignant pleural effusion. Chest 2001;119:1641–1646.

77. LIFSHITZ S, BUCHSBAUM H. The effect of paracentesis on serum proteins. Gynecol Oncol 1976;4:347–353.

78. BERKOWITZ K, BUTENSKY M, et al. Pulmonary function changes after large volume paracentesis. Am J Gastroenterol 1993;88(6):905–907.

79. PANOS M, MOORE K, et al. Single, total paracentesis for tense ascites: sequential hemodynamic changes and right atrial size. Hepatology 1990;11(4):662–667.

80. REYNOLDS T. Renaissance of paracentesis in the treatment of ascites. Adv Intern Med 1990;35:365–374.

81. LEE SY, PORMENTO JG, KOONG HN. Abdominal paracentesis and thoracocentesis. Surg Laparosc Endosc Percutan Tech 2009;19:e32–e35.

82. PFEIFLE C, HOWELL S, et al. Totally implantable system for peritoneal access. J Clin Oncol 1984;2(11):1277–1280.

83. NAUMANN R, ALVAREZ R, et al. The Groshong catheter as an intraperitoneal access device in the treatment of ovarian cancer patients. Gynecol Oncol 1993;50(3):291–293.

84. ARMSTRONG DK, BUNDY B, WENZEL L, et al. Gynecologic Oncology Group. Intraperitoneal cisplatin and paclitaxel in ovarian cancer. N Engl J Med 2006;354(1):34–43.

85. WALKER JL, ARMSTRONG DK, HUANG HQ, et al. Intraperitoneal catheter outcomes in a phase III trial of intravenous versus intraperitoneal chemotherapy in optimal stage III ovarian and primary peritoneal cancer: a Gynecologic Oncology Group study. Gynecol Oncol 2006;100(1):27–32.

86. IVY JJ, MELISSA GELLER M, et al. Outcomes associated with different intraperitoneal chemotherapy delivery systems in advanced ovarian carcinoma: a single institution's experience. Gynecol Oncol 2009;114:420–423.

Chapter 4

Fluids, Electrolytes, and Nutrition

Howard Silberman, MD and Matthew Powers, MD

FLUID AND ELECTROLYTE HOMEOSTASIS

In healthy persons, the fluid and electrolyte composition of the body is maintained by a variety of physiologic processes within a narrow range of normal, despite wide, variation in consumption of salt and water. However, the homeostatic mechanisms involved are frequently disrupted by surgical illness as well as by operative therapy so that fluid and electrolyte balance becomes a key element in perioperative care.

Total body water (TBW) is distributed between the intracellular and extracellular compartments. The latter is subdivided into the interstitial and vascular (plasma) spaces. TBW as a proportion of body weight decreases with increasing body fat since fat contains little water. The composition of the body fluid compartments is presented in Table 4.1. The distribution of water between the intracellular fluid (ICF) and extracellular fluid (ECF) compartments is determined by the concentration of osmotically effective particles within each of these compartments, which are separated by the functionally semipermeable cell membrane. Whereas all solutes contribute to body fluid osmolality, only those solutes whose movement is relatively restricted by cell membranes have the capacity to cause water to move from one body compartment to the other. This capacity to cause water to move is called *effective osmolality* or *tonicity*, and those solutes that contribute to tonicity are called *osmotically effective* solutes.[1]

The intracellular and extracellular compartments each have one primary solute that is limited to that compartment and therefore is the major determinant of its effective osmotic pressure (Fig. 4.1). In the extracellular space, sodium salts are the principal effective osmoles and, therefore, act to hold water in that compartment.[2] In contrast, potassium is the major intracellular ion, and thus, with its associated anions, exerts the major osmotic force tending to hold water within the cells. Although the cell

Gynecologic Oncology: Evidence-Based Perioperative and Supportive Care, Second Edition.
Edited by Scott E. Lentz, Allison E. Axtell and Steven A. Vasilev.
© 2011 John Wiley & Sons, Inc. Published 2011 by John Wiley & Sons, Inc.

Table 4.1   Body Fluid Compartments

Total Body Water	Body Weight (%)	Percentage of Total Water (%)
	60	100
Intracellular	40	67
Extracellular	20	33
Intravascular	5	8
Interstitial	15	25

From Reference 117.

membrane is in fact permeable to both sodium and potassium ions, these ions are able to act as effective osmoles because they are restricted to their respective compartments by the Na–K–ATPase pump in the cell membrane.[2] While the movement of the major intracellular and extracellular ions, as well as proteins, is restricted, water is freely diffusible. Thus, osmotic forces are the prime determinant of water distribution in the body because they underlie the movement of water across cellular membranes in such a manner as to achieve osmotic equilibrium (i.e., equal osmolalities) between all body compartments. If the tonicity of one fluid compartment changes, e.g., by the addition of water or hypertonic saline solution to the extracellular compartment, water will move across the separating cellular membrane in an amount exactly necessary to reestablish osmotic equilibrium. The osmolality at the new equilibrium will be higher or lower than the normal body fluid osmolality of approximately 290 mOsm/kg H_2O, depending on the direction of water movement.

The addition of an osmotically *ineffective* solute, such as urea, to the ECF compartment results in an increase in the *osmolality* of both the ECF and ICF

						195 meq/L		180+ meq/L	
153 meq/L	153 meq/L		149 meq/L	149 meq/L		Cations		Anions	
Cations	Anions		Cations	Anions		K	156	HPO_4	95
Na 142	Cl 102		Na 145	Cl 113				SO_4	20
	HCO_3 26			HCO_3 31				HCO_3	10
	SO_4 1			SO_4 1					
K 4	HPO_4 2		K 4	HPO_4 2		Na	10	Protein	55
Ca 5	Organic acids 6					Ca	3		
Mg 2	Protein 16			Protein 2		Mg	26		
Plasma			Interstitial fluid			Intracellular fluid			

Figure 4.1   Electrolyte composition of the major fluid compartments. (From Reference 4, p 4.)

compartments, as urea permeates freely across cell membranes, but there is no change in body fluid *tonicity* and therefore no movement of water.

Tonicity is calculated from the measured concentration of all of the *effective* solutes in ECF.[1] ECF tonicity can be estimated from the following expression:

$$\text{Tonicity (mOsm/kg)} = (2 \times S_{Na}) + \frac{S_G}{18}, \tag{4.1}$$

where S_{Na} and S_G are the serum sodium and the serum glucose concentrations, respectively. S_{Na} (mEq/L or mmol/L) is multiplied by 2 to take into account the osmotic pressure exerted by the anions (largely chloride and HCO_3^-) that accompany sodium. S_G(mg/dL) is divided by 18 to convert to mmol/L. Thus,

$$\text{Normal tonicity} = (2 \times 140) + \frac{90}{18} = 285 \text{ mOsm/kg}. \tag{4.2}$$

In contrast to tonicity, body fluid osmolality is a function of all solutes, effective or ineffective. Plasma osmolality (P_{OSM}) can be calculated as follows:

$$P_{OSM} \text{ (mOsm/kg)} = (2 \times S_{Na}) + \frac{S_G}{18} + \frac{BUN}{2.8}, \tag{4.3}$$

where BUN is the blood urea nitrogen (mg/dL) and is divided by 2.8 to convert to mmol/L. Thus,

$$\text{Normal osmolality} = (2 \times 140) + \frac{90}{18} + \frac{14}{2.8} = 290 \text{ mOsm/kg}. \tag{4.4}$$

Movement of water across cell membranes in response to a change in ECF tonicity (i.e., effective osmolality) results in a reciprocal change in cell volume. Thus, ECF hypertonicity leads to cell shrinkage or dehydration, and ECF hypotonicity leads to cell swelling or edema.[1] Similarly, deviations from normal tonicity produce a change in the volume of hypothalamic osmoreceptor cells, which in turn stimulates alterations in thirst (the major mechanism controlling water intake) and antidiuretic hormone (ADH) secretion (the major factor controlling water excretion). When the addition of impermeable solutes (effective osmoles) produces a rise in plasma osmolality above a threshold of approximately 280 mOsm/kg, the osmoreceptor cells shrink, resulting in a progressive stimulus to ADH release. When plasma osmolality reaches about 290–292 mOsm/kg, an ADH level (5 pg/mL) is reached that causes the maximal renal antidiuretic effect, with resultant water reabsorption in the renal collecting tubules yielding a maximum urine concentration of 1000–1200 mOsm/kg (Fig. 4.2).[3]

Sodium, as the primary extracellular effective solute, is the major osmotic stimulus to ADH release and, therefore, the major determinant of ECF volume in normal persons. The narrow range of plasma sodium concentration responsible for the

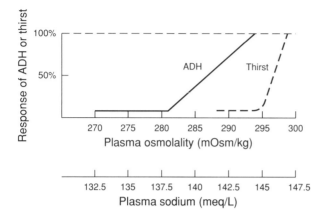

Figure 4.2 Comparative activities of ADH and thirst as a function of plasma osmolality and plasma sodium concentration. (From Reference 3, p 83.)

spectrum of ADH response is 137–145 mEq/L (Fig. 4.2).[3] As ECF osmolality falls in response to water absorption, osmoreceptor cell volume increases, and the stimulus to ADH secretion decreases. ADH secretion is completely inhibited at an ECF osmolality of 280 mOsm/kg.

Osomoreceptors also regulate thirst, but, compared to ADH release, higher thresholds for osmolality and sodium concentration (295 mOsm/kg and 145 mEq Na/L) are required to induce a response (Fig. 4.2). In clinical practice, it is important to recognize that the thirst response, which is the only physiologic mechanism that increases water intake, is abrogated in patients unable to drink because of illness, anesthesia, or postoperative ileus.

While this osmoregulatory system is the homeostatic mechanism maintaining fluid balance in normal persons, large, pathologic changes in volume generally produce a corresponding change in effective circulating volume, which in turn affects superior vena caval, atrial, arterial, and renal arteriolar baroreceptors. *Effective circulating volume* (ECV) is that portion of the ECF that is within the arterial system and that perfuses the tissues and generates the pressure that affects the baroreceptors. A reduction in ECV results in a fall in the perfusion pressure and stretch in the region of the baroreceptors. This, in turn, results in a cascade of homeostatic events that tends to restore ECV and perfusion pressure. The intrarenal baroreceptors, located primarily in the juxtaglomerular apparatus of the afferent arteriole, affect volume by influencing the activity of the renin–angiotensin–aldosterone system (Fig. 4.3).[2] In contrast to the intrarenal baroreceptors, the extrarenal receptors respond to decreased ECV by stimulating the sympathetic nervous system (Fig. 4.4) and inhibiting release of atrial natriuretic peptide (ANP).

Enhanced sympathetic tone tends to reverse the fall in perfusion pressure, and, as a result of renin and aldosterone release, tubular reabsorption of sodium and water increases circulating volume. Reduced atrial distention, or stretch, as a result of diminished ECV, removes the stimulus to increased urinary sodium and water loss normally induced by ANP, and thus renal sodium and water reabsorption is enhanced. Although ADH secretion is primarily controlled by the osmoreceptors,

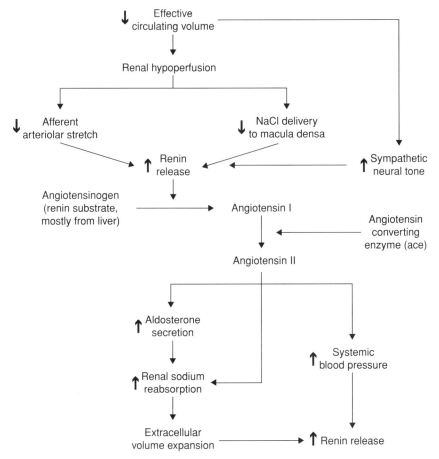

Figure 4.3   Renin–angiotensin–aldosterone system. (Modified after Reference 2, p 29).

decreased ECV also stimulates ADH secretion by activating nonosmolal, volume-sensitive receptors for ADH release.[2]

Thus, the renal control of sodium and water excretion is the final common pathway by which homeostatic mechanisms maintain normal ECV. When ECV is low, renal sodium and water reabsorption increases, and when ECV is high, sodium and water diuresis ensues. ECV is not easily measured, but ECV depletion can be diagnosed by demonstrating renal Na^+ retention as evidenced by a urinary Na^+ concentration below 25 mEq/L in the absence of diuretic therapy or intrinsic renal disease.[2]

In normal persons, ECV and ECF volume are directly proportional. In certain diseases, however, a dissociation between these two volumes occurs. For example, decreased ECV in the face of increased ECF volume is observed in congestive heart failure (decreased pressure at baroreceptors), arteriovenous fistulas (decreased pressure at baroreceptors), and advanced portal cirrhosis (ascites, arteriovenous fistulas).

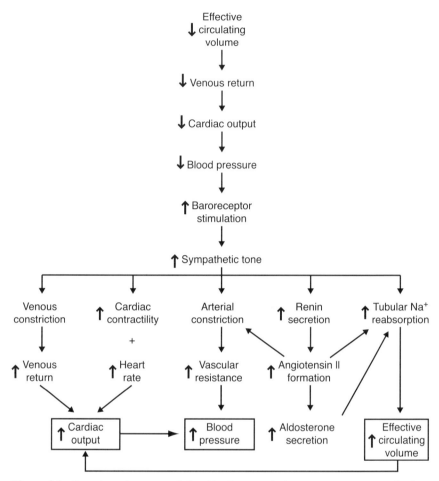

Figure 4.4   Hemodynamic responses induced by the sympathetic nervous system as a result of decreased effective circulating volume. (From Reference 2, p 267.)

Low ECV despite elevated ECF is seen also in surgical patients with interstitial extravasation ("third-space" loss) due to peritonitis, intestinal obstruction (bowel wall edema, transudation of fluid into bowel lumen), pancreatitis (retroperitoneal fluid extravasation), sepsis (capillary leak), extensive retroperitoneal dissection, major fractures, and thermal injuries.

The normal distribution of extracellular sodium and the normal 3:1 ratio of water between the intravascular (plasma) and interstitial spaces (Table 4.1) is maintained as a result of the movement of these substances between the two spaces at the level of the capillaries and postcapillary venules. The forces ("Starling forces") governing the net transcapillary sodium and water distribution (J_v) include (1) the hydrostatic pressure within the capillary (P_c) and the interstitium (P_i) and the osmotic pressure in the capillary (Π_c) and the interstitium (Π_i) (Fig. 4.5).[3] In contrast to the cell

CAPILLARY DRIVING FORCES

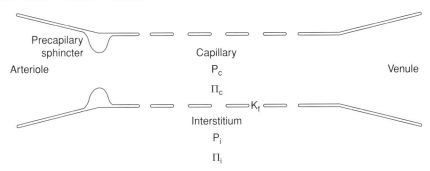

CAPILLARY PRESSURE GRADIENTS

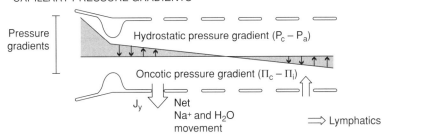

Figure 4.5   Forces governing transcapillary sodium and water distribution. (From Reference 3, p 5.)

membrane, the capillary wall is permeable to sodium salts and glucose so that the plasma proteins are the only effective osmoles because they move across the capillary wall only to a limited degree.

The *colloid osmotic pressure* or the *plasma oncotic pressure* denotes the sum of the contributions of the various fractions of the plasma proteins to osmotic pressure. Thus, 75% of the total colloid osmotic pressure results from the albumin fraction and 25% from the globulins. Fibrinogen makes a negligible contribution (Fig. 4.6). The *Gibbs-Donnan effect* causes the colloid osmotic pressure of the plasma to be greater than that caused by the proteins alone. This results from the fact that at physiologic pH 7.4, proteins have a negative charge and therefore behave as anions. This electronegativity is balanced by cations, mainly sodium, which contribute to the total osmotic pressure.[2,4] The hydrostatic pressure within the capillary diminishes from the arterial end to the venous end. Consequently, fluid moves into the interstitium at the arterial end, and reabsorption of about 90% of the filtrate occurs at the venous end. The net effect across the capillary is a small gradient (0.3 mm Hg) favoring filtration into the interstitium. This interstitial filtrate is normally returned to the circulation by the lymphatics (Table 4.2).

In clinical practice, pathologic conditions may arise (e.g., increased capillary hydrostatic pressure) resulting in an increase in net filtration into the interstitium that exceeds the limit of lymphatic drainage and edema supervenes (Table 4.3). Conversely, if the capillary pressure falls significantly, net reabsorption of the fluid

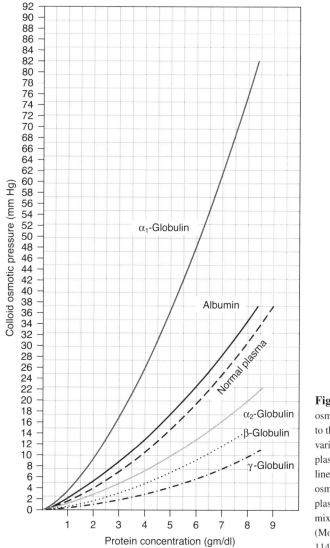

Figure 4.6 Colloid osmotic pressure in relation to the concentration of various fractions of the plasma proteins. The dashed line shows the colloid osmotic pressure of normal plasma proteins, which are a mixture of the others. (Modified after Reference 114.)

into the capillaries occurs ("transcapillary filling"), and the plasma volume increases at the expense of the interstitial compartment.[5,6]

ACID–BASE HOMEOSTASIS

Under normal conditions, the H^+ concentration and, therefore, the pH of the ECF vary little from the normal values of 40 nmol/L and 7.4, respectively, despite the continuous addition of endogenously produced acids and bases. Thus, the daily metabolism of

Table 4.2   Exchange of Water between the Intravascular (Plasma) and Interstitial Compartments

	Arterial End of Capillary	Venous End of Capillary	Mean
Forces tending to move fluid out of capillary (mm Hg)			
Capillary hydrostatic pressure	30	10	17.3
Negative interstitial hydrostatic pressure	3	3	3.0
Interstitial colloid osmotic pressure	8	8	8.0
	41	**21**	**28.3**
Forces tending to move fluid into capillary (mm Hg)			
Plasma oncotic pressure	28	28	28.0
Net force	13 mm Hg out of capillary	7 mm Hg into capillary	0.3 mm Hg out of capillary

Modified after Reference 118, p 189.

carbohydrates and fats generates 15,000 mmol of CO_2, from which carbonic acid is formed. In addition, non-carbonic acids and bases result from the metabolism of proteins and other substances. Non-carbonic acids are derived primarily from the oxidation of sulfur-containing amino acids (methionine and cysteine), cationic amino acids (arginine and lysine), and hydrolysis of dietary biphosphate, H2PO4−. Metabolism of anionic amino acids (glutamate and aspartate) and organic anions (such as citrate and lactate) is the major source of alkali.[2]

Acid–base homeostasis involves three major processes: (1) chemical buffering by the extracellular and intracellular buffer systems, (2) regulation of the P_{CO_2} in the blood by alveolar ventilation, and (3) control of the plasma bicarbonate concentration by changes in renal hydrogen ion excretion.[2] *Buffers* are aqueous systems that tend to minimize changes in pH when small amounts of acid or base are added. The body buffers are primarily a mixture of weak and therefore poorly dissociated acids and their salts. H^+ ions added in the form of a strong acid combine with anions from the salt component of the buffer to form a weakly dissociated acid, which consequently yields fewer hydrogen ions than the strong acid originally added. As a result, the fall in pH is diminished. The bicarbonate/carbon dioxide buffer system is the major extracellular buffer system. Other, quantitatively less important, buffers in the ECF include inorganic phosphate and the plasma proteins.

The bicarbonate/carbon dioxide buffer system is described by the following equation:

$$H^+ + HCO_3^- \leftrightarrow H_2CO_3 \leftrightarrow H_2O + \underset{\substack{\text{aqueous} \\ \text{phase}}}{CO_2} \leftrightarrow \underset{\substack{\text{gas} \\ \text{phase}}}{CO_2} \tag{4.5}$$

Table 4.3   Causes of Edema

I. Increased capillary pressure
   A Excessive kidney retention of salt and water
   B High venous pressure
      1. High failure
      2. Local venous block
      3. Failure of venous pumps
         (a) Paralysis of muscles
         (b) Immobilized parts of body
         (c) Failure of venous valves
   C Decreased arteriolar resistance
      1. Excessive body heat
      2. Paralysis of sympathetic nervous system
      3. Effects of vasodilator drugs

II. Decreased plasma proteins
   A Loss of proteins in urine (nephrosis)
   B Loss of protein from denuded skin areas
      1. Burns
      2. Wounds
   C Failure to produce proteins
      1. Liver disease
      2. Serious protein or caloric malnutrition

III. Increased capillary permeability
   A Immune reactions that cause release of histamine and other
     immune products
   B Toxins
   C Bacterial infections
   D Vitamin deficiency, especially vitamin C
   E Prolonged ischemia
   F Burns

IV. Blockage of lymph return
   A Blockage of lymph nodes by cancer
   B Blockage of lymph nodes by infection, especially with
     filaria nematodes
   C Congenital absence of or abnormality of lymphatic vessels

---

From Reference 118, p 303.

This buffer system is very effective because the P_{CO_2}, reflecting the concentration of CO_2 in the gas phase, can be regulated by changes in alveolar ventilation. The functions of this buffer system are quantitatively expressed in the Henderson-Hasselbach equation, which defines the pH in terms of the ratio of bicarbonate and carbonic acid present in the blood:

$$pH = pK + \log \frac{HCO_3^-}{H_2CO_3}, \tag{4.6}$$

where pK, the dissociation constant for this buffer system, has been measured to equal 6.1.

To maintain a normal body pH of 7.4, the ratio of bicarbonate to carbonic acid must remain 20:1, as depicted:

$$7.4 = 6.1 + \log \frac{27 \text{ mEq/L}}{1.35 \text{ mEq/L}}$$

$$7.4 = 6.1 + \log 20 \qquad \frac{20}{1}$$

$$7.4 = 6.1 + 1.3$$

As long as the 20:1 ratio is maintained, regardless of the absolute values, the pH remains 7.4. When an acid, such as H_2SO_4, is added to the system, Equation 4.5 is driven to the right by mass action:

$$H_2SO_4 + 2NaHCO_3 \rightarrow Na_2SO_4 + 2H_2CO_3 \qquad (4.7)$$

$$2H_2CO_3 \rightarrow 2H_2O + 2CO_2 \qquad (4.8)$$

Thus, HCO_3^- concentration decreases and aqueous CO_2 and hence alveolar CO_2 increase. The resultant rise in P_{CO_2} triggers an increase in alveolar ventilation, which immediately eliminates CO_2 in an amount exactly necessary to restore the HCO_3^- : H_2CO_3 ratio to 20:1.

These compensatory responses in the ECF compartment to minimize changes in pH are accompanied by analogous responses in the cells since a portion of the H^+ ions added to the ECF enter the cells. To maintain electroneutrality, H^+ ions enter the cells in exchange for intracellular Na^+ and K^+. In erythrocytes, electroneutrality is maintained by the concomitant entrance of Cl^- and H^+ ions into the cell (Fig. 4.7). Within cells, the primary buffers are proteins and organic and inorganic phosphates; hemoglobin is the main buffer in erythrocytes. In addition, bone represents an important site of acid–base buffering. Bone can take up excess H^+ ions in exchange for

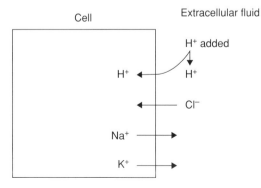

Figure 4.7 Effect of an HCl load on extracellular Cl^-, Na^+, and K^+. As H^+ enters the cells to be buffered, either Cl^- follows H^+ into the cells or intracellular Na^+ and K^+ leave the cells and move into the ECF. These ion shifts are reversed when H^+ ions are removed from the ECF. (Modified after Reference 2, p 316.)

surface Na^+ and K^+, and pH is also controlled by the dissolution of bone mineral, which results in the release of buffer compounds into the ECF. These compounds include $NaHCO_3$ and $KHCO_3$ initially and then $CaCO_3$ and $CaHPO_4$. It should be recognized that transcellular exchange of H^+ for K^+ observed in severe metabolic acidemia may result in clinically significant hyperkalemia.[2]

Although the various buffer systems minimize changes in pH consequent to the addition of acid or alkali to the ECF, the excess H^+ ions or HCO_3^- ions added must still be excreted by the kidney to prevent progressive depletion of the body buffers.[2] Thus, the renal contribution to acid–base balance consists mainly of reabsorption of normally filtered HCO_3^-, about 4300 mEq/day, and the generation of new HCO_3^- to replace alkali lost in the stool or consumed in neutralizing acid produced by cellular metabolism or an exogenous acid load. These functions are accompanied by the tubular secretion of H^+ ions. H^+ available for secretion is generated within the renal tubular cell from the reaction of CO_2 with H_2O to form H_2CO_3 and then H^+ + HCO_3^-. This reaction is catalyzed by carbonic anhydrase.[1,2]

The HCO_3^- ion formed in the reaction is reabsorbed into the peritubular blood. In the proximal tubular cells, H^+ is secreted into the tubular lumen (i.e., into the urine) in exchange for Na^+, and HCO_3^- moves from the tubular cells into the peritubular capillary blood accompanied by Na^+. In the cells of the collecting tubule, H^+ ion is secreted by active transport into the lumen (urine) or is secreted in exchange for K^+. Here, HCO_3^- ions in the collecting tubule cell move into the peritubular capillary blood in exchange for Cl^- (Fig. 4.8). In either case, the H^+ secreted into the tubular lumen may combine with filtered HCO_3^-, with NH_3, or with urinary buffers such as HPO_4^-, citrate, acetate, or creatinine, forming "titratable" acid. If the secreted H^+ ions combine with filtered HCO_3^-, the net effect is HCO_3^- reabsorption; if the secreted H^+ ions combine with urinary buffers or NH_3, new HCO_3^- is added to the ECF, and the plasma HCO_3^- concentration rises (Fig. 4.9). These processes are reversed in the face of an alkali load.

The rate of tubular acid secretion is substantially regulated by the pH of the ECF. When pH $<$ 7.4, hydrogen ion secretion can increase several fold with a concomitant increase in ECF HCO_3^- concentration. Conversely, at an ECF pH $>$ 7.4, hydrogen ion secretion into the urine diminishes, and sodium bicarbonate loss in the urine is increased as a result of secretion of bicarbonate and decreased reabsorption. These very efficient mechanisms available for the excretion of bicarbonate, however, are diminished in the presence of decreased ECV, chloride depletion, or hypokalemia. The latter are common clinical conditions most often associated with prolonged vomiting or loss of gastric juice by nasogastric aspiration, producing metabolic alkalosis. Under these circumstances, the homeostatic mechanisms tending to restore volume prevail over those tending to relieve alkalosis.

Thus, decreased ECV triggers angiotensin and aldosterone release, which in turn stimulates reabsorption of urinary Na^+ and water. Angiotensin activates Na^+ reabsorption in exchange for H^+ secretion in the proximal renal tubule. Aldosterone promotes Na^+ reabsorption accompanied by Cl^- or in exchange for either K^+ or H^+. In the face of hypokalemia, exchange for H^+ prevails. In addition, hypokalemia stimulates the movement of H^+ into cells in exchange for intracellular K^+, producing

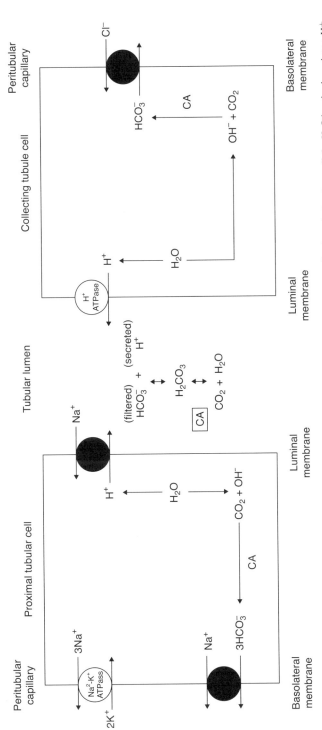

Figure 4.8 Major cellular and luminal events in bicarbonate reabsorption in the proximal tubule and the collecting tubules. Intracellular H_2O breaks down into a H^+ ion and a OH^- ion. The latter combines with CO_2 to form HCO_3^-, via a reaction catalyzed by carbonic anhydrase (CA). In the proximal tubule, the H^+ is secreted into the lumen by the Na^+–H^+ exchanger, whereas the HCO_3^- is returned to the systemic circulation primarily by a Na^+–$3HCO_3^-$ cotransporter. These same processes occur in the collecting tubules, although they are respectively mediated by an active H^+-ATPase pump in the luminal membrane and a Cl^-–HCO_3^- exchanger in the basolateral membrane. The secreted H^+ ions combine with filtered HCO_3^- to form carbonic acid (H_2CO_3) and then $CO_2 + H_2O$, which can be passively reabsorbed. This dissociation of carbonic acid is facilitated when luminal carbonic anhydrase (CA in box) is present, as in the early proximal tubule. The net effect is HCO_3^- reabsorption, even though the HCO_3^- ions returned to the systemic circulation are not the same as those that were filtered. Although not shown, the collecting tubule cells also have H^+–K^+–ATPase pumps in the luminal membrane that are primarily involved in K^+ reabsorption. (Modified after Reference 2, p 330.)

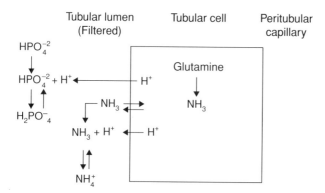

Figure 4.9 Formation of titratable acids and NH_4^+. (From Reference 25, p 689.)

a fall in intracellular pH. Low pH in the renal tubular cells triggers renal urinary acidification further enhancing Na^+ reabsorption in exchange for H^+. When Cl^- depletion coexists, less Cl^- ion is available to accompany the renal Na reabsorption stimulated by low ECV. An increased proportion of Na^+ reabsorption must, therefore, be associated with exchange for H^+ to maintain electroneutrality. All of these responses enhance renal urinary acidification and explain the "paradoxical" aciduria observed in hypochloremic, hypokalemic alkalosis and the perpetuation of the alkalosis ("contraction alkalosis") until ECV and plasma potassium and chloride levels are returned to normal.[2-4]

Analysis of Acid–Base Derangements

Acid–base derangements may be due to (1) disturbances that primarily affect alveolar ventilation, thereby producing abnormalities in arterial P_{CO_2} (Table 4.4) or (2)

Table 4.4 Causes of Respiratory Disturbances

Acidosis (Hypoventilation)	Alkalosis (Hyperventilation)
Airway obstruction	Central nervous system disorders
Foreign body, pneumonia, emphysema, laryngospasm	Injury, tumor, stroke, anxiety
Central nervous system depression	Hypoxia
Narcotics, anesthetics, injury, tumor	Adult respiratory distress syndrome, pulmonary embolus, atelectasis, anemia
Thoracic injury	Mechanical ventilation
Pneumothroax, flail chest, tracheal tear	Excess tidal volume and/or rate
Mechanical ventilation	Hypermetabolism
Inadequate rate and/or tidal volume, increased dead space	Fever, injury sepsis
Miscellaneous	Miscellaneous
Congestive heart failure, myopathy, severe obesity	Congestive heart failure, salicylate intoxication, cirrhosis

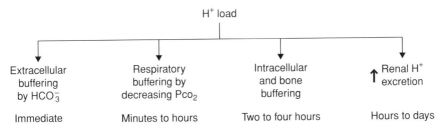

Figure 4.10   Sequential response to a H^+ load, culminating in the restoration of acid–base balance by the renal excretion of the excess H^+. (Modified after Reference 2, p 362.)

diseases that primarily affect the pH of the ECF and, therefore, the plasma HCO_3^- concentration. Respiratory acidosis and respiratory alkalosis, characterized by high and low P_{CO_2} levels, respectively, can be partially compensated by renal mechanisms that produce secondary changes in plasma HCO_3^- concentration. Metabolic acidosis and metabolic alkalosis, characterized by low or high plasma HCO_3^- concentration, respectively, each trigger a sequence of compensatory responses over time, including secondary changes in alveolar ventilation and, hence, in arterial P_{CO_2} levels (Fig. 4.10 and Table 4.5).

In acute, uncompensated acid–base disturbances, determining the nature of the derangement is simplified because only the P_{CO_2} *or* the HCO_3^- concentration is abnormal. In patients with changes in both the P_{CO_2} *and* the HCO_3^- concentration, the abnormalities may reflect partial compensation for primary respiratory or primary metabolic illness (Table 4.6)[7] or, alternatively, may reflect separate, coexistent respiratory and metabolic disorders producing a mixed acid–base derangement.

Since treatment is based on the underlying pathology, it is necessary to determine the respiratory and metabolic components in a given patient. Arterial blood gas analysis, including pH, P_{CO_2}, and HCO_3^- concentration, gives the requisite information for diagnosis. Primary changes in P_{CO_2}, acute or chronic, are associated with corresponding changes in pH and HCO_3^- concentration (Table 4.7).[8] For example, for each acute 10 mm Hg deviation of P_{CO_2} above or below a normal value of 40, the pH changes in the opposite direction by approximately 0.07 units. These relationships permit determination of pH and $HCO3^-$ values that can be attributed exclusively to a given P_{CO_2} level. pH and HCO_3^- values outside the range expected with this P_{CO_2} level reflect the metabolic component of the acid–base disturbance. For example, a patient with acute respiratory distress has the following arterial blood gases:

$$P_{CO_2} = 70 \text{ mm Hg}$$
$$pH = 7.10$$
$$HCO_3^{--} = 21 \text{ mEq/L}$$

Respiratory acidosis alone producing a P_{CO_2} of 70 should be associated with a pH of 7.19–7.23 and an HCO_3^- level of 26–29 mEq/L (Table 4.7). The lower actual values in this patient indicate a concomitant metabolic acidosis.[8]

Table 4.5 Summary of Acid–Base Disorders

	Defect	Common Causes	$\dfrac{BHCO_3}{H_2CO_3}$	Compensation
Respiratory acidosis	Retention of CO_2 (decreased alveolar ventilation)	Depression of respiratory center by morphine CNS injury Pulmonary disease: emphysema, pneumonia	↑Denominator Ratio less than 20:1	Renal Retention of bicarbonate, excretion of acid salts, increased ammonia formation Chloride shifts into red cells
Respiratory alkalosis	Excessive loss of CO_2 (increased alveolar ventilation)	Hyperventilation: emotional disturbances, severe pain, assisted ventilation, encephalitis	↓Denominator Ratio greater than 20:1	Excretion of bicarbonate, retention of acid salts, decreased ammonia formation
Metabolic acidosis	Retention of fixed acids or loss of base bicarbonate	Diabetes, azotemia, lactic acid accumulation, starvation	↓Numerator Ratio less than 20:1	Pulmonary (rapid): increased rate and depth of breathing Renal (slow): as in respiratory acidosis
Metabolic alkalosis	Loss of fixed acid salts Gain of base bicarbonate Potassium depletion	Vomiting or gastric suction with pyloric obstruction Excessive intake of bicarbonate Diuretics	↑Numerator Ratio greater than 20:1	Pulmonary (rapid): decreased rate and depth of breath[a] Renal (slow): as in respiratory alkalosis

[a]Compensation limited by the fall in po_2 associated with decreased ventilation.

Table 4.6 Respiratory and Metabolic Components of Acid Base Disorders

	Acute (Uncompensated)			Chronic (Partially Compensated)		
	pH	pco_2 (respiratory component)	Plasma HCO_3 (metabolic component)	pH	pco_2 (respiratory component)	Plasma HCO_3 (metabolic component)
Respiratory acidosis	↓↓	↑↑	N	↓	↑↑	↑
Respiratory alkalosis	↑↑	↓↓	N	↑	↓↓	↓
Metabolic acidosis	↓↓	N	↓↓	↓	↓	↓
Metabolic alkalosis	↑↑	N	↑↑	↑	↑?	↑

From Reference 7, p 59.

The metabolic component of an acid–base derangement is often reported in blood gas analyses in terms of *base deficit* or *base excess*, indicating metabolic acidosis or metabolic alkalosis, respectively. In performing blood gas analysis, the respiratory component is eliminated by equilibrating the arterial blood sample at 38°C in a gas with a Pco_2 of 40 mm Hg and a Po_2 of 100 mm Hg. This allows calculation of the *standard bicarbonate*, and from this value, the base excess or base deficit, representing the metabolic component of the abnormality, can be determined. The various causes of acid–base disturbances are outlined in Tables 4.8–4.11.

The metabolic acidoses can be divided into two groups by determining the *anion gap*:

$$\text{Anion gap} = [Na^+] - ([Cl^-] + [HCO_3^-]) \tag{4.9}$$

Table 4.7 Acute and Chronic Changes in Pco_2, Arterial pH, and $HCO_3{}^-$

	Arterial pH		$HCO_3{}^-$	
pco_2 (mm Hg)	Acute	Chronic	Acute	Chronic
15	7.61–7.74		15–21	
20	7.55–7.66		18–23	10–14
25	7.49–7.59		20–24	13–16
30	7.45–7.53	7.38–7.51	21–26	17–23
35	7.40–7.48		22–27	
40	7.37–7.44	7.37–7.51	23–27	23–31
45	7.33–7.39		24–28	
50	7.31–7.36	7.35–7.44	25–28	27–35
60	7.24–7.29	7.33–7.44	25–28	31–40
70	7.19–7.23	7.30–7.42	26–29	
80	7.14–7.18	7.28–7.39	26–29	
90	7.09–7.13		27–29	
100		7.24–7.35		42–54

From Reference 8, p 338.

Table 4.8   Causes of Respiratory Acidosis

Alveolar hypoventilation
  Central nervous system depression
    Drug induced
    Sleep disorders
    Obesity hypoventilation ("Pickwickian syndrome")
    Cerebral ischemia
    Cerebral trauma
  Neuromuscular disorders
    Myopathies
    Neuropathies
  Chest wall abnormalities
    Flail chest
    Kyphoscoliosis
  Pleural abnormalities
    Pneumothorax
    Pleural effusion
  Airway obstruction
    Upper airway
      Foreign body
      Tumor
      Laryngospasm
      Sleep disorders
    Lower airway
      Severe asthma
      Chronic obstructive airway disease
      Tumor
  Parenchymal lung disease
    Pulmonary edema
      Cardiogenic
      Noncardiogenic
    Pulmonary emboli
    Pneumonia
    Aspiration
    Interstitial lung disease
  Ventilator malfunction
Increased CO_2 production
  Large caloric loads (enteral or parenteral nutrition)
  Malignant hyperthermia
  Intense shivering
  Prolonged seizure activity
  Thyroid storm
  Extensive thermal injury (burns)

From Reference 9, p 716.

Table 4.9   Causes of Respiratory Alkalosis

Central stimulation
   Pain
   Anxiety
   Ischemia
   Stroke
   Tumor
   Infection
   Fever
   Drug induced
      Salicylates
      Progesterone
      Analeptics (doxapram)
Peripheral stimulation
   Hypoxemia
   High altitude
   Pulmonary disease
      Congestive heart failure
      Noncardiogenic pulmonary edema
      Asthma
      Pulmonary emboli
   Severe anemia
Unknown mechanism
   Sepsis
   Metabolic encephalopathies
Iatrogenic
   Ventilation induced

From Reference 9, p 720.

The normal value is 10–15 mEq/L. The "gap" represents anions not routinely measured in blood electrolyte determinations and thus reflects the sum of the serum proteins, sulfate, inorganic phosphate, and organic acids present in low concentrations. Acidosis associated with a high anion gap is generally secondary to increases in endogenously produced acids (e.g., lactic acidosis or ketoacidosis), decreases in renal excretion of acids (e.g., renal failure), or ingestion of toxins (Table 4.10).[9]

FLUID AND ELECTROLYTE THERAPY

A variety of crystalloid and colloid preparations for parenteral administration are available to maintain homeostasis in fasting individuals, to replace ongoing losses, or to treat existing derangements. Commonly used preparations are given in Tables 4.12 and 4.13.

Table 4.10   Causes of Metabolic Acidosis

Increased anion gap
  Increased production of endogenous nonvolatile acids
    Renal failure
      Acute
      Chronic
    Ketoacidosis
      Diabetes
      Starvation
    Lactic acidosis
    Mixed
      Nonketotic hyperosmolar coma
      Alcoholism
    Inborn errors of metabolism
  Ingestion of toxin
    Salicylate
    Methanol
    Ethylene glycol
    Paraldehyde
    Toluene
    Sulfur
    Rhabdomyolysis
Normal anion gap (hyperchloremic)
  Increased gastrointestinal losses of HCO_3^-
    Diarrhea
    Anion exchange resins (cholestyramine)
    Ingestion of $CaCl_2$ or $MgCl_2$
    Fistulae (pancreatic, biliary, or small bowel)
    Ureterosigmoidostomy or obstructed ileal loop
  Increased renal losses of HCO_3^-
    Renal tubular acidosis
    Carbonic anhydrase inhibitors
    Hyperaldosteronism
  Dilutional
    Large amounts of bicarbonate-free fluids
  Total parenteral nutrition (chloride salts of amino acids)
  Increased uptake of chloride-containing acids
    Ammonium chloride
    Lysine hydrochloride
    Arginine hydrochloride

From Reference 9, p 717.

Maintenance Therapy

In order to preserve fluid and electrolyte homeostasis for brief periods (e.g., 7–10 days), patients receive infusions of water, sodium, and potassium, usually as the chloride salts, in amounts approximating losses measurable in the urine and stool and

Table 4.11 Causes of Metabolic Alkalosis

Chloride sensitive
 Gastrointestinal
  Vomiting
  Gastric drainage
  Chloride diarrhea
  Villous adenoma
 Renal
  Diuretics
  Posthypercapnic
  Low chloride intake
 Sweat
  Cystic fibrosis
Chloride resistant
 Increased mineralocorticoid activity
  Primary hyperaldosteronism
  Edematous disorders (secondary hyperaldosteronism)
  Cushing's syndrome
  Licorice ingestion
  Bartter's syndrome
 Severe hypokalemia
Miscellaneous
 Massive blood transfusion
 Acetate-containing colloid solutions
 Alkaline administration with renal insufficiency
  Alkali therapy
  Combined antacid and cation exchange resin therapy
 Hypercalcemia
  Milk-alkali syndrome
  Bone metastases
 Sodium penicillins
 Glucose feeding after starvation

From Reference 9, p 720.

insensible losses from the lungs and skin. Urine volume averages 0.5–1.0 mL/kg/hour; stool water is approximately 250 mL/day. Insensible losses average about 10 mL/kg/day and are increased 10% for each degree of fever above 37°C.[10] The requirement for sodium is in the range of 1–2 mEq/kg/day and for potassium approximately 0.5–1.0 mEq/kg/day. Because normal kidneys can conserve or excrete as necessary to preserve fluid and electrolyte balance, normal persons have an enormously broad tolerance for salt and water. Therefore, homeostasis can be maintained with a wide variety of fluid and electrolyte formulations. However, for practical purposes, administration of maintenance fluid volumes in accordance with body weight, as indicated in Table 4.14, simplifies order writing (the calculations outlined in the table apply to patients from infancy to old age). If the volume calculated is provided as dextrose (glucose) 5% in sodium chloride 0.2% with the addition of potassium

Table 4.12 Commonly Used Parenteral Infusion Solutions

	Approximate pH	mOsm/L	kcal/L	Na mEq/L	K mEq/L	Ca mEq/L	Cl mEq/L	Lactate mEq/L
Dextrose 5% in water	4.3	253	170[a]					
Dextrose 10% in water	4.3	505	340[a]					
Dextrose 5% in sodium chloride 0.2%	4.4	320	170[a]	34			34	
Dextrose 5% in sodium chloride 0.45%	4.4	405	170[a]	77			77	
Dextrose 5% in sodium chloride 0.9%	4.4	560	170[a]	154			154	
Sodium chloride 0.45%	5.6	154		77			77	
Sodium chloride 0.9%	5.6	308		154			154	
Dextrose 5% in lactated Ringer's solution	5.0	530	170[a]	130	4	3	109	28
Lactated Ringer's solution	6.3	275		130	4	3	109	28

[a]Based on caloric value of 1G monohydrated glucose, 3.4 kcal.

chloride, 20mEq/L, then the infusion will meet the maintenance fluid and electrolyte requirements outlined above. Thus, a 70-kg patient would receive a daily infusion of 2500 mL of $D_5$0.2% NaCl containing 20 mEq/L of KCl, calculated as follows:

1st 10 kg of body weight	1000 ml (100 × 10)
2nd 10 kg of body weight	500 ml (10 × 50)
Remaining 50 kg of body weight	1000 ml (50 × 20)
	2500 ml

This regimen would deliver 85 mEq of sodium (34 mEq/L × 2.5 L = 85 mEq) providing 1.2 mEq/kg and 50 mEq of potassium (20 mEq/L × 2.5 L = 50 mEq) providing 0.7 mEq/kg. The electrolytes are provided in a 5% dextrose solution to avoid hypotonic infusions but, more importantly, to meet the energy requirements of the brain and the other glucose-dependent glycolytic tissues (erythrocytes, leukocytes,

Table 4.13 Plasma Expanders and Colloid Preparations

	Approximate pH	mOsm/L	kcal/L	Na mEq/L	Cl mEq/L
Human albumin					
1. Human albumin 25%				130–160	
2. Human albumin 5%				130–160	
Plasma protein fraction, 5%					
1. Plasmanate				130–160	
2. Plasmatein				130–160	
3. Proteinate				130–160	
Dextrans and starch					
1. Dextran 75, 6% in dextrose 5%	4	253	170		
2. Dextran 75, 6% in sodium chloride 0.9%	4.5	309		154	154
3. Dextran 70, 6% in sodium chloride 0.9%	4.5–7	300		154	154
4. Dextran 40, 10% in dextrose 5%	3–7	309	170		
5. Dextran 40, 10% in sodium chloride 0.9%	3.5–7	317		154	154
6. Hetastarch, 6% in sodium chloride 0.9%	3.5–7	310		154	154

active fibroblasts, certain phagocytes, peripheral nerves). When insufficient glucose in prescribed, the required energy substrate is derived by means of protein catabolism and gluconeogenesis. This protein-sparing effect of glucose is maximally achieved with about 100–150 g of glucose providing about 400 kcal. No further benefit in protein economy accrues, even with higher caloric intake in the absence of dietary protein.

The maintenance fluid and electrolyte regimen outlined here is satisfactory for most surgical patients who must fast for up to 7–10 days. If oral intake must be withheld for more than 7–10 days, a complete nutritional program should be considered in order to provide additional energy, a protein source, vitamins, essential fatty acids, and sufficient macro- and micronutrients so that energy, protein, and mineral balance can be achieved (infra vide).

Table 4.14 Maintenance Fluid Requirements

Body Weight	Fluid Required
For the first 10 kg (0–10 kg)	100 mL/kg/day
For the second 10 kg (11–20 kg)	Add 50 mL/kg/day
For each kilogram over 20 kg	Add 20 mL/kg/day[a]

[a]For elderly patients or patients with cardiac disease, reduce this amount to 15 mL/kg/day.

Fluid Resuscitation

The fluid preparation chosen to replace ongoing volume losses or replete existing deficits depends on the nature and composition of the loss as well as its rapidity and hemodynamic consequences. Intravascular volume deficits due to moderate blood loss or third-space extravasation associated with acute peritonitis, bowel obstruc tion, sepsis, burns, or extensive operative dissection can be managed with available crystalloid or colloid preparations (Tables 4.12 and 4.13). However, despite years of study, controversy remains concerning the relative merits and drawbacks of crystalloid and colloid infusions. The 2008 update from the *Surviving Sepsis Campaign*, an international effort to improve outcomes in severe sepsis, has given an equal recommendation for fluid resuscitation with either colloids or crystalloids.[11]

In contrast to colloid infusions, crystalloids are rapidly equilibrated throughout the *entire* ECF compartment, and consequently greater volumes are necessary to achieve equivalent *intravascular* volume expansion. This rapid equilibration has the apparent benefit of restoring interstitial space deficits that accompany intravascular losses, but excess interstitial water may result in peripheral edema, depending on the amount of the crystalloid infusion. The additional volume of crystalloid fluid compared to the volume of albumin required to achieve similar resuscitation goals appears less than previously thought.[12] In the *Saline Versus Albumin Fluid Evaluation* (SAFE) trial, the appropriate ratio of albumin administered to saline was determined to be approximately 1:1.4, indicating that larger volumes of crystalloids were not required to meet similar resuscitation end points.[12, 13] Reabsorption of the excess interstitial space fluid into the vascular space as the acute illness resolves may result in pulmonary congestion, in the absence of careful hemodynamic monitoring. In response to clinical concerns that fluid resuscitation with large, rapid infusions of crystalloid solutions will increase the incidence of cardiopulmonary dysfunction, adult respiratory distress syndrome, and the requirement for ventilatory support, advocates of crystalloid resuscitation cite data indicating no increased incidence of these problems when the fluid therapy is appropriately monitored by hemodynamic parameters.[6, 14]

In contrast, colloid infusions have the theoretical advantage that much smaller volumes can replete the intravascular space and, therefore, resuscitation is more rapid. This advantage is based on the fact that colloid preparations have a greater capacity to remain in the intravascular space unless the underlying disease is associated with increased microvascular permeability. In addition, as a result of increased plasma colloid oncotic pressure, interstitial fluid may be drawn into the intravascular space thereby reducing interstitial edema and producing an amount of volume expansion that may actually exceed the quantity of colloid infused. However, in the presence of increased microvascular permeability (as in severely traumatized patients with sepsis) extravasation of intravascular colloid into the pulmonary interstitium may result in increased, rather than decreased, interstitial edema, thereby causing or aggravating the adult respiratory distress syndrome.[15]

Commercially available colloid preparations include blood-derived products (albumin and plasma protein fraction), products from bacterial sources (the dextrans), and synthetic products (hetastarch) (Table 4.13). Albumin and plasma protein fraction are heated to 60°C for at least 10 hours to minimize the risk of transmitting the hepatitis viruses. Plasma protein fraction contains about 88% albumin and 12% globulins. Dextrans are colloid preparations of glucose polymers that are produced by the bacterium *Leuconostoc meserentoides*. The two most widely used products are dextran 70 (average molecular weight 70,000) and dextran 40 (average molecular weight 40,000). Dextran 70 is generally preferred for volume expansion because dextran 40 is more rapidly eliminated.[9, 14] These agents are associated with a dose-related hemostatic defect resulting from a decrease in platelet aggregation and adhesiveness. Infusions exceeding 20 mL/kg/day can interfere with blood typing and have been associated with renal failure. Anaphylactic reactions have also been described.[9, 14] Hetastarch (hydroxyethyl starch) is an artificial colloid composed almost entirely of amylopectin. Sporadic cases of coagulopathy have been described, but coagulation studies are usually unaffected by infusions of 1–2 L. The volume-expanding capacity of the various colloids appears to be comparable.[9]

In 2004, the SAFE Study investigators[12] published the results of a randomized clinical trial comparing the effect of 0.9% normal saline versus 4% albumin in nearly 7000 critically ill patients requiring intravascular fluid resuscitation. The data revealed no significant differences between the groups with respect to 28-day mortality, incidence of organ failure, intensive care unit length of stay, or duration of mechanical ventilation or renal replacement therapy. The study found that albumin administration was safe and equally as effective as crystalloid. However, in their subgroup analysis, treatment with albumin was associated with trends toward decreased mortality in septic patients ($p = 0.09$) and increased mortality in trauma patents ($p = 0.06$), especially those with traumatic brain injury.

In 2007, the SAFE Study investigators conducted a *post hoc* study to further evaluate the previously noted trend to higher mortality in traumatic brain injury patients resuscitated with albumin compared to those resuscitated with saline.[16] At 24 months' follow-up, patients with severe traumatic brain injury receiving 4% albumin were found to have impaired functional neurologic outcomes and an elevated mortality compared to those assigned to receive saline. These results demonstrate an advantage of saline over albumin in resuscitating patients with traumatic brain injury.

Hypertonic Saline

Various investigators have reported successful resuscitation using hypertonic saline in patients suffering hemorrhage, endotoxic shock, trauma, and burns. A survival benefit has been observed in some but not all studies comparing this form of therapy with isotonic fluid resuscitation.[6, 14, 17] Hypertonic solutions have greater volume expanding capacity than isotonic crystalloid solutions because of the osmotic gradient mobilizing fluids from the intracellular to extracellular compartments, and drawing fluid from the interstitial space to the intravascular space. In their review of the current status of hypertonic saline resuscitation, Oliveira et al.[18] showed that patients resuscitated with hypertonic saline have increased myocardial contractility, reduced tissue edema, improved microcirculation and blood viscosity, and immunomodulation. The immunomodulatory and metabolic effects of small-volume, 3% hypertonic saline resuscitation in hypovolumic shock have been associated with attenuated end-organ damage and decreased inflammatory response.[19]

Hypertonic saline fluid resuscitation has been studied extensively in the setting of traumatic brain injury, but the findings have been inconsistent.[17,20,21] Some studies show better control of intracranial pressure and improved neurological outcome with hypertonic infusions compared to physiologic crystalloid infusions. However, Copper et al.[20] compared prehospital treatment with rapid infusion of 250 mL of 7.5% saline with an infusion of 250 mL of Ringer's and found no difference in long term neurological outcomes between the two treatment regimens. The timing and concentration of the hypertonic saline administration continues to be investigated.

Replacement of Gastrointestinal Losses

Patients with abnormal losses of fluids and electrolytes from the gastrointestinal tract require fluid and electrolytes in amounts necessary to meet maintenance requirements, replete deficits, and to replace ongoing losses. Modest volume losses extending over brief periods may be treated with standard fluid preparations with an electrolyte composition that approximates losses. Normal kidneys will adjust to compensate for minor disparities in electrolyte composition between the infusate and the gastrointestinal loss. The volume and electrolyte content of the various gastrointestinal secretions are presented in Table 4.15. Gastric losses can be managed with a solution of 0.45%–0.9% NaCl in 5% dextrose containing 20 mEq KCl/L. Bicarbonate-containing secretions generally can be replaced with lactated Ringer's solution in 5% dextrose; 10–20 mEq KCl should be added to each liter. When losses are sustained or massive, more precise replacement is required. In such patients, an

Table 4.15   Volume and Electrolyte Content of Gastrointestinal Fluid Losses[a]

	Na^+ (mEq/L)	K^+ (mEq/L)	Cl^- (mEq/L)	HCO_3^- (mEq/L)	Volume (mL)
Gastric juice, high in acid	20 (20–30)	10 (5–40)	120 (80–150)	0	1000–9000
Gastric juice, low in acid	80 (70–140)	15 (5–40)	90 (40–120)	5–25	1000–2500
Pancreatic juice	140(115–180)	5 (3–8)	75 (55–95)	80 (60–110)	500–1000
Bile	148 (130–160)	5 (3–12)	100 (90–120)	35 (30–40)	300–1000
Small-bowel drainage	110 (80–150)	5 (2–8)	105 (60–125)	30 (20–40)	1000–3000
Distal ileum and cecum drainage	80 (40–135)	8 (5–30)	45 (20–90)	30 (20–40)	1000–3000
Diarrheal stools	120 (20–160)	25 (10–40)	90 (30–120)	45 (30–50)	500–17000

[a]Average values/24 hour with range in parentheses.
Reference 119, p 100.

aliquot of draining fluid is analyzed for electrolyte content, and additions to a standard preparation are made in the pharmacy so that the infusate matches the electrolyte content of the draining secretions. Excessive replacement should be avoided not only to prevent pulmonary congestion and edema but also because the additional fluid infused may actually further stimulate digestive secretions, the so-called "third kidney effect" of the gastrointestinal tract.[22] In this situation, a positive feedback cycle is initiated in which excessive parenteral infusion leads to increased gastrointestinal secretions, which in turn are replaced by ever greater parenteral volumes. This vicious cycle is identified by progressively increasing gastrointestinal secretions accompanying a concomitant diuresis. Although oliguria may occur, usually an increasing urine output is the cue to reduce the replacement volume.

Analysis of Fluid and Electrolyte Status

Assessment of fluid and electrolyte status is based on history, physical examination, serum electrolyte levels, urine values including volume, concentration and sodium content, and, if necessary, hemodynamic parameters such as central venous pressure, pulmonary capillary wedge pressure, and cardiac output. Important features in establishing a diagnosis of hypovolemia or dehydration include a history of external losses such as vomiting, profuse diarrhea, tube or fistula drainage, or polyuria; the presence of acute conditions associated with third-space extravasation such as acute peritonitis or pancreatitis; or the use of diuretics or vigorous purging as in surgical bowel preparation. In addition, patients with complex problems often undergo a series of diagnostic tests that require that the patient refrain from eating or drinking for a period of time preceding the test. A prolonged sequence of such tests is a subtle and often unrecognized basis for hypovolemia. The magnitude of the deficit can be estimated from such physical findings as tachycardia, hypotension, peripheral vasoconstriction, and oliguria, which occur promptly when there are large acute fluid losses. Decreased tissue turgor and intraocular pressure are manifestations of more chronic, ongoing negative fluid balance (Table 4.16). Laboratory findings in dehydration include rising hematocrit, increasing serum urea concentration, high urinary specific gravity, and low urinary sodium level (see later). Low central venous and pulmonary capillary wedge pressures confirm the diagnosis. The effect of dehydration on acid–base status is determined from serum electrolyte and arterial blood gas values, as discussed previously.

Volume overload also is an important finding in surgical patients and is manifest by cardiac gallop, dyspnea, rales, and dependent edema. A history of cardiac, renal, or liver disease may establish the etiology of the hypervolemia.

Preoperative Fluid Management

Anesthetic and operative risk is increased among patients arriving in the operating room with fluid or electrolyte derangements. For example, hypotension is frequently observed in dehydrated patients on the induction of general anesthesia. The effect

Table 4.16   Signs of Fluid Loss (Hypovolemia)

Sign	Fluid Loss (Expressed as Percentage of Body Weight)		
	5%	10%	15%
Mucous membranes	Dry	Very dry	Parched
Sensorium	Normal	Lethargic	Obtunded
Orthostatic changes	None	Present	Marked
In heart rate			> 15 bpm ↑[a]
In blood pressure			> 10 mm Hg ↓
Urinary flow rate	Mildly decreased	Decreased	Markedly decreased
Pulse rate	Normal or increased	Increased > 100 bpm	Markedly increased > 120 bpm
Blood pressure	Normal	Mildly decreased with respiratory variation	Decreased

[a]bpm, beats per minute.
From Reference 9, p 691.

of hypovolemia is magnified by the vasodilatation and myocardial depression associated with inhalation anesthetics. The interruption of normal baroreceptor reflexes by anesthesia abruptly reverses the increased vascular resistance and tachycardia that compensates for volume depletion in the awake patient. Therefore, patients must be assessed preoperatively and appropriate treatment prescribed to render the patient euvolemic.

Many patients undergoing elective surgery do not require any preoperative intervention; refraining from eating or drinking for 12 hours prior to surgery has no discernible adverse consequences. On the other hand, patients with significant fluid and electrolyte abnormalities should be treated preoperatively; the time devoted to such resuscitative therapy depends on the urgency of the proposed operation. Patients undergoing diagnostic studies or treatments such as surgical bowel preparation, known to predispose to negative fluid balance, should receive parenteral infusions on the preoperative day to avoid fluid and electrolyte deficits. Lactated Ringer's solution or a solution of 0.45% NaCl and 5% dextrose, each containing 20 mEq of KCl/L, in volumes necessary to meet maintenance requirements as well as to replace losses, is generally satisfactory.

Intraoperative Fluid Management

The goals of intraoperative fluid therapy are to correct any remaining preexisting deficits, supply maintenance fluids and electrolytes, and replace blood loss, evaporative losses, and third-space extravasation. Patients with normal hemoglobin concentrations prior to operation can sustain losses of 10%–20% of their blood volume (approximately 500–1000 mL) without transfusions; crystalloid or colloid replacement suffices. Blood is administered for greater losses or when the hemoglobin level

Table 4.17   Redistribution and Evaporative Surgical Fluid Losses

Degree of Tissue Trauma	Additional Fluid Requirement
Minimal (e.g., herniorrhaphy)	0–2 mL/kg/hour
Moderate (e.g., cholecystectomy)	2–4 mL/kg/hour
Severe (e.g., bowel resection)	4–8 mL/kg/hour

From Reference 9, p 697.

or the hematocrit falls below 7–10 g/dL or 21%–30%, respectively. In elderly patients or those with significant cardiac disease, blood transfusion is recommended when the Hgb concentration falls below 10 g/dL.[9]

Evaporative losses are proportional to the size of the operative wound, the surface area of the body cavity exposed, and the duration of the surgical procedure. In addition, evaporative losses are aggravated by the peripheral vasodilatation associated with regional and general anesthesia. "Third-space" extravasation represents an internal redistribution of fluids resulting in a decrease in the functional volume of the ECF compartment but not a loss of fluid from the body. Interstitial fluid increases in areas of surgical dissection, trauma, or inflammation. In abdominal surgery, fluid collects in the lumen and in the wall of the small bowel, and transudation of fluid across serosal surfaces results in the accumulation of free fluid in the peritoneal cavity. Again, the decrease in functional ECF volume is proportional to the magnitude of tissue injury, inflammation and surgical dissection, and the surface area of the affected tissues.

Evaporative and third-space losses are estimated and replaced continuously during the operation. During an abdominal operation, Shires[7] recommends infusion of 500–1000 mL/hour with a balanced salt solution. Morgan et al.[9] have estimated requirements in relation to the magnitude of the operation (Table 4.17). Over aggressive fluid treatment must be avoided due to the risk of fluid overload and pulmonary congestion in the postoperative period.

Intraoperative fluid management is monitored in the usual way, measuring hemodynamic parameters such as pulse and blood pressure, and urine output. Invasive monitoring with central venous or Swan-Ganz catheter is indicated when major fluid shifts are anticipated or occur unexpectedly intraoperatively.

Postoperative Fluid Management

Considerations in the 24-hour period immediately following operation include maintenance therapy, treatment of any residual deficits, and replacement of ongoing losses (e.g., nasogastric suction, drainage tubes) and continuing third-space extravasation. The latter is most commonly observed in patients with massive peritonitis or extensive retroperitoneal dissection, as in ruptured aortic aneurysm. Potassium supplements are generally withheld on the operative day because a mild hyperkalemia is routinely observed after operation, due in part to release of potassium from dissected or injured tissues.[5] More importantly, potassium is withheld because the status of kidney function is unknown in the first hours following operation, even when urine volume is apparently normal. In the event of impaired renal function, hyperkalemia is a life-threatening abnormality. The likelihood of renal impairment correlates with the magnitude of the operation, the amount of blood loss, and the occurrence of episodes of hemodynamic instability and hypotension. Occasionally, however, potassium supplements are required, primarily when marked hypokalemia occurs or when borderline low potassium levels are observed in patients receiving digitalis preparations. If postoperative renal function is normal, potassium supplements may be started on the first or second postoperative day.

In the immediate postoperative period, measurement of urinary output is the primary method of monitoring fluid status. The goal of fluid therapy is to achieve urinary output of at least 0.5 mL/kg/hour.

Reabsorption of Sequestered Losses

Later in the postoperative course, as inflammatory conditions resolve and areas of injury and dissection heal, third-space sequestered fluid is reabsorbed into the vascular space. This autotransfusion, which often begins as early as the third postoperative day, may result in significant fluid overload with pulmonary congestion, tachycardia, gallop rhythm, and edema. In patients with conditions associated with large third-space extravasation, reabsorption should be anticipated by restricting fluids, and diuretics are occasionally indicated.

Analysis of Oliguria

Low urine volume in the early postoperative period is a common clinical problem usually, but not always, due to volume depletion. The differential etiology is presented in Table 4.18. The intraoperative record of fluid administration and estimated losses may or may not be helpful in the analysis. History, physical examination, electrocardiogram, arterial blood gases, and irrigation of the urinary catheter to establish patency can readily eliminate most of the causes of postoperative oliguria except hypovolemia and renal failure. Tachycardia, hypotension, and peripheral vasoconstriction with cold extremities support the diagnosis of volume depletion. A low hemoglobin concentration or hematocrit level is consistent with unreplaced blood loss, but these indices do not reliably reflect the extent of acute hemorrhage. An unexpectedly high hemoglobin or hematocrit level suggests unreplaced crystalloid losses. In clinical practice, the commonest diagnostic (and therapeutic) approach to differentiate hypovolemia from renal failure is to rapidly administer a fluid challenge of 250–500 mL of balanced salt solution, or transfuse blood, if indicated. Increased urine output establishes the diagnosis of volume depletion, but a failure to respond may reflect a residual large volume deficit unaffected by only 250–500 mL of fluid or, alternatively, acute renal failure. In this setting, another fluid challenge may be ordered if the lungs remain clear. Blood chemistry and urine studies are also helpful in distinguishing oliguria due to hypovolemia or renal failure (Table 4.19). When the diagnosis remains in doubt, central pressure monitoring is useful. When

Table 4.18 Etiology of Postoperative Oliguria or Anuria

A. Prerenal causes
 1. Volume depletion
  (a) Unreplaced or ongoing blood loss
  (b) Unreplaced or ongoing external loss of body fluids
  (c) Unreplaced or ongoing third space extravasation
 2. Other causes of decreased effective circulating volume
  (a) Congestive heart failure
  (b) Myocardial infarction
  (c) Pericardial tamponade
  (d) Acute pulmonary embolism
  (e) Advanced hepatic cirrhosis
  (f) Arteriovenous fistula
  (g) Hypotension
    1. Hypovolemia (see A1)
    2. Anesthetic agents
    3. Narcotics or other drugs
  (h) Peripheral vasodilation due to bacteremia
 3. Increased renovascular resistance
  (a) Anesthesia
  (b) Surgical operation
  (c) Hepatorenal syndrome
 4. Bilateral renovascular obstruction
 (a) Embolism
 (b) Thrombosis

B. Renal causes: acute renal failure

C. Postrenal causes: obstructive uropathy
 1. Bilateral ureteral obstruction or injury
 2. Prostatic hypertrophy or other cause of bladder outlet obstruction
 3. Pelvic hematoma
 4. Urethral obstruction
 5. Malfunctioning urinary catheter

Table 4.19 Laboratory Values in the Analysis of Oliguria

	Prerenal	Renal
Urine specific gravity[a]	>1.020	1.010
Urine osmolality[a] (mOsm/kg)	>500	< 400
Urine sodium (mEq/L)	<20	> 40
BUN/serum creatinine	>15	< 10
Urine/plasma creatinine	>40	< 20
Urine/plasma urea	>8	< 3
Fractional excretion of filtered sodium (FE_{Na})[b]	<1	> 2

[a]Interpretation invalid in presence of glucosuria or proteinuria.
[b]$FE_{Na} = $ (U/P Na) (100)/(U/P Cr).

filling pressures are low, fluid administration is continued until values are normalized. Hypovolemia and acute renal failure can coexist initially, since hypovolemia, especially when associated with hypotension, may be the etiologic background for the development of intrinsic renal injury. Under these circumstances, oliguria will persist despite volume repletion and fluid restriction must then be prescribed (see later).

Fluid and Electrolyte Management of Postoperative Renal Failure

In the presence of renal failure, fluid and electrolyte administration is markedly restricted. Dextrose, 5% in water, is provided at a daily maintenance rate of 10 mL/kg, to cover insensible losses. Additional fluid and electrolytes are infused to replace other significant ongoing losses, including any urine output, but potassium is withheld. Central venous or left atrial pressure monitoring is invaluable in the assessment of fluid requirements when significant fluid shifts are anticipated. Restriction of fluid and potassium is of utmost importance since it is frequently desirable to delay hemodialysis in the newly postoperative patient as long as possible because of the dangers inherent in the use of heparin usually required for the extracorporeal circuit. On the other hand, surgical operations produce a catabolic state resulting in accelerated azotemia and hyperkalemia so that dialysis is generally required by the second postoperative day. Marked hyperkalemia is the most common reason for earlier dialysis, but fluid overload, often manifest by hypertension, is another important indication.[23] Life-threatening hyperkalemia must be treated emergently while dialysis is being arranged. The pharmacologic management is presented in Table 4.20.

Analysis and Management of Hyponatremia

Low serum sodium concentration may be due to a variety of causes (Fig. 4.11). Hyponatremia can occur in patients with increased, near-normal or decreased ECF volume; increased, near-normal, or decreased total body sodium;[24] and it may be associated with hypotonic, isotonic, or hypertonic serum. Nevertheless, hyponatremia, defined as a plasma sodium concentration below 135 mEq/L, usually reflects hypotonicity. It is the latter condition that is primarily responsible for the neurologic manifestations of severe hyponatremia, since low plasma tonicity induces the movement of water into cells, including brain cells, and water intoxication.[2]

Despite a wide array of potential conditions that may underlie hypotonic hyponatremia in surgical patients, the usual causes are (1) extrarenal losses such as vomiting, diarrhea, and third-space extravasation, producing ECF volume depletion, (2) the more subtle but perhaps more common condition of modest volume expansion due to free water retention, or (3) volume expansion and sodium retention due to an edematous disorder, such as congestive heart failure, or portal cirrhosis. Distinguishing between these conditions is important since the treatment, volume repletion in

Table 4.20 Emergency Treatment of Hyperkalemia

Method/Agent	Dose	Onset of Effect
1. Antagonism of membrane actions of potassium		
A. Calcium	10 mL of calcium gluconate infused IV over 2–3 minutes with EKG monitoring. Can repeat after 5 minutes if EKG changes of hyperkalemia persist.	Within 5 minutes
B. Hypertonic saline (if hyponatremic)	As needed to increase serum sodium.	
2. Increased potassium entry into cells		
A. Glucose and insulin	IV administration of 10 units of regular insulin and 50 g glucose. Also may use continuous infusions of glucose and insulin: 500 mL 10% glucose with 10 units of regular insulin.	Within 30 minutes
B. Sodium bicarbonate	1 ampule (44.6 mEq) of 7.5% $NaHCO_3$ infused IV over 5 minutes. May repeat in 30 minutes.	Within 30–60 minutes
C. B$_2$-adreneric agonists	Albuterol, 10–20 mg by nebulizer or 0.5 mg IV	Within 30 minutes
D. Hypertonic saline (if hyponatremic)		
3. Removal of the excess potassium		
A. Cation-exchange resin (Kayexalate)	20 mg Kayexalate orally with 100 mL of 2% sorbitol solution; or retention enema containing 50 g Kayexalate, 50 mL of 70% Sorbitol, and 100–150 mL tap water. Can repeat orally every 4–6 hour. Can repeat enema every 2–4 hour.	Variable

Modified after Reference 2, pp 913–918.

the first and volume restriction, sometimes with concomitant loop diuretics, in the latter two, are diametrically opposed.

In volume-depleted patients, hyponatremia ("hypotonic dehydration") usually reflects partial volume repletion due to oral water consumption induced by the thirst mechanism or, among hospitalized patients, parenteral infusion of hypotonic solutions. These patients have a low concentration of urinary sodium (<10 mEq/L). Treatment consists of volume and sodium repletion.

In contrast to these volume-depleted surgical patients with a deficit in total body sodium, hyponatremia may be observed in postoperative or trauma patients as a result of excessive free water retention due to increased ADH secretion. Increased ADH secretion unrelated to the usual stimuli of hyperosmolality or hypovolemia is

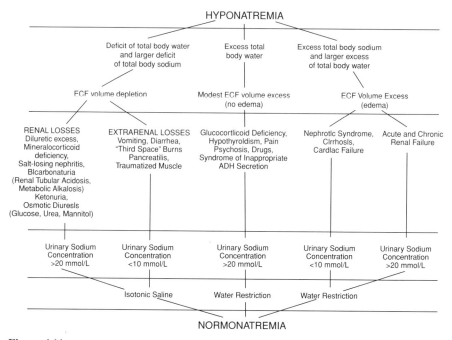

Figure 4.11 Analysis and management of hyponatremia. (From Reference 115, p 117.)

commonly observed for 2–5 days after major surgery.[2] The ADH response appears to be mediated by pain afferents that directly stimulate the hypothalamus. The hyponatremia observed under these circumstances may be aggravated by infusion of hypotonic solutions. These patients have high urinary sodium values (>20 mEq/L). The hyponatremia generally responds to fluid restriction.

Certain drugs have also been associated with free water retention and antidiuresis, presumably by increasing ADH activity, just as seen in postoperative patients. Of particular interest for oncologists is the association of hyponatremia with the antineoplastic agents vincristine, vinblastine, and cyclophosphamide. It is particularly important to anticipate potential acute hyponatremia in patients receiving intravenous cyclophosphamide because these patients are often vigorously hydrated to avert urologic complications, such as hemorrhagic cystitis.[2] Hyponatremia due to free water retention has also been observed in patients with a wide array of tumors, including cancer of the lung, duodenum, pancreas, ureter, bladder, prostate; thymoma; lymphoma; and Ewing's sarcoma. The mechanism is thought to be tumor production of ectopic ADH.

Finally, oxytocin, a hormone synthesized in the hypothalamus and released from the neurohypophysis, as is ADH, also has significant antidiuretic activity. Infusion of oxytocin in dextrose and water, to stimulate labor in pregnant women, has resulted in water retention, severe hyponatremia, and seizures in both mother and fetus. These complications can be avoided by restricting water consumption and preparing the hormone infusion in isotonic saline rather than in dextrose and water.[2]

When severe clinical manifestations of hypotonic hyponatremia supervene, urgent therapy with hypertonic saline is required to raise ECF tonicity and thereby ameliorate cerebral edema, the major underlying pathology. The morbidity and mortality of this condition are influenced by several factors: (1) the severity and rate of development of the hyponatremia, (2) the age and gender of the patient, and (3) the nature and magnitude of the underlying disease. The very young, the very elderly, women, and alcoholics appear to be at particular risk. Neurologic symptoms usually do not occur until body tonicity falls below 250 mOsm/kg, corresponding to a serum sodium concentration of 125 mEq/L. At this level of hypotonicity, anorexia, nausea, and malaise may develop. At sodium levels of 110–120 mEq/L, headache, lethargy, confusion, agitation, and obtundation can be seen. Seizures and coma may occur when serum sodium falls below 110 mEq/L.[25]

Symptomatic hypotonic hyponatremia that develops acutely, within several days, should be treated aggressively with 3%–5% hypertonic saline infused at a rate necessary to increase serum sodium concentration about 1–2 mEq/L/hour, until a sodium level of 120–125 mEq/L is reached. Chronic hypotonicity that develops over many days or weeks is more safely treated by increasing serum sodium levels no more than 0.5 mEq/L/hour.[25] In patients at risk of developing pulmonary edema due to volume overload (such as those with congestive heart failure), loop diuretics are administered to achieve negative fluid balance and 3% saline is infused concomitantly to replace urinary sodium losses while the fluid status is closely followed. In addition, careful monitoring during hypertonic saline infusion is mandatory because, despite the dangers of severe hyponatremia and hypotonicity, overly rapid correction may also be harmful, leading to central pontine myelinolysis, a severe neurologic disorder.[2]

To estimate the amount of sodium required to increase the serum concentration to a safe level of 125 mEq/L, the deficit per liter is multiplied by the TBW.[2] The latter is approximately 60% of body weight. Thus, the sodium required for a 70-kg patient with serum sodium of 110 mEq/L can be calculated as follows:

$$\text{Sodium required} = (125 - 110)(70 \times 0.6)$$
$$= 15 \times 42$$
$$= 630 \text{ mEq}$$

Pseudohyponatremia

Isotonic hyponatremia is an artifactual reduction of plasma sodium concentration due to paraproteinemia or hypertriglyceridemia. These substances do not contribute to osmolality but do produce an increase in plasma volume (but not plasma water). *Hypertonic hyponatremia* is associated with hyperglycemia or the administration of hypertonic substances, such as mannitol, which induce water movement out of the cells across a transcellular osmotic gradient. The initial effect is a dilutional hyponatremia. Later, when significant osmotic diuresis ensues, hypernatremia will develop.

Analysis and Management of Hypernatremia

Hypernatremia, defined as a serum sodium concentration greater than 145 mEq/L, may be due to a variety of causes (Fig. 4.12), but, regardless of etiology, it always implies coexistent hypertonicity of all body fluids and intracellular volume contraction.[25] This condition may arise from a pure water deficit so that the total body sodium remains normal. ECF contraction occurs, but clinical hypovolemia is unusual because the loss is significantly compensated by a shift of water from the intracellular space to the ECF compartment. Among cancer patients, this mechanism of hypernatremia is observed primarily in those with *secondary neurogenic diabetes insipidus* due to suprasellar and intrasellar tumors, primary or metastatic, or in those with *nephrogenic diabetes insipidus* due to hypokalemia or hypercalcemia (the major electrolyte abnormalities associated with a defect in renal concentrating capacity) or due to various drugs such as the antineoplastic agents vinblastine, ifosfamide, and cisplatinum, certain antibiotics such as amphotericin, gentamicin, and methicillin, or even angiographic dye.[2, 24] Finally, essentially pure water deficits are also observed when insensible losses from the skin are increased by fever or exercise and in patients with a tracheostomy who are breathing unhumidified air.

Hypernatremia may also be caused by loss of sodium and water but with a relatively greater loss of water. Here, total body sodium falls and symptomatic hypovolemia may supervene. Profuse sweating due to exercise or evaporative loss from burns may result in hypernatremia by this mechanism, but in oncologic patients, the more common causes are gastrointestinal losses of hypotonic secretions, such as nasogastric tube drainage, vomitus, or diarrhea; and osmotic diuresis due to mannitol, hyperglycemia, or, occasionally, urea.

Glucosuria, which develops when serum glucose levels reach 180–200 mg/dL, induces an osmotic diuresis resulting in an obligatory excretion of large volumes of salt-poor urine so that free water loss greatly exceeds sodium loss. As discussed previously, the initial increase in serum tonicity due to hyperglycemia will result in dilutional hyponatremia as intracellular water moves into the extracellular compartment. However, as osmotic diuresis continues, volume depletion and hypernatremia supervene. Sustained hyperglycemia with massive osmotic diuresis will eventually produce neurologic manifestations such as confusion, disorientation, lethargy, and finally hyperosmolar coma. Treatment is aimed toward reducing blood sugar and volume repletion with 0.45% sodium chloride solution. Potassium supplements may be required as resuscitation proceeds.

Intake of high protein, hyperosmolar enteral or parenteral feeding solutions may induce a urea diuresis resulting in azotemia, hypernatremia, and low ECF volume. These effects, especially common in those patients unable to drink or communicate thirst, can be averted when feedings provide at least 7 mL of free water per gram of dietary protein.[3, 26]

The magnitude of free water deficit when hypernatremia occurs with negligible or minimal sodium loss can be estimated by assuming that the total body osmoles

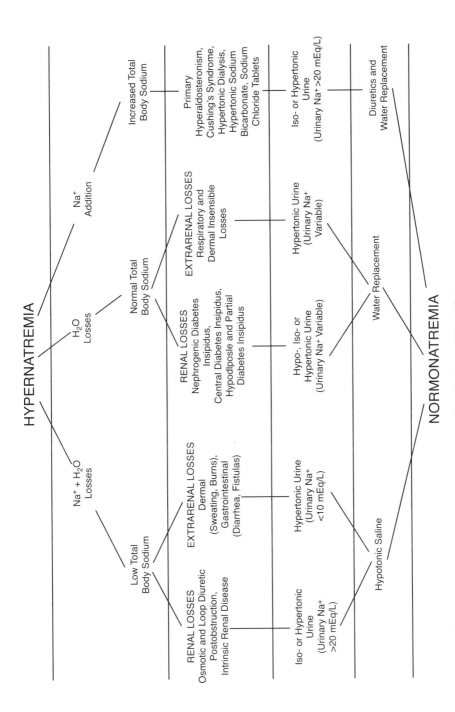

Figure 4.12 Analysis and management of hypernatremia. (From Reference 115, p 117.)

105

remain unchanged.[2, 24] For example, in a 60-kg patient with a serum sodium of 160 mEq/L, the water deficit can be estimated as follows:

1. Normal total body water (TBW) = $(60 \times 60\%) = 36$ L

2. Total body osmoles = TBW $\times$ P_{osm}

    Since the P_{osm} is primarily determined by the plasma Na^+ concentration and its accompanying anions,

    Total body osmoles $\cong$ TBW $\times$ 2$[Na^+]$

3. $\qquad\qquad \cong 36L \times 280$

    $\qquad\qquad \cong 10080$ mOsm

4. Current total body water $\cong \dfrac{10080}{2 \times 160} = 31.5$ L

5. Water deficit $\cong 36 - 31.5 \cong 4.5$ L

The water deficit is corrected with an infusion of 5% dextrose provided over at least 48 hours. Rapid replacement of large water deficits carries the risk of acute cerebral edema. In general, no more than half the estimated deficit should be replaced during the first 24 hours.[24, 25]

Management of Metabolic Acidosis

The causes of metabolic acidosis have been outlined previously (Table 4.10). In surgical patients, the common causes are gastrointestinal bicarbonate loss and lactate accumulation due to impaired tissue perfusion.

Significant gastrointestinal bicarbonate loss, which may be due to diarrhea (including that associated with most colonic villous adenomas) or pancreatic or biliary drainage or fistulas, produces a hypokalemic, hyperchloremic metabolic acidosis with a normal anion gap. Treatment is directed at reducing or eliminating the underlying problem and restoring volume with electrolyte solutions containing bicarbonate or bicarbonate-yielding anions, such as lactate. Potassium supplements are required since correction of the acidosis tends to decrease the plasma potassium concentration. Ongoing losses should be replaced with lactated Ringer's solution; saline infusions are inappropriate since they will aggravate the acid–base abnormality.

Lactic acidosis, with an increased anion gap, is usually the result of hypoxia due to inadequate tissue perfusion and circulatory failure. The primary therapeutic approach is to reverse shock and restore hemodynamic stability. Volume resuscitation alone may be sufficient to correct the acidosis in hemorrhagic shock. Use of vasopressors to treat hypotension in the face of volume depletion may worsen the acidosis.

The acute treatment of metabolic acidosis associated with an increased anion gap with intravenous sodium bicarbonate may be deleterious, especially in conditions associated with impaired tissue perfusion. Paradoxical intracellular acidosis and hypertonicity have been observed.[24, 25]

Bicarbonate therapy is indicated for severe degrees of acidosis, when pH falls below 7.2, especially after cardiac arrest, when partial correction of pH may be essential to preserve or restore myocardial function. The goal is to increase pH to 7.2 to 7.3 by administering one or two ampoules of bicarbonate (44.5–50 mEq/ampoule) initially and basing the need for additional bicarbonate on serial blood gas analyses.[9]

Management of Metabolic Alkalosis

Vomiting or nasogastric suction, especially in the face of gastric outlet obstruction, is the common setting for the development of metabolic alkalosis in surgical patients. Hypokalemia and hypochloremia accompany the alkalosis. In addition, a small subset of patients with colonic villous adenomas produce an acidic hyperchloremic diarrhea resulting in alkalosis.

Until the underlying problem is corrected, reversal of the metabolic abnormality requires volume repletion with sodium chloride; potassium replacement is also a key feature of therapy. In the absence of sufficient supplemental potassium, paradoxic aciduria will develop and alkalosis will persist.

Management of Ascites

Portal hypertension due to liver disease (such as alcoholic cirrhosis) or due to postsinusoidal obstruction (as an acute right-sided heart failure and Budd-Chiari syndrome) produces an increase in capillary hydrostatic pressure that may result in the transudation of fluid from the intravascular to the extravascular department and then into the peritoneal cavity from the surfaces of the liver, bowel, and mesentery, and hence the formation of ascites. Factors that promote the development of ascites in portal hypertension include hypoalbuminemia and a resultant reduction in plasma colloid osmotic pressure, renal sodium retention, and water retention. The pathogenesis of the sodium and water retention observed in cirrhosis is not firmly established but vasodilatation, which results in reduced ECV and, therefore, resultant activation of the renin-angiotensin system with increased aldosterone secretion, appears to be a major determinant.[24, 27]

First-line treatment of patients with cirrhosis and ascites consists of sodium restriction (2000 mg/day) and diuretic therapy with spironolactone and furosemide. Fluid restriction is no longer recommended unless serum sodium is less than 120–15 mEq/L. An initial therapeutic paracentesis is indicated in patients with tense ascites. Options for patients refractory to this standard medical regimen include (1) serial therapeutic paracenteses, (2) liver transplantation, (3) transjugular intrahepatic portasystemic shunt (TIPS), and (4) peritoneovenous shunt.[27, 28]

In cancer patients with ascites, the pathogenesis of the fluid accumulation in about one-third of patients is associated with portal hypertension or lymphatic obstruction, as in cases of massive liver metastases or lymphoma, respectively. Here the ascitic fluid is often cytologically negative for malignant cells and the ascites responds to the same treatment found effective in cirrhotic patients. In the remaining patients, the fluid is cytologically positive. It appears that the intraperitoneal tumor secretes a substance, probably vascular endothelial growth factor (VEGF), responsible for the increased capillary permeability that leads to decreased capillary oncotic pressure, increased net capillary filtration, and ultimately the accumulation of ascitic fluid, the reabsorption of which is inhibited by tumor-produced lymphatic obstruction. In the absence of a component of portal hypertension, malignant ascitic fluid elaborated from tumor-involved peritoneal surfaces generally has been regarded as resistant to diuretic therapy and to sodium and fluid restriction.[29] Pockros et al.[30] studied nine patients with ascites associated with peritoneal carcinomatosis. The patients received a diet providing 44 mEq sodium per day. Spironolactone, alone or in combination with furosemide, was given in increasing doses until a desired weight loss of 0.5 kg/day was achieved. Pretreatment renin and aldosterone levels were normal. No significant decrease in the volume of ascites was observed. Seven of the nine patients, however, had a decrease in plasma volume, producing symptomatic hypotension in one patient and renal dysfunction in two. The authors concluded that diuretics should not be used to treat malignant ascites.

Repeated paracenteses may provide symptomatic relief. A percutaneously placed intraperitoneal catheter may allow intermittent drainage by the patient or caregiver in an outpatient setting. Other palliative options include peritoneovenous shunting and intraperitoneal chemotherapy.[29]

PARENTERAL AND ENTERAL NUTRITION

The crystalloid and colloid preparations discussed above are effective in maintaining or restoring fluid and electrolyte homeostasis indefinitely, and when they are supplied in 5% glucose solution, the energy requirements of the glycolytic tissues, primarily the brain, are met. However, such solutions do not provide the energy and protein sources necessary for metabolic processes, growth or homeostasis, tissue repair, maintenance of body temperature, immunologic responses, or physical activity. In fasting patients, energy requirements can be met temporarily from endogenous calorie stores, but protein requirements cannot, because there are no protein reserves; each molecule of protein serves a specific nonfuel function, either as an enzyme or as a contractile protein.[26]

Potential endogenous energy sources for fasting patients include glycogen, protein, and fat. Glycogen stores are limited and totally dissipated within the first 1–3 days of fasting. Body protein represents a large potential energy source, but protein catabolism to provide energy (gluconeogenesis) is associated with some functional or structural loss. Fat is the main fuel reserve, and the length of survival during starvation correlates with the quantity of fat stores present at the onset of the fast. In the initial stages of starvation, adipose triglycerides provide about 85% of energy requirements, but as starvation proceeds, protein catabolism in both the skeletal and visceral compartments increases, with increasing compromise of body function as protein–fuel conversion continues. As lipid stores are depleted protein catabolism will effect even the essential proteins of the heart, lungs, blood cells, other vital tissues, and the immune system.[26]

Among patients requiring surgical therapy, the presence of nutritional deficits is of clinical importance because a substantial body of information attests to a strong association between the existence of such deficits and the occurrence of postoperative morbidity and mortality.[31] In 1936, Studley[32] observed a 10-fold increase in postoperative mortality among patients with intractable peptic ulcer disease who had sustained a preoperative weight loss of 20% or more. In 1944, Cannon and associates[33] reported the etiologic relationship between protein malnutrition, immune deficiencies, and an increased incidence of infection in experimental animals. In 1955, Rhoads and Alexander[34] demonstrated an association between postoperative infections and poor nutritional status and depressed serum albumin levels in patients. More recent observations also indicate a correlation between parameters that are influenced by nutritional status and postoperative morbidity and mortality. Thus, Mullen and associates[35] found that serum albumin levels < 3 g/dL and transferrin levels <220 mg/dL are associated with a significant increase in the incidence of postoperative complications. Similar adverse effects are observed when patients exhibit impaired reactivity to a panel of standard skin test antigens. A nearly eightfold increase in postoperative mortality and a fourfold increase in postoperative sepsis were reported by Pietsch and associates[36] among surgical patients who failed to react to any of five antigens before undergoing operation. Furthermore, when sequential skin testing indicates an improvement in immune reactivity, a reduced incidence of complications is observed.

Smale and associates[37] used a "prognostic nutritional index" (PNI) to quantify the probability that various deficits in putative nutritional indices will have an adverse effect on postoperative outcome. The PNI* is a computer-generated regression equation designed to predict the risk of postoperative complications which takes into account the serum albumin and transferrin concentrations, triceps skinfold thickness, and delayed hypersensitivity skin test reactivity. A group of 159 cancer patients scheduled for elective curative or palliative surgery were categorized according to their PNI values. Those deemed at high risk for the development of complications because of malnutrition (defined as PNI $\geq$ 40%) actually experienced a 5.7-fold increase in postoperative morbidity. Twenty-nine percent of high risk patients died; there was no mortality among the low risk group (PNI < 40%).

The influence of serum albumin concentration and body weight on the postoperative course of patients with operable colorectal cancer was studied by Hickman and associates.[38] Morbidity and mortality rates were significantly higher in patients with low albumin levels or low body weight. When both abnormalities were present, the complication rate exceeded 70% and the mortality rate was 42%.

Generally, crystalloid solutions containing 5% glucose are appropriate to maintain fluid and electrolyte homeostasis in fasting, well-nourished patients when

---

*PNI (%) = 158 − 16.6(ALB) − 0.78(TSF) − 0.20(TFN) − 5.8(DH), where ALB is the serum albumin concentration (g/dl); TSF is the triceps skinfold thickness (mm); TFN is the serum transferrin level (mg/dl); and DH is the delayed hypersensitivity skin test reactivity to any one of three recall antigens (mumps, *Candida*, streptokinase-streptodornase) graded 0 (nonreactive), 1 (<5 mm induration), or 2 ($\geq$5 mm induration).

resumption of normal oral diet is anticipated in 5–10 days. Providing approximately 400 kcal as glucose will meet the energy requirements of the glycolytic tissues thereby limiting gluconeogenesis and achieving maximal protein sparing until lipid stores are depleted. On the other hand, special nutritional support, enteral or parenteral feedings, is indicated for the following groups of patients:

1. Initially well-nourished patients unable to resume oral diets after 5–10 days of fasting.

2. Initially well-nourished patients with clinical conditions known to preclude oral diets for 5–10 days (e.g., acute hemorrhagic pancreatitis, short-bowel syndrome, mid-gut fistulas).

3. Initially malnourished patients unable to meet calorie and protein requirements with oral diets.

Patients unable to meet nutritional requirements by normal or enriched oral diets may receive enteral (tube) feedings or total parenteral nutrition using preparations formulated to replete deficits and provide all required nutrients.

Essential Components of Nutrient Preparations

The essential ingredients of enteral and parenteral preparations designed to meet all known nutritional requirements include nonprotein calories, utilizable nitrogen for protein synthesis, minerals, essential fatty acids, trace elements, and vitamins. Meeting the therapeutic goal of homeostasis (nitrogen equilibrium) or growth or nutritional repletion (positive nitrogen balance) depends on a variety of factors, most important among which are the levels of energy and nitrogen consumption.[39] At any given level of protein or nitrogen intake, nitrogen balance progressively improves to some maximum level as caloric intake increases from levels below requirements to levels exceeding requirements.[40] Maximum protein sparing and optimal utilization of dietary protein is achieved when the energy sources include at least 100–150 g of carbohydrate daily. As previously discussed, the requirement for this minimum amount of carbohydrate is based on its unique ability to satisfy the energy requirements of glycolytic tissues, including the central nervous system, erythrocytes, leukocytes, active fibroblasts, and certain phagocytes. The remaining energy requirements of most individuals can be met equally effectively by carbohydrate, fat, or a combination of these two.

At any given level of energy intake, nitrogen balance improves as nitrogen consumption increases. This dose–response relationship is curvilinear and the nitrogen balance plateaus at higher dosages of nitrogen intake.[40] To avoid the limiting effects of calories on nitrogen or of nitrogen on calories, nutrient solutions are prepared so that the nitrogen content bears a fixed relationship to the nonprotein calories provided. In studies of normal, active young men fed orally, optimal efficiency was achieved at a calorie:nitrogen ratio of approximately 300–350 kcal to 1 g of nitrogen.[40, 41] However, protein economy decreases during most serious illnesses, and nitrogen losses increase; therefore, dietary protein requirements rise. Nitrogen equilibrium or retention can usually be achieved, however, by approximately doubling the quantity of nitrogen required by a normal man at any given level of caloric intake. Thus, a calorie:nitrogen ratio of 150:1 is thought optimal for seriously ill patients, although the ratio actually may range between 100:1 and 200:1.[40]

Minerals required in amounts exceeding 200 mg per day include sodium, potassium, calcium, magnesium, chloride, and phosphate. These macronutrients are essential for the maintenance of water balance, cardiac function, mineralization of the skeleton, function of nerve, muscle, and enzyme systems, and energy transformation. In addition, protein utilization is affected by the availability of sodium, potassium, and phosphorus in the diet; nitrogen accretion is impaired when any of these mineral nutrients is withdrawn. Nutritional repletion evidently involves the formation of tissue units containing protoplasm and ECF in fixed proportion and with fixed elemental composition.[42] Thus, the retention of 1 g of nitrogen is characteristically associated with the retention of fixed amounts of phosphorus, potassium, sodium, and chloride.

Linoleic acid is the primary essential fatty acid for humans, and consequently it must be provided in order to avoid chemical and clinical evidence of deficiency. Linoleic acid requirements are generally met when a fat emulsion is used to provide at least 4% of calories as linoleic acid.[26]

Micronutrients, or trace elements, presently recognized as essential for humans include iron, iodine, cobalt, zinc, copper chromium, manganese, and possibly selenium. Cobalt is supplied as vitamin B_{12}, and iron is generally withheld because of poor marrow utilization in critical or chronic illness. The remaining trace elements are routinely supplied in the nutrient solution.

Finally, all the water soluble and fat soluble vitamins are also provided. Vitamin K may be withheld or dosage modified on an individual basis depending on the prothrombin time and any clinical indication for anticoagulation.[43,44]

Estimating Nutrient Requirements

The calorie requirement is usually estimated from simple formulas that are adjusted for activity and stress (Tables 4.21–4.23). Protein requirements can likewise be estimated from balance studies measuring nitrogen losses in various illnesses (Fig. 4.13). It appears that the requirements for essential amino acids and protein

Table 4.21 Caloric Requirements: Estimation of Resting Metabolic Expenditure (RME) from Harris-Benedict Equations (HBE)[a]

For men	RME (kcal/day) = 66.4730 + 13.7516 (W) + 5.0033 (H) − 6.7550 (A)
For women	RME (kcal/day) = 65.5095 + 9.563 (W) + 1.8496 (H) − 4.6756 (A)

W = body weight in kilograms; H = height in centimeters; A = age in years.
[a]Predicts RME for *normal* men and women. Correction factors must be applied for sick persons (see Table 4.22).
From Reference 26, p 91.

Table 4.22   Correction Factors for Estimating Caloric
Requirements of Hospitalized Patients from Harris-Benedict
Equations[a]

Clinical Condition	Correction Factor[b]
Nutritional status	
Normal	1.3[c]
Depleted	1.5[c,d]
Fever	1.0 + 0.13 per C
Elective surgery	1.0–1.2
Peritonitis	1.2–1.5
Soft tissue trauma	1.14–1.37
Multiple fractures	1.2–1.35
Major sepsis	1.4–1.8
Major head injury (with steroids)	1.4–2.0
Major head injury (without steroids)	1.4
Thermal injury[e]	
0%–20%	1.0–1.5
20%–40%	1.5–1.85
40%–100%	1.85–2.05
Starvation (adults)	0.70

[a]Total nonprotein energy requirement is estimated from the product of
correction factors × HBE.
[b]Correction factors apply to men and women. Figures represent maximal
increases and must be adjusted as recovery and convalescence proceed.
[c]Provides allowance for minimal activity above resting.
[d]Estimates additional requirement to achieve anabolism when accompanied
by optimal protein intake.
[e]Percent body surface burned.
Adapted form Reference 26, p 94.

for malnourished or hospitalized patients approximate those of a normally growing
10- to 12-year-old child (Table 4.24). Hence, a protein intake of 1.0–1.5 g/kg of
ideal body weight comprised of at least 25% essential amino acids has been recommended.[26, 45] Requirements for trace elements and vitamins are outlined in Tables 4.25
and 4.26.

Table 4.23   Caloric Requirements: Empiric Method

Clinical Status	Ideal Body Weight (kcal/kg)
Basal state	25–30
Maintenance (ambulatory)	30–35
Mild stress and malnutrition	40
Severe injuries and sepsis	50–60
Extensive burns	80

From Reference 26, p 95.

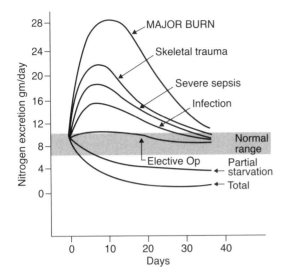

Figure 4.13   Catabolic response to serious illness. The increased nitrogen excretion and, therefore, nitrogen requirement for homeostasis depend on the magnitude of the insult. (From Reference 116.)

Formulating Nutrient Preparations

The specific nutrient requirements for a given individual depend on the initial nutritional and metabolic status of the patient and his or her underlying disease process.

Table 4.24   Essential Amino Acids and Total Protein Requirements for Normal Persons

	Adults		Boys 10–12 years	
Amino Acid	mg/kg	%TPR[a]	mg/kg	%TPR[a]
Histidine[b]	(12)	(1.6)	(19)	(1.9)
Isoleucine	10	1.3	28	2.8
Leucine	14	1.9	44	4.4
Lysine	12	1.6	44	4.4
Methionine + cystine	13	1.7	22	2.2
Phenylalanine + tyrosine	14	1.9	22	2.2
Threonine	7	0.9	28	2.8
Tryptophan	3.5	0.5	3.3	0.3
Valine	10	1.3	25	2.5
Total EAA[c] without histidine	83.5	11.1	216.3	21.8
Total EEA[c] including histidine	95.5	12.7	235.3	23.8
Total protein requirement[d] (g/kg)	0.75		1.0	

[a] %TPR, proportion of total protein requirement (high quality protein) supplied as given amino acid.
[a] Estimated requirement for histidine, which apparently is essential for adults and children as well as infants.
[a] EAA, essential amino acids.
[a] The level of intake of high quality protein that will meet the needs of nearly all normal persons.
Based on data from *Energy and Protein Requirements*, World Health Organization, 1985.
From Reference 26, p 99.

Table 4.25   Trace Element Requirements[a]

Chromium	10–15 mcg
Copper	0.3–0.5 mg
Iodine	1–2 mcg/kg
Manganese	60–100 mcg
Zinc	2.5–5.0 mg
Selenium	20–60 mcg

[a]Daily intravenous maintenance allowances for adults with normal initial values.
Modified after References 120 and 39.

Although the precise requirements for each nutrient can be determined by metabolic balance studies and direct or indirect calorimetry, such techniques are generally not employed in routine clinical practice. Instead, on the basis of data from clinical investigations applying such balance studies to patients with various diseases, injuries, and degrees of stress, requirements can be accurately estimated as presented above in Tables 4.21–4.26. As a result of these estimates, it is possible to formulate basic nutrient solutions of essentially fixed composition that can be used to meet the needs of most patients by varying only the volume of the basic formulation and by making appropriate adjustments in electrolyte administration. As discussed above, in clinical practice the caloric requirement is usually estimated from simple formulas which are adjusted for activity and stress. Although nitrogen requirements can likewise be determined or estimated, nitrogen needs are usually met as a consequence of the fixed calorie:nitrogen ratio, 100:1 to 200:1, of the nutrient solution. Thus, as the volume of solution prescribed is increased to meet increased caloric demands, the additional nitrogen requirements, which generally parallel the rising caloric needs, are likewise

Table 4.26   Vitamin Requirements[a]

Thiamine (B_1)	6 mg
Riboflavin (B_2)	3.6 mg
Niacin (B_3)	40 mg
Folic acid	600 mcg
Pantothenic acid (B_5)	15 mg
Pyridoxine (B_6)	6 mg
Cyanocobalamin (B_{12})	5 mcg
Biotin	60 mcg
Ascorbic acid (C)	200 mg
Vitamin A	3300 IU
Vitamin D	200 IU
Vitamin E	10 IU
Vitamin K	150 mcg

[a]Daily intravenous allowances for adults.
Based on Food and Drug Administration requirements. Reference 121.

met. Although such standard preparations can be used to satisfy the needs of most individuals, fluid-restricted patients, severely hypermetabolic patients, or those with renal or hepatic failure may require special nutrient formulations.

Enteral Nutrition (Tube Feedings)

The feasibility of enteral nutrition depends on the presence of sufficient functioning small bowel to allow the absorption of provided nutrients. Among patients meeting this criterion, suitable candidates include those in whom oral consumption is inadequate or contraindicated. Anorexia, weakness, lethargy, nausea, or oral inflammation are examples of factors contributing to poor oral intake. In addition, patients with diseases associated with markedly increased nutritional requirements, such as major burns, trauma, and sepsis, may be unable to eat enough to meet demands but often can be successfully nourished with the continuous administration of high calorie, high protein tube feedings. Patients in whom oral intake is contraindicated but who nevertheless may be candidates for enteral feeding include those who have certain neurologic disorders, including some patients following a cerebrovascular accident, and sometimes those who are comatose, stuporous, or extremely lethargic. Patients unable to eat because of oral, pharyngeal, esophageal, or proximal gastrointestinal conditions such as facial or jaw injuries, obstructing lesions, dysphagia, proximal enterocutaneous fistulas, or recent surgery, also may be candidates for tube feedings delivered distal to the lesion. In addition, enteral nutrition may be indicated for patients with certain gastrointestinal disorders, and who may benefit from an elemental diet, because such a diet is often unpalatable when taken orally.

Enteral feedings are contraindicated in patients at high risk for pulmonary aspiration and in patients with peritonitis, intestinal obstruction, paralytic ileus, gastrointestinal hemorrhage, or intractable vomiting or diarrhea. In addition, enteral feedings are likely to produce a salutary effect in the management of only the most proximal and distal intestinal fistulas. In the treatment of other fistulas, parenteral nutrition is preferred, since enteral feedings will usually increase fistulous output with concomitant fluid and electrolyte disturbances and skin breakdown. In addition, enteral feedings are not recommended in the presence of severe malabsorptive states or in the early stages of short bowel syndrome because the adequate absorption of nutrients is unlikely in these circumstances. Finally, enteral nutrition is contraindicated when a properly managed trial of such therapy fails to meet the nutritional goals, aggravates the underlying condition, or is associated with pulmonary aspiration or unmanageable diarrhea.[26]

Formulation of Enteral Feeding Products

A wide variety of liquid feeding preparations are presently available that differ in their content and source of protein, carbohydrate, and fat as well as in their osmolality, caloric density, sodium content, and residue.[26,46] Amino acids may be derived from intact protein in the form of pureed meat, eggs, or milk; from intact protein provided as semipurified isolates from milk, soybean, or eggs; from hydrolyzed protein with supplementary amino acids; or may be provided as purified free amino acids. Early formulations utilized glucose or sucrose as the carbohydrate source were high in osmolality. The current use of starches, dextrins, and glucose oligosaccharides reduces the number of active chemical components and hence the osmolality because the latter is a colligative property. The content of fat varies considerably among liquid feeding preparations; most contain long-chain fats, such as corn oil, soy oil, and safflower oil. However, some products contain medium chain triglycerides (MCTs), which are not dependent on pancreatic lipase or bile salts for digestion; they pass through the intestinal epithelium directly into the portal system as free fatty acids.

Commercially available, nutritionally complete formulations may be classified as follows:

A Polymeric formulas containing lactose with nitrogen supplied as intact protein.

B Polymeric formulas without lactose with nitrogen supplied as intact protein and/or protein isolates.

C Lactose-free diets with nitrogen supplied as hydrolyzed protein or amino acids ("peptide" or "elemental" formulas).

These formulations are designed to be nutritionally complete and, therefore, supply essential fatty acids and all the minerals, including trace elements, and vitamins (except vitamin K) necessary to meet the requirements of *normal* persons when sufficient volume is provided to meet caloric and protein requirements. Products contain vitamin K in variable amounts, and its presence must be considered in patients receiving oral anticoagulants. Supplements of essential fatty acids, minerals, and vitamins may be required by patients with malabsorption, marked gastrointestinal losses, increased demands associated with critical illness, or a preexisting deficiency state.

Preparations providing intact protein require effective digestive and absorptive processes for utilization and are therefore suitable only for patients with sufficient gastrointestinal function. In contrast, formulations providing utilizable nitrogen in the form of free amino acids or di- or tripeptides plus amino acids ("elemental" or "peptide" diets) may be suitable for patients with a variety of disorders of the small intestine or with severe insufficiency of the exocrine pancreas, because these preparations demand no digestive effort on the part of the handicapped alimentary tract and require only a minimal mucosal surface for absorption.

Formulations low in lactose are frequently indicated because of a high incidence of lactase deficiency in normal adults. In addition, bowel disease, fasting, starvation, protein depletion, and total parenteral nutrition have been associated with the development of temporary lactase deficiency.[47] Lactose consumption by affected patients may result in osmotic diarrhea, bloating, gas, and abdominal cramps.[48]

Long-chain triglycerides require pancreatic lipase, bile salts, and an adequate absorptive mucosal surface for satisfactory assimilation. Consequently, formulations containing long-chain triglycerides as a major energy source should be restricted in patients with severe exocrine pancreatic insufficiency, cholestatic jaundice, severe mucosal abnormalities, or short bowel syndrome.[49] In contrast, MCTs may be beneficial as they are well absorbed in such patients. When prescribed, MCTs should be introduced into the diet slowly to avoid nausea, vomiting, and diarrhea. In addition, because MCTs are ketogenic, administering these to diabetic, ketotic, or acidotic patients may be undesirable.[50–52] MCTs do not provide essential fatty acids.[52]

Site of Nutrient Delivery

Nutrients may be infused into the stomach, duodenum, or jejunum. *Intragastric feedings* have the advantage that the osmotic load reaches the duodenum in gradual fashion, limiting the incidence of the dumping syndrome. However, pulmonary aspiration is the major complication to be avoided, so that candidates for intragastric feedings must be alert with gag and cough reflexes intact, and gastric emptying should be normal. Suitable patients should have conditions that allow them to assume the semi-Fowler position (30° upright) for the duration of tube feeding therapy. Thus, intragastric feedings are contraindicated in comatose, stuporous, or lethargic patients, in severely debilitated or weak patients, in those with endotracheal or tracheostomy tubes, and in those with persistently high gastric residual volumes. Candidates for enteral nutrition who have a condition making intragastric feeding inadvisable can often be successfully managed by introducing nutrient solutions more distally.

   Duodenal feedings have the advantage that the pyloric sphincter is interposed between the nutrient solution and the tracheobronchial tree so that the incidence of aspiration is reduced although not eliminated. The disadvantage is that the symptoms of the dumping syndrome are more frequent.

   Jejunal feedings are generally not subject to regurgitation and therefore the risk of pulmonary aspiration is least associated with nutrients infused here. Jejunal feedings also enable patients with more proximal disease of the alimentary tract to receive enteral nutrition. In addition, the paralytic ileus associated with abdominal surgery affects primarily the stomach and colon; therefore, safe and effective enteral nutrition can sometimes be provided in the immediate postoperative period when the feedings are delivered directly into the jejunum. Finally, jejunostomy feedings induce less pancreatic stimulation than intragastric or intraduodenal diets and therefore may have a specific advantage in patients with inflammatory diseases of the pancreas. In contrast to these advantages of jejunal feedings, symptoms of the dumping syndrome associated with hyperosmolar nutrient solutions are more common with this method than with intragastric delivery.

Access to the Alimentary Tract

Enteral feedings are infused through tubes placed into the stomach, duodenum, or jejunum. Intubation can be achieved using nasal, percutaneous,[52–55] laparoscopic,[56–58] or open surgical methods. Intubation of the stomach, duodenum, or occasionally, the jejunum with a feeding tube of appropriate length passed through the nose is satisfactory for most hospitalized patients for whom the eventual resumption of oral feeding is anticipated. The correct position of the tube should be confirmed radiographically. When proper positioning is difficult, placement can be facilitated by direct endoscopic guidance. The discomfort of prolonged nasal intubation can be obviated by the creation of a tube cervical pharyngostomy in the occasional patient in whom percutaneous or laparoscopic placement may be technically difficult because of extensive intra-abdominal adhesions or carcinomatosis,[59, 60]

Prescribing Therapy

The specific nutrient formulation to be administered is chosen in relation to the patient's clinical status, the digestive and absorptive function of the small intestine, and the anatomic site selected for infusion. Additional considerations include the patient's caloric requirements and fluid and electrolyte status. The commercially available nutritionally complete products have a total caloric density, including both nonprotein and protein calories, varying between 1 and 2 kcal/mL. Fluid-restricted patients or those with high caloric requirements should receive a product with a high caloric density. Conversely, dehydrated patients or those with ongoing fluid losses require more fluid and therefore should receive more dilute formulations.

Expert opinions vary as to the optimal technique for initiating therapy. Patients commonly experience abdominal discomfort and diarrhea of varying severity during the initial phases of therapy. These symptoms have been attributed (without thorough study) to the rapid infusion of high osmolal solutions. Consequently, it has been customary to initiate enteral feedings with the continuous infusion of small volumes of diluted formula; others, however, recommend starting with full-strength formula. At the University of Southern California the volume of full-strength solution that will meet calorie and protein demands is determined. Then the enteral feeding formulation selected is diluted to one-third strength, placed in an enteral feeding container, and delivered continuously to the patient in the semi-Fowler position (30° upright). Infusion is begun at a rate of 50 mL/hour. Thereafter, the rate of administration is increased in increments of 25 mL/hour every 12 hours, so that by 24–36 hours, a rate that will provide the predetermined volume generally has been attained. As therapy proceeds, the patient is observed for manifestations of intolerance, such as abdominal cramps, diarrhea, glucosuria, and in the case of intragastric feedings, gastric retention. The presence of any of these findings early in the course of therapy is an indication to slow the rate of advancement to allow a longer period of adaptation. Until sufficient volume of solution is tolerated, supplemental intravenous fluid may be required to maintain water and electrolyte balance. After the dilute solution is administered for 24 hours at full volume with no manifestations of intolerance, the concentration of the nutrient is increased to two-thirds strength for 12–24 hours and finally to full strength without alteration in volume.

As previously discussed, hyperosmolar nutrient solutions may be associated with hypernatremic dehydration. Consequently, patients are allowed to freely consume clear liquids if feasible. In other patients, especially those unable to express thirst, free water should be given and can be provided with the tube feedings. Water is conveniently administered when the feeding bag is changed, usually every 8 hours.

Thus, 100–200 mL of water can be administered over 30 minutes every 8 hours through the feeding tube. This arrangement has the advantage that the tube is flushed after each container of liquid formula is administered, thus reducing the incidence of tube occlusion.

Continuous, around-the-clock delivery of liquid formula diets is generally preferred to intermittent, bolus feedings. Greater total daily volumes are tolerated with less gastric retention and fewer manifestations of gastrointestinal intolerance.[26]

Complications

Enteral nutrition is often prescribed without appropriate attention to technique or protocol because it is widely assumed that tube feedings are associated with few complications. In fact, complications are common, though often minor when promptly recognized and treated. The reported overall incidence of morbidity is quite variable, apparently reflecting the intensity of observation and care and the definition of terms. Cataldi-Betcher and associates[61] reported a complication rate of 11.7% among 253 patients studied, including an incidence of diarrhea (more than three liquid stools a day) of only 2.3%. In contrast, Heymsfield and associates[62] found that diarrhea occurred in up to 20% of patients. Silk and associates[49] reported that signs of gastrointestinal intolerance developed in 25% of their patients. Up to half of their patients developed metabolic abnormalities (hypokalemia, hypophosphatemia) and 40% had derangements of liver indices (alkaline phosphatase, transaminase) during the course of enteral nutrition.

Potential complications may be classified as mechanical, gastrointestinal, or metabolic and infectious (Table 4.27). Pulmonary aspiration of the feeding formula has emerged as the most common serious, potentially fatal complication of enteral nutrition.[26] Reported incidence is highly variable (0%–95%) depending on the population of patients studied and the definition of aspiration. Chemical evidence of aspiration is more common than clinically significant aspiration. Factors that increase the risk of this complication include mental obtundation, poor cough or gag reflexes, feeding in the supine position, impaired gastric emptying, an artificial airway, and gastroesophageal reflux. The latter may be induced or aggravated by feeding tubes, especially those of large diameter, traversing the gastroesophageal junction.

Total Parenteral Nutrition

Total parenteral nutrition (TPN) refers to a variety of methods by which all required nutrients can be provided intravenously independent of alimentary tract function. TPN is extremely effective, even life-saving, therapy for patients with medical conditions in which alimentary tract nutrition, either by mouth or by feeding tube, is inadequate or inadvisable.

The efficacy of TPN was established in a series of now-classic, modern-day animal experiments in which Rhoads, Dudrick, Wilmore, Vars, and their associates at the University of Pennsylvania demonstrated normal growth and development of

Table 4.27   Potential Complications During Enteral Nutrition

Mechanical	Gastrointestinal	Metabolic and Infectious
Depressed cough	Abdominal cramping	Congestive heart failure
Dysphagia	Abdominal distension	Disorder of calcium, magnesium, phosphorus
Esophageal erosions	Aggravation of primary disease	Essential fatty acid deficiency
Esophageal reflux	Diarrhea	Fluid and electrolyte disturbances
Esophagitis	Malabsorption	Hypercapnia and respiratory failure
Increased airway secretions	Nausea and vomiting	Hyperglycemia and hypoglycemia
Otitis media	Pneumatosis intestinalis	Hyperosmolar nonketotic coma
Nasopulmonary intubation		Hypoprothrombinemia
Parotitis		Inadvertent intraperitoneal infusion
Pharyngitis		Inadvertent intravenous infusion
Pneumothorax		Liver abnormalities
Pulmonary aspiration		Microbial growth in formula
Rhinitis		Prerenal azotemia
Tube dislodgement		Vitamin deficiencies
Tube obstruction		Warfarin resistance
		Zinc and copper deficiency

From Reference 26, p 147.

beagle puppies fed exclusively by vein after weaning.[63–65] The animals received a hypertonic infusate of glucose, protein hydrolysates, vitamins, and minerals through a central venous catheter. These investigators subsequently reported comparable results in humans: normal growth and development in children, nitrogen equilibrium in normal adults, and nutritional repletion in malnourished individuals.[63–65]

Formulating Nutrient Solutions

In current practice, nutrient solutions designed for parenteral administration are formulated to provide nonprotein calories as carbohydrate or a combination of carbohydrate and lipid. Glucose is the carbohydrate of choice since it is the normal physiologic substrate; it naturally occurs in blood; and it is abundant, inexpensive, and readily purified for intravenous administration. Glucose can be given in high concentrations and in large amounts that are well tolerated by most patients after a period of adaptation. Other carbohydrates such as fructose, sorbitol, xylitol, and maltose have been evaluated experimentally, but each has disadvantages that preclude clinical application at the present time. Glucose for parenteral infusion is commercially available in concentrations from 5% to 70% and is provided as glucose monohydrate with a caloric density of 3.4 kcal/g. Although isotonic (5%) solutions of glucose are available, concentrated glucose solutions are necessary in parenteral nutrition protocols in order to provide required calories in physiologic volumes of fluid.

Lipid is the alternative clinically useful nonprotein caloric source. Fat emulsions derived from soybean oil and safflower oil were approved for use in the United States in 1975 and 1979, respectively. The soybean oil emulsions had been used in Europe for nearly 20 years prior to their introduction in the United States. Currently employed fat emulsions are derived from soybean oil or are mixtures of soybean oil emulsion and safflower oil emulsion. The use of lipid emulsions in intravenous feeding regimens is attractive because of the high caloric density of fat (9 kcal/g) and because they are isotonic solutions that can, therefore, provide many calories in relatively small volumes via peripheral veins. Although early experience with lipids using the cottonseed oil emulsion Lipomul was unsatisfactory because of the toxicity of that preparation, fat emulsions derived from soybean oil and safflower oil have proven safe for clinical use. These newer preparations are purified plant oils emulsified in water. Egg phospholipids are added to regulate the size of the fat particles, stabilize the emulsion, and prevent fusion of the oil drops. Glycerol is added to make the emulsion isotonic, since oil and water emulsions have no osmolal effect. The resulting fat droplets have characteristics that are similar to those of naturally occurring chylomicrons found in the circulation after absorption of dietary lipid from the small intestine. Thus the particle size and the plasma elimination characteristics of these fat emulsions appear comparable to those of chylomicrons.[66, 67]

Studies of the elimination kinetics of soybean emulsion triglycerides indicate that at very low concentrations the rate of removal from the plasma is dependent on the triglyceride concentration. Above a certain critical concentration representing saturation of binding sites of lipoprotein–lipase enzymes, a maximum elimination capacity is reached that is independent of concentration. This maximum elimination capacity is influenced by the clinical state of the patient. It is increased during periods of starvation, after trauma, and in severely catabolic states.[67, 68] The infusion of fats is associated with an increase in heat production and oxygen consumption, a decrease in respiratory quotient, and the appearance of carbon 14 (^{14}C) in the expired air of patients receiving ^{14}C-labeled fat. These observations indicate that the infused fats are in fact used for energy. Soybean oil and soybean–safflower oil emulsions are available in 10%, 20%, and 30% concentrations and are mixtures of neutral triglycerides of predominantly unsaturated fatty acids. The major component fatty acids are linoleic, oleic, palmitic, and linolenic. The total caloric value of the 10% emulsions, including triglyceride, phospholipid, and glycerol, is 1.1 kcal/mL. The corresponding values for the 20% and 30% emulsions are 2 and 3 kcal/mL, respectively. In each of these preparations, approximately 0.1 kcal/mL of the total caloric value is derived from the added glycerol.

All nutrient solutions must provide at least 100–150 g of glucose per day to meet the needs of the glycolytic tissues, as described above. The proportional distribution of glucose and fat to provide the remaining required nonprotein calories apparently can be widely variable with the expectation of achieving the same nutritional goals. Commonly cited guidelines suggest that fat should not provide more than 30% of nonprotein calories and that the daily dosage of fat not exceed 2.5 g/kg in adults.[69] However, evidence-based reports indicate infusions providing over 80% of nonprotein calories as fat and daily dosages of as much a 12 g fat/kg/day have been tolerated with clinical benefit and no adverse effects.[70–72]

Consequently, protocols for solution preparation vary from institution to institution. Practical considerations in choosing the amount of glucose and the amount of fat relate primarily to the route of administration and to the fluid status of the patient. Parenteral nutrition solutions providing all nonprotein calories as glucose are highly concentrated and require central venous administration (see below). As an increasing proportion of the caloric content of the nutrient solution is provided by an isotonic fat emulsion, the content of glucose is thereby reduced, and, consequently, the concentration of the resultant solution falls. Nutrient solutions with an osmolarity not exceeding approximately three times normal serum levels can be successfully infused through peripheral veins;[73] more concentrated solutions must be infused centrally. Parenteral nutrition solutions are formulated in accordance with one of three commonly used protocols: the glucose-based system, the lipid-based system, and a three-in-one system of variable composition.

The nutrient solution prescribed for a 24-hour period usually is prepared in single container in a pharmacy under strict aseptic conditions. Manufacturing pharmacies responsible for preparing solutions for many patients often employ automated, computerized compounding apparatus, which is programmed to add the specified nutrient components to the infusion container.

THE GLUCOSE SYSTEM

This is the original carbohydrate-based system developed by Dudrick and his associates at the University of Pennsylvania.[64] The nutrient solution is prepared by the admixture of equal volumes of 50% glucose and 8.5% crystalline amino acids and the addition of appropriate electrolytes, vitamins, and trace elements (Table 4.28). One liter of such a solution provides 850 nonprotein kcal, and approximately 7 g of nitrogen, equivalent to 44 g protein. Consequently, the solution has a calorie:nitrogen ratio of about 120:1. The nitrogen content and the calorie: nitrogen ratio will vary slightly depending upon the brand of amino acid solution used. Because of the osmolar contribution of each of the constituents, this nutrient solution has a final concentration of approximately 2000 mOsm/L. Such a solution can never be safely infused through peripheral veins; consequently, the glucose system must be delivered into a central vein where the infusate is immediately diluted. Vascular access is usually through a percutaneously placed subclavian venous catheter or, for short-term use, a peripherally inserted central venous catheter ("PICC line"). Other routes (e.g., via jugular, saphenous, or femoral veins) are used occasionally with variable success. The incidence of morbidity associated with establishing and maintaining central venous access is influenced by the site and technique of insertion of the venous cannula and the diligence with which the apparatus is managed during the course of nutrition therapy.

Table 4.28   The Glucose System[a,b,c,d]

50% Glucose	500 mL
8.5% Amino acids	500 mL
Sodium (as acetate)	25 mEq
Sodium (as chloride)	5 mEq
Sodium (as phosphate)	14.8 mEq
Potassium (as chloride)	40 mEq
Phosphate (as sodium salt)	11.1 mM
Magnesium sulfate	8 mEq
Calcium gluconate	5 mEq

[a]Composition per liter.
[b]Provides 850 nonprotein kcal and 7.1 g nitrogen per liter.
[c]Trace elements and vitamins are provided daily (see Tables 4.25 and 4.26).
[d]Electrolyte additives based on Travasol as amino acid source.
From Reference 39, p 132.

Because of the high concentration of glucose in this form of parenteral nutrition, therapy should begin gradually to allow adaption and thereby avoid hyperglycemia. Generally, on the first day, a patient receives 1 L of nutrient solution, which is infused at a constant rate over the full 24-hour period. Blood and urine glucose levels are monitored frequently, and if this initial rate of infusion is well tolerated, the volume prescribed is increased from day-to-day until the volume infused meets the caloric requirement of the individual patient. For the average patient, the nutritional requirements as well as the requirements for fluid and electrolytes are usually met by 2.5 L/day of the nutrient solution, providing 2125 nonprotein kcal.

Infusion of the glucose system at a constant rate is a critical feature of safe practice since abrupt changes in the rate of delivery may be associated with marked fluctuations in blood sugar levels. The constant rate of infusion is most efficiently achieved by using an infusion pump. At the conclusion of therapy, the rate of infusion should be tapered gradually over several hours to avoid hypoglycemia. When infusion must be abruptly terminated, a solution of 10% glucose is substituted for the nutrient solution.

THE LIPID SYSTEM

The system of TPN based on glucose as the major caloric source is simple in concept and the least expensive, but patients' glucose metabolism must be closely monitored, and administration of the infusate requires technical expertise to achieve and maintain the central venous access necessary for safe treatment. The use of lipid emulsions as the major caloric source is attractive because of the high caloric density and isotonicity of these products. These considerations have logically led to the preparation of nutrient solutions based on fat as the major caloric source, with the goal of providing all required nutrients by peripheral vein. An example of such a lipid-based system

Table 4.29   The Lipid System[a,b,c,d,e]

10% Fat emulsion	500 mL
50% Glucose	100 mL
8.5% Amino acids	350 mL
Sodium (as acetate)	35 mEq
Sodium (as chloride)	5 mEq
Sodium (as phosphate)	6 mEq
Potassium (as chloride)	40 mEq
Phosphate (as sodium salt)[e]	4.5 mM
Magnesium sulfate	8 mEq
Calcium gluconate	5 mEq
Heparin sodium	1000 U
Distilled water	q.s.ad 1000 mL

[a]Composition per liter.
[b]Provides 720 nonprotein kcal and 5.0 g nitrogen per liter.
[c]Trace elements and vitamins are provided daily (see Tables 4.25 and 4.26).
[d]Electrolye additives are based on Travasol as amino acid source.
[e]Aproximately 7 mM additional phosphorus derived from fat emulsion.
From Reference 39, p 127.

of TPN is presented in Table 4.29.[73] This nutrient solution was devised with the aim of maximizing caloric and amino acid content without producing a solution with a concentration that would preclude safe peripheral venous administration. Each liter provides 720 nonprotein kcal and 5.0 g of nitrogen, equivalent to 31 g of protein. The calorie:nitrogen ratio is 144:1. The nitrogen content of the solution will vary slightly, depending upon the amino acid product used in its preparation. As with the glucose system, sufficient volume is given to meet measured or estimated caloric requirements. The safety and efficacy of nutrient solutions utilizing lipid as the major caloric source were established by Jeejeebhoy and associates[72] in their landmark investigation of lipid-based TPN in which 83% of nonprotein calories were supplied as fat. As many as 5 L daily of the lipid system described here have been infused for periods of weeks to months without apparent adverse effect.

THE THREE-IN-ONE SYSTEM

Innumerable nutrient solutions can be prepared with a distribution of glucose and lipid calories that differs from the two systems described above. Although there is no established biological advantage of differing proportions of fat and glucose as long as the minimum 100–150 g of carbohydrate are supplied, many clinicians prefer a profile of nutrients that mimics the optimal oral diet. Such a three-in-one system calls for the admixture of the three major nutrient components (amino acids, glucose, and lipids) such that carbohydrate provides approximately 65%–85% of nonprotein calories and lipid approximately 15%–35% (Table 4.30).[69, 74]

Table 4.30   A Three-in-One System[a,b,c,d]

50% Glucose	300 mL
10% Fat emulsion	300 mL
10% Amino acids	400 mL
Sodium (as acetate)	25 mEq
Sodium (as chloride)	5 mEq
Sodium (as phosphate)	14.8 mEq
Potassium (as chloride)	40 mEq
Phosphate (as sodium salt)	1.1 mM
Magnesium sulfate	8 mEq
Calcium gluconate	5 mEq

[a]Composition per liter.
[b]Provides 840 nonprotein kcal and 6.8 g nitrogen per liter.
[c]Trace elements and vitamins are provided daily (see Tables 4.25 and 4.26).
[d]Electrolyte additives based on Travasol as amino acid source.
From Reference 39, p 128.

However, altering the lipid system described here by increasing the glucose content would have certain nonnutritional effects. Thus, a solution with a higher proportion of glucose calories could be produced by replacing some of the fat emulsion with isotonic glucose. The concentration of the final solution would remain unchanged, but a much greater total volume would be required to provide the same number of calories. If the substitution were made with hypertonic glucose, as called for in the three-in-one system described in Table 4.30, the final concentration of the nutrient solution would be so increased as to require central venous administration, thereby losing the advantage of peripheral venous delivery.

COMPLICATIONS OF PARENTERAL NUTRITION

Morbidity associated with intravenous feedings may be related to drug toxicity, difficulties with vascular access, sepsis, or metabolic derangements.

Drug Toxicity

Adverse reactions to the components of parenteral nutrition solutions are uncommon. Although glucose is virtually nontoxic, the hypertonic solutions employed in the glucose system of TPN may be associated with potentially serious complications usually related to alterations in blood glucose levels. Currently used solutions of synthetic amino acids provide all of the nitrogen in the form of free L-amino acids and, in contrast to previously used protein hydrolysates, no potentially toxic ammonia or peptide products are present. Toxicity associated with the intravenous infusion of the currently available fat emulsions also has been minimal. The most frequent acute adverse reactions are fever, sensations of warmth, chills, shivering, chest or back pain, anorexia, and vomiting. Similarly, adverse reactions associated with chronic infusions of fat emulsions are also quite uncommon. Anemia and alterations in blood coagulation have been observed during treatment, but the etiologic relationship to lipid infusions has been unconfirmed. The most serious adverse effects have been observed in infants and children. The "fat overload" syndrome associated with the older cottonseed emulsion has rarely been observed with the newer current preparations. Nevertheless, several reports have been published[75] in which children receiving fat emulsions have developed marked hyperlipidemia, gastrointestinal disturbances, hepatosplenomegaly, impaired hepatic function, anemia, thrombocytopenia, prolonged clotting time, elevated prothrombin time, and spontaneous bleeding. These findings resolved when the fat emulsion was withdrawn.

Complications of Vascular Access

The lipid-based system of parenteral nutrition can be infused through the ordinary peripheral venous cannulae used for the administration of crystalloid solutions. Local phlebitis and inflammation from infiltration and cutaneous extravasation occur with about the same frequency as that associated with the infusion of nonnutrient solutions. In contrast, a central venous catheter is required for infusion of the highly concentrated glucose and three-in-one systems. Insertion and maintenance of such catheters may be associated with a variety of complications. Complications that may occur during the placement of the catheter include improper advancement of the catheter tip into one of the jugular veins or the contralateral innominate vein, instead of into the superior vena cava. In addition, air embolization or cardiac arrhythmias may occur. Percutaneous jugular or subclavian cannulation may rarely result in an injury to an adjacent anatomic structure, such as the brachial plexus, great vessels, or thoracic duct. Pneumothorax, usually resulting from inadvertent entrance into the pleural cavity, is probably the most common complication of attempted subclavian catheterization and has been reported to occur in about 2%–3% of attempts in large series. Late complications after successful central catheterization may include air embolism, catheter occlusion, central vein thrombophlebitis, and catheter-related sepsis.

Systemic Sepsis

Sepsis attributable primarily to the administration of parenteral nutrition should be an infrequent complication in modern practice. A variety of factors may contribute to the development of this complication. Hyperglycemia, which may be induced or aggravated by nutrient infusions, has been associated with sepsis in critically ill patients. In addition, patients requiring TPN are often inordinately susceptible to infection because of serious illness, malnutrition, and chronic debilitation—all conditions associated with impaired immune responses. Patients receiving immunosuppressive therapy, cytotoxic drugs, or corticosteroids are likewise susceptible to infection. These drugs as well as prolonged administration of broad-spectrum antibiotics may subject patients to sepsis from unusual, ordinarily saprophytic, microorganisms.

In addition to these patient-related factors, several specific TPN-related factors contribute to the pathogenesis of sepsis. The various components of the nutrient solution can become contaminated during manufacture or at the time of component admixture in the hospital pharmacy. The ability of the nutrient solution to support microbial growth is well established, but with present techniques of solution preparation sepsis from contamination should be rare. The vascular access apparatus appears to be the most common source of TPN-associated sepsis. Contamination may take place when the infusion catheter is inserted, when containers of the nutrient solution are changed, when intravenous tubing is replaced, when in-line filters are inserted, or when the intravenous cannula is used for measurement of central venous pressure, blood sampling, or the infusion of medication or blood products. In addition, to-and-fro motion of a subclavian catheter due to inadequate fixation will allow exposed portions of the catheter to enter the subcutaneous tract leading to the vein, which may result in infection. Hematogenous contamination of the infusion catheter may occasionally occur following bacteremia secondary to a distant focus of infection. More commonly, however, catheter-related sepsis is due to contamination of the catheter by organisms colonizing the skin surrounding the catheter insertion site. The incidence of sepsis varies greatly in reported series, but in recent years TPN has been administered with very low rates of infection. This improving trend is evidently due to adherence to rigid protocols of practice, and the employment in many hospitals of a dedicated, multidisciplinary team to manage the nutritional therapy. With this approach, TPN-related sepsis occurs in about 3% of patients receiving the glucose system. This complication is much less common among patients receiving the lipid-based system of parenteral nutrition through a peripheral vein.[26]

Metabolic Complications

A variety of metabolic derangements have been observed during the course of TPN. These derangements may reflect preexisting deficiencies, or they may develop during the course of parenteral nutrition as a result of an excess or deficiency of a specific component in the nutrient solution. As would be expected, the standard solutions may not contain the ideal combination of ingredients for a given individual. In fact, adverse effects from an excess or deficiency of nearly every component of nutrient solutions have been described. Consequently, patients must be carefully monitored so that the content of the nutritional solution can be adjusted during the course of therapy. For example, minor alterations in electrolyte content are often necessary.

Abnormalities of blood sugar are the most common metabolic complications observed in patients receiving TPN. Hyperglycemia may be associated with critical illness independent of nutrient infusions. However, patients receiving the glucose-rich glucose and the three-in-one systems are particularly susceptible to elevated blood sugar levels. In addition, hyperglycemia may manifest when the full caloric dosage of the glucose and three-in-one systems is inappropriately given initially and later if rates of infusion are abruptly increased. In addition, glucose intolerance may be a manifestation of overt or latent diabetes mellitus, or it may reflect reduced pancreatic insulin response to a glucose load—a situation commonly observed during starvation, stress, pain, major trauma, infection, and shock. Hyperglycemia also may be a reflection of the peripheral insulin resistance observed during sepsis, acute stress, or other conditions that are accompanied by high levels of circulating catecholamines and glucocorticoids. Decreased tissue sensitivity to insulin is also associated with hypophosphatemia, and hyperglycemia has been observed in patients with a deficiency of chromium. The latter trace metal probably acts as a cofactor for insulin. The incidence of hyperglycemia can be minimized by initiating therapy gradually with either of the two glucose-rich systems. Full dosage should be achieved over a 3-day period, during which time adaption to the glucose load takes place. In addition, careful metabolic monitoring during this period will disclose any tendency to hyperglycemia. Subsequently a constant rate of infusion is maintained. An inadvertent decrease in the rate of the infusion should not be compensated by abrupt increases in rate because such "catching up" is not allowed. When hyperglycemia supervenes despite these precautions, the etiology is sought. The common cause of hyperglycemia after a period of stability is emerging sepsis, the overt manifestations of which may not appear for 18–24 hour after development of elevated glucose levels.

Moderate hyperglycemia is controlled initially by subcutaneous or intravenous administration of insulin; the TPN infusion is continued at the usual rate. Subsequently, the appropriate amount of insulin is added to the TPN solution during its aseptic preparation in the pharmacy. Providing insulin in the TPN solution has the advantage that inadvertent alterations in the rate of glucose delivery are automatically accompanied by appropriate adjustments in the amount of insulin administered. Patients with hyperglycemia complicated by massive diuresis, dehydration, neurologic manifestations, or the syndrome of hyperosmolar nonketotic coma are managed by immediate termination of the TPN infusion, fluid resuscitation, and insulin administration.

In contrast to the problem of hyperglycemia, blood sugar levels decrease when the rate of infusion of the glucose system is abruptly reduced. Symptomatic hypoglycemia is most likely to occur when the reduction of the infusion rate had been preceded by an increased rate. When the glucose system is to be discontinued electively, the rate of delivery should be tapered gradually over several hours. Patients who are hemodynamically unstable or who are undergoing surgery should not receive TPN, since fluid resuscitation may be inadvertently carried out using the TPN solution. Therefore, the TPN infusion is discontinued abruptly in such patients and hypoglycemia is averted by infusing a solution of 10% glucose. Hypoglycemia may also reflect an excessive dosage of exogenous insulin. This most commonly occurs as a result of failure to recognize the resolution of peripheral insulin resistance and the associated decreased insulin requirement when the provoking condition responds to therapy.

Serum lipid profiles, which are routinely monitored during treatment with the lipid system, commonly reveal elevations of free fatty acids, cholesterol, and triglycerides However, adverse clinical effects are uncommon.[72, 76] Nevertheless, triglyceride levels exceeding 400 mg/dL should be avoided since hypertrigylceridemia of this magnitude may be associated with an increased risk of pancreatitis, immunosuppression, and altered pulmonary hemodynamics.[69]

Deficiencies of the major intracellular ions may occur in the catabolic state since the protein structure of cells is metabolized as an energy source, intracellular ions are lost, and the total body concentration of these ions, including potassium, magnesium, and phosphate, are decreased. Furthermore, during nutritional repletion, these ions, derived from the serum, are deposited or incorporated in newly synthesized cells. When supplementation of these ions in nutrient solutions is insufficient, hypokalemia, hypomagnesemia, and hypophosphatemia ensue. Serum levels of these substances should be measured regularly during TPN since such monitoring will disclose deficiencies before the clinical manifestations develop. Symptoms of hypokalemia are unusual when serum levels of potassium exceed 3.0 mEq/L. Asymptomatic hypokalemia can be managed by increasing the potassium supplement added to the nutrient solution at the time of preparation. When cardiac arrhythmias or other significant symptoms develop, the rate of TPN infusion should be tapered promptly while serum glucose levels are monitored closely and an intravenous infusion of potassium chloride is begun.

Intracellular consumption of inorganic phosphate during the synthesis of proteins, membrane phospholipids, DNA, and ATP may produce a striking deficit in the serum phosphate level after only several days of intravenous feedings devoid of or deficient in phosphate. Symptoms of hypophosphatemia may occur when serum phosphate levels fall to 2 mg/dL. However, severe manifestations are particularly apt to occur as levels fall below 1 mg/dL. These include acute respiratory failure, marked muscle weakness, impaired myocardial contractility, severe congestive cardiomyopathy, acute hemolytic anemia, coma, and death. Hypophosphatemic patients who are asymptomatic can be managed by increasing the phosphate supplement in the nutrient solution. Symptomatic patients or those with serum phosphate levels less than 1 mg/dL should be repleted intravenously through a separate infusion line. Parenteral nutrition should be stopped, and a 10% glucose solution should be infused to avert hypoglycemia. Since intracellular phosphate consumption depends on caloric intake, withdrawing TPN alone often results in an increased serum phosphate level within 24 hour.

A variety of adverse effects comprising the *refeeding syndrome* have been associated with the rapid induction of the anabolic state in severely malnourished, cachectic patients using standard nutrient solutions.[26, 77] Cardiac decompensation, the most serious feature of the syndrome, may be due to overhydration and salt retention in the face of starvation-induced low cardiac reserve. Hypophosphatemia, consequent to rapid refeeding, is another important contributing factor to cardiac failure. Rapid nutritional repletion also is implicated in producing deficits of the other major intracellular ions, magnesium and potassium, as well as acute deficiencies of vitamin A (associated with night blindness), thiamine (associated with the high output cardiac failure of beriberi, Wenicke's encephalopathy, and lactic acidosis), and zinc (associated with diarrhea, cerebellar dysfunction, dermatitis, impaired wound healing, and depressed immunity). Refeeding alkalosis also has been described. To avoid the refeeding syndrome in the chronically starved patient, parenteral nutrition should be introduced more gradually than usual, perhaps reaching the full caloric and protein requirements over the course of 5–7 days.[26]

Healthy or malnourished individuals who receive a constant parenteral infusion of a fat-free, but otherwise complete diet eventually develop clinical and biochemical manifestations that are completely reversed by the administration of linoleic acid. Thus, the syndrome of essential fatty acid deficiency in humans is due principally, if not exclusively, to a lack of linoleic acid. Exogenous linolenic acid is required by some species, but its essentiality for man is unproven. The most commonly recognized manifestation of linoleic acid deficiency is an eczematous desquamative dermatitis largely but not always confined to the body folds. Other clinical findings may include hepatic dysfunction, anemia, thrombocytopenia, hair loss, and possibly impaired wound healing. Growth retardation has been observed in infants. Fatty acid deficiency is treated by the administration of linoleic acid, usually by infusing one of the currently available fat emulsions. Patients receiving the glucose-based system of parenteral nutrition should be treated prophylactically by providing 4% of calories as linoleic acid. This requirement is usually met by infusing 1 L per week of a 10% fat emulsion.

Abnormalities in bone metabolism have been observed in patients receiving parenteral nutrition for prolonged periods, especially in home treatment programs. Such metabolic bone disease includes the common disorders of osteoporosis and osteomalacia and is characterized by hypercalciuria, intermittent hypercalcemia, reduced skeletal calcium, and low circulating parathormone levels. The clinical features have included intense periarticular and lower extremity pain. The pathogenesis of this syndrome is obscure, but hypotheses include an abnormality of vitamin D metabolism and aluminum toxicity.[78–80] Most recently, vitamin K deficiency has been considered an etiologic factor since it has been recognized that this condition increases the risk of osteoporosis and fractures and that these risks can be reduced with vitamin K therapy. Vitamin K also appears to be necessary for the synthesis of a diverse group of proteins involved in calcium homeostasis.[43,44,81,82] These findings have lead to the recent recommendation to routinely add vitamin K to TPN solutions, as discussed above.

NONNUTRITIONAL EFFECTS OF PARENTERAL NUTRITION

Effects on the Stomach

Gastric acid secretion is significantly increased during the initial period of treatment with the glucose system, but the duration of this effect is unknown. The acid secretory response observed is due primarily to the infusion of crystalline amino acids, and this effect of amino acids on gastric secretion is virtually abolished by the concurrent intravenous infusion of a fat emulsion. The effect of chronic TPN on gastric secretory function is less clear. Chronic parenteral nutrition in animals has been associated with decreased antral gastrin levels and atrophy of the parietal cell mass.

This observation is consistent with anecdotal clinical reports in which gastric hyposecretion has been observed in patients receiving long-term parenteral nutrition at home.[83]

Effects on the Intestinal Tract

Morphologic and functional changes occur in the small intestine and the colon when nutrition is maintained exclusively by vein. A significant reduction in the mass of the small and large intestine occurs, and there is a marked decrease in mucosal enzyme activity. Enzymes affected include maltase, sucrase, lactase, and peroxidase. These changes are not in response to intravenous nutrition per se but reflect the need for luminal nutrients for maintenance of normal intestinal mass and function. The mechanism by which food exerts a trophic effect is at least in part endocrine in that intraluminal contents stimulate the release of enterotrophic hormones such as gastrin.[26, 84, 85]

Effects on the Pancreas

Similar morphologic and functional atrophy of the pancreas is observed during the course of parenteral nutrition. In contrast to the effect of fat consumed orally, intravenous lipids do not stimulate pancreatic secretion.[26, 86]

Effects on the Liver

Transient derangements of liver function indices occur in the majority of patients receiving parenteral nutrition regardless of the proportion of glucose and lipid.[87, 88] Similar abnormalities also have been observed in patients receiving enteral nutrition (tube feedings).[49, 89] The etiology of these changes is uncertain and probably multifactorial. One hypothesis is that glucose and protein infusions in amounts exceeding requirements may contribute to these changes. In addition, an infectious etiology, perhaps related to the underlying condition requiring nutritional support, has been suggested, since oral metronidazole has been reported to reverse the changes in some patients. Administration of ursodesoxycholic acid also has been associated with improvement of TPN-related cholestasis,[90] In any case, the clinical course associated with the liver changes is nearly always benign so that TPN need not be discontinued. Nevertheless, patients receiving TPN for several years or more are at greater risk for developing severe or chronic liver disease, but again the etiologic relationship is unclear.[87]

Effects on the Respiratory System

Fuel oxidation is associated with oxygen consumption and carbon dioxide production. Oxygenation and carbon dioxide elimination are normal pulmonary functions.

Consequently, patients with respiratory failure receiving aggressive nutritional support may not be able to meet these demands of fuel metabolism. It is particularly important to avoid infusing calories in amounts exceeding requirements since this aggravates the problem, increases tidal volume, respiratory rate, and Pco_2, and offers no nutritional benefit.[91]

INDICATIONS FOR PARENTERAL NUTRITION

Although the clinical benefits derived from nutritional substrates infused intravenously appear equivalent to those derived from substrates absorbed from the alimentary tract, feeding through the alimentary tract is preferable when feasible because this route of administration is less expensive, less invasive, and, most importantly, is associated with a significantly lower incidence of infectious complications.[92] Nevertheless, many hospitalized patients have conditions in which alimentary tract nutrition either by mouth or tube feeding is inadequate, inadvisable, or would require an operative procedure (e.g., gastrostomy or jejunostomy) to establish access. It is for these patients that parenteral feeding should be considered. Normally nourished patients unable to eat for as long as 7–10 days generally do not require parenteral nutrition. The protein-sparing effect of 100–150 g of glucose provided in a 5% solution is sufficient. Patients in this category include those undergoing gastrointestinal surgery in whom only several days of ileus are anticipated postoperatively. However, if the resumption of adequate intake is not imminent after 7–10 days, parenteral feedings are recommended. In contrast, normally nourished patients should receive TPN promptly when initial evaluation discloses gastrointestinal dysfunction that is expected to persist beyond 7–10 days. In addition, malnourished or markedly hypercatabolic patients (e.g., those with severe burns, sepsis, or multiple trauma) with gastrointestinal dysfunction are given parenteral nutrition immediately.

In some patients, parenteral feedings have benefits in addition to improved nutrition. When all nutrients are provided intravenously, a state of bowel rest can be achieved in which the mechanical and secretory activity of the alimentary tract declines to basal levels (supra vide). These nonnutritional effects may be beneficial in the management of gastrointestinal fistulas and acute inflammatory diseases such as pancreatitis and regional enteritis. Parenteral nutrition may also be useful as a "medical colostomy." Thus, the reduction or elimination of the fecal stream associated with intravenous feedings may benefit patients with inflammation or decubitis ulcers adjacent to the anus or an intestinal stoma or fistula.

Any preexisting acute metabolic derangement should be treated before parenteral nutrition is begun. In addition, TPN should not be used during periods of acute hemodynamic instability or during surgical operations since the nutrient solution may be used inadvertently for fluid resuscitation. Parenteral nutrition is not indicated for patients with malnutrition due to a rapidly progressive disease that is not amenable to curative or palliative therapy.

COMPARING METHODS OF TPN

Factors to be considered in comparing the glucose system, the lipid system, and the three-in-one system of parenteral nutrition include the composition and nutrient value of the three systems, the relative efficacy of glucose and lipid calories, and the ease and safety of administration.

Comparative Composition of Parenteral Nutrition Systems

As outlined in Table 4.31, the lipid system provides fewer calories and less nitrogen per unit volume than the glucose and three-in-one systems. Thus, greater volumes of the lipid system are required to provide an isocaloric and isonitrogenous regimen. On the other hand, the lower osmolarity of the lipid system permits safe peripheral venous administration of all required nutrients, whereas the higher concentration of the other two systems mandates central venous infusion.

Glucose versus Lipid as a Caloric Source

The relative impact of glucose and lipid calories on nitrogen retention or body composition has been the subject of extensive investigation often with disparate conclusions, depending on the subset of patients studied.[26] However, the preponderance of evidence supports the conclusion that the two caloric sources are of comparable value in their effect on nitrogen retention in normal persons or in chronically ill, malnourished patients. The major study supporting this conclusion is that of Jeejeebhoy and associates,[72] who observed that optimal nitrogen retention with the lipid system requires a period of about 4 days to establish equilibrium, after which nitrogen balance is positive to a comparable degree with both the glucose and lipid systems. More recent data now attest to the equivalent efficacy of lipid as a major caloric source in critically illness and sepsis.[93–95]

Table 4.31   Comparison of Parenteral Nutrition Systems

	Glucose System	Lipid System	Three-in-One System
Carbohydrate calories	850 kcal/L	220 kcal/L	540 kcal/L
Lipid calories	0 kcal/L	500 kcal/L	300 kcal/L
Caloric density	0.85 kcal/mL	0.72 kcal/mL	0.84 kcal/mL
Nitrogen provided	7.1 g/L	5.0 g/L	6.8 g/L
Protein equivalent	44 g/L	31 g/L	42.5 g/L
Calorie:nitrogen ratio	120:1	144:1	124:1
Concentration (approximate)	2000 mOsm/L	900 mOsm/L	1500 mOsm/L

From Reference 39, p 132.

Ease and Safety of Administration

The glucose and three-in-one systems require central venous administration. Percutaneously inserted central venous catheters must be placed by physicians and peripherallyinserted central venous catheters (PICC) by physicians or specially trained nurses under sterile conditions. Insertion and use of central catheters may be associated with certain complications discussed previously that are not seen with the peripherally administered lipid system.

The ordinary venous cannulae used for infusion of the lipid system can be easily inserted at the bedside and maintained by ward personnel. While a central venous catheter requires special care and attention to prevent catheter sepsis, best provided by a dedicated team, the cannulae used in the lipid system require the same simple care as those used in the peripheral venous administration of crystalloid solutions. The peripherally infused lipid system is rarely associated with systemic sepsis.[26, 73]

SELECTING THE TPN REGIMEN

For many patients, the nutritional requirements can be met equally well by any of the TPN systems discussed. The selection in these cases is often based on nonnutritional factors such as the experience of the physician, ease of administration, and anticipated duration of therapy. On the other hand, there are subsets of patients requiring intravenous nutritional support who have associated or concurrent medical conditions that influence the choice of treatment. '

Fluid Restriction

The lipid system described here has the lowest caloric and nitrogen content per unit volume of the three standard regimens (Table 4.31). Thus, a greater volume has to be infused to provide the same nutrients. Fluid restriction is facilitated, therefore, by prescribing the more concentrated glucose or three-in-one system. For patients who must be severely fluid restricted, these two systems may be modified by substituting 70% glucose and 10%–15% amino acids for the 50% and 8.5% preparations, respectively, in order to supply equivalent nutrient content in a smaller volume. The recently available 30% fat emulsion, providing 3 kcal/mL, may prove useful in designing additional TPN regimens for fluid-restricted patients.

Acute Myocardial Ischemia

In some studies, lipid infusions have been associated with elevated circulating free fatty acid levels. The effect of the latter on patients with acute myocardial ischemia is controversial, but there is evidence that arrhythmias may be precipitated and the area of ischemic damage may be extended in patients with acute myocardial infarctions.[96–98] In view of these data, the glucose system is recommended in this group of patients.

Glucose Intolerance

It appears that hyperglycemia due to stress or diabetes mellitus is more easily managed if less glucose is infused, as in the three-in-one and lipid systems.[99–101]

Hyperlipidemia

Lipid infusions are contraindicated in patients with conditions in which the metabolism of endogenous lipids is abnormal; therefore, the glucose system the glucose system is prescribed.

Pulmonary Disease

In patients with pulmonary insufficiency, it is particularly important that lipogenesis induced by excess glucose be avoided because it results in an increase in total CO_2 production, which may in turn lead to elevated P_{CO_2} values. In addition, significantly less CO_2 is produced during the metabolism of isocaloric amounts of lipid compared to glucose. Thus, increasing the proportion of lipid calories in the nutrient solution, as in the three-in-one and lipid systems, may facilitate the clinical management of patients with chronic pulmonary insufficiency and hypercarbia.[102–104] In contrast, impaired pulmonary function has been observed when patients with acute respiratory distress syndrome receive lipids infusions. The adverse effects reported include decreased P_{O_2} and compliance and increased pulmonary vascular resistance.[105]

HOME PARENTERAL NUTRITION

Methods of TPN have become sufficiently standardized and simplified that such care can now be safely and effectively provided at home on an ambulatory basis.[106, 107] Candidates for such home care include those in whom the acute underlying medical condition requiring initial hospitalization has resolved but who still require intravenous nutrition usually for a prolonged or indefinite period or even permanently. Patients with anorexia nervosa, Crohn's disease, short bowel syndrome, or severe hyperemesis gravidarum are among those who have been successfully managed with ambulatory TPN. Other candidates for home therapy include cancer patients with anorexia associated with chemotherapy or radiation therapy and patients with controlled enterocutaneous fistulas, radiation enteritis, or partial intestinal obstruction.

While the general principles of TPN outlined previously are applicable here, there are certain specific considerations in home care necessary to make this method safe, convenient, and practical. Home patients requiring prolonged treatment should receive their nutrient solution through a tunneled, cuffed, silicone rubber or polyurethane central venous catheter (Hickman-type catheter). Such catheters are of low thrombogenicity, and passing the cuffed catheter through a subcutaneous tunnel reduces the incidence of ascending infection. Central placement, usually through the subclavian vein or internal jugular vein, frees the patient's extremities from any apparatus. A PICC may provide satisfactory access for patients requiring treatment for short periods. Such patients may include those that may benefit from preoperative nutritional repletion or postoperative supplementation, or those patients with a condition expected resolve (e.g., postoperative ileus) or for which a trial of nonoperative management is indicated (e.g., partial small bowel obstruction).

While inpatient TPN is infused around the clock, home TPN is often infused in cyclic fashion, usually during sleeping hours, so that patients may be free of the infusion apparatus for part of the day. Patients must adapt to the more rapid hourly rates of infusion necessary to provide the required volume in a shorter period. Alterations of blood sugar, the commonest acute metabolic abnormalities, are best prevented by gradually increasing the rate of delivery over 1–2 hour at the beginning of therapy and tapering the rate over several hours at the conclusion of the daily treatment.

Finally, chronic TPN for months or years appears to be unmasking requirements for additional nutrients that are stored in significant quantities or that are required in minute amounts. For example, further investigation may indicate requirements for molybdenum, taurine, and probably other micronutrients.

COMPARISON OF ENTERAL AND PARENTERAL NUTRITION

The preponderance of data derived from controlled, prospective studies in humans indicates that the nitrogen economy is supported to the same extent when equivalent nutrients are provided intravenously or by continuous infusion into the alimentary tract.[26]

Nevertheless, when both enteral and parenteral feedings are feasible and safe, enteral feeding is the preferred method of nutrition support primarily because this method is associated with a reduced incidence of infectious morbidity, cost, and possibly length of hospital stay. However, no significant difference in mortality between the two routes of nutritional support has been observed.[108, 109]

Nutritional Support in Cancer Patients

Malnutrition is a frequent accompaniment of malignant disease, and when it occurs, prognosis is adversely affected.[26] Smale and associates[37] documented a significant increase in postoperative morbidity and mortality among those deemed at high risk because of malnutrition. DeWys and associates[110] analyzed the effect of weight loss on the survival of patients scheduled to receive chemotherapy for various lesions. For patients with nearly every tumor type, weight loss was associated with a statistically significant reduction in survival.

The malnutrition observed in cancer patients is related not only to the anorexia and metabolic derangements associated with the *cancer cachexia syndrome*[77,110,111] but also to the adverse nutritional consequences of the antineoplastic therapy prescribed, including paralytic ileus, nausea, vomiting, mucositis, and diarrhea. Although the effectiveness of nutritional support may be limited in patients with the cancer cachexia syndrome, recommendations have been made for the administration of parenteral or enteral nutrition primarily to treat or prevent malnutrition and its complications when effective antitumor therapy is available. Routine adjunctive nutrition therapy is not recommended because specific oncologic benefits have not been demonstrated. However, nutrition therapy has an indirect oncologic benefit in repleting patients with a degree of inanition so severe as to otherwise preclude administration of optimally aggressive antitumor therapy. In addition, adjunctive parenteral or enteral feedings may be indicated to prevent malnutrition in patients receiving a course of therapy known to produce anorexia or other significant side effects that would preclude normal oral intake. Such aggressive nutritional support usually is not indicated for patients for whom no effective antitumor therapy is available.

Parenteral Nutrition as an Adjunct to Surgery

Smale et al.[37] reported that 6 or more days of preoperative parenteral nuitrition was associated with a 2.1-fold reduction in all postoperative complications, a 2.9-fold reduction in major sepsis, and a 2.7-fold reduction in mortality among poorly nourished, high risk cancer patients. Current guidelines call for 7–14 days of preoperative nutritional support in patients with moderate or severe malnutrition.[111]

Parenteral Nutrition as an Adjunct to Chemotherapy

Adjunctive nutrition therapy is often advisable in severely depleted patients because nutritional repletion may enable such patients to receive aggressive chemotherapy that would otherwise be contraindicated because of fear of complications from malnutrition and inanition.[112] Unfortunately, however, randomized trials have failed to demonstrate a survival benefit or a diminution of chemotherapy-associated toxicity attributable to nutritional support therapy.[111]

Parenteral Nutrition as an Adjunct to Radiation Therapy

Malnutrition occurring in patients undergoing radiation therapy may be a result of the underlying malignant disease but may also be associated with or aggravated by the treatment itself. Thus, radiation therapy may be associated with loss of taste, anorexia, and dysphagia or nausea, vomiting, and diarrhea secondary to radiation enteritis. Some patients may obtain marked relief of symptoms when they receive nutrients intravenously and refrain from oral intake. In addition, adjunctive parenteral nutrition may be able to stabilize or improve body weight and reduce delays in initiating or carrying out a planned course of radiotherapy because of inanition. However, the major finding in prospective, randomized trials is that adjunctive TPN does not enhance the efficacy of radiotherapy. No improvement has been demonstrated in antitumor response or local control, in tolerance to treatment, or in the incidence of complications of therapy.[26, 113]

REFERENCES

1. HUMES HD, COX MCL. Principles of the renal regulation of fluids and electrolytes. In: KELLY WN, editor. Textbook of Internal Medicine. 3rd ed. Philadelphia, PA: Lippincott-Raven Company; 1997. p 49–55.
2. ROSE BD, POST TW. Clinical Physiology of Acid-Base and Electrolyte Disorders. 5th ed. New York: McGraw-Hill; 2001.
3. COGAN MG. Fluid and Electrolytes: Physiology and Pathophysiology. Norwalk, CT: Appleton and Lange; 1991.
4. GOODWIN CW Jr. Fluid and electrolyte balance and disorders of acid-base. In: LEVINE BA, COPELAND EM III, HOWARD RJ, SUGARMAN H, WARSHAW AL, editors. Current Practice of Surgery. New York: Churchill Livingstone; 1993. Part II, Chapter 6, p 1–27.
5. MOORE FD. Metabolic Care of the Surgical Patient. Philadelphia, PA: WB Saunders; 1959.
6. SHIRES GT, BARBER AE, ILLNER HP. Current status of resuscitation: solutions including hypertonic saline. Adv Surg 1995;28:133–170.
7. SHIRES GTIII. Fluid and electrolyte management of the surgical patient. In: BRUNICARDI FC, editor. Schwartz's Principles of Surgery. 9th ed. New York: McGraw-Hill; 2010.
8. BOYSEN PG, KIRBY RR. Acid-base problem solving. In: CIVETTA JM, TAYLORS RW, KIRBY RR, editors. Critical Care. Philadelphia, PA: JB Lippincott; 1988. p 335–339.
9. MORGAN G Jr, MIKHAIL MS, MURRAY MJ. Clinical Anesthesiology. 4th ed. New York: McGraw-Hill; 2006.
10. HAYES MA. Water and electrolyte therapy after operation. N Engl J Med 1968;278(19):1054–1056.
11. DELLINGER RP, LEVY MM, CARLET JM, et al. Surviving sepsis campaign: international guidelines for management of severe sepsis and septic shock: 2008. Crit Care Med 2008;36(1):296–327.
12. FINFER S, BELLOMO R, BOYCE N, et al. A comparison of albumin and saline for fluid resuscitation in the intensive care unit. N Engl J Med 2004;350(22):2247–2256.
13. PEREL P, ROBERTS I. Colloids versus crystalloids for fluid resuscitation in critically ill patients. Cochrane Database Syst Rev 2007; (4):CD000567.
14. RATNER LE, SMITH GW. Intraoperative fluid management. Surg Clin North Am 1993;73(2):229–241.
15. VELANOVICH V. Crystalloid versus colloid fluid resuscitation: a meta-analysis of mortality. Surgery 1989;105(1):65–71.
16. MYBURGH J, COOPER DJ, FINFER S, et al. Saline or albumin for fluid resuscitation in patients with traumatic brain injury. N Engl J Med 2007;357(9):874–884.
17. TYAGI R, DONALDSON K, LOFTUS CM, et al. Hypertonic saline: a clinical review. Neurosurg Rev 2007;30(4):277–289; discussion 289–290.
18. OLIVEIRA RP, VELASCO I, SORIANO F, et al. Clinical review: hypertonic saline resuscitation in sepsis. Crit Care 2002;6(5):418–423.
19. VINCENZI R, CEPEDA LA, PIRANI WM, et al. Small volume resuscitation with 3% hypertonic saline solution decrease inflammatory response and attenuates end organ damage after controlled hemorrhagic shock. Am J Surg 2009;198(3):407–414.
20. COOPER DJ, MYLES PS, MCDERMOTT FT, et al. Prehospital hypertonic saline resuscitation of patients with hypotension and severe traumatic brain injury: a randomized controlled trial. JAMA 2004;291(11):1350–1357.
21. PINTO FC, CAPONE-NETO A, PRIST R, et al. Volume replacement with lactated Ringer's or 3% hypertonic saline solution during combined experimental hemorrhagic shock and traumatic brain injury. J Trauma 2006;60(4):758–763; discussion 763–754.
22. BERRY RE. The "third kidney" phenomenon of the gastrointestinal tract. A complication of parenteral fluid therapy and intestinal trauma. Arch Surg 1960;81:193–204.
23. SILBERMAN H. Renal failure and the surgeon. Surg Gynecol Obstet 1977;144(5):775–784.

24. Schrier R. Renal and Electrolyte Disorders. 6th ed. Philadelphia, PA: Lippincott Williams & Wilkins; 2003.

25. Weisberg L, Szerlip H, Cox MCL. Approach to the patient with altered sodium and water homeostasis. In: Kelley W, editor. Textbook of Internal Medicine. 2nd ed. Philadelphia, PA: JB Lippincott; 1992. p 839–848.

26. Silberman H. Parenteral and Enteral Nutrition. 2nd ed. Norwalk, CT: Appleton & Lange; 1989.

27. Hou W, Sanyal AJ. Ascites: diagnosis and management. Med Clin North Am 2009;93(4):801–817, vii.

28. Runyon BA. Management of adult patients with ascites due to cirrhosis: an update. Hepatology 2009;49(6):2087–2107.

29. Kammula US. Malignant ascites. In: De Vita VT Jr, Lawrence TS, Rosenberg SA, editors. Cancer: Principles and Practice. 8th ed. Philadelphia, PA: Lippincott Williams & Wilkins; 2008. p 2533–2539.

30. Pockros PJ, Esrason KT, Nguyen C, et al. Mobilization of malignant ascites with diuretics is dependent on ascitic fluid characteristics. Gastroenterology 1992;103(4):1302–1306.

31. Silberman H. The role of preoperative parenteral nutrition in cancer patients. Cancer 1985;55(1 Suppl):254–257.

32. Studley HO. Percentage of weight loss: a basic indicator of surgical risk in patients with chronic peptic ulcer. JAMA 1936;106:458–460.

33. Cannon PR, Wissler RW, Woolridge RL, et al. The relationship of protein deficiency to surgical infection. Ann Surg 1944;120(4):514–525.

34. Rhoads JE, Alexander CE. Nutritional problems of surgical patients. Ann NY Acad Sci 1955;63(2):268–275.

35. Mullen JL, Gertner MH, Buzby GP, et al. Implications of malnutrition in the surgical patient. Arch Surg 1979;114(2):121–125.

36. Pietsch JB, Meakins JL, MacLean LD. The delayed hypersensitivity response: application in clinical surgery. Surgery 1977;82(3):349–355.

37. Smale BF, Mullen JL, Buzby GP, et al. The efficacy of nutritional assessment and support in cancer surgery. Cancer 1981;47(10):2375–2381.

38. Hickman DM, Miller RA, Rombeau JL, et al. Serum albumin and body weight as predictors of postoperative course in colorectal cancer. J Parenter Enteral Nutr 1980;4(3):314–316.

39. Silberman H. Nutrition, parenteral. In: Webster JG, editor. Encyclopedia of Medical Devices and Instrumentation. Vol. 5, 2nd ed. Hoboken, NJ: Wiley-Interscience; 2006. p 124–134.

40. Wilmore DW. Energy requirements for maximum nitrogen retention. In: Greene HL, Holliday MA, Munro HN, editors. Clinical Nutrition Update: Amino Acids. Chicago, IL: American Medical Association; 1977. p 47–57.

41. Calloway DH, Spector H. Nitrogen balance as related to caloric and protein intake in active young men. Am J Clin Nutr 1954;2(6):405–412.

42. Rudman D, Millikan WJ, Richardson TJ, et al. Elemental balances during intravenous hyperalimentation of underweight adult subjects. J Clin Invest 1975;55(1):94–104.

43. Bern M. Observations on possible effects of daily vitamin K replacement, especially upon warfarin therapy. J Parenter Enteral Nutr 2004;28(6):388–398.

44. Helphingstine CJ, Bistrian BR. New Food and Drug Administration requirements for inclusion of vitamin K in adult parenteral multivitamins. J Parenter Enteral Nutr 2003;27(3):220–224.

45. Ziegler TR. Parenteral nutrition in the critically ill patient. N Engl J Med 2009;361(11):1088–1097.

46. Chen Y, Peterson SJ. Enteral nutrition formulas: which formula is right for your adult patient? Nutr Clin Pract 2009;24(3):344–355.

47. Levine GM, Deren JJ, Steiger E, et al. Role of oral intake in maintenance of gut mass and disaccharide activity. Gastroenterology 1974;67(5):975–982.

48. Stephenson LS, Latham MC. Lactose intolerance and milk consumption: the relation of tolerance to symptoms. Am J Clin Nutr 1974;27(3):296–303.

49. Silk DBA. Nutritional Support in Hospital Practice. Oxford: Blackwell Scientific Publications; 1983.

50. BACH AC, BABAYAN VK. Medium-chain triglycerides: an update. Am J Clin Nutr 1982;36(5):950–962.

51. GORDON EE, DUGA J. Experimental hyperosmolar diabetic syndrome. Ketogenic response to medium-chain triglycerides. Diabetes 1975;24(3):301–306.

52. SUCHER K. Medium chain triglycerides: a review of their enteral use in clinical nutrition. Nutr Clin Pract 1986;1:146–150.

53. COPE C, DAVIS AG, BAUM RA, et al. Direct percutaneous jejunostomy: techniques and applications—ten years experience. Radiology 1998;209(3):747–754.

54. DAVIES RP, KEW J, WEST GP. Percutaneous jejunostomy using CT fluoroscopy. Am J Roentgenol 2001;176(3):808–810.

55. EVANS AL, UBEROI R. CT-guided jejunostomy tube insertion. Am J Roentgenol 2005;185(5):1369.

56. DUH QY, SENOKOZLIEFF-ENGLEHART AL, CHOE YS, et al. Laparoscopic gastrostomy and jejunostomy: safety and cost with local vs general anesthesia. Arch Surg 1999;134(2):151–156.

57. GRONDONA P, ANDREANI SM, BARR N, et al. Laparoscopic feeding jejunostomy technique as part of staging laparoscopy. Surg Laparosc Endosc Percutan Tech 2005;15(5):263–266.

58. HAN-GEURTS IJ, LIM A, STIJNEN T, BONJER HJ. Laparoscopic feeding jejunostomy: a systematic review. Surg Endosc 2005;19(7):951–957.

59. GRAHAM WP III, ROYSTER HP. Simplified cervical esophagostomy for long term extraoral feeding. Surg Gynecol Obstet 1967;125(1):127–128.

60. KENT MS, AWAIS O, SCHUCHERT MJ, et al. Cervical pharyngostomy: an old technique revisited. Ann Surg 2008;248(2):199–204.

61. CATALDI-BETCHER EL, SELTZER MH, SLOCUM BA, et al. Complications occurring during enteral nutrition support: a prospective study. J Parenter Enteral Nutr 1983;7(6):546–552.

62. HEYMSFIELD SB, ERBLAND M, CASPER K, et al. Enteral nutritional support. Metabolic, cardiovascular, and pulmonary interrelations. Clin Chest Med 1986;7(1):41–67.

63. DUDRICK SJ, RHOADS JE. New horizons for intravenous feeding. JAMA 1971;215(6):939–949.

64. DUDRICK SJ, WILMORE DW, VARS HM, et al. Long-term total parenteral nutrition with growth, development, and positive nitrogen balance. Surgery 1968;64(1):134–142.

65. WILMORE DW, DUDRICK SJ. Growth and development of an infant receiving all nutrients exclusively by vein. JAMA 1968;203(10):860–864.

66. HALLBERG D. Therapy with fat emulsion. Acta Anaesthesiol Scand Suppl 1974;55:131–136.

67. MCNIFF BL. Clinical use of 10% soybean oil emulsion. Am J Hosp Pharm 1977;34(10):1080–1086.

68. HALLBERG D. Studies on the elimination of exogenous lipids from the blood stream. The effect of fasting and surgical trauma in man on the elimination rate of a fat emulsion injected intravenously. Acta Physiol Scand 1965;65(1):153–163.

69. MIRTALLO J, CANADA T, JOHNSON D, et al. Safe practices for parenteral nutrition. J Parenter Enteral Nutr 2004;28(6):S39–S70.

70. BLANCHARD R, GILLESPIE D. Some comparisons between fat emulsion and glucose for parenteral nutrition in adults at the Winnipeg Health Sciences Center. In: MENG H, WILMORE D, editors. Fat Emulsions in Parenteral Nutrition. Chicago, IL: American Medical Association; 1976. p 63–64.

71. HADFIELD J. High calorie intravenous feeding in surgical patients. Clin Med 1966;73:25–30.

72. JEEJEEBHOY KN, ANDERSON GH, NAKHOODA AF, et al. Metabolic studies in total parenteral nutrition with lipid in man. Comparison with glucose. J Clin Invest 1976;57(1):125–136.

73. SILBERMAN H, FREEHAUF M, FONG G, et al. Parenteral nutrition with lipids. JAMA 1977;238(13):1380–1382.

74. MIRTALLO J. Parenteral formulas. In: ROMBEAU JL, ROLANDELLI RH, editors. Clinical Nutrition: Parenteral Nutrition. 3rd ed. Philadelphia, PA: WB Saunders; 2001:118–139.

75. HANSEN LM, HARDIE BS, HIDALGO J. Fat emulsion for intravenous administration: clinical experience with intralipid 10%. Ann Surg 1976;184(1):80–88.

76. EISENBERG D, SCHMIDT B, SILBERMAN H. Safety and efficacy of lipid-based TPN: I Effects of 20% fat emulsion on serum lipids and respiratory functions. J Parenter Enteral Nutr 1982;6:586.

77. RUSSELL MK, STEIGER E. Specialized nutritional support for cancer patients. In: SILBERMAN H, SILBERMAN AW, editors. Principles and Practice of Surgical Oncology: Multidisciplinary Approach to Difficult Problems. Philadelphia, PA: Lippincott Williams & Wilkins; 2010. p 51–58.

78. FUHRMAN MP. Complication management in parenteral nutrition. In: MATARESE LE, GOTTSCHLICH MM, editors. Contemporary Nutrition Support Practice: A Clinical Guide. 2nd ed. Philadelphia, PA: Saunders; 2003.

79. KLEIN GL, TARGOFF CM, AMENT ME, et al. Bone disease associated with total parenteral nutrition. Lancet 1980;2(8203):1041–1044.

80. SHIKE M, HARRISON JE, STURTRIDGE WC, et al. Metabolic bone disease in patients receiving long-term total parenteral nutrition. Ann Intern Med 1980;92(3):343–350.

81. BUCHMAN AL, MOUKARZEL A. Metabolic bone disease associated with total parenteral nutrition. Clin Nutr 2000;19(4):217–231.

82. HAMILTON C, SEIDNER DL. Metabolic bone disease and parenteral nutrition. Curr Gastroenterol Rep 2004;6(4):335–341.

83. KOTLER DP, LEVINE GM. Reversible gastric and pancreatic hyposecretion after long-term total parenteral nutrition. N Engl J Med 1979;300(5):241–242.

84. MAGNOTTI LJ, DEITCH EA. Mechanisms and significance of gut barrier function and failure. In: ROLANDELLI RH, BANKHEAD R, BOULLATA JI, COMPHER CW, editors. Clinical Nutrition: Enteral and Tube Feeding. 4th ed. Philadelphia, PA: Elsevier Saunders; 2005. p 23–31.

85. TILSON MD. Pathophysiology and treatment of short bowel syndrome. Surg Clin North Am 1980;60(5):1273–1284.

86. GRUNDFEST S, STEIGER E, SELINKOFF P, et al. The effect of intravenous fat emulsions in patients with pancreatic fistula. J Parenter Enteral Nutr 1980;4(1):27–31.

87. SHATTUCK KE, KLEIN GL. Hepatobiliary complications of parenteral nutrition. In: ROMBEAU JL, ROLANDELLI RH, editors. Clinical Nutrition: Parenteral Nutrition. 3rd ed. Philadelphia, PA: WB Saunders; 2001. p 140–156.

88. WAGNER WH, LOWRY AC, SILBERMAN H. Similar liver function abnormalities occur in patients receiving glucose-based and lipid-based parenteral nutrition. Am J Gastroenterol 1983;78(4):199–202.

89. KWAN V, GEORGE J. Liver disease due to parenteral and enteral nutrition. Clin Liver Dis 2004;8(4):893–913, ix–x.

90. KRAWINKEL MB. Parenteral nutrition-associated cholestasis—what do we know, what can we do? Eur J Pediatr Surg 2004;14(4):230–234.

91. ASKANAZI J, ROSENBAUM SH, HYMAN AI, et al. Respiratory changes induced by the large glucose loads of total parenteral nutrition. JAMA 1980;243(14):1444–1447.

92. GRAMLICH L, KICHIAN K, PINILLA J, et al. Does enteral nutrition compared to parenteral nutrition result in better outcomes in critically ill adult patients? A systematic review of the literature. Nutrition 2004;20(10):843–848.

93. DE CHALAIN TM, MICHELL WL, O'KEEFE SJ, et al. The effect of fuel source on amino acid metabolism in critically ill patients. J Surg Res 1992;52(2):167–176.

94. DRUML W, FISCHER M, RATHEISER K. Use of intravenous lipids in critically ill patients with sepsis without and with hepatic failure. J Parenter Enteral Nutr 1998;22(4):217–223.

95. GARCIA-DE-LORENZO A, LOPEZ-MARTINEZ J, PLANAS M, et al. Safety and metabolic tolerance of a concentrated long-chain triglyceride lipid emulsion in critically ill septic and trauma patients. J Parenter Enteral Nutr 2003;27(3):208–215.

96. Editorial: free fatty acids and arrhythmias after acute myocardial infarction. Lancet 1975;1(7902):313–314.

97. JONES JW, TIBBS D, MCDONALD LK, et al. 10% Soybean oil emulsion as a myocardial energy substrate after ischemic arrest. Surg Forum 1977;28:284–285.

98. OPIE LH, TANSEY M, KENNELLY BM. Proposed metabolic vicious circle in patients with large myocardial infarcts and high plasma-free-fatty-acid concentrations. Lancet 1977;2(8044):890–892.

99. BAKER JP, DETSKY AS, STEWART S, et al. Randomized trial of total parenteral nutrition in critically ill patients: metabolic effects of varying glucose-lipid ratios as the energy source. Gastroenterology 1984;87(1):53–59.

100. MEGUID MM, SCHIMMEL E, JOHNSON WC, et al. Reduced metabolic complications in total parenteral nutrition: pilot study using fat to replace one-third of glucose calories. J Parenter Enteral Nutr 1982;6(4):304–307.

101. WATANABE Y, SATO M, ABE Y, et al. Fat emulsions as an ideal nonprotein energy source under surgical stress for diabetic patients. Nutrition 1995;11(6):734–738.

102. ASKANAZI J, NORDENSTROM J, ROSENBAUM SH, et al. Nutrition for the patient with respiratory failure: glucose vs. fat. Anesthesiology 1981;54(5):373–377.

103. SHERMAN SM. Parenteral nutrition and cardiopulmonary disease. In: ROMBEAU JL, ROLANDELLI RH, editors. Clinical Nutrition: Parenteral Nutrition. 3rd ed. Philadelphia, PA: WB Saunders; 2001. p 335–352.

104. SILBERMAN H, SILBERMAN AW. Parenteral nutrition, biochemistry and respiratory gas exchange. J Parenter Enteral Nutr 1986;10(2):151–154.

105. LEKKA ME, LIOKATIS S, NATHANAIL C, et al. The impact of intravenous fat emulsion administration in acute lung injury. Am J Respir Crit Care Med 2004;169(5):638–644.

106. STEIGER E. Consensus statements regarding optimal management of home parenteral nutrition (HPN) access. J Parenter Enteral Nutr 2006;30(1 suppl):S94–S95.

107. STEIGER E. JONATHAN E Rhoads lecture: experiences and observations in the management of patients with short bowel syndrome. J Parenter Enteral Nutr 2007;31(4):326–333.

108. LIPMAN TO. Grains or veins: is enteral nutrition really better than parenteral nutrition? A look at the evidence. J Parenter Enteral Nutr 1998;22(3):167–182.

109. MCCLAVE SA, MARTINDALE RG, VANEK VW, et al. Guidelines for the provision and assessment of nutrition support therapy in the adult critically ill patient: Society of Critical Care Medicine (SCCM) and American Society for Parenteral and Enteral Nutrition (ASPEN). J Parenter Enteral Nutr 2009;33(3):277–316.

110. DEWYS WD, BEGG C, LAVIN PT, et al. Prognostic effect of weight loss prior to chemotherapy in cancer patients. Eastern Cooperative Oncology Group. Am J Med 1980;69(4):491–497.

111. AUGUST DA, HUHMANN MB. ASPEN. clinical guidelines: nutrition support therapy during adult anticancer treatment and in hematopoietic cell transplantation. J Parenter Enteral Nutr 2009;33(5):472–500.

112. COPELAND EM III, MACFADYEN BV Jr, LANZOTTI VJ, et al. Intravenous hyperalimentation as an adjunct to cancer chemotherapy. Am J Surg 1975;129(2):167–173.

113. DONALDSON SS. Nutritional support as an adjunct to radiation therapy. J Parenter Enteral Nutr 1984;8(3):302–310.

114. OTT H. Calculation of the colloidal osmotic serum pressure from the protein spectrum, and the average molecular weight of serum protein fractions. Klin Wschr 1956;34:1079–1083.

115. BERL T, ANDERSON RJ, MCDONALD KM, et al. Clinical disorders of water metabolism. Kidney Int 1976;10:117–132.

116. LONG CL. Energy and protein needs in the critically ill patient. Contemp Surg 1980;16:29–42.

117. MULHOLLAND MW, LILLEMOE KD, DOHERTY GM, et al. (Editors). Greenfield's Surgery: Scientific Principles and Practice. 4th ed. Philadelphia, PA: Lippincott Williams and Wilkins; 2006. p 215.

118. GUYTON AC, HALL JE. Textbook of Medical Physiology. 11th ed. Philadelphia, PA: Elsevier Saunders; 2006.

119. DOHERTY GM (ed). Current Diagnosis and Treatment: Surgery. 13th ed. New York: McGraw-Hill, 2010.

120. SRIRAM KS, LONCHYNA VA. Micronutrient supplementation in adult nutrition therapy: practical considerations. J Parenter Enteral Nutr 2009;33:548–562.

121. Fed Regist 2000;65:21200–212010.

Part Two

Perioperative Management of Gynecologic Surgery

Chapter 5

Preoperative Evaluation

Devansu Tewari, MD

INTRODUCTION

Preoperative assessment is an integral part of preparation for surgery and should be considered as important as the surgery itself. Unfortunately, the importance of attention to details in such preoperative evaluation has been underestimated. Instead, a battery of tests and evaluations are routinely and reflexively ordered without careful regard for the patient's history, cost, or discomfort and potential morbidity. As a result, estimates of more than $30 billion a year in health-care costs in the United States have been attributed to preoperative testing.[1] Some estimates have suggested that up to 60% of these routine testing procedures could be eliminated without adversely affecting outcomes.[2–4]

Advances in medicine and preoperative risk assessment have made surgery safer than ever before, creating an opportunity to tailor these tests to the individual. Creating such an environment depends on a systematic history and physical examination for patients undergoing an operative procedure and proceeding with evidence-based approaches to the selection of appropriate medical tests and evaluations. In this manner the provider can determine which patients may have contraindications for surgery, to help anticipate possible adverse outcomes and to guide postoperative management. The focus of this chapter will be to provide an evidence-based approach to the necessary preoperative studies often included, such as tests in chemistries, coagulation, and imaging. These recommendations are to serve as guidelines and should not replace sound clinical judgment.

THE IMPACT OF ROUTINE TESTING

Surgical texts in gynecology have differed over the years in their recommendations on routine testing.[5,6] Generally, tests in regard to complete blood count (CBC), electrolytes, and urinalysis have been generally recommended without clear evidence

Gynecologic Oncology: Evidence-Based Perioperative and Supportive Care, Second Edition.
Edited by Scott E. Lentz, Allison E. Axtell and Steven A. Vasilev.
© 2011 John Wiley & Sons, Inc. Published 2011 by John Wiley & Sons, Inc.

of their benefit. This has been exemplified in two large studies, one retrospective and the other prospective in which routine preoperative laboratory evaluations, when done as routine without any specific clinical indications, are of little clinical value.

Kaplan et al. retrospectively reviewed preoperative laboratory tests done at a single teaching hospital at the University of California, San Francisco, to assess their necessity.[2] Routine preoperative laboratory tests including CBC, platelet count, differential, prothrombin time (PT), partial thromboplastin time (PTT), electrolytes, creatinine (Cr), and glucose were retrospectively reviewed for medical indication and whether an abnormal result altered surgical or anesthetic management. Of the 2785 laboratory tests that were reviewed, 60% were ordered without any apparent specific medical conditions being present and were therefore defined as "un-indicated." The hemoglobin level as part of a CBC was deemed indicated in this study if the planned surgery was "potentially bloody" (i.e., vaguely defined as a procedure requiring preoperative cross matching). Of these un-indicated tests there were only four (0.22%) abnormal laboratory tests that were judged to be of clinical significance in which the result may possibly have altered surgical or anesthetic management. However, on further review of medical records, no alteration in management induced by these laboratory results was noted. Furthermore, Kaplan estimated that in his hospital where approximately 8600 procedures are performed each year, not performing this un-indicated battery of preoperative laboratory tests would result in 1 death in 100 years. However, this retrospective study identified only abnormal laboratory tests that may have delayed or canceled surgery, or altered anesthetic management. It did not or was not able to identify laboratory tests that may possibly have affected postoperative management. Such a retrospective study may have limitations in identifying such potential consequences.

Similarly, in a prospective study of 520 general, vascular, head and neck, and thoracic surgery patients, univariate and multivariate analyses were used in assessing the ability of electrolytes, glucose, blood urea nitrogen (BUN), creatinine (Cr), CBC, total protein/albumin/lymphocyte count (nutritional studies), coagulation studies, and urinalysis in predicting postoperative complications.[7] Overall, routine preoperative laboratory tests studied were of no minimal clinical value in predicting meaningful clinical complications. Although not confirmed by multivariate analyses, univariate analyses did suggest correlation between abnormal nutritional tests (total protein/albumin/lymphocyte count) and postoperative death. This, however, should not be interpreted that such tests should be obtained preoperatively for all patients, as the incidence of death is low and there are usually clinical findings that suggest a severely malnourished state. Although this study addressed the likelihood that preoperative tests may predict postoperative complications, it did not determine whether the laboratory tests may have altered perioperative management in any other way.

Blery et al. proposed a protocol of selectively obtaining preoperative labs under certain guidelines and evaluated such a protocol prospectively at a teaching hospital in Paris, France.[8] Clinical indications suspected by history for ordering preoperative laboratory tests are as follows:

Type and screen for major surgical procedures

Hemoglobin for major surgical procedures

PT/PTT for malignancy, hepatobiliary and bleeding disorders, or use of anticoagulants

Electrolytes for age above 70, renal disorder, diabetes, use of diuretics, digitalis, or corticosteroids

BUN/Cr for age above 70, renal disorder, diabetes, or use of diuretics

Glucose for diabetes or use of corticosteroids

Chest X-ray for cardiovascular or pulmonary disorders

Electrocardiogram (EKG) for age above 40 and for cardiovascular or pulmonary disorders

This protocol was employed over one year in which 3866 patients were enrolled. Upon discharge or after an appropriate postoperative period had lapsed, anesthesiologists were asked to review the hospital course to determine whether any of the above evaluations not obtained would have been "potentially useful." No perioperative deaths were attributed to omission of an evaluation. Furthermore, only 0.2% of omitted laboratory tests were deemed to have been potentially useful upon review of the perioperative course. One serious postoperative complication occurred in a 23-year-old man who was noted to have a cardiac arrhythmia and pulmonary edema after an appendectomy. A postoperative EKG revealed Wolff–Parkinson–White syndrome. Additionally, the authors felt that omission of tests may have hampered diagnosis or therapy in 10 other cases. However, half of these scenarios could have been avoided if a thorough history and physical examination was done. The protocol presented above served as a guideline, and in 18% of the cases, deviations from the guideline were made because of individual preferences of the attending physicians. No modification to this protocol was made during this prospective study and the authors concluded that no perioperative deaths could be attributed to omission of any tests. Nevertheless, the size of this study prevents one from concluding whether omission of any tests may have significantly increased perioperative morbidity. The authors felt their protocol was acceptable, but warned that it be used only as a guideline, and should not replace good clinical judgment.

LABORATORY TESTS

Coagulation Studies

The lack of clinical value for routine preoperative coagulation studies, specifically PT and PTT, has been established. In a prospective study of 282 patients, 4% of coagulation studies performed was abnormal. However, none of these abnormalities identified a clinically significant coagulopathy that altered patient management.[9] In a retrospective study of 480 patients who had PT and PTT performed without specific indications, 2.7% of these patients had abnormal results.[10] Only one of these patients had a bleeding complication; this patient underwent a second operation to control arterial bleeding. It is unclear whether this complication can be truly ascribed to the abnormal PTT. Others have similarly found no benefit.[11, 12] A review of the literature of 29 studies involving hemostasis tests showed no study comparing the health outcomes of patients undergoing these tests with those who did not, and therefore no benefit in obtaining PT and PTT as part of routine preoperative screening when a history and physical examination did not suggest a possible coagulopathy can be recommended.[13]

Complete Blood Count

Almost all agree that the hemoglobin/hematocrit portion of a preoperative complete blood count (CBC) is prudent prior to a major surgery regardless of whether such a test could be predictive of a potential postoperative complication. The value of a CBC extends beyond the ability to predict postoperative complications, providing information for intraoperative planning. However, how one acts on a hemoglobin level preoperatively or perioperatively is debatable. Traditional perioperative management dictated red blood cell transfusion for a hemoglobin level of less than 10 g/dL.[14, 15] Modern practice suggests that most patients with a hemoglobin level of around 10 g/dL rarely need blood transfusions and that other conditions such as the presence of signs and symptoms of anemia, coronary vascular disease, and baseline hemoglobin level should be taken into consideration. Moreover, evidence suggests that perioperative morbidity is not adversely affected by mild to moderate anemia if the patient remained normovolemic.[16] Findings from a systematic review of the literature of 29 studies regarding CBC testing preoperatively found no study comparing the health outcomes of patients who underwent the testing with those who did not.[13] As a result, no direct evidence exists that such testing would or could not result in improved clinical outcomes. Another review of 23 studies found that routine preoperative hemoglobin levels lead to a change in management of patients in 0.1%–2.7% of patients.[17] Clearly, the risk of bleeding from the procedure employed or the patient's own inherent risk factors of bleeding have to be factored in. But from a clinical evidence point of view the level of evidence supporting routine use is not warranted.

Complete Compatibility Testing (ABO, Rh, Antibody Screen, and Crossmatch)

With regard to preoperative preparation for possible blood product use, it is important to note that hospitals must maintain an inventory based on the amount of blood crossmatched (i.e., reserved) rather than the amount used. Therefore, some basic strategies ought to be considered for optimal resource utilization.[18, 19] This should be based on the probability of significant bleeding, preoperative hemoglobin value, and the knowledge of how rapidly red cell blood products can generally become available.

Complete compatibility testing (ABO, Rh, antibody screen, and crossmatch) in the absence of unexpected red cell antibodies can generally be performed in 1 hour. If an antibody screen is positive, this process can take twice as long or longer. However, if a "type and screen" procedure is performed preoperatively, the ABO/Rh/antibody status is already known intraoperatively. Assuming no antibodies are isolated, in the event of unanticipated transfusion need, the blood can become available within 10–15 minutes.

If a "type and screen" is not ordered preoperatively, type specific or emergency crossmatched blood can also rapidly be available. However, antibody screening is not performed in this circumstance, increasing transfusion reaction risk. If preoperative antibody screening reveals the presence of complex antibodies, it may be prudent to crossmatch several units of blood even in those patients who are at relatively low risk for significant blood loss. Generally, presence of antibodies in the recipient is more dangerous than in the donor, as the antibodies are diluted within the recipient's circulation during transfusion in the latter situation, minimizing the reaction.

Preparation for autologous blood use deserves special comment. National trends reflect the perception that autologous blood is safer than allogeneic blood during transfusion. Between 1989 and 1992 the overall transfusion rate decreased, but autologous blood donation increased by 60%.[20] Unfortunately, up to half of these units are never used. Additionally, transfusion is not risk-free with an estimated overall transfusion risk of 1 in 15,000–50,000 units.[21] Thus the benefits are not clear-cut. Cost analysis reveals that processing autologous blood is also significantly more expensive. Marginal analysis has demonstrated that costs range from $235,000 to $23 million per quality adjusted life year (QALY) gained using autologous blood.[22] Given the low donated autologous unit utilization rates, preoperative strategy should be based upon the likelihood of transfusion just as recommended for allogeneic blood product use. A complete discussion of transfusion medicine is beyond the scope of this chapter and the reader is referred elsewhere.[8]

Biochemistry/Electrolyte Tests (Sodium, Potassium, Creatinine, Blood Urea Nitrogen, Glucose)

Clearly, electrolyte abnormalities can impact both perioperative and postoperative care and would be relevant in individuals on diuretics, insulin, or other medications as well as those being treated for particular illnesses. However, abnormal values are uncommon in healthy individuals and routine screening rarely leads to clinical changes in management. A review of 8 different studies found that abnormal levels of sodium or potassium were seen in 1.4% of patients with abnormal levels of creatinine and BUN in up to 2.5% of patients with glucose abnormalities in nearly 52% of individuals tested.[17] A literature review of 9 different studies of routine biochemistry tests found that no paper existed comparing the health outcomes for patients who had preoperative testing versus those who did not and that when abnormal values were identified, rarely was clinical management changed.[13] So, although there is some clinical benefit in patients at risk for electrolyte abnormalities, it is clear in routine screening that very few changes in clinical management are seen and therefore ordering of such studies should be individualized to those patients not only at risk but in which their care may be modified.

Urinalysis

Routine screening of urine in the absence of symptoms has not been shown to provide any risk reduction to patients in the postoperative period in a systematic review of 11 studies. Another systematic review of 15 studies showed some evidence that abnormalities were associated with increased age and comorbidities, but the absence of comparing health outcomes for those patients with testing versus without testing means that there is no good evidence to lead to a recommendation of routine screening.[13]

ELECTROCARDIOGRAM

The routine use of electrocardiogram (EKG) preoperative screening in patients undergoing surgery has been controversial in terms of its actual clinical value in healthy individuals. Multiple recommendations and schemes have been applied, but the level of evidence pointing to an advantage in routine use has been limited and a subject of growing controversy. More recently, recommendations of screening have referred to the ASA (American Society of Anesthesiologists) classification system (Table 5.1) in which most studies looking at preoperative EKG use has not correlated it with the ASA class of patient.[13] A review of 29 studies found no studies comparing health outcomes for patients who underwent preoperative EKGs with patients who did not.[13] Although abnormal tests increased with age and comorbidities, there is no clear evidence that performing these studies would improve the clinical outcomes of these patients. Another review of 16 studies found that the predictive power of preoperative EKGs for postoperative cardiac complications in a noncardiopulmonary surgery was weak and no evidence was found to support its value in routine screening.[17] Table 5.2 outlines the practice guidelines put forth by the American College of Cardiology in conjunction with the American Heart Association along with the level of evidence used to develop them.[24] These recommendations are based on estimated surgical risk, a concept which is highly variable and poorly defined. The summary guidelines classify procedures into three categories: low, intermediate, and high risk. Low risk procedures are those such as ophthalmologic or superficial surgeries, those least likely to be associated with excess morbidity or mortality. Major vascular surgeries constitute the highest risk category, and all other procedures fall into the intermediate

Table 5.1 American Society of Anesthesiologists (ASA) Classification System

Class I	A normal healthy patient
Class II	A patient with mild systemic disease
Class III	A patient with severe systemic disease
Class IV	A patient with severe systemic disease that is a constant threat to life
Class V	A moribund patient who is not expected to survive without the operation
Class VI	A declared brain-dead patient whose organs are being removed for donor purposes

Table 5.2   General Recommendations for Preoperative Resting 12-lead EKG[a]

	Class I (Benefit >>> Risk)	Class IIa (Benefit >> Risk)	Class IIb (Benefit ≥ Risk)	Class III (Risk ≥ Benefit)
Level A Multiple (3–5) risk strata evaluated				
Level B Limited (2–3) risk strata evaluated	Patients with one clinical risk factor[b] undergoing vascular procedures	Patients with no clinical risk factors undergoing vascular surgical procedures	Patients with at least one clinical risk factor who are undergoing intermediate-risk procedures	Asymptomatic patients undergoing low risk surgical procedures
Level C Very limited (1–2) risk strata evaluated	Patients with known coronary artery disease, peripheral arterial disease, or cerebrovascular disease who are undergoing intermediate-risk surgical procedures			

[a]Adapted from Reference 24.
[b]Clinical risk factors are history of ischemic heart disease, congestive heart failure (currently compensated), or cerebrovascular disease; diabetes mellitus; renal insufficiency (creatinine ≥ 2.0 mg/dL).
EKG changes are defined as:
Nonspecific: T wave flattening; nonspecific ST segment sloping; small Q waves in inferior leads; premature ventricular or supraventricular contractions; old left bundle branch block, left anterior fascicular block, or right bundle branch block.
Significant: New ST or T wave changes compared to previous EKG; deep T wave inversions; ST segment depression of >1 mm (must be new and patient is not on digoxin); new pathologic Q waves; ST elevation or new left bundle branch block.
Cardiology consultation should be considered for patients with significant EKG findings.

category. This risk structure is modified by the surgical location and the extent of the procedure, requiring that the surgeon exercise clinical judgment in determining the need for further evaluation.

CHEST RADIOGRAPH

A study that could definitively determine the value of routine preoperative chest X-rays would be difficult to accomplish. Ideally, this would involve a prospective investigation in which patients are randomized to having a preoperative chest X-ray or no chest X-ray, followed by an analysis of health outcomes between the two groups. Such a definitive study would require large numbers of patients (>20,000).[25] Also contributing to the difficulty of such a study is the fact that clinical decisions based on chest X-ray findings are often subjective and individualized. For example, a particular chest X-ray finding may alter one surgeon's plan of management, whereas such a finding may have no effect on another's clinical plan. It would be virtually impossible for a prospective study to attempt to control or standardize widely different management styles.

Several retrospective studies, although limited by the adequacy of record charting as is common in retrospective chart reviews, have not been able to demonstrate much value of routine preoperative chest X-rays in the general patient population. The largest study was conducted by the Royal College of Radiologists, a multicenter study which surveyed the practice of obtaining routine preoperative chest X-rays in noncardiopulmonary surgical patients among eight hospitals in Great Britain.[26] Of the 10,619 patients involved in this survey, only 30% had a routine preoperative chest X-ray done. Practice variance was wide among the various institutions, ranging between 12% and 54%. The investigators in this study defined as their outcome the impact of an abnormal chest X-ray on the decision to operate or on the type of anesthesia used. Findings in this study suggested that the preoperative chest X-ray had little influence on either outcome. Regarding whether the preoperative chest X-ray may have altered the decision to operate, 96% of patients with a normal chest X-ray and 92% of patients with significant radiological abnormalities proceeded to surgery. The difference was not statistically significant. Similarly, chest X-ray findings did not seem to have an effect on the type of anesthesia used with 96% of patients with normal chest X-rays and the same percentage with abnormal chest X-rays undergoing inhalational anesthesia. However, the study design limits conclusions regarding whether a preoperative chest X-ray may have in any other way altered perioperative management.

Some have argued that preoperative chest X-rays are of value in serving as a baseline to which subsequent postoperative chest X-rays could be compared. Mendelson and colleagues attempted to address this question in a review of 369 general surgery patients.[26] Of this number, 65 had postoperative chest X-rays done. The authors reported that in approximately half of these cases (33), a preoperative chest X-ray was "essential" in making an accurate interpretation of the postoperative chest X-ray. Unclear in this study is whether an increased accuracy in interpreting the postoperative chest X-ray truly altered postoperative clinical management.

Another factor that could be evaluated is the likelihood of finding significant radiological abnormalities on preoperative chest X-rays done without any clinical indications. One study by Sagel revealed a 1% incidence of a serious radiological abnormality found on chest X-rays in patients under 30 years of age.[27] In patients 50–60 years of age, the incidence of significant abnormalities increased to approximately 20% and attained an even higher percentage with increasing age (Table 5.3). Tornebrandt and Fletcher reported a 37% rate of serious abnormal preoperative chest X-ray findings such as cardiomegaly, pulmonary venous hypertension, and emphysema in

Table 5.3 Risk of Clinically Significant Chest Radiograph
Abnormality by Age

Age	Number of Serious Abnormality	Percentage Abnormality
00–19	0/521	(0)
20–29	9/894	(1)
30–39	22/942	(2)
40–49	66/928	(7)
50–59	179/883	(20)
60–69	290/977	(30)
≥70	347/832	(42)

Adapted from Reference 27.

patients 70 years or older who had no other medical indications for having a chest
X-ray.[28] Rucker and colleagues proposed certain risk factors that could predict the
likelihood of having an abnormal preoperative chest X-ray[29] (Table 5.4). These risk
factors include age being above 60, history of cardiac or pulmonary disease, and signs
and symptoms of chest disease. Using their criteria, 905 patients from various surgical

Table 5.4 Risk Factors for Abnormal Chest Radiographs

Medical history
    Cancer at any site
    Valvular heart disease
    Stroke
    Myocardial infarction
    Angina
    Asthma
    Tuberculosis
    Chronic obstructive pulmonary disease
    Cigarettes
    Occupational exposures: asbestos, fumes, or ores
    Review of systems
    General: fever, chills, sweats, or weight loss
    Paroxysmal nocturnal dyspnea
    Orthopnea
    Class 3 or 4 dyspnea
    Angina

Physical findings
    Vital signs: fever, tachycardia, hypertension, or tachypnea
    Chest: abnormal breath sounds, abnormal adventitial sounds, or dullness
    Cardiovascular: severe murmurs, S3, or displaced point of maximum impulse

Adapted from Reference 29.

services including gynecology and general surgery were studied. Of the 368 patients who had no risk factors, only one patient had a significant abnormality (elevated diaphragm), and none of the patients in this low risk group had any postoperative pulmonary or cardiac complications.

In summary, available studies in the literature have been unable to support the use of routine, preoperative chest X-ray in the general patient population. Nevertheless, in certain patient populations at higher risk of having a clinically significant radiological abnormality on chest X-ray, such as the elderly, a preoperative chest X-ray may be of value. Certainly, patients with cardiopulmonary findings on history and physical examination should have a preoperative chest X-ray done. In these situations, chest X-rays would not be considered routine, which implies chest X-rays are obtained with no other indications other than as part of general presurgical preparation. There may be other reasons for obtaining a chest X-ray before surgery, such as in the evaluation of a patient with a newly diagnosed gynecological malignancy. The finding of distant metastasis may dramatically change the surgery planned. It is not within the scope of this chapter to discuss these circumstances.

PULMONARY FUNCTION TESTING

Pulmonary complications, such as atelectasis or pneumonia, are a frequent and important group of complications postoperatively with a generally reported incidence ranging between 6% and 60%.[31] Abdominal incisions, especially upper abdominal incisions, are frequently associated with pulmonary complications postoperatively.[31–34] No other class of surgery except for thoracotomy is associated with a higher frequency of pulmonary problems. A major factor accounting for the pathophysiology behind pulmonary complications after abdominal surgery is the decrease in lung volumes and flow rates that occur postoperatively.[33–35] This is felt to be secondary to diaphragmatic dysfunction from decreased phrenic nerve output following abdominal surgeries. Other risk factors that have been associated with postoperative pulmonary complications include history of cigarette smoking,[31,33–36] underlying respiratory disease,[36] obesity,[34] and prolonged anesthesia time of more than 3–3.5 hours.[31,33] Increasing age has been also associated with pulmonary complications. However, this is felt not to be a major independent risk factor. The higher rate of complications seen in older patients is probably due to a higher prevalence of chronic pulmonary disease and decreased pulmonary function in this population.[36]

A pulmonary function test or a spirometry is a common screening tool used in the evaluation of the respiratory system. The objective of this section is to review the literature assessing the value of spirometry in its ability to prevent or decrease pulmonary complications. Spirometry has been demonstrated to be of value in lung resection surgeries.[32] Due to the lack of studies specifically evaluating preoperative pulmonary function tests in gynecologic surgeries, this review will be directed toward studies focused on abdominal surgeries. One of the major difficulties in evaluating the role of spirometry is the subjectivity by which outcomes are assessed, which in this case would be pulmonary complications. The wide range of reported pulmonary complications ranging from 6% to as high as 80% underlies the lack of strict objective criteria by which pulmonary complications are defined and diagnosed.[31,37] Some authors have included as pulmonary complications clinically trivial situations such as the presence of "atelectasis" on chest X-ray without regard to the clinical situation of the patient, or simply a temperature elevation of 1–2°F postoperatively. Others, recognizing the difficulty in strictly defining pulmonary complications, have used instead clinically meaningful outcomes such as length of hospital stay or mortality secondary to respiratory complications as surrogate measures of pulmonary complications.

In order for spirometry to be of clinical value as a screening tool, it must first of all accurately predict those patients at risk for pulmonary complications. Secondly, there must exist some type of medical management that could be employed, depending on the results of the screening test, which could prevent those deemed at higher risk from developing pulmonary complications.

A widely cited study promoting the use of routine screening spirometry preoperatively in predicting those patients at risk for pulmonary problems was a 1962 report by Stein and colleagues..[37] In this study 63 patients scheduled for a variety of surgeries including dilatation and curettage, hysterectomy, bowel resection, and pneumonectomy underwent preoperative spirometry. On the basis of the results of spirometry, 33 patients were classified in the normal risk group and 30 were classified in the high risk category. Among the normal risk patients, only one was deemed to have developed a postoperative pulmonary complication, whereas among the patients in the high risk group, 21 were determined to have pulmonary complications. Limiting to only patients who had abdominal incisions, 9 patients had normal spirometry, none of whom developed pulmonary complications. Of the 14 patients who had abnormal spirometry, 11 developed pulmonary complications. Unfortunately, major criticisms of this study include the lack of objective information regarding the diagnosis and severity of pulmonary complications, and that assessors of pulmonary complications were not blinded to the preoperative spirometry result. Both of these conditions may have introduced significant potential for bias. Other subsequent papers addressing patients undergoing abdominal surgeries have similarly concluded that preoperative pulmonary function tests are of value as a screening tool.[37,39,40] However, all of these studies have methodological flaws that preclude drawing any firm conclusions. Postoperative pulmonary complications ranged between 14% and 76% in these reports. This wide range was due not only to differences in patient populations, but also to differences in types of outcomes assessed and varying definitions of pulmonary complications. For example, one study of 46 patients with only upper abdominal surgeries reported a 76% incidence of postoperative pulmonary complications including conditions such as the presence of atelectasis on chest X-ray.[37] Another study, a retrospective chart review, which defined outcomes of pulmonary complications as respiratory failure or death, reported spirometry was predictive of pulmonary complications. However, other factors such as the patient's age, serum albumin level, or PaO_2 were even more predictive than spirometry in this report.[40] One prospective study examined 100 "apparently normal" clinical subjects who underwent preoperative spirometry.[39] Among the 14% of patients who developed pulmonary complications, a higher percentage (57%) had an abnormal FEV1/FVC ratio compared to only 8% of the group of patients who did not develop complications. However, there were other confounding factors such as higher average age and higher frequency of upper abdominal incisions in the complications group which preclude drawing the conclusion that spirometry alone could accurately predict those at risk.

The second requirement before a screening test could be of clinical value is that clinical approaches or techniques exist which could be implemented to decrease the pulmonary complication rate. In a follow-up to his 1962 study on the predictive value of pulmonary function tests, Stein and Cassara in 1970 reported that the institution of preventive measures including cessation of smoking, bronchodilators, antibiotics, postural drainage, inhalation of humidified gases, and chest physiotherapy could decrease postoperative pulmonary complications.[40] In this study, patients with abnormal pulmonary function tests, according to the criteria in their 1962 paper, were randomized to either the treatment arm in which they received one or more of the above measures or the no-treatment arm. Patients in the treatment arm had fewer complications. However, the difference in complications was seen only in those who had thoracotomies. The number of patients who underwent abdominal surgeries were too small to make any statistically meaningful comparisons; five in the treatment arm, one of whom had a complication, compared to three in the no-treatment arm, one of whom also developed a complication. In addition, other problems with this study included a lack of strict stratification by type of respiratory maneuvers employed among the treatment group. Even in the no-treatment group, some patients received respiratory treatments based solely on physician preference.

Other better designed trials have sought to evaluate such interventions as expiratory maneuvers, positive pressure breathing, hyperventilation, and incentive spirometry.[42,43] Incentive spirometry was noted in prospectively randomized trials to be effective in decreasing respiratory complications. Some of the other maneuvers were noted to be of no value and at the same time to be associated with a higher risk of morbidity.[43] None of the respiratory maneuvers noted above were observed to be more efficacious than incentive spirometry in reducing the postoperative pulmonary complication rate (**Level I**). As a result, the general recommendation is that incentive spirometry should be advocated for all patients undergoing abdominal surgeries, especially upper abdominal surgeries, regardless of whether a patient is at higher risk for complications. This is due to the low cost, efficacy, and absence of associated morbidity attributable to incentive spirometry.[41] In other words, these characteristics of incentive spirometry obviate the need for a screening test to define a subpopulation of patients felt to be at higher risk.

In summary, although preoperative screening spirometry has been demonstrated to be clinically beneficial in the management of lung resection patients, its value in patients undergoing abdominal surgeries has not been clearly proven.[43] Studies have reported value of routine screening spirometry in nonthoracotomy procedures. Nevertheless, all have serious methodological problems that prevent drawing any firm conclusions. It is not clear that screening spirometry contributes any more predictive value beyond a careful history and physical examination alone. In addition, incentive spirometry should be universally utilized in all abdominal surgeries because of its efficacy, low cost, and lack of associated morbidity.

There is currently no support in the literature for the use of screening pulmonary function tests in the routine, general population. There may, however, be some subsets in the general population who may benefit from preoperative spirometry. Although not specifically studied in previously reported studies, some pulmonologists have recommended that preoperative spirometry be obtained in patients who have a significant history of cigarette smoking or underlying respiratory conditions. In these cases spirometry may aid in the assessment of pulmonary impairment and the information gained may have an impact on surgical and perioperative management.[33,34]

SUMMARY

One cannot overemphasize the value of a careful general history and physical examination focused on eliciting signs and symptoms that may alter surgical risk and management. The necessity of routine preoperative evaluations and the level of evidence in the literature supporting these recommendations are summarized in this chapter. No laboratory test or radiograph should be used as a substitute for a careful preoperative examination. At the same time, although studies have not proven certain tests to be clinically beneficial, the circumstances surrounding these studies in an individual patient may differ. Thus, the above recommendations should serve only as guidelines combining the best published evidence with solid clinical judgment and experience.

Strength of Evidence of Recommendations for Preoperative Evaluations

1. CBC should be obtained in all patients undergoing major surgery with significant risk of hemorrhage (**Levels III, II-3**).
2. Pregnancy test should be obtained in all female patients with reproductive potential (**Level III**).
3. PT/PTT should not be routinely obtained without indications, and are indicated preoperatively when there is a clinical concern for a coagulopathy (**Level II-2**).
4. There is no evidence to support routine electrolytes (**Level II-3**).
5. There is no evidence to support routine BUN/Cr (**Level II-3**).
6. There is no evidence to support routine urinalysis (**Level II-3**).
7. There is no evidence to support routine chest X-ray without underlying cardiovascular/pulmonary disease (**Level II-3**).
8. There is no evidence to support routine spirometry to be clinically beneficial without underlying pulmonary disease (**Levels III, II-3**).
9. Preoperative "type and crossmatch" vs. "type and screen" order should depend on the anticipated need for blood product use (**Level III**).

10. Resting EKG is recommended for all patients undergoing major vascular surgery and in intermediate-risk procedures on patients with known vascular disease (**Level II-1**).

11. Resting EKG should be considered for patients undergoing intermediate-risk procedures with at least one clinical risk factor (**Level II-3**).

REFERENCES

1. ROIZEN M. Preoperative patient evaluation. Can J Anesth 1989;36:S13–17.
2. KAPLAN EB, SHEINER LB, BOECKMANN AJ, et al. The usefulness of preoperative laboratory screening. JAMA 1985;253:3576–3581.
3. MACARIO A, ROIZEN MF, THISTED RA, et al. Reassessment of preoperative laboratory testing has changed the test-ordering patterns of physicians. Surg Gynecol Obstet 1992;175:539–543.
4. VELANOVICH V. The value of routine preoperative laboratory testing in predicting postoperative complications: a multivariate analysis. Surgery 1991;109:236–243.
5. THOMPSON JD, ROCK JA. TeLinde's Operative Gynecology. 8th ed. Philadelphia, PA:Lippincott-Raven; 1996. p 70–71.
6. GERSHENSON DM, DECHERNEY AH, CURRY SL. Operative Gynecology. Philadelphia, PA:WB Saunders; 1993. p 30.
7. WATSON-WILLIAMS EJ. Hematologic and hemostatic considerations before surgery. Med Clin North Am 1979;63:1165–1189.
8. BLERY C, SZATAN M, FOURGEAUX B, et al. Evaluation of a protocol for selective ordering of preoperative tests. Lancet 1986;1:139–141.
9. ROHRER MJ, MICHELOTTI MC, NAHRWOLD DL. A prospective evaluation of the efficacy of preoperative coagulation testing. Ann Surg 1988;208:554–557.
10. EISENBERG JM, CLARKE JR, SUSSMAN SA. Prothrombin and partial thromboplastin times as preoperative screening tests. Arch Surg 1982;117:48–51.
11. ROBBINS JA, ROSE SD. Partial thromboplastin time as a screening test. Ann Intern Med 1979; 90:796–797.
12. ROBBINS JA, MUSHLIN AI. Preoperative evaluation of the healthy patient. Med Clin North Am 1979;63:1145–1156.
13. National Institute for Clinical Excellence. Preoperative tests: the routine use of preoperative tests for elective surgery—Evidence, methods and guidance. June 2003. p 1–117.
14. Office of Medical Applications of Research. Summary of NIH Consensus Development Conference on perioperative red cell transfusion. Am J Hematol 1989;31:144.
15. HEUGHAN C, GRISLIS G, HUNT TK. The effect of anemia on wound healing. Ann Surg 1974;179: 163–167.
16. SILBERSTEIN LE, KRUSKALL MS, STEHLING LC, et al. Strategies for the review of transfusion practices. JAMA 1989;262:1993–1997.
17. Routine preoperative testing: a systematic review of the evidence [diagnosis-screening]. Database of abstracts of reviews of effectiveness. Vol. 3, Sept. 2002.
18. STEHLING L, LUBAN NLC, ANDERSON KC, et al. Guidelines for blood utilization review. Transfusion 1994;34:438–448.
19. WALLACE EL, SURGENOR DM, HAO HS, et al. Collection and transfusion of blood and blood components in the United States. Transfusion 1993;33:139–144.
20. National Heart, Lung, and Blood Institute Expert Panel on the Use of Autologous Blood. Transfusion alert: use of autologous blood. Transfusion 1995;35:703–711.
21. ETCHASON L, POTZ L, KEELER E, et al. The cost-effectiveness of preoperative autologous blood donations. N Engl J Med 1995;332:719–724.
22. MCCULLOUGH J. Transfusion Medicine. 1st ed. New York:McGraw Hill; 1998.

23. TAPE TG, MUSHLIN AI. The utility of routine chest radiographs. Ann Intern Med 1986;104:663–670.
24. FLEISHER LA, BECKMAN JA, BROWN KA, et al. ACC/AHA 2007 guidelines on perioperative cardio-vascular evaluation and care for noncardiac surgery: executive summary: a report of the American College of Cardiology/American Heart Association Task Force on Practice Guidelines (Writing Committee to Revise the 2002 Guidelines on Perioperative Cardiovascular Evaluation for Noncardiac Surgery). Circulation 2007;116:1971–1996.
25. Royal College of Radiologists. Preoperative chest radiology. Lancet 1979;2:83–86.
26. MENDELSON DS, KHILNANI N, WAGNER LD, et al. Preoperative chest radiography: value as a baseline examination for comparison. Radiology 1987;165:341–343.
27. SAGEL SS, EVENS RG, FORREST JV, et al. Efficacy of routine screening and lateral chest radiographs in a hospital-based population. N Engl J Med 1974;291:1001–1004.
28. TORNEBRANDT K, FLETCHER R. Pre-operative chest X-rays in elderly patients. Anaesthesia 1982;37:901–902.
29. RUCKER L, FRYE EB, STATEN MA. Usefulness of screening chest roentgenograms in preoperative patients. JAMA 1983;250:3209–3211.
30. HARMAN E, LILLINGTON G. Pulmonary risk factors in surgery. Med Clin North Am 1979;63: 1289–1298.
31. ZIBRAK JD, O'DONNELL CR, MARTON K. Indications for pulmonary function testing. Ann Intern Med 1990;112:763–771.
32. GARIBALDI RA, BRITT MR, COLEMAN ML, et al. Risk factors for postoperative pneumonia. Am J Med 1981;70:677–680.
33. TISI GM. Preoperative evaluation of pulmonary function. Am Rev Respir Dis 1979;119:293–310.
34. JACKSON CV. Preoperative pulmonary evaluation. Arch Intern Med 1988;148:2120–2127.
35. WIGHTMAN JAK. A prospective survey of the incidence of the incidence of postoperative pulmonary complications. Br J Surg 1968;55:85–91.
36. LATIMER RG, DICKMAN M, DAY WC, et al. Ventilatory patterns and pulmonary complications after upper abdominal surgery determined by preoperative and postoperative computerized spirometry and blood gas analysis. Am J Surg 1971;122:622–632.
37. STEIN M, KOOTA GM, SIMON M, et al. Pulmonary evaluation of surgical patients. JAMA 1962;181:765–770.
38. APPLEBERG M, GORDON L, FATTI LP. Preoperative pulmonary evaluation of surgical patients using the vitalograph. Br J Surg 1974;61:57–59.
39. FAN ST, LAU WY, YIP WC, et al. Prediction of postoperative pulmonary complications in esopha-gogastric cancer surgery. Br J Surg 1987;74:408–410.
40. STEIN M, CASSARA EL. Preoperative pulmonary evaluation and therapy for surgery patients. JAMA 1970;211:787–790.
41. CELLI BR, RODRIGUEZ KS, SNIDER GL. A controlled trial of intermittent positive pressure breath-ing, incentive spirometry, and deep breathing exercises in preventing pulmonary complications after abdominal surgery. Am Rev Respir Dis 1984;130:12–15.
42. BARTLETT RH, GAZZANIGA AB, GERAGHTY TR. Respiratory maneuvers to prevent postoperative pulmonary complications. JAMA 1973;224:1017–1021.
43. LAWRENCE VA, PAGE CP, HARRIS GD. Preoperative spirometry before abdominal operations. Arch Intern Med 1989;149:280–285.

Chapter 6

Postoperative Surveillance and Perioperative Prophylaxis

Harriet O. Smith, MD and Lejla Delic, MD

Excellence in gynecologic surgery depends on experience in a wide variety of operative techniques, and a working knowledge of the effects of anesthesia and surgical trauma on healthy and diseased organ systems. Perioperative morbidity is reduced, costs are minimized, and patient satisfaction is enhanced when the operative procedure selected is tailored to the patient's specific needs and limitations, the preoperative and postoperative counseling is supportive and comprehensive, and the intensity of perioperative surveillance is proportionate to previously recognized risk factors.

PHYSIOLOGICAL RESPONSES TO SURGERY (LEVEL II-2)

Changes associated with surgical trauma adversely affect practically every organ system of the human body. Particularly susceptible are the very young, the elderly, or patients with medical conditions that reduce tolerance to anesthetic and surgical stress. The metabolic response to surgery may be divided into: (1) an early *ebb phase*, characterized by hypovolemia and associated endocrine and sympathetic responses; (2) a *flow phase*, characterized by oxidation of muscle protein to supply glucose; and (3) the *convalescence phase*, which begins immediately postoperatively and may extend for 3–12 months.[1] The first 24 hours following surgery are the most hazardous: in one large study of 2153 consecutive operations, 80% of patients who experienced major morbidity or mortality began to deteriorate within 24 hours (**Level II-2**). With more aggressive management, major morbidity might have been prevented in 12% of these patients.[2]

The pathophysiological effects, and management, of surgical trauma may be categorized by the specific organ systems involved.

Gynecologic Oncology: Evidence-Based Perioperative and Supportive Care, Second Edition.
Edited by Scott E. Lentz, Allison E. Axtell and Steven A. Vasilev.
© 2011 John Wiley & Sons, Inc. Published 2011 by John Wiley & Sons, Inc.

Changes in Fluid and Electrolytes (Level II-1)

Total body water constitutes 50%–70% of the total body weight. It is dependent on lean body mass, or muscle, which decreases with age. Body fat contains little water. Consequently, at comparable weights, a young athletic woman will have 20%–30% more body water per kilogram than an elderly obese woman. Body water is dispersed into three functional compartments: the *intracellular volume compartment*, which comprises 40% of the body weight, and the *extracellular fluid compartment*, which comprises 20% of the body weight and is disproportionately distributed between the *plasma* and the *interstitial fluid compartment*. Plasma, the intravascular volume compartment, comprises only 5% of the body weight, and interstitial fluid (lymph, joint, and "third" spaced fluid) constitutes the remaining 15%. Body compartment protein and electrolyte composition and hydrostatic pressures vary significantly. Within cells the major cations are potassium and magnesium; phosphates and proteins are the principal anions. The total *ionic* concentration [milliequivalents/liter (mEq/L)] within plasma and interstitial fluid is considered the same for all practical purposes. The principal cation in the extracellular compartment is sodium, and chloride and carbonate are the principal anions. The total intracellular particulate concentration is 200 mEq/L, 1.3-fold higher than the extracellular compartment particle concentration. Differences in ionic composition between the cellular and extracellular compartments are maintained by semipermeable cell membranes, energy-dependent cell transport mechanisms, and transmembrane differences in electrical potential, particle charge, and oncotic pressure. Oncotic pressure is dependent on the total number of osmotically active particles in each compartment, usually 290–310 mOsm. *Effective oncotic pressure* reflects membrane impermeable particles such as plasma proteins and extracellular sodium. *Colloid oncotic pressure*, the effective osmotic pressure between plasma and interstitial spaces, plays a critical role in maintaining body water distribution between compartments.

Surgery, especially abdominal, is associated with a decline in total body protein, albumin, and total lymphocyte counts, which correlates with severity of blood loss, duration of surgery, and weight gain postoperatively. Perioperative hypoalbuminemia of some degree is almost universal, and results from crystalloid dilution, increases in capillary permeability and sequestration of albumin in interstitial fluid, and/or intraoperative loss. Postoperative albumin levels do not accurately reflect nutritional status (**Level II-2**).[3]

Fluid balance disturbances are divided into (1) volume changes: depletion, redistribution, and excess; (2) changes in extracellular sodium; and (3) compositional alterations, including changes in acid–base and departmental concentrations of potassium, magnesium, and calcium.[4] In surgical patients, volume depletion from poor intake, vomiting, nasogastric (NG) suction, diarrhea, or fistula drainage is the most common extracellular volume deficit (Table 6.1). A healthy 70-kg woman requires approximately 2000–2500 cc of fluid replacement per day.[4,5] Extra fluid is needed to compensate for increased extracellular fluid losses including perspiration losses, fever, and tachypnea, which increase insensible losses to approximately 1000–1500 cc/day. Ascites, pleural effusions, fluid sequestration into the bowel lumen, and extravasation into soft tissues are examples of "third" space losses that result from

Table 6.1   Average Losses Per Day[a]

	Volume (mL/ 24 hours)	Na (mEq/L)	K (mEq/L)	Cl (mEq/L)	HCO$_3$ (mEq/L)
Salivary	1500 (500–2000)	10 (2–10)	26 (20–30)	10 (8–18)	30
Stomach	1500 (100–4000)	60 (9–116)	10 (0–32)	130 (8–154)	–
Duodenum	100–2000				
Ileum	3000 (100–9000)	140 (80–150)	5 (2–8)	104 (43–137)	30
Colon	–	60	30	40	–
Pancreas	(100–800)	140 (113–185)	5 (3–7)	75 (54–95)	115
Bile	50–800	145 (131–164)	5 (3–12)	100 (89–180)	35

[a] Adapted from Reference 5.

malignancy-associated lymphatic obstruction, colloid oncotic pressure changes (hypoalbuminemia or excessive fluid or crystalloid resuscitation), extensive surgical dissection, or ileus. Bowel preps and poor oral intake aggrevate preoperative volume contraction. Volume excess is usually secondary to renal failure or excessive hydration.

Serum levels of sodium generally reflect body fluid tonicity because sodium is the principal ion responsible for the osmolarity of the extracellular space.[4] *Hypernatremia* is associated with efflux of water from the intracellular to the extracellular compartment, usually in response to acute water loss.[4] To maintain a normal plasma osmolality, renal free water clearance must equal the free water intake minus insensible losses. Generation of free water to dilute urine depends on an intact renal collecting system, normal suppression of Antidiuretic hormone (ADH), adequate renal profusion, and a normal glomerular filtration rate. *Hypertonic hyponatremia* results in the redistribution of body water from the intracellular space (Fig. 6.1), and is corrected with hydration with normal saline. Insulin therapy increases cellular uptake of glucose, thereby decreasing extracellular osmolality. *Hypotonic hyponatremia* may be associated with expanded, normal, or deficient total body water. Unless the rate of change in sodium concentration is quite rapid, symptoms are typically absent until sodium concentrations are severely abnormal or corrective measures are excessive. Thus, postoperative sodium concentrations should be checked frequently in patients at risk (**Level III**).[6, 7]

Cardiovascular and Thermoregulatory Effects

Effects of inhalation anesthetics on the endocrine stress response are agent- and dose-dependent, and include an increase in circulating catecholamines, ADH, Adrenocorticotrophic hormone (ACTH), and cortisol (**Level III**). Systemic blood pressure is maintained by factors that influence cardiac output (CO) as well as systemic vascular resistance, which reflects afterload. Peripheral vascular tone is regulated by receptors within the arterioles and the central nervous system. In response to surgical stress, norepinephrine and epinephrine are locally and/or systemically released, resulting in an increase in CO secondary to catecholamine-mediated inotropic and chronotropic

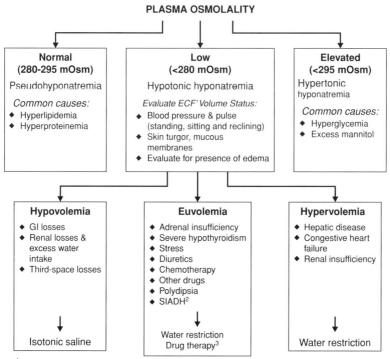

PLASMA OSMOLALITY

Normal (280-295 mOsm)	Low (<280 mOsm)	Elevated (<295 mOsm)
Pseudohyponatremia	Hypotonic hyponatremia	Hypertonic hyponatremia
Common causes: ♦ Hyperlipidemia ♦ Hyperproteinemia	*Evaluate ECF' Volume Status:* ♦ Blood pressure & pulse (standing, sitting and reclining) ♦ Skin turgor, mucous membranes ♦ Evaluate for presence of edema	*Common causes:* ♦ Hyperglycemia ♦ Excess mannitol

Hypovolemia	Euvolemia	Hypervolemia
♦ GI losses ♦ Renal losses & excess water intake ♦ Third-space losses	♦ Adrenal insufficiency ♦ Severe hypothyroidism ♦ Stress ♦ Diuretics ♦ Chemotherapy ♦ Other drugs ♦ Polydipsia ♦ SIADH[2]	♦ Hepatic disease ♦ Congestive heart failure ♦ Renal insufficiency
Isotonic saline	Water restriction Drug therapy[3]	Water restriction

[1]Extracellular fluid volume.
[2]Syndrome of inappropriate antidiuretic hormone secretion (urine Osm >200 mOsm/kg and elevated urinary sodium [>20 mEq/L] without other etiologies).
[3]Demeclocycline, lasix, increased salt intake.

Figure 6.1 Recognition and management of hyponatremia (level III). (Adapted from O'Shea MH. Fluid and electrolyte management. In: Woodley M, Whelan A, editors. Manual of Medical Therapeutics, 27th ed. Boston: Little, Brown, and Company, 1992, p 42–61.

effects. Venoconstriction further increases venous return, enhancing stroke volume (SV) and CO. In addition to the hypothalamic-hypophyseal-adrenal mechanisms, systemic blood pressure is regulated by the renin-angiotensin-aldosterone system. Renin release by the juxtaglomerular cells is mediated by a decrease in wall tension or sodium as well as by sympathetic activation. Renin converts angiotensinogen into angiotensin I, which, in turn, is converted into angiotensin II, a potent vasoconstrictor that stimulates aldosterone secretion from the renal cortex. Aldosterone increases sodium and water retention, resulting in increased venous return and consequently SV, CO, and blood pressure.[8, 9] Hypertension may also result from bladder distension, direct laryngoscopy/intubation, pain, and as a "rebound effect" from hypotension.[9] Inhalation agents alter cerebral blood flow by opposing direct (vasodilatation that results in increased cerebral blood flow) and indirect (decreased metabolism which reduces cerebral blood flow) mechanisms. Anesthetics attenuate cerebral autoregulation, which normally assures that cerebral blood flow does not fluctuate with changes in arterial blood pressure (**Level III**).[10]

All volatile anesthetics depress myocardial contractility. Compared with nitrous oxide or isoflurane, halothane and enflurane decrease CO by 20%–40%. Intravenous narcotics (e.g., morphine) induce hypotension, especially when given at rates above 10 mg/minute (1–4 mg/kg).[11] Fluctuations in the intraoperative mean arterial pressure of more than 20 mm Hg, congestive heart failure (CHF), myocardial infarction (MI), and renal failure are all significant predictors of major postoperative morbidity (**Level II-2**).[12] In patients with longstanding or newly diagnosed essential hypertension, blood pressure should be optimally controlled prior to elective surgery, and on the morning of the surgery, antihypertensives should be taken orally in usual doses. Although sedation preoperatively may prevent intraoperative hypotension, and oversedation may result in hypoxia and hypercapnia, and consequently significant hypertension, sedatives should be used cautiously in the lowest possible effective doses (**Level II-2**).[8, 9] Optimization of preload and afterload is especially important in patients with ventricular dysfunction; inotropic support guided by pulmonary artery catheterization may be warranted.[13]

Hypothermia, defined as a core temperature of less than 36°C, affects approximately 14 million patients annually and nearly 70% of patients requiring surgery (**Level III**).[14] Temperature regulation is under the control of the posterior hypothalamus, which receives signals from *core zone receptors* in the preoptic area of the hypothalamus as well as from the spinal cord, major vasculature, and viscera, and *shell zone receptors* within the skin. Hypothalamic response to hypothermia includes (1) activation of motor nerves responsible for shivering; (2) stimulation of catecholamine release, which induces vasoconstriction and consequently an increase in the basal metabolic rate; and (3) increased thyroxine secretion.[15] Hypothermia is an iatrogenic complication of surgery, resulting from prolonged exposure to a cold ambient environment and from the physiological effects of anesthesia. Anesthetic agents lower the basal metabolic rate, inhibit redirection of blood flow from the skin, and prevent shivering.[14] Even without shivering, a decrease in core body temperature of 0.3°–1.2°C increases oxygen consumption by approximately 92%; shivering may magnify this effect by as much as 500%. Oxygen demand is consequently increased at a time when pulmonary reserve is diminished, increasing the risks for arterial desaturation, which, in turn, increases heart rate, CO, and oxygen consumption.[14] In addition to patient discomfort, unintentional hypothermia is associated with transient hypoxia (a reduction in PaO_2 < 80 mm Hg) and a higher incidence of angina and myocardial ischemia in the early postoperative period.[15, 16] Coagulopathies secondary to impaired enzymatic reactions of the clotting cascade and/or impaired platelet function with or without thrombocytopenia often develop; hypothermia also predisposes to hypercoagulability, which increases the risk of pulmonary embolism (PE).[17]

Pulmonary Effects

All inhalation agents are respiratory depressants. Atelectasis has been demonstrated in approximately 50% of patients postoperatively (**Level II-2**).[18] During and following general anesthesia, gas exchange is impaired by paralysis of the chest wall and diaphragm, loss of the normal hypoxic drive to ventilation, and inhibition of hypoxic pulmonary vasoconstriction that serves to redirect oxygen to underventilated pulmonary segments.[19] Sighing, a physiological mechanism that reduces alveolar collapse, is also diminished by anesthesia and postoperative sedation (**Level II-2**).[20] Opioid analgesics slow the respiratory rate, decrease minute ventilation, and further reduce the functional residual capacity (FRC) to approximately 60% of the preoperative value.[21] Mucociliary action is inhibited, resulting in a reduced capacity to clear mucous secretions. Depressed macrophage, neutrophil, and lymphocyte function contribute to the increased risks of bacterial colonization and subsequent infection.[11] Reduced lung compliance and FRC result in microatelectasis and pulmonary shunting, further increasing the alveolar-arterial oxygen gradient. Compared with general anesthesia, epidural anesthesia offers several potential advantages: In the period immediately postoperatively, its blocking effects reduce plasma epinephrine release, thereby reducing oxygen consumption and consequently mixed oxygen saturation (**Level II-2**).[22,23] Although epidural anesthesia appears to provide superior pain relief, in a controlled randomized study of 150 patients, the incidence and severity of pulmonary complications following epidural anesthesia compared with parenteral morphine were not improved (**Level I**).[24]

Effects on Protein Catabolism and Immune Response

Following uncomplicated surgery, weight loss averages about 3 kg, and, in the absence of preexisting deficits, is usually restored within 3 months. Weight loss results from oxidation of fat and protein breakdown.[1] When carbohydrate intake is inadequate, glycogen stores are rapidly depleted and, to supply fuel essential for the brain and healing tissues, gluconeogenesis occurs at the expense of protein catabolism. The rate of metabolism is further accelerated in critically ill patients.[1] High dose inhalation anesthesia appears to reduce perioperative catabolism, and may be an important means of reducing perioperative morbidity in patients with preexisting protein deficits (**Level II-2**).[25] Protein loss does not account for postoperative fatigue, a syndrome found exclusively in humans, characterized by muscle weakness and fatigue for days or weeks following surgery. Although the mechanisms involved are poorly understood, there appears to be both a physiological and psychological basis.[1,25]

Systemically and at the site of tissue injury, mediators including cytokines, vasoactive amines, and arachidonic acid products act to increase protocoagulant activity, vascular permeability, and vasodilatation.[26] Following general surgery, there is an increase in total leucocyte count; function, however, as measured by directed motility (chemotaxis), serum opsonic activity, and ingestive capacity is depressed for hours to days.[27] Phagocytosis by monocytes and macrophages is also suppressed. Perioperatively, macrophages excrete a variety of factors including cytokines (IL-1, IL-6, TNF), which are the major mediators of the acute-phase response, as well as proteases, prostaglandin products, and interferon.[11,27] The effect of surgery on the release and activity of these mediators is under intense investigation. IL-6 is consistently elevated 4–6 hours postoperatively, and has been implicated in the pyrogenic response, and also in the stimulation of acute-phase protein production by hepatoma cells.[28] Transient increases in serum levels of IL-1β are consistently preceded by elevations in IL-6 levels[29]; however, since TNF, a potent pyrogenic cytokine implicated in septic shock, is not detected, a role for TNF in mediating the acute-phase response is doubtful.[28, 29] Complement activity, cell-mediated immunity, and humoral immunity may all be depressed, the severity of which is proportionate to the duration of anesthesia and surgical trauma.[27] The clinical significance of these physiological alterations has yet to be elucidated (**Level II-2**).[27, 28, 30]

Gastrointestinal Changes

Entry into the peritoneal cavity and/or the neuroinhibitory effects of general anesthesia result in a transient loss of gastrointestinal (GI) peristaltic activity termed *postoperative ileus* (POI) (**Level III**).[31] Symptoms of POI include bloating secondary to air swallowing, abdominal distension, emesis, and pain. Treatment is generally supportive and includes NG intubation and intravenous hydration. This self-limiting condition generally lasts for 1–3 days.[32] In uncomplicated POI, small intestinal transit recovers first with return of phase III activity of the interdigestive migrating motor reflex, followed by gastric and later colonic activity.[33] Resolution of POI is assessed clinically by auscultation of normoactive bowel sounds and by the passage of flatus and stool. *Paralytic ileus*, or complicated ileus lasting more than 3 days after surgery, is frequently associated with excessive intestinal manipulation, peritonitis, pancreatitis,[34] opiate administration (**Level II-2**),[35] and high vasopressin levels,[36] and probably reflects inhibition of small bowel activity.[34] Inhalation anesthetic agents, especially enflurane and halothane, but not nitrous oxide, suppress motor activity throughout the colon.[36] Although presentation and symptoms are similar, the pathophysiological mechanisms of paralytic ileus are poorly understood. Paralytic ileus must be distinguished from ileus resulting from intestinal obstruction and from mechanical ileus.

GENERAL PERIOPERATIVE PROPHYLAXIS

Medical History, Physical Examination, and Informed Consent

Preoperative medical history should include thorough investigation of the presenting complaint, past medical history including prescription and over-the-counter medications, and inquiry with respect to prior hospitalizations, exposure to general anesthesia, and all food and drug allergies. A complete review of systems and physical examination provide the basis for indicated laboratory and radiographic investigation as well as the need for consultation and collaborative management involving other clinical services. Informed consent should include, in layman's terms, a detailed discussion of the planned operative procedure, the potential risks and benefits, the likelihood of success or failure of the anticipated procedure, and treatment alternatives

Table 6.2   Guidelines for Informed Consent

1.	Define the disease process and its severity.
2.	Describe the planned operative procedure in understandable language.
	What organs will be removed or altered?
	What is the planned operative incision?
	How will intraoperative findings affect:
	The planned procedure?
	The extent of surgery?
	The need for blood products?
3.	Provide a discussion of the risks and potential complications of the proposed procedure.
	What is the probability of success or failure?
	What are the anesthetic risks?
	Define risks within the context of the patient's underlying physical condition.
4.	Describe the level of care anticipated in the immediate postoperative and recovery period.
	Will the patient require intensive care monitoring or ventilatory support?
	What is the anticipated length of hospitalization and convalescence?
	How will fertility and ovarian function be affected?
	Will special devices (e.g., prolonged urinary catheterization or central venous access, ostomy products) or medications be necessary, and for how long?
	What, if any, additional therapy would be required?
5.	List the treatment alternatives and their risks and benefits.
6.	Describe the usual course of the patient's disease if the proposed treatment is withheld.

(Table 6.2). A useful way to clarify misconceptions and improve rapport is to have the patient to keep a diary of her questions and concerns, and to address these issues preoperatively. Timely charting of relevant history, physical findings, and preoperative discussions cannot be overstressed. The patient's chart is a legal document and can be the physician's best testament to the quality of care rendered.

Laboratory Screening

Preoperative laboratory testing should be performed as indicated by a thorough assessment of the patient, including performance status, medical history, and complexity of the planned operative procedure. Routine laboratory screening (complete blood count, urinalysis, and electrocardiogram [ECG]) and chest X-ray are generally recommended in patients over 40 years of age, when extensive surgery is anticipated, and in patients with underlying medical disease or malignancy (Fig. 6.2). However, when performed routinely in healthy young patients undergoing ambulatory surgery, including hysterectomy, elective preoperative screening is costly, unlikely to affect outcome, and increases the probability that additional expensive and potentially harmful tests will be ordered (**Level II-2**).[38–41] Although intravenous pyelography (IVP) may be occasionally helpful (malignancy, extensive pelvic inflammatory disease,

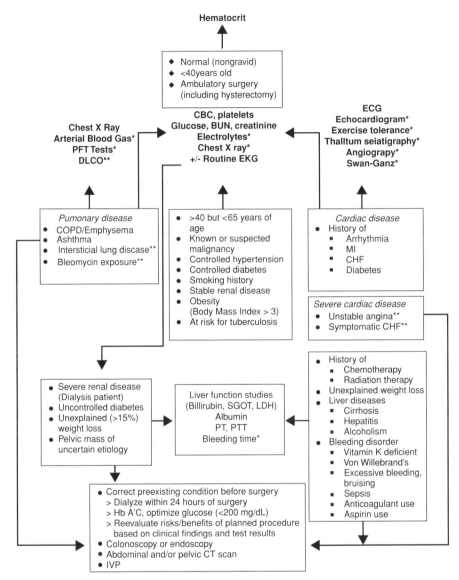

*Depending upon severity of clinical symptoms and/or physical findings.
**Test is indicated for specific indication as highlighted.

Figure 6.2   Guidelines for preoperative screening tests (levels II.2, III).[38–41]

or congenital anomalies of the genitourinary tract), the potential risks (reaction to contrast, nephrotoxicity, and radiation exposure), in addition to costs, prohibit obtaining IVPs routinely (**Level II-3**).[42–44] Following administration of contrast material, mild, generalized reactions including hives, pruritus, syncope, and GI symptoms are common, affecting 5%–10% of patients, and fatal anaphylactic reactions occur in approximately 1 per 14,000 procedures performed.[42] Prophylactic steroid administration may prevent life-threatening reactions in patients with a history of allergies to contrast material or seafood.[45] Intravenous contrast agents can also induce acute renal insufficiency by reducing renal blood flow, resulting in medullary ischemia.[46] In patients with chronic renal failure, intravenous hydration 12 hours before and after radiocontrast administration reduces this risk; mannitol or furosemide does not improve the protective effects of hydration alone.[47]

Perioperative Cardiac Assessment

The incidence of MI following noncardiac surgery is approximately 0%–0.7%[48]; a nonfatal infarction rate in patients over 40 years of age (with or without coronary artery disease) is approximately 0.15% (**Level II-2**).[49] Cardiac morbidity is a leading cause of perioperative death which is exceeded in frequency only by deaths from anesthetic or surgical complications (Table 6.3).[48] Goldman et al. developed a multifactorial index of independent factors associated with cardiac risk (Table 6.4).[49,50] Based on the stratification of these risks factors, the incidence of life-threatening or fatal myocardial morbidity was found to be I (1%), II (7%), III (14%), and IV (78%) (**Level II-3**).[50] Reinfarction rates are increased following vascular surgery (1%–15%) and previous MI (1%–7.7%), especially within the antecedent 3 months (0%–37%).[48] In recent years, aggressive hemodynamic monitoring has reduced the rate of reinfarction in patients to 1.9% overall and to 5.7% following a recent (<3 months) MI (**Level II-2**).[51] Noninvasive screening tests including preoperative exercise testing, dipyridamole-thallium scintigraphy, stress echocardiography, and ambulatory ischemia monitoring may be useful to identify patients at high risk for

Table 6.3 Perioperative Cardiac Morbidity (Noncardiac Surgery)[a]

Cardiac Complication	Estimated Incidence
Myocardial ischemia	
Preoperative	24%
Intraoperative	18–74%
Postoperative	27–38%
Myocardial infarction (MI)	
General population	0.1–0.7%
Prior MI	1.9–7.7%
Vascular surgery	1–15%
Recent MI (<3 months)	0–37%
Unstable angina	–
Congestive heart failure (CHF)	
Intraoperative	4.8%
Postoperative	14–40.5%
Cardiac death with perioperative MI	36–70%

[a] Adapted from Reference 48.

Table 6.4 Goldman Risk Factors for Postoperative MI (Noncardiac Surgery)[a]

Criteria	Points
S3 gallop or jugular venous distension on preoperative physical examination	11
MI within the previous 6 months	10
Premature ventricular beats (>5 per minute)	7
Rhythm other than sinus or premature atrial contractions on preoperative ECG	7
Age > 70 years	5
Emergency surgery	4
Site of surgery intrathoracic, intraperitoneal, or aortic	3
Significant valvular stenosis	3
Poor general medical condition[b]	3

[a] Adapted from Reference 50.
[b] Poor respiratory function (PaO_2 < 60 mm Hg or $PaCO_2$ > 50 mm Hg); significant electrolyte disturbances (K < 3.0 or HCO_3 < 20 mEq/L); renal insufficiency (BUN > 50 or creatinine > 3.0 mg/dL); liver dysfunction (increased SGOT, SGPT, chronic liver disease); chronically bedridden.

postoperative MI; in general, however, the cost–benefit ratio of these tests are prohibitive for routine screening.[52] Stratification of perioperative MI risks (Table 6.5) has been modified by Ashton[53] to take into account the three most important risk factors for perioperative MI: (1) recent MI (antecedent 3 months), (2) CHF, and (3) unstable angina (**Level II-2**). Cardiac evaluation other than preoperative ECG is not recommended for asymptomatic patients lacking a history or physical evidence of cardiovascular disease[52]; however, patients at high or intermediate risk[53] may benefit from aggressive perioperative evaluation including cardiac screening, preoperative cardiac consultation, and aggressive postoperative monitoring.

The Role of Other Perioperative Screening Tests

CT contrast studies, ultrasound, barium enema, upper GI studies, flexible proctosigmoidoscopy, and/or colonoscopy should be performed only in select cases for specific indications, such as symptoms or clinical findings suggestive of involvement of other organs within proximity to the planned operative field (e.g., advanced ovarian cancer or severe endometriosis). When the origin of a pelvic mass is uncertain, such as distinguishing diverticular disease or a GI tumor from an ovarian neoplasm, additional clinical or radiographic studies may be helpful (**Level III**).

Prevention of Surgical Wound Infection

Nosocomial bacteremias in the United States, 25% of which are accounted for by postoperative wound infections,[54] adversely affect approximately 200,000 patients each year, increasing morbidity and mortality, duration of hospital stay, additional

Table 6.5   Risk for Perioperative MI[a,b]

Risk Assessment[c]	Prevalence of CAD	Observed MI Rate	Cardiac Death Rate
Negligible: No evidence of atherosclerosis (AS), low atherogenic risk factor profile	Almost 0%	Unknown	0% (0/652)
Low risk: More than 75 years old, high AS risk index, no evidence of AS	5–30%	0% (0/256)	0.4% (1/256)
Intermediate risk: No evidence of CAD, history of CVA, vascular surgery, carotid bruit, TIA, claudication, atypical chest pain	30–70%	0.8% (2/260)	0.4% (1/260)
High risk: CAD, history of MI, abnormal ECG consistent with previous MI, atypical angina pectoris, angiographic evidence of significant CAD, or prior coronary bypass surgery	Nearly 100%	4.1% (13/319)	2.3% (7/319)

[a] Adapted from Reference 53.
[b] Risk assessment based upon preexisting coronary artery disease (CAD).
[c] Based on age, sex, smoking history, elevated blood pressure, abnormal glucose tolerance, elevated cholesterol, risk of cardiac event within 6 years ≥15%.

antibiotic use, and health care costs by up to $860 million each year (**Level II-2**).[55] The past 25 years have witnessed a dramatic reduction in the postoperative wound infection rate, mainly due to the use of prophylactic antibiotics. In contrast, indiscriminate use of antibiotics (prolonged use, three or more agent therapies, and timing) increases the risks of toxicity, allergic reactions, and overgrowth of resistant organisms.[58,59] Traditionally, risk for wound infection and need for prophylactic antibiotics was based on stratification by severity of wound contamination–clean, clean contaminated, contaminated, and dirty or infected, which carry an expected risk of infection of 2% or less, 5%–15%, 15%–30%, and over 30%, respectively.[58,59] Strictly defined, prophylactic antibiotics are given in the absence of contamination and infection to reduce the risks of perioperative infection; antibiotic use aimed at underlying infection are considered therapeutic antibiotics.[58] To achieve and maintain effective tissue levels, the first dose of parenteral antibiotic should be given within 60 minutes before the skin incision. If, however, fluoroquinolone or vancomycin prophylaxis is used, infusion should begin 120 minutes before the skin incision to account for antibiotic-associated reactions.[363] Repeated antibiotic doses should be given for prolonged operations at interval of two half-lives after the first dose. Furthermore, antibiotic dose should be adjusted on the basis of a patient's body mass index. For example, 2 g vs. 1 g of cefazolin in obese patients results in lower incidence of surgical site infection (SSI)[364] (**Level II-2**). To be effective, perioperative prophylaxis must be administered on schedule. A 1991 survey found that 83% patients undergoing abdominal or arterial surgery underwent inappropriate perioperative prophylaxis consisting of missed doses (35%), excessive duration (71%), or questionable agents (25%).[61] Established hospital guidelines with formal instruction of new surgical and anesthesia staff significantly reduce inappropriate antibiotic dosing, in particular with respect to prolonged administration, in up to 40% of cases.[61,62] According to the National Surgical Infection Prevention Project (**Level III**) that focused on the most commonly performed operations on Medicare patients, including colorectal surgery and abdominal and vaginal hysterectomy, for the majority of operations (single exception was cardiothoracic surgery) prophylaxis should end within 24 hours after the operation. This guideline is particularly important given the current ongoing battle with induction of bacterial resistance. Single antimicrobial is usually sufficient for most operations unless a coexisting infection is present or suspected[363] (**Level I**). Finally, the agent and dosing schedule should consist of the least expensive regimen that provides adequate protection.

Moreover, supplemental nonpharmacological measures such as intraoperative normothermia, supplemental oxygen, aggressive fluid resuscitation, and tight glucose control should not be forgotten as important steps in control of SSI[365–368] (**Levels I, II-2**).

Prophylaxis for Abdominal or Vaginal Hysterectomy

Significant febrile morbidity occurs in 20%–30% of abdominal and 30%–50% of vaginal hysterectomies. Although serious postoperative infections are uncommon after abdominal or vaginal hysterectomy (0%–1% vs. 1%–4%, respectively), prophylactic antibiotics are associated with a 5%–15% reduction in febrile morbidity.[73] Significant risk factors for infection include prolonged operative time, abdominal compared with vaginal surgery, premenopausal versus postmenopausal status, the absence of perioperative prophylactic antibiotics, and low socioeconomic status.[74] A meta-analysis inclusive of 25 prospective randomized studies published since 1971 found that patients not receiving antibiotic prophylaxis had significantly higher infection rates (21.2% compared with 9.0%, $p = 0.00001$); at least three drugs—cefazolin, metronidazole, and tinidazole—were found to be effective prophylactic agents. Based on these results, the authors proposed that the practice of withholding prophylactic antibiotics at the time of abdominal hysterectomy was no longer justifiable[75] (**Level I**).

For gynecologic oncology surgical procedures, skin, vaginal, or GI tract flora represents the most common source of endogenous pathogens. Endogenous skin pathogens include aerobic gram-positive cocci such as staphylococci or fecal flora if the incision is near the perineum or groin. If the vagina is incised intraoperatively, the surgical site will be exposed to polymicrobial aerobes and anaerobes. The same holds for GI flora: the high density of bacteria in the large intestine increases the risks for infectious complications in colorectal surgery or appendectomy due to appendicitis.[85] The most common pathogens involved in infectious morbidity following colorectal surgery include *Escherichia coli*, Klebsiella, Enterobacter, *B. fragilis*, Bacteroides sp., peptostreptococci, and Clostridia sp.[59] In the absence of obstruction, the proximal small bowel has no resident flora, and prophylaxis is unnecessary. With obstruction, the small bowel becomes contaminated with colonic flora and antibiotic prophylaxis is recommended.[59]

Due to low cost, long half-life, and low incidence of side effects and allergic reactions, cephalosporins are prophylactic antimicrobials of choice for most procedures, including abdominal and vaginal hysterectomies. In 1995, a randomized controlled trial published by Hemsell and colleagues found cefotetan to be superior to cefazolin as a single-dose prophylaxis in women undergoing elective abdominal hysterectomy.[369] Since then, other studies have reported that cefazolin and cefoxitin are acceptable alternatives with similar antimicrobial efficacy. In patients with immunoglobulin E mediated allergic reaction to cephalosporins, metronidazole or clindamycin in combination with gentamicin, quinolones, or aztreonam is an acceptable alternative[363,370] (**Level III**).

Although there are no recent trials focusing on prophylaxis in laparoscopically assisted hysterectomy, endogenous vaginal flora is also encountered with this surgical approach and therefore preoperative prophylaxis remains a reasonable option[370] (**Level III**).

Active bacterial vaginosis or trichomoniasis vaginitis at a time of hysterectomy increases the risk of postoperative vaginal cuff cellulitis[371] (**Level II-2**). In the open randomized controlled trial from Sweden, none of the 59 women with abnormal vaginal flora treated for at least 4 days with rectal metronidazole beginning just prior to surgery had postoperative vaginal cuff infections compared to 22 of 83 women (27%) in the "no treatment arm"[372] (**Level I**).

Several factors such as location of tumor, subclinical infections, malnutrition, and compromised immune response due to previous exposure to chemotherapy and pelvic radiation therapy may increase the risk of postoperative infections in patients undergoing radical pelvic surgery. As with other gynecologic oncology procedures, antibiotic prophylaxis with first-generation cephalosporins is adequate to prevent SSI. Broader spectrum coverage with multiple antibiotics was suggested as superior by Level III evidence (clinical experience, expert committee, descriptive studies), but as of today this has not been confirmed in large clinical trials.

Laparoscopy and Laparatomy

There are no trials to date that suggest a need for antibiotic prophylaxis for clean laparatomies that do not involve intestinal or vaginal resections. One randomized, placebo controlled study from Czechoslovakia also failed to show a benefit of cefazolin prophylaxis in women undergoing clean laparoscopic procedures[369,373] (**Level I**).

Bowel Preparation and Antibiotic Prophylaxis for Intestinal Surgery

Although mostly based on Level III evidence, mechanical bowel preparation has been a mainstay for prevention of infectious complications in colorectal surgery for more than a century. Based on clinical observational studies, mechanical bowel preparation reduces fecal mass and bacterial counts and ultimately decreases the risk of operative site infection. Furthermore, mechanical bowel preparation facilitates exposure and intestinal mobilization during laparoscopic surgery by cleansing the GI tract of feces and air.[378,379] In even as early as 1972, randomized controlled trials have painted a different picture: bowel preps are unnecessary, cumbersome, and time-consuming for patients, may increase risk of electrolyte disturbances and dehydration particularly in elderly, and may actually increase risk of intestinal wall inflammation[374-377] (**Level I**). Since then, multiple randomized controlled studies, meta-analyses, and Cochrane reviews have also questioned this dogma. In 2005, a Cochrane review of nine randomized studies with a total of 1592 patients suggested an increase in overall anastomotic leakage in a bowel prep group (6.2% vs. 3.2%; $OR = 2.03, p = 0.003$). In a subgroup analysis based on the location of the anastomosis—low anterior resection vs. other colon sites—this difference was not statistically significant[16] (**Level I**). Five additional trials were incorporated in a 2008 Cochrane review resulting in a total of 4821 participants admitted for elective colorectal surgery. Patients with colorectal cancer were also included in this review. No statistically significant difference between mechanical vs. no bowel prep group was found in regard to wound infection, mortality rate, peritonitis, other abdominal infections, or need for reoperation. Furthermore, in this analysis there was no statistically significant difference in a rate of overall anastomotic leakage (4.2% bowel prep vs. 3.4% no bowel prep; $OR = 1.1$) or leakage stratified by the anastomotic site—low anterior resection vs. colon surgery[379] (**Level I**). The latest meta-analysis published in February 2009 included 14 trials with a total of 2452 patients who had mechanical bowel prep and 2407 patients who did not. The primary outcome was anastomotic breakdown and secondary outcome "septic complications" such as wound infections and postoperative morbidity rates. Overall there was no statistically significant difference in the rate of anastomotic breakdown, wound infections, abdominal or pelvic postoperative abscess rate, extra-abdominal sepsis, reoperation, or death in patients with bowel prep vs. no bowel prep (**Level I**). On the other hand, "all SSI" rate was slightly higher in the bowel prep group: 15.7% vs. 14.58% in no bowel prep group ($OR = 1.4$, $p = 0.02$).[380] It should be noted that majority of trials in this analysis excluded rectal surgery and hence outcomes associated with rectosigmoid anastomosis.

In light of the above it can be concluded that prophylactic mechanical bowel preparation prior to open colorectal surgery does not improve patient outcomes. In regard to laparoscopic approach, debate is ongoing. Some experts argue that it is easier to manipulate bowel with solid matter and thusly visualize the field while the others argue quite the opposite (**Level III**).[378,379] Randomized controlled trials focusing on laparoscopic intestinal resection and anastomosis will be necessary to answer this question appropriately.

If mechanical bowel preparation is elected prior to laparoscopic procedures, available bowel cleansing methods include the following: clear liquid intake with cathartics and/or enemas the evening and morning before surgery until efflux is clear; Golitely[R]—an isotonic solution of polyethylene glycol, sodium sulfate, NaCl, and KCl that induces diarrhea within 3–4 hours following oral intake; and oral sodium phosphate solution such as Fleets Phospho Soda^R that induces diarrhea within 3–6 hours. It should be noted that most recently, oral sodium phosphate solution has been linked to an increased risk of acute phosphate nephropathy particularly in the elderly (>62 years of age), in patients with renal dysfunction or dehydration, or in patients who use medications that may affect renal function (e.g., ACE inhibitors, angiotensin receptor blockers, diuretics, nonsteroidal anti-inflammatory drugs [NSAIDs]).[381,382] Therefore, oral sodium phosphate bowel preparation should be used with caution and avoided in patients at risk of renal failure (**Level II-2**). Most patients will tolerate bowel preps but not without side effects such as fullness, cramps, nausea, and vomiting; occasionally NG tube placement and/or antiemetics are necessary to complete an adequate prep. Furthermore, it should be noted that poor oral intake and multiple bowel cleansing for tests and for the surgical preparation predispose the patient to hypovolemia, the extent of which is often underestimated. In patients with little cardiac reserve, hypovolemia may induce clinically significant increases in cardiac work, hypotension, as well as increase in operative blood loss. Adequate pre- and intraoperative hydration helps to reduce these adverse effects. For patients at increased risk, potassium levels should be checked early on the morning of surgery and losses replaced (**Level II-3**).

Antibiotic Prophylaxis   In addition to mechanical bowel cleansing, infectious morbidity following colorectal surgery is significantly reduced by oral, parenteral, or a combination of oral and parenteral antibiotic prophylaxis, especially when the duration of surgery exceeds 3.5–4 hours (**Level II-2**).[89] By reducing bacterial counts,[90] oral antibiotics reduce the risks of postoperative wound infection from 43% to 9% compared with mechanical bowel cleansing alone.[90] The "gold standard" is oral prophylaxis, which consists of neomycin combined with either erythromycin or metronidazole, 1 g each at 1 p.m., 2 p.m., and 11 p.m. the evening before surgery, after completion of bowel cleansing.[90,91] The use of intravenous agents including cefoxitin, ceftriaxone/metronidazole, or cefotaxime/metronidazole in addition to oral prophylaxis has recently become a more common practice. Although some studies have demonstrated no benefit,[92] others have found that systemic agents significantly reduce infection rates compared with oral agents used alone.[93–96] When oral agents were not given, cefotaxime/metronidazole was found to be superior prophylaxis compared with aztreonam/metronidazole, presumably because azetreonam provides little activity against gram-positive organisms; in this study, *staphylococcus* was found to be the major organism involved in postoperative surgical sepsis and abscess formation.[97] Intravenous antibiotics should also be given when surgery is delayed beyond 12 hours past the last oral antibiotic dose. When there is insufficient time to complete an oral bowel preparation, parenteral prophylaxis should be extended to cover gram-negative bacilli and anaerobic organisms. Options include the addition of clindamycin or metronidazole with an aminoglycoside, or cefoxitin (2 g), that is continued for 24 hours postoperatively. Contaminated cases involving fecal spillage should be treated with broad-spectrum antibiotic therapy, which is continued for a full therapeutic course.

Other Indications for Antibiotic Prophylaxis

Endocarditis Prophylaxis   According to the latest AHA (the American Heart Association) guidelines from 2007, there is no published data that demonstrates evidence of an increased risk of infectious endocarditis during GI or GU tract procedures, antibiotic prophylaxis is not recommended for this patient population[383] (**Level II-1**). Only patients with an ongoing GI or GU tract infection or those who receive antibiotics to prevent wound infection associated with GI or GU tract procedure may have a higher risk of intermittent or sustained enterococcal bacteremia. In the absence of overt GI or GU tract infection, the risk of sustained enterecoccus bacteremia associated with these procedures is less than 5%. Patients at highest risk of adverse outcomes associated with endocarditis usually have the following cardiac conditions: prosthetic valves or prosthetic material used for valve repair; history of infectious endocarditis; congenital heart disease including unrepaired cyanotic congenital heart disease, with or without palliative shunts and conduits, completely repaired congenital heart disease with prosthetic material during the first 6 months after the procedure, repaired congenital heart disease with residual defects at the site or adjacent to the site of a prosthetic device; cardiac transplantation and cardiac vulvopathy. As per AHA 2007 guidelines prophylaxis with ampicillin, amoxicillin, piperacillin, or vancomycin (in patients with penicillin allergy) should be used only for these highest risk patients who have an established GI or GU tract infection or who would have received antibiotic prophylaxis to prevent wound infection or sepsis associated with GI or GU tract procedure[383] (**Level II-1**).

Intensive-Care Patients and Special Considerations   Critically ill patients are especially susceptible to hospital-acquired infections. Predisposing factors include altered resistance of the digestive tract and oropharynx, underlying disease, advanced age, medical and surgical interventions, prolonged ICU admissions, and altered immune response (**Level II-2**).[99–101] Nosocomial colonization of the oropharyngeal and digestive system in mechanically ventilated patients approaches 70%–90%, and over 60% of colonized patients subsequently become infected (**Level I**).[102] Pathogens involved are predominantly gram-negative microorganisms (*Enterobacteriaceae* or *Pseudomonas* species). Oral tobramycin, amphotericin B, and polymixin E reduce endotracheal and GI colonization, and in critically ill patients requiring ICU admission and ventilatory support, reduced nosocomial infection rates by 60.7% (**Level I**).[102] The use of nystatin "swish and swallow" (5–10 cc of nystatin [100,000 U/cc]) prophylactically has been found to reduce the incidence of *Candida* wound infection and systemic candidiasis (**Level II-1**)[103] and should be used routinely in patients with granulocytopenia, on broad-spectrum antibiotics, or following radical pelvic or GI procedures.

Neutropenic patients who develop fever are at high risk for infection that, without appropriate therapy, may rapidly develop into sepsis and death. Broad-spectrum beta-lactam-antibiotic/beta-lactamase-inhibitor combinations such as ticarcillin/clavulanate, alone or in combination with aminoglycosides, are the agents of choice for neutropenic fever.[81] Klastersky et al. demonstrated that, in combination with an aminoglycoside, extended-spectrum penicillins (azlocillin, meszlocillin, and pipercillin) compared with extended-spectrum cephalosporins (cefoxtaxime, moxalactam, cefoperazone) are more active against gram-negative bacteremias in febrile granulocytopenic patients (**Level I**).[104]

Whenever possible, antibiotics should be directed against the specific organism(s) involved, and should be given for the shortest possible effective time. Healthy intestinal mucosa functions as a protective barrier to prevent bacteria from invading the host. When the normal endogenous microflora is altered by prolonged antibiotic use, endotoxemia, impaired host defenses, or injury, bacteria within the GI tract can pass through the epithelial mucosa to infect mesenteric lymph nodes, a process known as bacterial translocation (**Level II-3**).[99, 105, 106] Translocation of pathogens contributes to the development of sepsis syndrome, septic shock, and multiorgan failure which carries a mortality rate (30%–100%).[107, 108] Intravenous antibiotics, especially clindamycin, cephalosporins, and ampicillin (or amoxicillin), are frequently associated with the development of diarrhea and/or pseudomembraneous colitis.[109–116] Alteration in the normal gut flora from antibiotic use or bowel preps permits the overgrowth of a gram-positive anaerobic bacillus, *Clostridium difficile*. Heat-resistant spores produced by the organism are very hearty, and may persist in the environment for years. Infection is by oral-fecal contamination. Diarrhea and colitis result from colonization of the colon by toxin-producing strains of *C. difficile*; strains incapable of producing toxins are not pathogenic. Although fewer than 1% of healthy adults are carriers, approximately 25% of adults recently treated with antibiotics are colonized with *C. difficile*, and most carriers remain asymptomatic.[110, 114] Although the treatment of asymptomatic carriers is not recommended, colonized health-care providers may be an important source of infection in hospitalized and immunocompromised patients.[116] Other factors that increase susceptibility include chemotherapy, severe debilitation, and hospitalization.[109, 110, 112, 113, 116] Reported outbreaks of this organism in intensive care units (ICUs) involving patients not receiving antibiotics emphasize the nosocomial nature of this infection and the importance of vector transmission (bed pans, floors, toilets, and shelves where bedpans are stored).[114] *C. difficile* infection usually presents with mild to moderate diarrhea, occasionally accompanied by lower abdominal cramping. Most patients lack systemic symptoms including fever or chills, and other than slight tenderness in the lower abdomen, physical examination is normal. Severe colitis with or without pseudomembrane formation may occur, and it is associated with profuse, debilitating diarrhea, abdominal pain, and distention. Rarely, patients present with an acute abdomen and fulminant, life-threatening colitis. These patients are acutely ill, with lethargy, fever, abdominal pain, marked abdominal distension, and toxic megacolon. A history of recent antibiotic use, and the presence of *C. difficile* toxins (toxin A or B) in the stool, confirms the diagnosis.[116] Although lower abdominal endoscopy (proctosigmoidoscopy/colonoscopy) is the only diagnostic test for pseudomembranous colitis, it is expensive, invasive, insensitive (51%–55%), and should be avoided when fulminant colitis is present because of the risk of perforation.[110] Whenever possible, the first step in treatment is discontinuation of antibiotics, and in mild cases this is the only intervention required.[116] Since life-threatening toxic megacolon[115] or bowel perforation has been associated with their use, in addition to the potential risks of increased metronidazole systemic absorption, reducing its effectiveness, antiperistaltic agents (e.g., Lomotil, G.D. Searle and Co, Chicago, IL) should be avoided alone or in conjunction with antibiotic therapy.[112] When symptoms are persistent or severe, or when antibiotic therapy must be continued, the treatment of choice is oral metronidazole (250 mg four times per day), or vancomycin (125 mg four times per day) when symptoms persist or metronidaxole is not tolerated. More severe symptoms require intravenous hydration, and when patients cannot tolerate oral medication because of ileus or recent abdominal surgery, they may be effectively treated with metronidazole (but not vancomycin) intravenously.[111, 116] Alternative agents include bacitracin, anion-exchange resins, rifampin, and ciprofloxacin (but not norfloxacin). In most instances, symptomatic relapses should be treated with metronidazole or vancomycin rather than second-line therapy, and asymptomatic colonization in patients with a history of *C. difficile* diarrhea do not require retreatment. For those patients who must receive antibiotic therapy, antimicrobial agents, infrequently or rarely associated with *C. difficile*, such as aminoglycosides, bacitracin, metronidazole, or quinolones, should be considered (**Level II-2**).[111, 116]

Prevention of Venous Thromboembolism

Major risk factors predisposing to the development of venous thromboembolism (VTE) as defined by Virchow's triad include hypercoagulability, venous stasis, and vessel injury. Compared with patients without malignant disease, active cancer increases risk of thrombotic events by 4.1-fold and chemotherapy by 6.5-fold.[384, 385] This increased baseline risk of venous thromboembolic disease may be further compounded by the presence of other risk factors commonly identified in patients with malignancy (Table 6.6 and 6.7).[386]

Following gynecologic surgery, the majority of pulmonary emboli arise from venous thrombosis of the deep lower extremity leg and pelvic veins. Using I

Table 6.6   Risk Factors for VTE

Age 60 years or older[387–389]
Race: VTE risk is increased in African American population and
  decreased in Asian-Pacific islanders[390]
History of VTE[389, 391]
Inherited or acquired thrombophilia[392–395]
Cancer site (pancreas, lung, ovary, stomach, brain, renal,
  lymphoma)[386, 390, 395, 396]
Initial 3–6 months after diagnosis[386, 390, 391, 395]
Metastatic disease[389, 395]
Elevated prechemotherapy platelet count (>350,000)[386, 391, 396]
Erythropoiesis-stimulating agents[397]
Immunomodulator, antiangiogenesis, and hormonal therapy (e.g.,
  thalidomide, bevacizumab, tamoxifen)[398–402]
Surgery[385]
Radiation[389, 391]
Presence of central venous catheters[385, 389, 391]

Table 6.7 Risk Factors for Deep Venous Thrombosis[117–119,121] (Level II-2)[a]

Risk Factor	Etiology	Comment
Older age	Activation of peripheral vascular system; increased venous stasis	Risk increases exponentially above 50 years of age
Malignancy	Increased thromboplastin and other procoagulants produced by malignant tissues; direct tumor extension or compression of veins	Increases risk —three- to fivefold
Immobility; operative time	Venous dilation and stasis; reduced mechanical fibrinolysis	
Obesity	Increased venous stasis; impaired fibrinolytic activity	
Varicose veins	Increased venous stasis; minor varicosities not significant	Increases risk twofold
Pregnancy; oral contraceptives[b]	Increased factor VII and X activity and platelet aggregation; decreased anti-thrombin III activity	Increases risk four- to sevenfold; Dissipates 6–8 weeks after discontinuation of pregnancy or contraceptive use
Previous thromboembolic event		Increases risk two- to threefold
Surgery/trauma	Venous stasis; activation of coagulation system	Risk dependent on length of surgery and type of procedure performed. Risk with gynecologic surgery: 7–45%
Hypercoagulable states; inherited risk factors	Deficiencies of protein S, C, anti-thrombin III; antiphospholipid antibody syndromes	
Smoking	Nicotine-induced reduction in venous stasis; improved fibrinolysis	Increases risk threefold

[a] Adapted from Reference 118.
[b] Postmenopausal hormone replacement therapy does not alter coagulation factors.

125-fibrinogen uptake tests, it has been demonstrated that the thrombotic process usually starts in the calf veins (**Level II-2**). The majority of thrombi within the calf veins remains localized and resolve spontaneously. However, approximately 20% propagates into the proximal thigh and pelvic veins, and about 50% develops into pulmonary emboli, the majority of which are not fatal.[121–123] Thrombosis may originate in the pelvic veins, but this is usually in association with trauma to the veins, such as occuring at the time of a lymphadenectomy. In the absence of perioperative prophylaxis, the incidence of deep venous thrombosis (DVT) in surgical setting is approximately 20% and the incidence of PE is 1%–2%. Following gynecologic surgery, the incidence of fatal pulmonary emboli is estimated to be 0.01%–0.87%, and accounts for approximately 40% of all postoperative deaths.[121, 124, 125] In general, VTE is the number one preventable cause of death in hospitalized patients. Two-thirds of patients die from pulmonary emboli within half an hour of the onset of symptoms, and approximately 80% of pulmonary emboli occur in the absence of clinical signs of peripheral venous thrombosis.[126] Since the majority of pulmonary emboli arise from thrombi developing in the deep veins of the pelvis or legs, prevention of thromboembolic events should be aimed at the cause, alterations in coagulability, and venous stasis (Fig. 6.3).

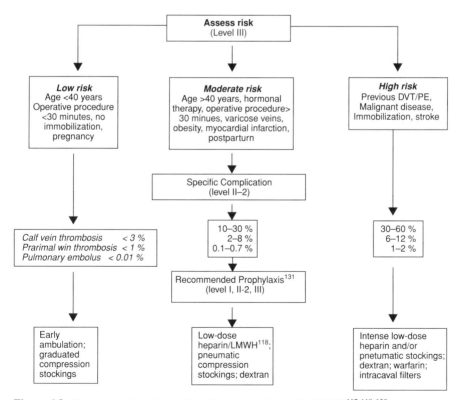

Figure 6.3   Deep venous thrombosis risk and prophylaxis (Levels I, II-2, III).[117, 118, 138]

VTE in cancer patients results in greater in-hospital mortality rate (with or without metastatic disease), threefold greater risk of fatal PE, threefold greater risk of VTE recurrence, and twofold greater risk of bleeding complications while on anticoagulation therapy.[403,404] Extrapolating from a Danish registry of more than 34,000 cancer patients and their mortality data, cancer patients with concurrent VTE have 1-year survival rate of 12% vs. 36% for cancer patients without VTE.[405] Two major methods for postoperative VTE prophylaxis in cancer patients include mechanical calf compression devices and pharmacological agents (Table 6.8). Physical measures that decrease venous stasis, such as intermittent pneumatic compression (IPC) stockings, have been shown to decrease incidence of DVT postoperatively **(Level I)**.[135–137] In a controlled study of 107 patients undergoing surgery for gynecologic malignancy VTE was reduced threefold with use of external pneumatic compression device before induction of anesthesia and during the first 5 postoperative days. (34.6% patients with VTE in a control group vs. 12.7% in a treated group p < 0.05) **(Level II-1)**.[406] Three randomized controlled trials and one retrospective study focusing on gynecologic surgical patients showed that incidence of postoperative DVT (ranging between 1% and 6.5%) was similar when either IPC stockings, unfractionated heparin (UFH), or low molecular weight heparin (LMWH) alone was used **(Level I)**.[407–410] IPC as a single-agent prophylaxis may be sufficient to lower the incidence of DVTs; however, none of these studies have shown effectiveness of IPC as a single-agent prophylaxis in decreasing the incidence of PE and its subsequent morbidity and mortality in cancer patients. Furthermore, among patients in whom IPC was used as a single-agent prophylaxis there was a subgroup at "higher risk" of IPC failure. These "high risk patients" characterized as having two or more risk factors (60 years or older, prior history of VTE, active cancer diagnosis) could have benefited from a combined prophylaxis approach.[410] Subsequently, Martino and colleagues have shown that IPC alone is not sufficient for VTE prophylaxis in patients with cancer who were undergoing major abdominal surgery: 4.1% incidence of PE vs. 0.3% in patients with benign disease (OR = 13.8, p < 0.001) **(Level II-3)**.[411] Combined method for VTE prophylaxis was also found to be more effective in a Cochrane review of 19 studies including the highest risk population undergoing colorectal cancer surgery: dual-agent prophylaxis with mechanical and pharmacological therapy (low dose UFH) was four times more effective for VTE prevention than low dose UFH alone.[412]

Pharmacological VTE prophylaxis for surgical and cancer patients has been investigated in several large clinical trials. Initial trials focused on low dose UFH followed by trials on LMWH (enoxaparin and dalteparin). Most recently, studies on indirect factor Xa inhibitor fondaparinaux were published (Table 6.9).[413]

Low dose UFH has been extensively studied in cancer patients. In 1975 an international multicenter trial that included 953 patients with malignancy reported a decrease in frequency of postoperative PE from 0.8% in the control group to 0.1% in the group that received subcutaneous doses of unfractionated heparin after a variety of elective major surgical procedures.[414] Meta-analysis published in 1988 showed that low dose of UFH was also efficient as postoperative DVT prophylaxis in general surgical patients: in 919 patients with malignant disease (data pooled from 10 trials)

Table 6.8 Perioperative Thromboembolism Prophylaxis

Method	Dose	Indications	Mechanism	Drawbacks	Benefits
Low dose heparin	5000 IU/IM 2 hours pre-op and q 12 hours post-op[b,127]	Moderate risk	Increased AT-III activity; inactivation of factors Xa, thrombin; possibly coats endothelial walls; decreases thrombogenesis	Bleeding complications[127]; wound hematomas[141], ↑transfusions[139]; ↑retroperitoneal drain output; thrombocytopenia[118]	Decreased risk of DVT from 7%–45% to 6.2%–11.9%[142]; easy to administer and highly effective
LMWH[c]	2500 IU/IM 2 hours pre-op and daily for 7–10 days[130]	Moderate to high risk	Similar to heparin	High DVT rates[118]; ↑bleeding complications especially with doses >5000 IU/day[118,143]	Single daily injection effective as low dose heparin[132,143]; fewer bleeding complications[142] Probably not as effective as heparin[143]
DHE[d]	0.5 mg post-op 2 hours pre-op and twice daily post-op[b]	Not recommended	Selective venoconstrictor; decreases venous stasis	Vasoconstrictive complications: bowel necrosis, vascular spasm, skin/muscle necrosis, many contraindications[145]	
DHE and heparin/LMWH	0.5 mg post-op and 5000 IU H or 1500 IU/IM LMWH[143] 2 hours pre-op and daily post-op	High risk			No more effective than low dose heparin, or LMWH[135,143]

(Continued)

Table 6.8 (*Continued*)

Method	Dose	Indications	Mechanism	Drawbacks	Benefits
Dextran 70[e]	1 L IV/q 6 hours at onset of surgery; effects last 7 days	Moderate to high risk	↑Microcirculation; antiplatelet activity; increases fibrinolysis; alters factors V, VIII[117]	↑Risks for CHF, renal failure, bleeding complications, allergic reactions, anaphylaxis (0.001–0.1%)[142]; avoid use with heparin	Volume expander; probably as effective as heparin[117,135]
Pneumatic compression stockings	Placed at induction of anesthesia	Moderate to high risk	↑Venous flow velocity; decreases venous stasis[146]	Patient discomfort rare	As effective as heparin, even in high risk patients; few or no contraindictions[137]

[a] High risk patients may alternatively be treated with one or two 5000 IU q 8 hours preoperatively and q 8 hours postoperatively for 7–10 days.[139]
[b] Postoperative administration.
[c] Low molecular weight heparin.
[d] Dihydroergotamine.
[e] Alternatively, Dextran 70, 500 m/IV every 4 hours daily for 2–5 days after surgery.
[f] Contraindicated in pregnancy, hypertension, coronary artery disease, renal failure, or in patients using β-adrenergic antagonists or dopamine.

Table 6.9 National Comprehensive Cancer Network recommendations for inpatient VTE prophylaxis

Agent	Mechanism of Action	Dosing
Unfractionated heparin	Inactivates thrombin and activated coagulation factors (IX, X, XI, XII, and plasmin) while potentiating effects of antithrombin Inhibits conversion of fibrinogen to fibrin	5000 U SQ every 8 hours
Low molecular weight heparins	Inhibit factor Xa and thrombin (IIA) with higher ratio of antifactor Xa to antifactor IIA activity	
○ Enoxaparin		40 mg SQ daily
○ Dalteparin		5000 U SQ daily
○ Tinzaparin		4500 IU SQ daily
Fondaparinux	Synthetic heparin pentsaccharide analog Selectively inhibits factor Xa via antithrombin-mediated mechanism	2.5 mg SQ daily

low dose UFH reduced incidence of postoperative DVT from 30.6% in the control group to 13.3% in the treated group.[415] Low dose UFH should be administered at a dose of 5000 U subcutaneously 2 hours before surgery and then every 8 hours after surgery for VTE prevention in cancer patients (**Level I**). Earlier trials focused on dosing regimens of UFH have shown that in cancer patients UFH is ineffective when administered at a dose of 5000 U every 12 hours.[408] On the other hand, when given every 8 hours UFH decreased DVT incidence from 19% in a control group to 4% in a treatment group[409] (**Level I**).

Subsequently, multiple trials confirmed similar efficacy of LMWH and UFH in the prevention of VTE in patients with cancer (**Level I**). One such trial, ENOXACAN I, a prospective, double-blind, randomized multicenter trial, evaluated the use of LMWH 40 mg SQ daily vs. UFH 5000 U subcutaneously every 8 hours for 8–12 days postoperatively in patients over 40 years of age undergoing elective curative abdominal or pelvic surgery for cancer. Primary outcome was incidence of VTE detected by mandatory bilateral venography or pulmonary scintigraphy at 30 days or 3 months. Enoxaparin and UFH were equally effective in reducing episodes of early onset VTE (14.7% vs. 18.2%) and were both associated with a similar risk of bleeding and other complications.[416] Most recently, fondaparinux, a selective indirect Xa inhibitor, was studied in the ARTEMIS trial which investigated incidence of VTE in placebo vs. treatment group of older acutely medically ill patients treated with 2.5 mg of subcutaneous fondaparinux daily. Fifteen percent of enrolled patients in this study had a current or past cancer diagnosis. VTE incidence was significantly lower in a treatment group (5.6% vs. 10.5% with an RR reduction of 46.7%, $p = 0.029$).[417]

Finally, results from two recent randomized controlled trials and one retrospective trial focusing on gynecologic cancer patient population suggested that prolonged postoperative VTE prophylaxis is more effective in reducing incidence of VTE, especially in the highest risk patients, i.e., patients with previous history of VTE, obesity, and who underwent major abdominal surgery leaving large residual disease burden (**Level I**). ENOXACAN II, a double-blind multicenter randomized study, evaluated short-term (6–10 days) vs. long-term (4 weeks) postoperative prophylaxis with enoxaparin in patients undergoing planned curative open surgery for abdominal or pelvic cancer. The primary end point was incidence of VTE between days 25 and 31 as detected by mandatory bilateral venography or sooner if symptoms of VTE developed. The rates of VTE were significantly reduced in patients who received 4 weeks of prophylaxis (4.8% in treatment group vs. 12% for patients who received 6–10 days of enoxaparin followed by placebo) ($p = 0.02$). This difference also persisted at a 3-month follow-up visit (5.5% vs. 1.8%) ($p = 0.01$). The incidence of major or minor bleeding complications was similar.[418] Similarly, a multicenter randomized European trial that investigated efficacy of prolonged thromboprophylaxis with 5000U of dalteparin daily for 4 weeks after a major abdominal surgery reported a decrease in VTE incidence from 16.3% in a short-term (7 days) prophylaxis group to 7.3% in a prolonged prophylaxis group (RR reduction 55%, $p = 0.012$). More than half of the patients in each group underwent surgery for malignancy, with colorectal resection being the most common surgical procedure. For the majority of patients, surgery was curative. The incidence of bleeding complications was once again similar.[419] It should be noted that both ENOXACAN II and the European trial used asymptomatic DVT diagnosed by means of venography as the primary end point for efficacy. Furthermore, majority of diagnosed DVTs were distal calf-vein DVTs, which, as noted previously, frequently resolve spontaneously.

Most recently, a retrospective case-control study focused on dual VTE prophylaxis with sequential compression devices and prolonged 2-week postoperative anticoagulation with either heparin TID or daily LMWH in gynecologic cancer patient population. In particular, prolonged dual prophylaxis was instituted in patients over 60 years of age, with malignancy and/or history of prior VTE episode. Prior to the universal dual protocol, VTE prophylaxis at this institution consisted of IPC only prior to induction of anesthesia and continued until discharge. The incidence of PE or DVT diagnosed within 6 weeks of surgery was calculated for the "prior to protocol" era and for "universal prolonged dual prophylaxis" era: 6.5% patients with VTE in the former vs. 1.9% in the latter group. There were no major differences in bleeding complications (**Level II-2**).[420]

Based on the above and other published evidence, current ASCO (American Society of Clinical Oncology) and ACCP (American College of Chest Physicians) consensus guidelines for cancer patients undergoing surgery advocate use of either low dose UFH every 8 hours or LMWH or fondaparinux daily, as early as possible for at least 7–10 days unless contraindicated (Grade 1A recommendation). Prolonged prophylaxis with LMWH administered for up to 4 weeks should be considered in high risk patients who are older, obese, have residual malignant disease, and/or a previous history of VTE. Mechanical IPC may be added to prophylaxis regimen in highest risk patients but should not be used alone unless anticoagulation is contraindicated.[386]

An alternative to anticoagulation in patients with high risk of both VTE and hemorrhage due to anticoagulation is fluoroscopic placement of vena cava filters preoperatively. Pulmonary complications are uncommon and similar in frequency to those of CVP placement i.e., pneumothorax, arrhythmias, and vascular injury; however, since clots may propagate above the filter, and patients may develop extensive venous thrombosis associated with debilitating leg edema, even when coincident anticoagulation is used, filters should be reserved for the high risk patient.[141]

GI Bleeding Prophylaxis

Bleeding within the upper GI tract secondary to stress ulcers and aggravated by NG intubation is a potentially life-threatening complication in perioperative patients. Histamine type 2 (H2) blockers such as ranitidine and cimetidine, and/or antacids, are frequently prescribed as prophylaxis against stress-induced bleeding.[148, 149] Antacids, which inhibit peptic activity, and H2 blockers, which inhibit gastric acid secretion, reduce bleeding risks by elevating gastric pH.[150, 151] Dose efficacy is dependent on the elevation of pH in the 3–5 range, which requires serial gastric pH determinations. Unfortunately, gastric acidity is an important physiological mechanism that prevents upper GI tract colonization with enteric pathogens, and may predispose to pneumonia. Hospital-acquired pneumonia, a complication of 0.5%–1% of all patients undergoing hospitalization, is the leading cause of death secondary to nosocomial infection.[152] Sucralfate is a weak buffer that probably acts through pepsin adsorption, mucosal protein binding, and cytoprotection.[153] In a comparative study of sucralfate and H2 blockers with/without antacids, sucralfate administration resulted in reduced gastric colonization by gram-negative bacteria that was associated with lower rates of hospital-acquired pneumonia and reduced mortality, without increasing the incidence of gastric bleeding (**Level I**).[154]

Adrenal Insufficiency and Steroid Prophylaxis

The stress of surgery leads to an increase of adrenal corticosteroids. With adrenal insufficiency, circulatory shock may result secondary to inability of the adrenal glands to produce the necessary glucocorticoids. Basal, daily adrenal cortisol production is the equivalent of hydrocortisone (30 mg) or prednisone (7.5 mg). Corticosteriods are given for a variety of medical conditions. Exogenous steroids may suppress the hypothalamic-pituitary-adrenal axis; doses equivalent to 20–30 mg of prednisone/day for at least 1 week are probably sufficient to produce adrenal suppression, and recovery of the adrenal glands may take up to 1 year.[155, 156] Cosyntropin, a synthetic ACTH, can be utilized in a dose of 25 U, intramuscularly or intravenously, as a stimulation test to assess the integrity of the hypothalamic-pituitary-adrenal axis. Cortisol levels are measured before and 60 minutes after the injection. Normal values, indicating sufficient adrenal reserve for the stresses of surgery, are an absolute rise in cortisol of 7 μg, a doubling of the baseline control value, or a stimulated value greater than 18 μg.[157] Patients with a history of suppressive dose of exogenous steroids within 1 year prior to surgery or those with an abnormal suppression test need perioperative stress doses of glucocorticoids. Traditionally, these doses have been four times the current steroid dosage.[158] Studies have demonstrated that the normal adrenal output of cortisol is about 75–150 mg/day in response to major surgery, and 50 mg/day during minor surgery, with cortisol secretion in the first 24 hours after surgery rarely exceeding 200 mg.[158] There is no data to support that administration of doses exceeding this amount is beneficial. After major surgery, plasma cortisol levels usually return to normal within 24–48 hours. Postoperative complications such as infection require continued administration of stress doses of glucocorticoids. As soon as the patient is able to tolerate oral intake, the preoperative steroid dose is resumed. A tapering of the steroid dose is probably not necessary unless the patient has been on prolonged, high doses of glucocorticoids (**Level II-3**).

High dose glucocorticoids may increase susceptibility to infection secondary to suppression of the immune response, and may have adverse effects on wound healing. Consequently, assessment of the hypothalamic-pituitary-adrenal axis is recommended whenever possible to avoid steroid administration. The current recommendation for major surgical corticosteroid stress dosage is the equivalent of hydrocortisone, 100 mg given intraoperatively and every 8 hours postoperatively for 24 hours.[159] Although these doses may be excessive, until lower doses of perioperative steroids have been evaluated in a large number of patients, physiological doses cannot be recommended (**Level II-3**).[158]

Splenectomized Patients

Splenectomy is rarely indicated as part of cytoreductive surgery for ovarian cancer, and is occasionally performed to control bleeding from capsular avulsion, usually resulting from traction in the course of total omentectomy.[160, 161] Splenectomized patients are at increased risks for left lower lobe atelectasis, thrombocytosis, and increased infection risks. In these patients, postoperative care should emphasize deep breathing exercises, broad-spectrum prophylactic antibiotics, and administration of 0.5 mL pneumococcal polyvalent vaccine (Pneumovax[R], Merck, Sharp & Dome). Thrombocytosis (platelet counts in the range of 625,000–1,221,000 mg/dL) has been reported in up to 66% of these patients and is usually detected 2–3 weeks postoperatively. Although it does not affect platelet counts, low dose heparin therapy is generally advocated in the immediate postoperative period, because of the risks for DVT and pulmonary embolus (**Level II-2**).[160]

GENERAL PROBLEMS IN POSTOPERATIVE MANAGEMENT

Initial Management in the Postoperative Recovery Room Area

Until the effects of anesthesia are reversed and function (physiological and mental) returns, adequate oxygenation, airway maintenance, frequent monitoring of vital signs, and correcting hypothermia are primary concerns. Untoward complications of anesthesia (neuromuscular blockade, hyperthermia, bronchospasm, or cardiovascular or respiratory insufficiency) should be recognized immediately and therapy instituted. Fluid, electrolyte, and blood product replacement are instigated based on vital signs, urinary output, and preexisting deficits or excesses. In addition to immediate replacement needs, postoperative orders (Fig. 6.4) define activity level, doses and frequency of analgesia and other medications, which physical parameters are to be measured and how often, and other care needs specific for each patient in the recovery area and after transfer to the wards. All hypothermic patients should be actively treated with warming therapy. Shivering can be suppressed by application of heat to the patients' skin, or with sedation (meperidine 15–25 mg intravenously). Traditional methods of warming patients (warmed cotton blankets, warmed intravenous fluids, and use of warm water mattresses) provide little benefit. Hypothermia may be successfully treated or prevented by the use of heated and humidified inspired gases, maintaining an ambient operating room temperature over 80°C whenever possible, use of radiant heat, and use of convective warming therapy consisting of a disposable plastic and tissue paper cover that is inflated with warm air from its heating unit (**Level II-2**).[14, 162]

In uncomplicated patients, recovery care is safely accomplished in 1–2 hours in a specifically designed unit. Criticaly ill patients requiring aggressive hemodynamic monitoring, inotropic agents, or ventilatory support should undergo postoperative recovery in an ICU supervised by a critical care team of doctors, nurses, nutritionalists, and respiratory therapists (**Level III**). When postoperative intensive unit care is anticipated, preoperative consultation with critical care team is preferable.

Fluid and Electrolyte Replacement

Immediately postoperatively, fluid, electrolytes, and/or blood product replacement is guided by clinical, and when indicated, laboratory assessment of the patient's postoperative volume status. The uncomplicated surgical patient who is NPO requires 2000–3000 cc/day to compensate for insensible losses and to maintain urinary output at approximately 1000–1500 cc/day (minimum 0.5 cc/kg/hour).[6] Solutions (Table 6.10) that also replace physiological and excess losses of sodium, potassium, magnesium, calcium, and glucose are commercially available.[163] Volume replacement should be based on the preoperative volume status, intraoperative losses and replacement, and compartmental shifts in cellular water that occur in response to surgical

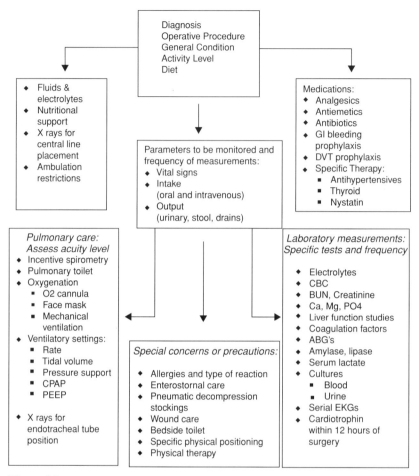

Figure 6.4   Postoperative orders (Levels II-2, II-3, III).

stress. Additional fluids are required to compensate for increased losses from postoperative fever, gastric suctioning, third space losses resulting from sequestration of fluid within the bowel lumen or actual losses, as from abrupt drainage of ascites. GI losses should be replaced based on the electrolyte and acid–base composition of the source of loss (Table 6.1). A solution that is isotonic with plasma with additional potassium and chloride is required to correct for gastric losses, whereas small intestinal losses (ileostomies, fistula, or obstruction) benefit from isotonic saline replacement with added sodium bicarbonate.[4,6] Diarrhea losses typically require replacement with hypotonic buffered solutions.[6] A useful guide for replacement is that approximately one third of the volume of isotonic fluid given will remain in the intravascular space, and the remainder will redistribute into the interstitium or within cells (**Level II-3**).

Postoperative *hyponatremia* most frequently results from fluid replacement in excess of water loss.[4] Additional causes include hyperglycemia, physiological and

Table 6.10   Composition of Common Parenteral Fluids[a]

	Cation (mEq/L)					Anion (mEq/L)			
Solution	Na+	K+	Ca+	Mg+	NH_{4+}	Cl−	HCO_{4-}	HPO^4_{3-}	Protein
Plasma	142	4	5	3	0.3	103	27	3	
Intracellular fluid	10	150		40		10		150	40
Ringer's lactate[b]	130	4	2.7			109	28*		
0.9% sodium chloride (normal saline)	154					154			
0.45% sodium chloride (half-normal saline)	77					77			
3% sodium chloride	513					513			
5% sodium chloride	855					855			
0.9% ammonium chloride	168					168			

[a]Modified from Reference 203.
[b]Lactate in solution is converted to bicarbonate.

pathological changes in renal water and sodium excretion, and CHF (Fig. 6.1). Management of hyponatremia usually requires isotonic fluid replacement or restriction, depending on the cause within the context of the extracellular fluid compartment (**Level II-3**).[5,6] *Hypernatremia* (serum sodium concentration above 150 mEq/L) is usually secondary to insufficient replacement of excess losses. Fever results in excess hypotonic losses through the skin and respiratory system of up to 1–1.5 L/day.[4] Renal losses may be increased in response to increased solute load resulting from high protein intake or hyperglycemia, diuretic therapy, acute and chronic renal insufficiency, a deficiency in ADH, or nephrogenic diabetes insipidis. Treatment depends on recognition of the underlying cause; as with hyponatremia, correction of hypernatremia should proceed slowly to avoid central nervous system dysfunction (**Level II-3**).

Hypokalemia is a frequent postoperative surgical problem that may be secondary to diuretics, other medications (digitalis, beta-agonists, aminoglycosides, high doses of some penicillins), and GI losses. Severe hypokalemia, or moderate in the patient at increased risk (digitalized patients, history of arrhythmias), can result in cardiac arrhythmia, cardiac arrest, muscular paralysis, and respiratory failure (**Level II-2**).[164] Although oral replacement of 40–60 mEq/day is preferred, intravenous replacement is safely accomplished with 20–40 mEq of potassium per liter of isotonic solution or, when more rapid replacement is advisable, given at a rate of up to 10 mEq/hour. In an ICU setting, severe and life-threatening hypokalemia may be safely replaced by using peripheral or ventral venous access to infuse KCl at a rate of 20 mEq/hour (**Level II-2**).[164] When volume restriction is essential, as little as 25–50 cc of compatible solution may be used for dilution.

Manifestations of severe hyperkalemia include weakness, paresthesias, respiratory failure, bradycardia, and cardiac arrhythmias that predispose to complete heart block, ventricular fibrillation, or asystole. ECG changes include ST segment depression, first-degree AV block, and widening of the QRS interval which, without treatment, may progress into a biphasic sinusoidal pattern, predicting impending asystole. Causes include decreased renal potassium excretion from intrinsic renal disease, hypoaldosteronism, medications (potassium sparing diuretics, neuromuscular blocking agents, heparin, etc.), adrenal insufficiency, excessive potassium administration, tissue destruction (burns, malignant hyperthermia, massive blood transfusion), and acidosis which results in shifts of intracellular potassium into the extracellular fluid compartment.[165] Treatment directed at shifting potassium to the intracellular compartment includes infusion with glucose and insulin (10 U regular insulin after one ampule of 50% glucose), sodium bicarbonate,[6] and albuterol.[166] When life-threatening (serum K > 7 mEq/L or associated with ECG changes), calcium gluconate, 10 mL of 10% solution, should be given intravenously over 2–5 minutes, with a second dose if indicated.[6] Calcium exchange resins, such as sodium polystyrene sulfonate, bind potassium in exchange for sodium within the GI tract, and are frequently used in patients with chronic renal disease. The usual dose is 15–30 g in 50–100 cc of 20% sorbitol. Oral administration is preferable to enemas; intestinal necrosis has been reported in patients receiving Kayexalate enemas, especially when preexisting diverticular disease or other colorectal pathology is present (**Level II-2**).[167] Chronic therapy for hyperkalemia includes dietary restriction and loop diuretics (**Level II-2**).

Nutritional Support

Critically ill and malnourished patients are at an increased risk for prolonged hospitalization and postoperative morbidity and mortality compared with healthy patients.[168–171] Postoperative nutritional support with central hyperalimentation has been found to effectively reverse compromised immunologic function that is frequently present in severely malnourished patients.[168] A standard nutritional assessment begins with dietary history, physical examination, and laboratory evaluation. Physical assessment of nutritional status includes the use of anthropometric measurements to estimate skeletal muscle, changes in body weight over time, creatinine-height index. Laboratory parameters include measurement of albumin, transferrin, thyroxine-binding prealbumin, somatomedin-C.[172] Oral feeding, or enteric nutrition via gastroduodenal or jejunal tubes, is preferable to central venous hyperalimentation (total parenteral nutrition (TPN)), as starvation disrupts indigenous GI tract microflora and allows for overgrowth of pathogenic gram-negative and aerobic bacteria.[104, 105, 173] Glutamine, a nonessential amino acid that is unstable in aqueous solutions, and for that reason, cannot be provided by standard TPN solutions, has been found to be important in preventing skeletal muscle catabolism,[174] which further supports the practice of intestinal feeding. Nevertheless, enteric feeding is frequently insufficient in critically ill patients because of problems with tube placement or subtle bowel dysfunction. Augmentation of enteric feeding with TPN in critically ill patients improves calorie delivery as well as helps maintain the integrity of the GI mucosa.[175]

Regardless of whether oral or intravenous nutrition is used, caloric, protein, and trace element requirements are the same. Basal metabolic requirements (BMR) for women may be calculated using the Harris–Benedict equation: BMR (kcal/day) = 65.5 + 9.6 (weight in kilograms) + 1.7 (height in centimeters) – 4.7 (age). Depending on energy expenditure, caloric needs are usually between 20 and 35 kcal/kg/day; the unstressed elderly female patient typically requires approximately 20 kcal/kg/day.[176] A rule of thumb is that approximately half of calories should be provided by fat (1 g of fat is equivalent to 9 kcal; 1 cc 10% intralipid provides 1.1 kcal) and the remaining half by carbohydrate (1 g CHO supplies 3.4 kcal; 1000 cc of 10% dextrose provides 340 kcal). Additional calories are indicated in patients who are severely malnourished or stressed; however, overzealous supplementation may result in hyperglycemia and hyperosmolar states that predispose the patient to respiratory failure.[177] Protein requirements should be based on nitrogen balance studies, and a positive nitrogen balance is the goal of therapy. Usually, 1.0–1.5 g of amino acids per kilogram of body weight is sufficient to maintain a state of positive nitrogen balance. Trace elements (zinc, copper, chromium, and manganese)[178] as well as electrolytes, calcium, magnesium, and phosphorus should also be provided (**Level II-2**).

Solutions with high osmotic loads require central venous access. In the past, septicemia was a common complication of central venous catheterization, reported in 6%–27% of patients (**Level II-2**).[179–181] The risk of central venous catheter infection is significantly reduced by adherence to strict aseptic maintenance of the catheter and limiting its use to TPN only[182] and to use of single-lumen compared with double-lumen catheters.[181] Other complications include arterial catheterization, air or catheter embolism, thrombosis, injury of the brachial plexus, pneumothorax, and mediastinal hematoma formation.[183] Very low doses of warfarin (2.5 mg daily) are effective in preventing central venous catheter thrombosis.[184] Although instillation of 5000 U of urokinase with one or two repeat doses is sufficient to relieve thrombosis in the majority of patients with permanent access catheters, persistent withdrawal occlusion may be effectively managed with high doses of urokinase infusion (250,000 U dissolved in 150 cc D5W infused over 90 minutes[185]) or a 12-hour infusion of urokinase at 40,000 U/hr.[183]

Pain Management

Despite effective agents and methods of delivery, postoperative pain remains a major source of postoperative morbidity, adversely affecting approximately 30%–40% of patients.[187] Analgesics are typically ordered on a p.r.n. (as needed) basis, and underdosing frequently occurs because of failure by the nursing staff to adequately assess the patients' requirements for analgesia, and, all too often, because patients are reluctant to ask for pain relief, as a certain amount of pain is expected.[188] Pain increases the risk for pulmonary complications as well as thromboembolic events.[189, 190] Patient-controlled anesthesia, which provides intravenous analgesia on demand, has become tremendously popular over the past several years, as it overcomes many of the delivery problems associated with p.r.n. orders.[191–194] Regardless of the analgesic agent selected, front-loading is necessary to provide adequate serum levels and sufficient analgesia immediately postoperatively.[187] Epidural anesthesia, compared with intramuscular administration of standard agents such as morphine, has also been demonstrated to reduce pulmonary dysfunction and provide superior pain relief[195–199]; however, costs for surveillance are significantly increased (**Level I**).

NSAIDs have gained popularity in the postoperative setting. These agents are safe in majority of patients, pain control comparable to narcotic analgesia is achieved, the frequency and intensity of drowsiness, nausea, and vomiting are reduced, and in some reports, the length of hospital stay is reduced[200–204]. Toradol[R] (Syntex Laboratories, Inc.), 30–60 mg load (intravenously or intramuscularly), followed by 15–30 mg every 6–8 hours for up to 5 days is the usual recommended dose; dose reductions or alternative agents are recommended for patients who are elderly, have impaired renal or hepatic function, or who are at significant risk for bleeding complications (**Level II-1**).[205]

Postoperative Nausea and Vomiting

Emesis, the most frequently reported "minor" complication of surgery, affects approximately 30% of patients, and is a major source of patient discomfort (**Level II-3**).[206] Multiple factors, including age, sex, operative procedure performed and duration, anesthetic agents, preoperative and postoperative opioids, anxiety, a history of motion sickness or previous postoperative nausea, and pain all affect the severity of perioperative nausea and vomiting. Anesthetics, especially nitrous oxide and cyclopropane compared with isoflurande, enflurane, halothane, and propofol are associated with higher rates of nausea and vomiting. Perioperative emesis is two- to fourfold more common in women, especially during the luteal phase, and abdominal and gynecologic surgery including laparoscopy are associated with higher rates of perioperative nausea and vomiting than many other surgical procedures.[206, 207] The vomiting reflex results from central or GI stimulation of the chemoreceptor trigger zone (CTZ) in the area postrema. Vagal afferents within the upper GI tract relay stimuli to the CTZ from chemoreceptors and mechanoreceptors that are triggered by intestinal manipulation or luminal distension.[208] Commonly used antiemetics include droperidol, metoclopramide, and hyosine, which effectively alleviate nausea and vomiting but may be associated with distressing extrapyramidal side effects.[206] Serotonin [5-hydroxytryptamine (5-HT)] appears to mediate emesis via activation of receptors, specifically, the 5-HT$_3$ receptor.[208, 209] Ondansetron, a 5-HT$_3$ receptor agonist, significantly reduces nausea and vomiting associated with chemotherapy as well as opioid administration. It is now licensed for the treatment of postoperative nausea and vomiting.[206, 210] Prophylactic ondansetron[210] is superior to both droperidol and metoclopramide in preventing nausea and vomiting following gynecologic surgery, and reduces the emetogenic effects of opioids administered postoperatively.[211]

Tubes and Drains

Open and Closed Suction Tubes and Drains

Surgical drains are commonly used to prevent seroma formation and to drain abscesses, blood, and lymphatic fluid. The Penrose drain, the prototype of an open drain,[212] functions by capillary action to facilitate drainage. However, open drains also permit ingress of bacteria that increases infection rates.[213] Consequently, closed suction drains are popular in breast and gynecologic surgery. Although closed suction drainage after lumpectomy and axillary node dissection significantly reduces the incidence and severity of seromas,[214] use of drains after radical hysterectomy has recently been challenged.[215] Modern surgical techniques such as use of hemaclips and electrocautery, prophylactic antibiotic therapy, and leaving the retroperitoneum open have reduced the incidence of pelvic lymphocysts following radical hysterectomy from 15%–49%[215] to 5% or less.[216, 217] When pelvic drainage is necessary, complications may be reduced by subfascial operative placement of the perforated portion of the drain to prevent peritubal extravasation, avoidance of irrigation solutions,[218] frequent drain "stripping" to remove clots, and removal within a few days of surgery (**Level II-2**).[219]

Lymphocysts usually develop within 3 weeks of surgery, but they have been described months or years following radical hysterectomy.[217] Observation is usually adequate therapy for small cysts (4–5 cm). Cysts may be managed by simple needle drainage, insertion of catheters using radiographic guidance,[217] sclerosis with povidone-iodine,[218] and as a final alternative, surgical excision (**Level II-2**).

Foley Catheter Care and Percutaneous Nephrostomies

Foley catheters are routinely inserted perioperatively in the operating room to facilitate examination under anesthesia, to document urinary output, and to minimize patient discomfort from urinary retention associated with anesthesia or immobility. The most common complication from foley catheter insertion is urinary tract infection, affecting approximately 3.9%–40% of patients.[221, 222] The incidence and severity of urinary tract infections are dramatically reduced by use of prophylactic antibiotics,[223] leaving the catheter in site for 1 day or less, and by avoiding the use of foley catheters entirely when clinically unnecessary.[221] Percutaneous nephrostomy tubes require peritubal dressing changes and irrigation with sterile saline once or twice a week. Tubes should be exchanged every 3 months or, preferably, whenever ureteral patency is established, with a universal stent that restores continuity with the bladder.

Nasogastric Decompression

Since its introduction in the 1920s and 1930s, prophylactic nasogastric (NG) decompression has become standard therapy following laparotomy for intestinal procedures and cholecystectomy, despite retrospective and prospective randomized studies condemning this practice (**Level I**).[224–231] Although NG tube placement reduces the frequency of emesis, postoperative nausea and vomiting is usually self-limited, and several randomized studies have found that NG tubes significantly increase discomfort and duration of hospitalization, costing on average, $1,500 per patient (**Level II-2**).[34,232] Early enteric feeding reduces the duration of POI and helps to restore the normal GI barrier mechanism (**Level I**).[233] There is no data to support the notion of routine NG suction until gastric output is under 1000–1500 cc/day. In uncomplicated patients, the routine use of NG tubes following gynecologic surgery is unnecessary and should be discouraged.

On busy gynecologic oncology services, NG tube drainage is often routine and excessively prolonged. "Indications" include ovarian staging and debulking with total omentectomy and/or splenectomy to reduce the risks of postoperative omental pedicle bleeding, extensive retroperitoneal dissection, and/or following intestinal surgery. The care of these patients may also be complicated by a history of prior radiation or chemotherapy, advanced disease, rapid reaccumulation of ascites, and peritonitis, which predispose to paralytic ileus or obstruction. Routine NG suction following gynecologic oncology surgery should be reevaluated in light of evidence in the surgical literature, where withholding their use postoperatively did not increase the incidence of anastomotic leaks, abdominal dehiscence, and/or paralytic or mechanical ileus (**Level II-2**).[224,225,228] These patients are particularly susceptible to gram-negative sepsis that may be precipitated by well-intended but potentially harmful interference with normal, physiologically protective GI barriers. In the absence of paralytic ileus or obstruction, NG tubes should be removed in the majority of these patients within 1–3 days of surgery (**Level II-2**).

Wounds, Wound Healing, and Infectious Complications

Wound infections, for the purpose of postoperative surveillance, are divided into incisional surgical site infections (SSI) and organ/space SSIs (**Level II-3**). Superficial incisional SSIs are infections that occur within 30 days of the operative procedure and involve only skin or subcutaneous tissue. One of the following must also be present: purulent drainage, positive culture from the wound, signs or symptoms of infection (heat, redness, or swelling), and a diagnosis of superficial infection by the attending physician. Stitch abscesses, infection of episiotomy or circumcision incision, and infected burn wounds are not considered superficial infections.[84, 234]

Deep incisional SSIs involve the deep soft tissues, including fascial and muscle layers, of the incision. Characteristics of deep incisional SSIs include purulent drainage that is not arising from an infected organ/space component of the surgical site, deep incisional dehiscence or surgical separation, or an abscess found on direct examination or using radiographic studies. Criteria for organ/space SSIs include infections in any organ or body space with purulent drainage, positive cultures, or identified by radiographic studies. Wound infections involving both deep and superficial sites are considered deep incisional SSIs.[84, 234]

Management of a suspected wound infection includes opening and cleaning the wound, debridement of any necrotic tissue, and wet to dry dressing changes with normal saline, until the wound granulates closed. Although these infections are usually self-limiting and resolve over time with sufficient wound care, they must be distinguished from necrotizing fasciitis, a life-threatening condition characterized by infection of the superficial and deep fascia with associated thrombus formation. Mortality rates of 8.7%–73% have been reported; morbidity and mortality are significantly reduced by early recognition, broad-spectrum antibiotic coverage, and operative debridement within 12 hours of diagnosis.[235] Intra-abdominal abscesses also require drainage, either by reoperation[236] or by CT scan directed drainage, in addition to broad-spectrum antibiotic therapy (**Level II-2**).

The most common complication following hysterectomy is febrile morbidity (oral temperature over 38°C on two or more occasions at least 6 hours apart during any consecutive 48-hour period, excluding the first 24 hours), often resulting from low grade infection at the vaginal cuff. Postoperative fever prolongs hospital stay and increases patient anxiety and discomfort; however, in the majority of cases, low grade fevers resolve spontaneously without antibiotic therapy.[237] Hysterectomy exposes the pelvic peritoneum and soft tissues to bacteria commonly residing in the vaginal vault, which are the most common organisms involved in infection.[63] Risk factors for the development of postoperative infections, including cuff infections, pelvic cellulitis or abscess, and/or abdominal wound infections following abdominal or vaginal hysterectomy, include the abdominal approach, an indigent population, duration of surgery, and estimated blood loss. However, menopausal status, obesity, recent antibiotic administration, and pathological diagnosis were not found to be significant risk factors, and, using multivariate analysis, the effect of blood loss was found to be insignificant when corrected for the length of surgery (**Level I**).[74]

Mild vaginal cuff inflammation is an expected complication of hysterectomy and generally resolves spontaneously. Pelvic cellulitis associated with fever, pelvic pain, and marked vaginal induration with or without a local collection of pus should be treated with broad-spectrum antibiotics aimed at the probable offending organisms. Since the vaginal vault flora is polymicrobial, antibiotic coverage should be sufficient to cover gram-positive, gram-negative, and anaerobic bacteria.[237, 238] Ampicillin/sulbactam has been found to be as effective in the management of soft tissue infections as metronidazole–gentamicin (**Level II-2**).[239] Although many antibiotic combinations have comparable efficacy, the therapeutic regimen should consist of different antibiotics than those given for surgical prophylaxis. If the cuff is fluctuant or a mass is palpable, the vaginal cuff should also be gently probed and opened with a blunt surgical instrument with or without placement of a drain (**Level II-3**).

Methods to prevent wound infection include perioperative antibiotic prophylaxis, hexachlorophene showers before surgery, avoiding or minimizing surgical shaving, reducing operative time and length of hospital stay, strict adherence to asepsis, and meticulous surgical technique (**Level II-3**).[240] Risk factors include advanced age, preexisting illness, diabetes mellitus, obesity, length of preoperative hospitalization, abdominal operations, malignancy, other sites of infection remote from the surgical incision, malnutrition, and cigarette smoking.[241] In one study of high risk patients, delayed primary closure (post op day 4) using vertical mattress technique and non-absorbable suture reduced the incidence of postoperative surgical wound infections from 23.3% to 2.1%.[242] Finally, the incidence of wound infection from contamination by vectors can be reduced by careful hand washing techniques and the use of gloves for surgical dressing changes. To reduce the risks of contamination of fresh surgical incisions, we have adopted the practice of morning wound care by individuals other than the operative team of the day.

Decubital Care

Decubitus ulcers are pressure sores that develop as a result of tissue ischemia due to continual pressure on the skin. The soft tissues are compressed between two hard surfaces—an underlying bony structure inside the body and a bed or chair outside the body. This causes occlusion of tissue capillary perfusion, leading to ischemia and necrosis.[243, 244] With the body in the reclining position, the greatest pressures are exerted over the sacrum and the heels.[245, 246] In the sitting position, pressure is concentrated over the ischial tuberosities; when lying on the side, pressure is greatest over the trochanter of the femur. Elevation of the head above 30 degrees increases pressure to the sacrum. Normally, capillary perfusion pressure is approximately 30 mm Hg.[246] Prolonged pressure greater than the vascular perfusion pressure may lead to pressure sores. There is an inverse relationship between amount of pressure and time needed to cause damage. Pressures on soft tissues above 45–50 mm Hg are likely to cause reversible damage, whereas pressures on soft tissues greater than 70 mm Hg applied for 2 or more hours lead to irreversible tissue damage (**Level II-2**).[247]

Patients at risk for the development of decubitus ulcers are those with decreased mobility, most commonly spinal injury and orthopedic patients.[243, 244] Individuals with impaired microvascular circulation, such as those with diabetes and peripheral vascular disease, are more susceptible to the development of pressure sores. Gynecologic surgery patients are also at risk, and careful positioning of patients during surgery to avoid pressure points is important to reduce the risks, which are further aggravated postoperatively by altered levels of consciousness and prolonged immobility. Tissue integrity and wound healing may also be enhanced by optimum nutrition, especially protein, ascorbic acid, and zinc replacement, maximizing tissue perfusion, and avoidance of anemia.[249,250] Hypotension reduces tissue perfusion and lowers the pressure necessary to occlude capillary blood flow.

Prevention is aimed at the four etiologic factors involved in the development of pressure sores: (1) shear forces, (2) friction, (3) moisture, and (4) compressive forces. Various pressure reduction devices such as foam, cushions, and special beds allow diffusion of pressure to surrounding tissue areas rather than concentrating force over small, susceptible areas. Sheep skin and egg crate mattresses are not very effective. Control of exposure time to pressure forces is achieved by turning patients in bed at least every 2 hours on a regular mattress.[245] Repositioning without sliding or rubbing, and keeping the patient dry, helps to reduce friction and shear forces which can predispose to tissue breakdown. Despite these preventative measures, approximately 9.2% of hospitalized patients, and up to 35% of critical care patients, develop pressure sores.[252,253] Pressure sores are staged or graded according to the depth of tissue destruction (**Level II-3**):

Stage I: Nonblanchable erythema of intact epidermis. Erythema of skin which does not resolve within 30 minutes of relief of skin pressure.

Stage II: Partial-thickness skin loss involving the epidermis with or without partial dermis involvement. The wound base is painful and free of necrotic tissue.

Stage III: Full-thickness skin loss penetrating through to the full-thickness dermis and involving subcutaneous tissues, but not underlying fascias, muscle layers, joints, or bones. The wound base is a shallow and nonpainful ulcer, and necrosis, exudates, sinus tract formation, and infection may be present.

Stage IV: Full-thickness skin loss with extension into underlying fascia, muscles, joints, or bones. The wound base has a nonpainful, deep crater; necrosis, tissue undermining, sinus tract formation, infection, and exudate may be present.[254]

Pressure sores may be treated by conservative and surgical methods. Stages I and II can usually be managed nonoperatively with pressure relief and cleansing of ulcerated area. Pressure relief may be best managed by pressure-redistributing/decreasing mattresses such as the Comfortex DeCube[R] mattress.[247,255] Localized treatment is aimed at debridement of necrotic areas and relief of infection. As necrotic tissue is usually colonized by skin flora only, debridement with application of a topical antibiotic, such as bacitracin or silver sulfadiazine, is generally adequate to clear local infection. Systemic antibiotics are not recommended unless cellulitis or osteomyelitis is present, as they may slow wound healing and promote resistant bacterial growth. Prompt treatment of these infectious processes is imperative, however, because bacteremia in association with pressure sores carries a 50% mortality rate.[256] Debridement can be accomplished surgically, mechanically, or chemically with enzymatic preparations. Whirlpools are helpful with large ulcers. The healing process may be accelerated once the ulcer is cleaned with the use of tissue growth factors such as platelet-derived growth factor.[257] In the absence of necrosis and infection, occlusive, semi-occlusive, and hydrocolloid wound dressings, including DuoDerm[R], Op-Site[R], and IntraSite[R], may be applied to create a physiological, wound-healing environment. Most ischial ulcers have a deep underlying cavity and small outlet and are best managed with saline gauze packing to allow healing from the bottom up; an abscess cavity may form if the outlet closes first. Surgery is the preferred threatment for Grade III and IV pressure sores over 2 cm in size (**Level II-2**).[248, 257] After the ulcer bed is clean and free of infection or necrosis, simple excision of devitalized tissue followed by closure, with or without the use of skin grafts, muscle flaps, or myocutaneous grafts, may be performed.

STOMAL CARE

The surgical management of gynecologic malignancies frequently requires intestinal surgery. Rubin et al., in a retrospective review, found that 10.4% of all laparotomies on a busy gynecologic oncology service were complicated by intestinal surgery.[258] In a 1992 summary of the complications of colostomy performed on patients with gynecologic cancer, Hoffman et al. found a 6.3% incidence of early complications, and a 15.3% incidence of delayed complications, that compared favorably with the 8%–27% complication rate reported in the surgical literature (**Level II-2**).[259] Common stomal complications are summarized in Table 6.11. Peristomal skin irritation, the most common early stomal complication, affects approximately 42.1% of all ostomies,[260] occurs three times more frequently in ostomies created at unmarked

Table 6.11 Peristomal and Stomal Complications[258–262] (Level II-3)

Early Complications	Late Complications	Dermatologic Complications
Bleeding	Prolapse/ parastomal herniation	Caput medusae
Necrosis	Stenosis	Allergic dermatitis
Mucocutaneous separation	Retraction	Irritant dermatitis
Ostomy wound infection	Tumor involvement	Folliculitis
Melanosis coli	Site choice problems	Hyperplastic (Pseudoverrucous) lesions
Partial stomal obstruction		Infectious
		Candida
		Bacterial
Peritonitis/sepsis		Mucosal transplantation
		Preexisting dermatoses
		Dermatomyositis
		Psoriasis
		Pemphigus
		Mycosis fungoides

sites, and is usually the result of improper site selection, suboptimum stomal construction, or inadequate peristomal skin protection.[260, 261] Management directed to the specific etiology includes avoidance of irritants and adhesive products, topical treatment of yeast and other infections, steroidal creams, control of diarrhea, and avoidance of trauma.[261] Stomas that are flushed or retracted, on soft abdomens, or have deep peristomal creasing are particularly difficult management problems, and may cause significant emotional distress and social incapacitation. Treatment options include the creation of convexity using belts, inserts, or faceplates, and custom-made abdominal supports. Surgical revision is sometimes accomplished by stomal mobilization and advancing the loop of bowel so that a stoma can be created without tension.[262] More frequently, laparotomy with additional intestinal resection is required. In a series of 123 patients undergoing 156 colostomy revisions, Allen-Mersh and Thomson[262] achieved a 63% success rate after one or more attempts. However, because a high failure rate was anticipated, morbidly obese and "frail" patients were excluded (**Level II-2**). Ileostomies and ileal and jejunal conduits have higher complication rates than colostomies or transverse colon conduits; ostomies constructed in the course of resection of gynecologic pelvic malignancies have also been associated with higher complication rates.[260] Our patients frequently have comorbid conditions that increase the risks for peristomal complications; therefore, the gynecologic surgeon must be especially attuned to the construction and management of intestinal stomas, as prevention is clearly preferable to repair (Table 6.12). Prior to surgery, ostomy site selection and patient education should be performed by a trained enterostomal nurse. Within the context of the individual's psychosocial needs, dietary restrictions, and physical limitations, thorough perioperative counseling regarding stomal care improves adjustment to enterostomal lifestyle changes. Skin site problems are reduced by careful preoperative site selection, delineating skin folds and pannus creases with the patient in various positions. Other surgical options include use of turnbull ostomies for additional mesenteric length, transverse colon conduits in heavily radiated patients, and placement of the colostomy and mucous fistula at separate skin sites. Seromuscular to fascial tacking sutures may increase local infection rates and fistula formation (**Level II-3**).[260]

Table 6.12   Guidelines for Stomal Construction[258–262] (Level II-3)

Preoperative counseling by a trained enterostomal nurse.
Assess the abdominal wall in supine, sitting, and standing positions.
Avoid skin folds, scars, belt lines, bony protruberances, and incisions.
Place all stomas through the rectus muscle.
Avoid fecal spillage into the peristomal space.
Stomas should be placed without tension.
Adequately mobilize intestinal segment with mesenteric blood supply.
Avoid trimming peristomal fat and epiploic appendages.
Mature stomas primarily using mucosubcutaneous closures.
Apply peristomal protection.

SPECIAL MANAGEMENT CONSIDERATIONS IN THE HIGH RISK SURGICAL PATIENTS

Early recognition of potentially life-threatening complications such as hemorrhage, intestinal perforation, or sepsis reduces morbidity and mortality. In physiologically compromised patients, critical care units capable of intensive hemodynamic monitoring and cardiorespiratory support have dramatically improved survival.

Surgical Complications

Perioperative Bleeding and Blood Component Therapy

Perioperative bleeding requiring transfusion complicates approximately 8% of vaginal hysterectomies and 15% of abdominal hysterectomies for benign disease. When radical abdominal hysterectomy and pelvic exenterative procedures are performed, the average blood loss is 1500 and 3000 cc, respectively.[263] It has been estimated that about 60% of all blood transfused in the United States is given to surgical patients.[264] Because oxygen-carrying capacity is met in most healthy women by a hemoglobin of 7 g/dL, the concept of empiric transfusion at a hemoglobin level of 8, 9, or 10 mg/dL is no longer justifiable.[265] Loss of approximately 20% of blood volume is equivalent to 1500 cc blood loss in a 70-kg individual, and is not associated with a significant reduction in oxygen-carrying capacity or ventricular filling pressures when appropriate crystalloid resuscitation is provided. In the absence of preexisting coagulation defects, duration of surgery (>3 hours), pelvic malignancy with associated extensive dissection, and surgical expertise are the most important factors that affect blood loss. Most healthy gynecologic patients require a preoperative type and screen only, as crossmatching in the absence of antibodies can be completed in under an hour in most hospitals. Preoperative crossmatch is routine, however, for patients with significant cardiopulmonary disease, preexisting anemia, or when extensive abdominal or pelvic dissection is anticipated (**Level III**).

Blood component therapy specific for the component needed has replaced transfusion with whole blood as the standard of care. Adverse effects of the transfusion of blood products include infection, alloimmunization, and transfusion reaction.[265] An acute hemolytic reaction occurs in 1 per 6000 U transfused, and is associated with a 1:17 mortality rate, or 1 in 100,000 U.[266] Prior to blood product transfusion, correct identification of each unit of blood and the patient receiving the product should be checked by two trained personnel. All blood products should be administered through filtered lines with normal (9.0%) saline without electrolyte or drug additives. Other crystalloid solutions should be avoided because of the risks of hemolysis, agglutination, and/or clotting.[265] Warming is indicated when the volume infused exceeds 50 mL/kg/hour to prevent cardiac-induced hypothermia, and in the presence of cold agglutinin disease, using an in-line blood warmer. Packed red blood cells (RBCs) have a volume of 200–250 mL, a hematocrit of 70%, and, combined with crystalloid therapy for volume expansion, are the component of choice for hemorrhagic shock.

Whole blood or packed RBCs with fresh frozen plasma (FFP) in a 4:1 ratio are appropriate when blood loss exceeds 25% of the blood volume. Platelet transfusions are indicated in the presence of severe thrombocytopenia and platelet dysfunction, and may be indicated after massive transfusion (10 U/24 hours in a 70-kg individual). One unit of platelet concentrate will usually increase the count of a 70-kg patient by 5000–10,000/mm.[267] FFP is indicated for patients with disseminated intravascular coagulation, severe liver disease, massive transfusion, coumadin therapy reversal, and specific clotting disturbances when the specific factor concentrate is not available. FFP transfusion should be based on coagulation studies that generally should be repeated and checked after every 5–10 U of blood transfused. FFP is never indicated for volume expansion, nutritional support, or prophylactically with massive blood transfusion (**Level III**).[268]

Cryoprecipitate is concentrated FFP in a small volume of 10–15 mL (one bag per 5 kg in a 70-kg individual). Because cryoprecipitate represents pooled factor components from multiple donors, risk of infection is significantly increased. Cryoprecipitate is reserved for deficiencies in factor VIII, von Willebrand factor, fibrinogen factor XIII, and fibronectin. If disseminated intravascular coagulation is suspected based on massive transfusion and persistence of significant bleeding and oozing, FFP rather than cryoprecipitate is the component of choice.[269]

GI Injury, Paralytic Ileus, and Intestinal Obstruction

Because serosal injuries are rarely documented, it is difficult to document the incidence of laceration injuries encountered in gynecologic surgery. Obese patients have a 2.5-fold greater risk of injury.[270] Other factors that increase risk for injury and for which preoperative bowel preparation is strongly recommended include previous abdominal surgery, pelvic inflammatory disease, endometriosis, and pelvic malignancies.[271] Thermal injuries complicate 1%–2% of all laparoscopic surgical procedures and are often not recognized until the patient presents with peritonitis 4–7 days postoperatively. Management consists of prompt surgical exploration, wide resection (3–5 cm) of the thermal burn, and reanastomosis whenever feasible (**Level II-2**).[271]

Intestinal obstruction complicates only about 0.2% of surgical procedures for benign gynecologic conditions. In contrast, nearly half of patients with ovarian malignancies and 3% of patients with other gynecologic cancers experience this complication. Obstruction usually involves the small bowel (77% of cases).[270, 272] In the Western world, adhesions following general surgical and gynecologic procedures are the most common cause, and precede the obstructive event by an average of 6–10 years.[273–276]

Differentiating between paralytic ileus and complete obstruction is critical, as ileus and partial small bowel obstruction will resolve in approximately 80% of postoperative patients with medical management.[261] However, unrecognized ischemia and strangulation increase risks of peritonitis, perforation, sepsis, and death. Complete history and physical examination are crucial for appropriate decision making (Fig. 6.5). Both conditions are characterized by volume contraction resulting from "third"

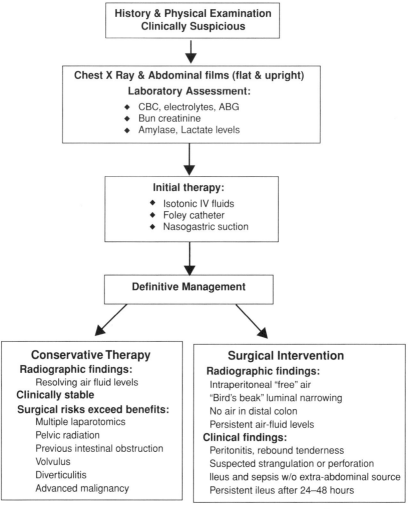

Figure 6.5 Intestinal Obstruction – diagnosis and management (level II-2).[271–276]

spacing into the intestinal lumen. Metabolic alkalosis may result from NG losses and is often associated with respiratory acidosis; metabolic acidosis is an ominous finding indicative of cellular ischemia. Initial management consists of volume resuscitation with isotonic crystalloid solutions, electrolyte and blood product replacement based on laboratory findings, and nutritional support. Radiographic findings consistent with partial or complete obstruction include "bird's peak" luminal narrowing, air–fluid levels, and absence of air in the distal colon. In the absence of recent celiotomy, intraperitoneal "free" air on upright abdominal films or chest X-ray signifies perforation. Broad-spectrum antibiotics should be administered for associated abscess and perioperatively.

Proximal small bowel obstruction frequently presents with bilious vomiting, upper abdominal and/or generalized abdominal pain, and high pitched hyperactive bowel sounds. Patients with partial obstruction who are likely to respond to conservative management usually do so within 24 hours of presentation (**Level II-2**). In one large series, 75% of patients managed conservatively with clinical improvement within 24 hours ultimately avoided surgery, compared with only 5% of patients with no improvement after 48 hours.[276] Laparotomy is indicated in patients who fail to respond after 48 hours of conservative management to prevent ischemia or perforation. As obstruction progresses, NG drainage may become feculent, reminiscent of distal obstruction; a suddenly "quiet" abdomen with fever, leukocytosis, or leukopenia is an ominous finding associated with strangulation or ischemia from mesenteric arterial or venous thrombosis. Surgical management should be conducted in consultation with a general surgical specialist or gynecologic oncologist, and consists of lysis of adhesions, adequate mobilization, isolation of the involved intestinal segment, and resection with primary anastomosis or bypass. Surgical stapling devices shorten operative time and improve blood supply and may reduce risks of anastomotic leaks or strictures.

Large bowel obstruction is common in the elderly, and often results from fecal impaction, diverticular disease, and benign or malignant luminal tumors. Pseudoobstruction and volvulus can often be managed conservatively with colonoscopy. Clinical findings include generalized abdominal distension, feculent vomiting, and fever with leukocytosis and left shift. Surgical management with resection and primary reanastomosis frequently is impossible because of fecal contamination. Operative management may require extirpation of both intestinal loops and protective colostomy.

Risks for intestinal obstruction, primary or repetitive, are reduced by meticulous operative management. Adhesion formation can be minimized by gentle handling of bowel and peritoneal surfaces, sharp dissection, meticulous hemostasis, careful repositioning of bowel in an anatomical position, use of omentum or peritoneum to cover denuded surfaces or to fill pelvic defects, use of delayed absorbable suture, gentle and limited intestinal packing with moist laparotomy pads, and avoidance of foreign body contamination, including cotton fibers from sponges and talc from surgical gloves.[271–274]

Medical Conditions Requiring Special Surveillance

Diabetes Mellitus

Diabetes mellitus, a group of closely related disorders characterized by insulin insufficiency that results in hyperglycemia, is the most common endocrine disease that the gynecologist is likely to encounter. Over 11 million Americans are affected; of these, approximately half will undergo one or more operations in their lifetime, usually after the age of 50.[277] Clinical manifestations are variable, and depend on disease duration and severity. Symptoms at onset include polyuria, polydipsia, and weight loss that, without appropriate intervention, progress to ketoacidosis or nonketotic hyperosmolar syndrome.[278] Longstanding diabetes adversely affects multiple organ systems and is characterized by microvascular insufficiency resulting in the development of cardiovascular disease, diabetic retinopathy, neurological deficits, GI disturbances, and peripheral neurovascular impairment that predisposes to lower extremity skin ulcerations, infection, tissue necrosis, and fracture (**Level III**).[278]

Vascular disease related to diabetes is the single most important risk factor for perioperative morbidity and mortality. Over half of diabetics ultimately succumb to complications of cardiovascular disease.[279] Cardiovascular complications are the leading cause of mortality in diabetic patients, accounting for approximately 30% of perioperative deaths.[280] The rates of postoperative morbidity are highest among patients undergoing coronary artery bypass surgery and patients with severe renal insufficiency, with an increase in average hospitalization stay by 30%–50%.[281] Although the extent of ischemia and infarction is comparable in patients with and without angina, diabetics have a significantly higher incidence of painless myocardial ischemia perioperatively, increasing the probability of progression to irreversible injury.[282] Hyperglycemia in patients undergoing coronary artery bypass surgery has been reported to significantly reduce the ratio of the arterial partial pressure of oxygen to the inspired oxygen gradient as well as elevate the alveolar-arterial oxygen gradient to levels consistent with significant pulmonary dysfunction.[283] Nevertheless, with optimal preoperative assessment and perioperative control, patients with diabetes mellitus have similar rates of surgical complications as patients without diabetes.[284] Thus, the surgeon's responsibility prior to elective surgery is to adequately assess the patient to determine the extent of organic manifestations, correct existing hyperglycemia, and stabilize any related electrolyte disturbances. This evaluation includes a complete history, physical examination, and laboratory testing including electrolytes, glucose, BUN, creatinine, preoperative cardiovascular screening proportionate to cardiovascular involvement, and endocrine consultation where appropriate.

The stress response is characterized by metabolic alterations that affect the rate of hepatic glucose production and peripheral glucose disposal. Cortisol and glucagon accelerate hepatic gluconeogenesis, whereas adrenaline stimulates glycogenolysis; increased glucose production coupled with relative insulin resistance results in hyperglycemia.[285] Postoperative hyperglycemia is not indicative of diabetes; surgical stress and its associated glucose load reduce both the number and the affinity of insulin receptors, a possible mechanism for physiological insulin resistance that accompanies surgical stress.[286] In uncomplicated cases, insulin resistance is reversible by administration of insulin that, coupled with nutritional supply sufficient to meet metabolic demands, effectively preserves body protein and energy stores.[287] Hyperglycemia also lowers serum insulin levels, an effect counterbalanced and exceeded by the glycogenic effects of adrenaline, glucagon, growth hormone, and cortisol.[288] In the absence of insulin, the metabolic effects of these hormones include glycogenolysis; once glycogen stores are depleted, protein catabolism and lipolysis ensue.[285, 289] The consequences of this hyperosmotic load include diuresis, potentially resulting in hypotension and decreased cellular perfusion, ketoacidosis, and redistribution of potassium from within cells to the extracellular space. Insulin therapy reverses hyperkalemia by stimulating sodium and potassium exchange via the adenosine triphosphate Na^+–K^+ pump mechanism.[285] Both hyperglycemia and hypoglycemia may induce significant neurological damage, especially in patients at greatest risk.[285,289] Altered mental consciousness, often the most sensitive indicator of brain function, cannot be assessed intraoperatively, when the patient is at greatest risk of hypoxia.[279] Thus, operative management includes adjusting insulin infusion based on the results of frequent blood glucose sampling every 2 or 3 hours to keep the serum glucose in the range of 120–250 mg/dL.[285]

Hyperglycemia (>240–250 mg/dL) impairs wound healing by altered leukocyte function including impaired phagocytosis, chemotaxis, and ability to kill bacteria, and inhibition of collagen synthesis, fibroblast formation, and neovascularization.[289] Risks of wound infection, gram-negative and staphylococcal pneumonia, and gram-negative and β-hemolytic streptococcal septicemia are increased, probably in association with impaired neutrophil function.[289,290] Thromboembolic complications are common in diabetic patients secondary to increased levels of thromboxane-mediated platelet activation, which is partially reversible with metabolic control as well as with the administration of low dose aspirin therapy (**Level II-2**).[291]

When surgery is elective, diabetes should be optimally controlled prior to the operative procedure. Elevated glycosylated hemoglobin levels have been found to accurately reflect the level of diabetic control within the antecedent 2 or 3 months (**Level II-2**).[291] Long-acting oral glycosemic agents should be discontinued at least 36 hours prior to surgery; shorter acting agents such as glyburide (Micronase[R], Diabeta[R]) and glipizide (Glucotrol[R]) should be withheld the day prior to surgery to reduce the risks of hypoglycemia (**Level II-3**).[285]

Although it is generally agreed that perioperative hyperglycemia should be prevented, the ideal method to accomplish this is controversial. Traditionally, on the morning prior to surgery, approximately one half to two thirds of the usual insulin dose is administered in combination with low dose carbohydrate infusion such as D5W at 100–125 cc/hour to prevent hypoglycemia and ketosis.[293] Alternatively, the patient may be maintained by a low dose dextrose infusion along with an insulin drip at 1–2 U/hour to maintain a serum glucose level in the 120–180 mg/dL range,[281,293,294] followed postoperatively by subcutaneous insulin titrated to severity. As serum glucose determinations are only reflective of glucose levels at the time they were drawn, it is important that levels be checked frequently and acted upon promptly. Severe hyperglycemia with associated ketosis, metabolic acidosis, and hyperkalemia is managed by aggressive volume replacement, intravenous insulin infusion, and laboratory-directed replacement of potassium and phosphate. In complicated patients requiring prolonged nutritional support, continuous insulin infusion may be administered in parenteral nutrition. In insulin-dependent diabetes, as soon as oral nutritional replacement is tolerated, enteric feeding should be supplemented by the combination of regular and intermediately acting insulin, which peak in activity 3 and 10 hours, respectively, after administration.[288]

Cardiac Insufficiency

While the reported incidence of perioperative MI varies widely, ranging from <1% following minor, low risk procedures and exceeding 10% with vascular procedures,[53] the risk of fatality (36%–70%) emphasizes the seriousness of this complication.[295] Although it is recommended that patients over 70 years of age or with a history of cardiovascular disease be followed postoperatively with serial ECGs, the ECG is an insensitive and nonspecific tool for the diagnosis of perioperative MI. Over half of perioperative MIs are diagnosed on or before the third postoperative day. Measurement of MB creatine kinase has been the marker of choice for the detection of cardiac ischemia, although false positives may result from skeletal muscle injury. Serum CK-MB bands in excess of 5% of the serum CK, or greater than 50 IU per liter, are considered diagnostic of perioperative MI.[296] An elevated CK-MB 6–9 hours postoperatively that remains elevated, with one or more confirmatory studies (new Q waves on ECG and/or a positive myocardial pyrophosphate scan), enhances the predictive value of serum CK-MB.[297] The serum level of cardiac troponin I, a regulatory protein produced only within the myocardium, is a highly sensitive (100%) and specific (99%) marker for MI that avoids the high false positives (19%) associated with CK-MB measurement (**Level I**).[295]

The ACC/AHA (American College of Cardiology/American Heart Association) task force in 1990 published guidelines of recommended indications for diagnostic procedures and therapeutic interventions including triage and transport, ECG monitoring, invasive hemodynamic monitoring, antiarrhythmic therapy, and thrombolytic therapy, which are based on classification of risk.[298] In uncomplicated MI, basic support includes oxygen therapy to alleviate hypoxemia; nitroglycerin to reduce preload and improve epicardial blood flow, morphine sulfate to alleviate pain, reduce preload and afterload, and decrease myocardial oxygen demand; and recognition and management of arrhythmias. Invasive hemodynamic monitoring including balloon flotation right heart catheters and/or arterial pressure catheters is indicated for patients with hemodynamic instability manifested by hypotension (systolic <80 mm Hg) requiring presser agents, cardiogenic shock, pulmonary edema, and severe or progressive CHF (**Level II-2**).[298] The case fatality rate for acute MI in patients receiving thrombolytic therapy is 10%–15%, significantly reduced from the 30%–50% mortality rates from perioperative MI.[53] However, because surgery or trauma within 2 weeks is a relative contraindication to thromboembolytic therapy,[298] coronary angioplasty, which has been associated with success rates comparable to thrombolysis, may be a viable alternative in the high risk postoperative patient.[53]

CHF following surgery is a particularly ominous finding. In a series of 15 patients developing postoperative CHF, 5 patients (33%) developed pulmonary edema, including 4 patients (26.7%) with concomitant myocardial ischemia; 7 patients (46.7%) had evidence of postoperative myocardial ischemia. Risk factors associated with postoperative CHF included diabetes mellitus, age over 70 years, less than 500 mL intake or urine output in the 24 hours preceding surgery, and preexisting cardiac disease (**Level II-2**).[299]

Pulmonary Complications

The most common respiratory complications following hospitalization or surgery are nosocomial infections of the respiratory tract, affecting 0.5%–5.0% of all hospitalized patients (**Level II-2**).[300] There appears to be no significant difference in the incidence of nosocomial pneumonia on surgical compared with medical services (approximately 75–80 cases per 10,000 patient discharges). Approximately half of hospital-acquired pneumonia are caused by gram-negative organisms.[301] The most common organisms involved in nosocomial pneumonia (12%–22%) include Pseudomonas sp., Staphylococcus sp., Klebsiella sp., and Enterobacter sp., while the frequency of other organisms less commonly isolated, including Serratia sp., Candida sp., Haemophilus sp., and Acinetobacter sp., are in the order of 4%–9% of cases.[301–303] In normal individuals, death associated with gram-negative bacteremia is only 10%, compared with high mortality rates (45%–70%), from nosocomial infection.[304]

Hypoventilation in the immediate postoperative period predisposes to the development of atelectasis, which is characterized by collapse of the small airways, resulting in intrapulmonary venous shunting as well as entrapment of bacteria (**Level II-2**). Atelectasis is the most common cause of postoperative fever within the first 24 hours of surgery. There is no evidence that antibiotic therapy reduces the probability of pneumonia in high risk patients; rather, empiric antibiotic use predisposes to the development of resistant organisms.[300, 305] Uncomplicated atelectasis should be treated with early ambulation and incentive spirometry. Persistent fever and leukocytosis associated with rales and/or rhonchi on clinical examination and with purulent sputum production signify the development of pneumonia, which is confirmed by pulmonary infiltrates on chest X-ray.[305] In hospitalized patients, antibiotic therapy should cover both gram-positive and gram-negative organisms until cultures are available. Choice of antibiotic coverage should depend on a number of high risk factors including whether or not the patient is or has recently been intubated, aspiration is suspected, systemic manifestations of sepsis are present, and recent antibiotic therapy.[300, 305] In uncomplicated patients, single-agent therapy aimed at pneumococcal or Haemophilus sp. is usually sufficient, with therapy continued for approximately a week, and until after clinical and chest X-ray findings have abated. For patients in the ICU, vancomycin in doses of 2–4 g/day is frequently used.[300] When aspiration is suspected, and in patients on mechanical ventilation, coverage is often extended to include anaerobic flora. Aminoglycoside dosing in high risk patients (patients with significant metabolic derangement, sepsis, or renal failure) should be based on pharmacokinetics as well as peak and trough levels, to prevent either overdosing and associated ototoxicity and nephrotoxicity or underdosing, resulting in inadequate tissue levels. For patients with normal renal function, doses of gentamicin or tobramicin should be in the 3–5 mg/kg/day range, whereas elderly patients and patients with renal dysfunction require major dose reductions and/or interval spacing between doses. Third-generation penicillins and cephalosporins are preferred in patients with renal insufficiency; however, when *Pseudomonas* is suspected, single-agent therapy with these agents is inadequate because of the rapid development of resistance to these agents when they are used alone.

Risks for all forms of respiratory dysfunction including nosocomial pneumonia are dramatically increased by the presence of pulmonary compromise, as measured by alterations in ventilation, lung water content, perfusion, and resistance to infection.[20] Ventilation may be impaired by structural defects (scoliosis, kyphosis), mechanical uncoupling (effusions, hemorrhage, pneumothorax), muscular weakness (severe malnutrition, ventilatory paralysis, chronic muscular diseases), conditions that increase the work of breathing (abdominal distension from ascites or pregnancy, obesity), imbalance in nutritional supply and demand (thyroid disease, hypoperfusion states), and conditions that restrict lung movement (pulmonary edema, pulmonary fibrosis, adult respiratory distress syndrome [ARDS]).[20] Increased lung water, which may result from alterations in permeability (ARDS, aspiration, sepsis) or hemodynamic alterations (CHF, valvular heart disease), increases the risk of hypoxia resulting from ventilation–perfusion mismatch. Any condition that reduces immune function, such as use of steroids, smoking, or *chronic obstructive pulmonary disease* (COPD), increases the risk of postoperative infection. Although controversy exists as to the potential risk of H-2 blockers and the development of pneumonia,[154] use of these agents to prevent GI hemorrhage continues to be advocated in some ICUs.[305]

Patients with COPD and hypoxemia/hypercapnia are particularly susceptible to postoperative complications and/or requirements for postoperative ventilatory support (**Level II-2**).[306, 307] Preoperative interventions that reduce infection risks include cessation of smoking, use of bronchodilators, antibiotic coverage when a purulent cough is present, chest physical therapy with postural drainage, nebulizers, and control of CHF.[20] Postoperatively, meticulous attention to pulmonary toilet and incentive spirometry are imperative in these patients.

For many years, ventilation has been routinely quantified using pulmonary function tests and arterial blood gas determinations. Predictors of postoperative atelectasis include a reduction in the maximal breathing capacity to 50% or less of predicted, FEV1 of less than 1 L, forced vital capacity (FVC) of less than 70% predicted, and FEV1/FVC of less than 65% of the predicted value. Low serum oxygenation (PaO_2 < 60 mm Hg) and carbon dioxide retention ($PaCO_2$ > 45 mm Hg) are also predictive of postoperative complications.[308] Despite their routine use, there is little evidence that preoperative spirometry and pulmonary exercise testing improve the sensitivity of history and physical examination in identifying patients at risk for postoperative pneumonia, prolonged hospitalization, or death, with the exception of patients undergoing lung resection.[309, 310]

Asthma is a common condition in the Western world, affecting approximately 5% of the population; the incidence appears to be increasing. Asthma is an inflammatory disease characterized by infiltration of the airways with inflammatory cells (**Level III**). Chronic asthma is also associated with bronchial hyperresponsiveness that is induced by inflammatory cell mediators. The treatment of choice includes the use of inhalant steroids (up to 2 mg/day) and β2-adrenergic agents. Anticholinergic agents are equally effective as β2-adrenergic agents; there appears to be no therapeutic advantage to combining these agents (**Level II-2**).[306] In adults, chronic use of inhalant steroids in recommended doses (up to 2 mg/day) does not appear to be associated with adrenal insufficiency. When severe, refractory asthma, and acute asthmatic exacerbations are encountered, the immediate treatment of choice includes inhalant and intravenous steroids rather than intravenous theophylline, which, although it is a useful adjunctive agent in asthmatics, appears to have no effect on inflammatory cell-mediated hyperresponsiveness.[311]

Renal Disease

Acute renal failure is a complication affecting only approximately 2%–5% of all hospitalized patients. Surgery, however, with its associated hemodynamic and neuroendocrine changes, is second only to decreased renal perfusion as the cause of acute renal failure, and accounts for 18%–47% of all cases.[313–315] Development of acute renal failure in one case control study was associated with a 6.2 to 1 risk in death.[316] Although isolated acute renal failure carries a mortality rate of only approximately 10%, multiorgan system failure is more common; renal failure in association with multisystem organ failure (three or more organ systems) carries a mortality rate of over 90%.[314] Significant risk factors for the development of postoperative renal failure include hypertension, diabetes mellitus, volume depletion, aminoglycoside use, CHF, radiocontrast exposure, and septic shock (**Level II-3**).[316–320]

Acute renal failure may be divided into three main categories: (1) *prerenal azotemia*, which is reversible renal failure caused by decreased effective arterial blood flow to the kidneys; (2) *intrinsic renal disease*, which accounts for approximately 30% of cases of acute renal failure in hospitalized patients; and (3) *obstructive uropathy*, which accounts for approximately 10% of all cases arising on inpatient services. Prerenal azotemia may be caused by induction anesthesia, severe volume overload resulting in CHF and shunting of blood flow away from the kidneys, or sepsis. A serum BUN to creatinine ratio of 40:1 is considered indicative of prerenal azotemia, although other conditions such as sepsis, urea absorption from GI bleeding, and steroid use may also elevate serum urea nitrogen levels.[315]

The most common cause of intrinsic renal disease, accounting for more than 90% of cases, is *acute tubular necrosis* that usually develops in association with ischemia or nephrotoxin use, and is frequently aggravated by perioperative hypotension.[308] In patients with preexisting hypertension or diabetes, Charlson et al. found that continuous infusion of 300 cc or more per hour of isotonic solutions significantly reduced the risk of postoperative renal insufficiency. Because decompensated CHF was found to be associated with a 36% rate of postoperative renal dysfunction, the authors strongly advised against elective surgery in these patients until cardiac function improved.[317] Renal dysfunction associated with aminoglycoside therapy is related to dose, dosing intervals, duration of therapy, previous use of aminoglycoside therapy, use of other nephrotoxic agents such as intravenous contrast materials, volume status, and host factors. In the adult population, the incidence of nephrotoxicity from a single therapeutic cycle of aminoglycosides is approximately 5%–10%, and is the fourth leading cause of renal failure, after hypoperfusion, surgery, and administration of radiographic contrast.[303, 309] Another uncommon, but life-threatening, cause of operative renal failure is malignant hyperthermia and associated disorders. Malignant hyperthermia, an autosomal dominant pharmacogenetic disorder of the musculoskeletal system instigated by exposure to certain anesthetic agents including isoflurane and succinylcholine, is characterized by rhabdomyolysis, hyperthermia, generalized muscle rigidity, and renal failure. Prior to the use of dantrolene, which has reduced mortality rates to approximately 10%, the mortality from this condition approached 80%.[320]

Causes for obstructive uropathy in the postanesthetic period include the anticholinergic effects of certain anesthetics and antihistamines that can cause acute urinary retention, especially in patients with diabetes mellitus. Ureteral obstruction may result from retroperitoneal hematoma formation and iatrogenic ureteral injury in the course of pelvic surgery. Patients with advanced cervical cancer or a pelvic mass with hydronephrosis and partial ureteral obstruction may have renal dysfunction disproportionate to the serum creatinine; postoperative obstructive diuresis may induce profound hypotension that further predisposes to acute tubular necrosis.

Factors that reduce the risk of acute renal failure in surgical patients include maintaining an adequate volume status preoperatively, intraoperatively, and postoperatively, avoidance of nephrotoxic agents whenever possible, and documenting the existing level of renal function prior to surgery. When contrast studies are essential, hydration with isotonic saline solution before and after the procedure reduce the risks of renal dysfunction in patients at increased risk (**Level II-3**).[47]

Chronic renal failure is characterized by fluid retention, disturbances in electrolyte function, hematologic and coagulation abnormalities including a normocytic normochromic anemia, and increased bleeding time probably in association with reduced factor VIII in the serum of uremic patients. In a study of over 300 chronic dialysis patients, the overall operative mortality was 3 in 312 procedures (0.96%), with an operative mortality following major surgery of 2%, although a high complication rate (68%) was also reported.[321] Management consists of performing renal dialysis within 24 hours of surgery and correcting any existing problems of volume overload and/or electrolyte disturbances. Postoperatively, patients are at high risk for fluid overload, arrhythmias, respiratory decompensation, and shunt thrombosis. Analgesic and sedative doses must be decreased to reduce deterioration in respiratory and mental function. The most common electrolyte disturbance is hyperkalemia, which, in a report by Pinson et al., developed postoperatively in 19% of all patients with renal failure. Contributing factors included massive blood transfusion and elevations in preoperative serum potassium levels.[321] Insulin in glucose is more effective than epinephrine or bicarbonate solutions in reducing hyperkalemia[322]; in postoperative patients, however, the most effective management of hyperkalemia is dialysis.[321] When surgery is elective, recombinant human erythropoietin (500 U/kg) may elevate the hematocrit by as much as 10% within 3 weeks and may significantly reduce transfusion requirements.[323] Conjugated estrogen therapy results in a prolonged (14-day) improvement in the bleeding time in patients with chronic renal failure, compared with the short-term effects of more commonly used agents including cryoprecipitate or desmopression.[324] Postoperatively, patients on chronic dialysis therapy are also at increased risk for infection, most commonly *Staphylococcus aureus*, followed by *S. epidermidis* and *E. coli*, that partly results from alterations in neutrophil and monocyte function.[325]

Liver Disease

Although there is no evidence that currently used anesthetic agents are direct hepato-toxins, all agents reduce hepatic blood flow, resulting in decreased oxygen uptake by the liver and splanchnic organs.[326] Additionally, other factors associated with surgery including hypotension, blood loss, use of vasoactive drugs, surgical manipulation of abdominal viscera, and hypoxemia reduce hepatic blood flow and contribute to the morbidity associated with preexisting significant hepatobiliary disease.[327] Sedatives, narcotics, neuromuscular blocking agents must be used with caution in these patients because of reduced metabolic clearance that may result in severe respiratory depression and/or result in requirements for prolonged postoperative ventilation. In addition to increased risk for increased morbidity and mortality from exacerbated hepatic dysfunction, patients with significant liver failure are at increased risk for bleeding complications resulting from coagulopathies, renal failure, and pulmonary compromise from ascites or coexisting derangement in hemodynamic function. In managing a patient with liver disease, it is imperative that the risks of morbidity be weighed against the potential operative risks; thus, a thorough preoperative assessment, including history, physical examination, and laboratory investigation, including prothrombin time, partial thromboplastin time, albumin, total and direct bilirubin, and transaminases be obtained prior to surgery.

Acute and chronic viral hepatitis, alcoholic liver disease, and cirrhosis are among the most common conditions associated with liver dysfunction. Active viral hepatitis is felt to be a contraindication to elective surgery.[327] However, surgery is well tolerated in chronic persistent hepatitis, which is characterized by mild persistent elevations in serum aminotransferases, and does not progress to cirrhosis. In contrast, chronic active hepatitis associated with portal inflammation and marked elevations in serum aminotransferase and bilirubin levels may develop into cirrhosis. Preoperative liver biopsy is usually necessary to determine the level of hepatic injury.[326] Mild elevations in hypothrombinemia can be corrected with one or serial (3-day) injections of Vitamin K (10 mg) intramuscularly.[328, 329] Cirrhosis is an irreversible condition of the liver characterized by parenchymal necrosis, nodular regeneration, and fibrosis. Severe metabolic derangement (hyponatremia, hypoalbuminemia, glucose intolerance, prolonged protime/partial thromboplastin times) may be present. Clinical findings may include weight loss, nausea and vomiting, gynecomastia, and ascites. Although more data is available regarding operative risks for cirrhosis compared with liver disease from other causes, most of the available literature is retrospective, consisting of anecdotal reports or studies with small patient numbers.[326] The best predictor of tolerance to surgery is the Child's Classification (**Level II-2**).[330–332] In patients with Child's Class A (no evidence of encephalopathy or ascites, a normal serum albumin, and elevations in bilirubin or prothrombin time less than two times normal values), surgery is usually well tolerated. In patients with Child's Class B or C (ascites, encephalopathy, marked elevations in bilirubin levels and prothrombin time, and hypoalbuminemia), the substantial risks of operative morbidity and mortality must be carefully weighted against the expected benefits of surgery.

Thyroid Disease

Hyperthyroidism Hyperthyroidism, most commonly secondary to Grave's disease, is a state of increased metabolic rate secondary to increased levels of thyroid hormone. Increased thyroid function can also occur in association with gestational trophoblastic disease as a result of circulating thyroid stimulator secreted by trophoblastic tissue. The effects of surgery and anesthesia on thyroid function is very complex; laboratory evaluation may not completely reflect the thyroid status, as chronic illness or surgery can inhibit the conversion of T4 to T3, with a shift to conversion to reverse T3. Recognition of the hyperthyroid state is imperative, and relies upon careful clinical assessment as well as laboratory data. Thyroid storm, defined as extreme hyperthyroidism with cardiovascular collapse, can be precipitated by an operative procedure in 10%–32% of insufficiently treated patients.[159,333,334] Elective surgery should be postponed, awaiting return to the euthyroid state (**Level II-3**).

Treatment of hyperthyroidism includes medications and/or ablative therapy with radioactive iodine or surgery. Propylthiouracil and methimazole interfere with thyroid hormone production (**Level II-3**). The starting dose of propylthiouracil is 100 mg po three times daily; in severely symptomatic patients, 150–200 mg is recommended.[334] Methimazole is administered in a starting dose of 30 mg/day; up to 90 mg/day may be required. Methimazole is contraindicated in pregnancy. Clinical response to these antithyroid medications takes weeks to months as their mode of action is on the production of hormone, whereas release of stored hormone is minimally effected. Consequently, thyrotoxic symptoms are managed with beta-blockers, such as propranolol, 10–20 mg every 6 hours, increased to up to 320 mg every 6 hours, to decrease the heart rate to less than 90 beats per minute.[159,333,334] Propranolol can also be given slowly intravenously, 2–10 mg every 6 hours.[159] An alternative is diltiazem, a calcium channel blocker, initiated at 30 mg every 6 hours, with gradual increase to up to 360 mg per day, to control symptoms.[334] Iodide is used to treat patients in thyroid storm, patients undergoing emergency surgery, and patients with significant underlying cardiovascular disease; iodide interferes with treatment with radioactive iodine. It is given as SSKI, 1–2 drops BID.[51] Finally, dexamethasone, 2 mg IV or by mouth every 6 hours, or hydrocortisone, 100 mg IV or orally every 8 hours, which inhibits the release of thyroid hormones and peripheral conversion of T4 to T3, can be used in the management of thyroid storm.[159,333,334] In the postoperative period, antithyroid medications can be withheld for several days until oral intake is possible. If this period is prolonged, these medications may be administered via NG tube.[159]

Hypothyroidism Decreased thyroid function is associated with decreased metabolic rate, decreased serum T4, and elevated TSH. The diagnosis may be subtle, but should be suspected in patients with symptoms of weight gain, cold intolerance, constipation, bradycardia, edema, especially of the hands and the face, and delayed deep tendon reflexes. Underlying cardiac disease may be masked by hypothyroidism (**Level II-3**).[159,333,334]

Elective surgery should be postponed several months until thyroid medication, levothyroxine (1.6 μg/kg/day; usual dose 0.10–0.125 mg/day), renders the patient euthyroid. To avoid the complications of angina and cardiac arrhythmia, in elderly patients and patients at greatest risk, therapy should begin at a lower dose, with gradual dose escalation as clinical evidence of myxedema resolves and thyroid function improves (**Level II-3**).[334,335] The final dose is determined by TSH and T4 levels. Serious illness, including surgery, can precipitate myxedema coma, an illness characterized by hypotension, hypothermia, hyponatremia, hypoglycemia, and respiratory difficulties. Cardiomegaly and pericardial effusion can also develop.[159,333,334] This disease is treated with intravenous levothyroxine (200–500 μg) followed by levothyroxine 100 μg intravenously per day.[334] Following most gynecologic procedures, thyroid medication can be safely withheld until the patient is tolerating oral intake. However, if the recovery interval becomes unduly prolonged, levothyroxine may be given intravenously or via NG tube.[159]

Pituitary Insufficiency and Hypoparathyroidism

Hypopituitarism is a rare disorder that may develop secondary to profound systemic hypotension and infarction of portions of the pituitary gland (**Level II-3**).[335] Particularly susceptible are lactotropes and gonadotropes, which account for lack of milk production that characterizes Sheehan's syndrome, and subsequent alterations in reproductive function.

The parathyroid gland mediates calcium balance between the intravascular and extravascular spaces and the bone via parathyroid hormone (PTH) and calcitonin. PTH increases serum calcium, mainly by increasing bone resorption and renal reabsorption.[336] Hypercalcemia most commonly is caused by primary hyperparathyroidism secondary to adenoma, hyperplasia, or carcinoma. Malignancies, such as breast cancer that has metastasized to bones, and ovarian cancer (e.g., small cell carcinoma and clear cell adenocarcinoma), with malignant production of PTH-like peptides, are causes of increased serum calcium that are likely to be encountered on a gynecologic service. Although hypercalcemia is asymptomatic in approximately half of affected patients, preoperative chemistry screening should identify the patient with asymptomatic elevated serum calcium, and appropriate evaluation should establish the diagnosis. When primary hyperparathyroidism is diagnosed, elective surgery should be delayed until treatment is initiated to avoid the risks of hypercalcemic parathyroid crisis, which is characterized by marked dehydration and coma. Unfortunately, the only effective therapy is parathyroidectomy. After correcting calcium, phosphate, magnesium, and electrolyte disturbances in collaboration with endocrine and surgical consultants, the preferred surgical management may involve a multidisciplinary approach, combining parathyroidectomy with the gynecologic procedure under the same anesthetic.

Hypercalcemic patients undergoing nonelective surgery or those with malignant hypercalcemia are managed with measures that increase calcium excretion and decrease bone calcium resorption.[336] Acute management is initiated when serum calcium levels are greater than 12 mg/dL; lower serum levels can usually be managed expectantly. Simple hydration with 1–3 L of isotonic solution will generally effectively lower serum calcium levels. After sufficient hydration, lasix diuresis may also be beneficial; however, urine electrolytes should be obtained prior to diuretic administration if kidney disease is the suspected etiology.

Hypocalcemia can occur as a consequence of renal failure, hypoparathyroidism, abnormal serum magnesium levels, pancreatitis, tumor lysis syndrome, and multiple citrated blood transfusions.[336] Calcium replacement is administered as calcium gluconate 10% in ampules containing 90 mg elemental calcium per 10 mg. Magnesium levels must be evaluated and replaced if indicated in order to correct hypocalcemia. The most common cause of decreased serum calcium is hypoalbuminemia; for every 1 g/dL decrease in albumin, serum calcium will decrease by 0.8 mg/dL.[336] An ionized serum calcium level, or correction for low albumin, should be performed before initiation of calcium repletion.

Surgery in Pregnant Patients

During pregnancy, 0.75%–2.2% of women undergo surgery for nonobstetrical indications.[337,338] Morbidity and mortality, both maternal and fetal, are dictated by severity of preexisting disease and are not adversely affected by pregnancy. Surgery during the first and second trimesters has been associated with a slight, but significant, increase in spontaneous abortion.[337] In the largest study published till date, an increase in preterm delivery, low and very low birth weight infants, as well as intrauterine growth retardation was reported, with no increase in the rate of stillbirths (**Level II-2**).[337] Fortunately, multiple studies have demonstrated no increase in congenital anomalies associated with operative procedures during pregnancy, even when surgery is performed in the first trimester, which is considered the period of greatest risk because of ongoing organogenesis.[338–340]

Beginning at about 16 weeks estimated gestational age (EGA), perioperative fetal heart rate (FHR) monitoring is indicated, with continuous monitoring of FHR and uterine activity once fetal viability (24 weeks) is reached, so that tocolytics may be given where appropriate.[340] Beta-mimetics use is not recommended in patients with cardiovascular disease. Magnesium sulfate, another commonly used tocolytic, has been associated with pulmonary edema as well as with decreasing respiratory effort. In preterm pregnancies (EGA less than 32 weeks), the antiprostaglandin indomethacin can be safely used with little toxicity, but should be avoided in later gestations because of risks of premature closure of the ductus. The loading dose is 60 mg given orally or per rectum, followed by 25–50 mg every 6–8 hours for total 24 hours.[341] Prophylactic perioperative hydroxyprogesterone has not been demonstrated to be of any benefit in prevention of fetal wastage.[342] If the adnexa containing the corpus luteum is removed prior to the 10th week of pregnancy, however, hormonal support becomes essential. Progesterone in oil, 100 mg intramuscularly per day, should be given until hormonal production by the corpus luteum is superceded by placental hormonal production, which predominates at approximately 10 weeks gestation.[343] Continuous fetal assessment with heart rate monitoring after 24 weeks is important, as maternal blood pressure, pulse, and oxygen status as determined by pulse oximetry may not reflect uterine perfusion and fetal status.[344] Because fetal physiology is exquisitely sensitive to changes in maternal ventilation or hemodynamic status, changes in fetal heart rate may indicate maternal compromise long before changes in maternal vital signs become apparent.

Surgery in the Elderly

Our society is continuing to age. It is estimated that 21% of the U.S. population, approximately 53 million people, are over 55 years of age and 31.5 million are over 65. By 2050, approximately 21.7% are expected to be over 65 years of age, and women will constitute the majority of these patients. Today, there are 19 million women over 65 years of age.[345] About 50% of all cancers are detected in patients within this age group (**Level II-2**).[346]

Until recently, few reports existed in the literature that provided data regarding the perioperative care or morbidity of surgery in the elderly. Genitourinary (GU) cancers, including cancer of the bladder, breast, ovary, cervix, and uterus, are significantly more likely to be diagnosed at advanced stages in older patients.[347] There is an inverse relationship between frequency in gynecologic examinations and Pap smears with advancing age, which supports the premise that inadequate screening among the elderly is a major factor in failure to diagnose gynecologic cancers at early, potentially treatable stages.[348, 349] The increased side effects of cytotoxic chemotherapy and/or radiation therapy in elderly patients often require major reductions in dose, which, in part, accounts for the higher incidence of treatment failures in elderly patients, including those with local disease only.[350, 351] Several studies have confirmed that surgery can safely be accomplished, even in the very elderly, although the rate of perioperative morbidity is increased proportionate to age and preexisting health.[348, 349] With the advent of critical care surveillance, even ultraradical surgery including ovarian debulking, radical hysterectomy, and pelvic exenteration may be safely accomplished with acceptable morbidity in older patients who are otherwise in good health.[350, 351]

Nevertheless, blood loss, morbidity, length of hospital stay, and multiorgan failure are complications that are significantly increased with surgery in the elderly. Coronary artery disease, CHF, and malignancy with its associated immunological suppression and malnutrition, and other preexisting diseases predispose the elderly to more perioperative complications by virtue of organ system dysfunction. Wound complications and skin breakdown are increased in older patients.[360] Recovery in muscle strength including handgrip and respiratory muscle strength is significantly reduced in the elderly, and may contribute to the development of atelectasis, pneumonia, and DVTs that are major contributors to morbidity and mortality in these patients.[361, 362] Reduced morbidity and mortality require a thorough preoperative assessment of preexisting medical diseases with appropriate perioperative medical and intensive care consultation as needed.[356]

REFERENCES

1. HILL GL, DOUGLAS RG, SCHROEDER D. Metabolic basis for the management of patients undergoing major surgery. World J Surg 1993;17:146–153.
2. GAMIL M, FANNING A. The first 24 hours after surgery. Anaesthesia 1991;46:712–715.
3. SUN H, ILES M, WEISSMAN C. Physiologic variables and fluid resuscitation in the postoperative intensive care unit patient. Crit Care Med 1993;21:555–561.
4. SHIRES GT, CANIZARO PC, LOWRY SF. Fluid, electrolyte, and nutritional management of the surgical patient. In: SCHWARTZ SI, SHIRES GT, SPENCER FC, STORER EH, editors. Principles of Surgery. 4th ed. New York: McGraw-Hill; 1984. p 45–80.
5. SHIRES GT, CANIZARO PC. Fluid and electrolyte management of the surgical patient. In: SEBASTIAN DC JR, editor. Textbook of Surgery. 14th ed. Philadelphia, PA: WB Saunders Company; 1991. p 57–76.
6. O'SHEA MH. Fluid and electrolyte management. In: WOODLEY M, WHELAN A, editors. Manual of Medical Therapeutics. 27th ed. Boston: Little, Brown and Company; 1992. p 42–61.
7. DEFRONZO RA, THIER SO. Pathophysiologic approach to hyponatremia. Arch Intern Med 1980;140:897–902.
8. LEVI R. Therapies for perioperative hypertension: pharmacodynamic considerations. Acta Anaesthesiol Scand 1993;37(S99):16–19.
9. HEUSER D, GUGGENBERGER H, FRETSCHNER R. Acute blood pressure increase during the perioperative period. Am J Cardiol 1989;63:26C–31C.
10. AKEN HV, HEMELRIJCK JV. The influence of anesthesia on cerebral blood flow and cerebral metabolism: an overview. Agressologie 1991;32:303–306.
11. LAYON JA. Physiologic effects of anesthesia in the critically ill. In: CIVETTA JM, TAYLOR RW, KIRBY RR, editors. Critical Care. Philadelphia, PA: JB Lippincott; 1988. p 145–156.
12. CHARLSON ME, MACKENZIE CR, GOLD JP, et al. Intraoperative blood pressure: what patterns identify patients at risk for postoperative complications? Ann Surg 1990;212:567–580.
13. KOLANSKY DM, COHEN LS. Chapter 14. Immediate postoperative management. In: FRANKL WS, BREST AN, editors. Valvular Heart Disease: Comprehensive Evaluation and Treatment. Cardiovasc Clin 1992;23:277–291.
14. AUGUSTINE SD. Hypothermia therapy in the postanesthesia care unit: a review. J Post Anesth Nurs 1990;5(4):254–263.
15. OSGUTHORPE SG. Hypothermia and rewarming alter cardiac surgery. AACN Clin Issues Crit Care Nurs 1993;4(2):276–292.
16. FRANK SM, BEATTLE C, CHRISTOPHERSON R, et al. Unintentional hypothermia is associated with postoperative myocardial ischemia. Anesthesiology 1993;78:468–476.
17. DANZL DF, POZOS RS. Current concepts: accidental hypothermia. N Engl J Med 1994;331:1756–1760.
18. STRANDBERG AA, TOKICS L, BRISMAR B, et al. Atelectasis during anaesthesia and in the postoperative period. Acta Anaesthesiol Scand 1986;30:154–158.
19. JONES JG, SAPSFORD DJ, WHEATLEY RG. Postoperative hypoxaemia: mechanisms and time course. Anaesthesia 1990;45:566–573.
20. PETT SB JR, WERNLY JA. Respiratory function in surgical patients: perioperative evaluation and management. Surg Annu 1988;20:311–329.
21. MEYERS JR, LEMBECK L, O'KANE H, et al. Changes in functional residual capacity of the lung after operation. Arch Surg 1975;110:576–583.
22. HOSODA R, HATTORI M, SHIMADA Y. Favorable effects of epidural analgesia on hemodynamics, oxygenation and metabolic variables in the immediate post-anesthetic period. Acta Anaesthesiol Scand 1993;37:469–474.
23. LICKER M, SUTER PM, KRAUER F, et al. Metabolic response to lower abdominal surgery: analgesia by epidural blockade compared with intravenous opiate infusion. Eur J Anaesthesiol 1994;11:193–199.
24. JAYR C, MOLLIE A, BOURGAIN JL, et al. Postoperative pulmonary complications: general anesthesia with postoperative parenteral morphine compared with epidural anesthesia. Surgery 1988;104:57–63.

25. GIESECKE K, KLINGSTEDT C, LJUNGOVIST O, et al. The modifying influence of anaesthesia on postoperative protein catabolism. Br J Anaesth 1994;72:697–699.
26. SCHULZE S. Humoral and neural mediators of the systemic response to surgery. Dan Med Bull 1993;40:365–377.
27. SALO M. Effects of anaesthesia and surgery on the immune response. Acta Anaesthesiol Scand 1992;36:201–220.
28. PULLICINO EA, CARLI F, POOLE S, et al. The relationship between the circulating concentrations of interleukin 6 (IL-6), tumor necrosis factor (TNF) and the acute phase response to elective surgery and accidental injury. Lymphokine Res 1990;9:231–238.
29. BAIGRIE RJ, LAMONT PM, KWAITKOWSKI D, et al. Systemic cytokine response after major surgery. Br J Surg 1992;79:757–760.
30. LENNARD TWJ, SHENTON BJ, BORZOTTA A, et al. The influence of surgical operations on components of the human immune system. Br J Surg 1985;72:771–776.
31. BOWLING, TE. Does disorder of gastrointestinal motility affect food intake in the post-surgical patient? Proc Nutr Soc 1994;53:151–157.
32. CLEVERS GJ, SMOUT AJ. The natural course of postoperative ileus following abdominal surgery. Neth J Surg 1989;41:97–99.
33. WALDHAUSEN JHT, SHAFFREY ME, SKENDERIS II BS, et al. Gastrointestinal myoelectric and clinical patterns of recovery after laparotomy. Ann Surg 1990;211(6):777–785.
34. LIVINGSTON EH, PASSARO EP. Postoperative ileus (Review Article). Dig Dis Sci 1990;35:121–132.
35. INGRAM DM, CATCHPOLE BN. Effect of opiates on gastroduodenal motility following surgical operation. Dig Dis Sci 1981;26:989–992.
36. MITCHELL A, COLLIN J. Vasopressin effects on the small intestine: a possible factor in paralytic ileus? Br J Surg 1985;72:462–465.
37. CONDON RE, COWLES V, EKBOM GA, et al. Effects of halothane, enflurane, and nitrous oxide on colon motility. Surgery 1987;101:81–132.
38. JOHNSON H JR, KNEE-IOLI S, BUTLER TA, et al. Are routine preoperative laboratory screening tests necessary to evaluate ambulatory surgical patients? Surgery 1988;104:639–645.
39. VELANOVICH V. The value of routine laboratory testing in predicting postoperative complications: a multivariate analysis. Surgery 1991;109:236–243.
40. ROHRER JM, MICHELOTTI MC, NAHRWOLD DL. A prospective evaluation of the efficiency of pre-operative coagulation testing. Ann Surg 1988;208:554–557.
41. ROIZEN MI. Preoperative evaluation. In: MILLER RD, editor. Anesthesia. Vol. 1, 4th ed. New York: Churchill Livingstone; 1994. p 827–882.
42. MUSHLIN AI, THORNBURY JR. Intravenous pyelography: the case against its routine use. Ann Intern Med 1989;111:58–70.
43. SIMEL DL, MATCHAR DB, PISCITELLI JT. Routine intravenous pyelograms before hysterectomy in cases of benign disease: possibly effective, definitely expensive. Am J Obstet Gynecol 1988;159:1049–1053.
44. PISCITELLI JT, SIMEL DL, ADDISON WA. Who should have intravenous pyelograms before hysterectomy for benign disease? Obstet Gynecol 1987;69:541–545.
45. LASSER EC, BERRY CC, TALNER LB, et al. Pretreatment with corticosteroids to alleviate reactions to intravenous contrast material. N Engl J Med 1987;317:845–849.
46. HEYMAN SN, BREZIS M, EPSTEIN FH, et al. Early renal medullary hypoxic injury from radiocontrast and indomethacin. Kidney Int 1991;40:632–642.
47. SOLOMON R, WERNER C, MANN D, et al. Effects of saline, mannitol, and furosemide on acute decreases in renal function induced by radiocontrast agents. N Engl J Med 1994;331:1416–1420.
48. MANGANO DT. Perioperative cardiac morbidity. Anesthesiology 1990;72:153–184.
49. GOLDMAN L. Cardiac risk factors and complications in non-cardiac surgery. Medicine 1978;57:357–370.
50. GOLDMAN L, CALDERA DL, NUSSBAUM SR, et al. Multifactorial index of cardiac risk in noncardiac surgical procedures. N Engl J Med 1977;297:845–850.

51. RAO TLK, JACOBS KH, EL-ETR AA. Reinfarction following anesthesia in patients with myocardial infarction. Anesthesiology 1983;59:499–505.

52. GOLDMAN L. Assessment of perioperative cardiac risk (Editorial). N Engl J Med 1994;330:707–709.

53. ASHTON CM. Perioperative myocardial infarction with noncardiac surgery. Am J Med Sci 1994;308(1):41–48.

54. NICHOLS RE. Surgical wound infection. Am J Med 1991;91(Suppl 3 B):54–64.

55. MAKI DG. Nosocomial bacteremia: an epidemiologic overview. Am J Med 1981;70:719–732.

56. LEAPER DJ. Prophylactic and therapeutic role of antibiotics in wound care. Am J Surg 1994;167:15S–20S.

57. EHRENKRANZ NJ, BLACKWELDER WC, PFAFF SJ, et al. Infections complicating low-risk cesarean sections in community hospitals: efficacy of antimicrobial prophylaxis. Am J Obstet Gynecol 1990;162:337–343.

58. PAGE CP, BOHNEN JMA, FLETCHER JR, et al. Antimicrobial prophylaxis for surgical wounds. Arch Surg 1993;128:79–88.

59. LUDWIG KA, CARLSON MA, CONDON RE. Prophylactic antibiotics in surgery. Annu Rev Med 1993;44:385–393.

60. CULVER DH, HORAN CT, GAYNES RP, et al. Surgical wound infection rates by wound class, operative procedure, and patient risk index. Am J Med 1991;91:152S–157S.

61. DROBRZANSKI S, LAWLEY DI, MCDERMOTT I, et al. Research and reports: the impact of guidelines on perioperative antibiotic administration. J Clin Farm Ther 1991;16:19–24.

62. DELLINGER EP, GROSS PA, BARRETT TL, et al. Quality standard for antimicrobial prophylaxis in surgical patients. Clin Infect Dis 1994;18:422–427.

63. STEIN GE. Patient costs for prophylaxis and treatment of obstetric and gynecologic surgical infections. Am J Obstet Gynecol 1991;164:1377–1380.

64. ORR JW, SISSON PF, PATSNER B, et al. Single-dose antibiotic prophylaxis for patients undergoing extended pelvic surgery for gynecologic malignancy. Am J Obstet Gynecol 1990;162: 718–721.

65. HAGAR WD, RAPP RP, BILLETER M, et al. Choice of antibiotic in nonelective cesarean section. Antimicrob Agents Chemother 1991;35:1782–1784.

66. GALASK RP. The challenge of prophylaxis in cesarean section in the 1990s. J Reprod Med 1990;35:1078–1081.

67. LANG R, SHALIT I, SEGAL J, et al. Maternal and fetal serum and tissue levels of ceftriaxone following preoperative prophylaxis in emergency cesarean section. Chemotherapy 1993;39:77–81.

68. CHANG PL, NEWTON ER. Predictors of antibiotic prophylactic failure in post-cesarean endometritis. Obstet Gynecol 1992;80:117–122.

69. FEJGIN MD, MARKOV S, GOSHEN S, et al. Antibiotic for cesarean section the case for "true" prophylaxis. Int J Gynaecol Obstet 1993;43:257–261.

70. MCGREGOR JA, FRENCH JI, MAKOWSKI E. Single-dose cefotetan versus multidose cefoxitin for prophylaxis in cesarean section in high-risk patients. Am J Obstet Gynecol 1986;154:955–960.

71. KRISTENSEN GB, BEITER E-C, MATHER O. Single-dose cefuroxime prophylaxis in non-elective cesarean section. Acta Obstet Gynecol Scand 1990;69:497–500.

72. VON MANDACH U, HUCH R, MALINVERNI R, et al. Ceftriaxone (single dose) versus cefoxitin (multiple doses): success and failure of antibiotic prophylaxis in 1052 cesarean sections. J Perinat Med 1993;21:385–397.

73. SWARTZ WH. Prophylaxis of minor febrile and major infectious morbidity following hysterectomy. Obstet Gynecol 1979;54:284–288.

74. SHAPIRO M, MUNOZ A, TAKGER IB, et al. Risk factors for infection at the operative site after abdominal or vaginal hysterectomy. N Engl J Med 1982;307:1661–1666.

75. MITTENDORF R, ARONSON MP, BERRY RE, et al. Avoiding serious infections associated with abdominal hysterectomy: a meta-analysis of antibiotic prophylaxis. Am J Obstet Gynecol 1993;169:1119–1124.

76. CAMPILLO F, RUBIO JM. Comparative study of single-dose cefotaxime and multiple doses of cefoxitin and cefazolin as prophylaxis in gynecologic surgery. Am J Surg 1992;164:12S–15S.

77. STIVER HG, BINNS BO, BRUNHAM RC, et al. Randomized, double-blind comparison of the efficacies, costs, and vaginal flora alterations with single-dose ceftriaxone and multidose cefazolin prophylaxis in vaginal hysterectomy. Antimicrob Agents Chemother 1990;34:1194–1197.

78. SEVIN BU, RAMOS R, LICHTIGER M, et al. Antibiotic prevention of infections complicating radical hysterectomy. Obstet Gynecol 1984;64:539–545.

79. CARTANA J, CORTES J, YARNOZ MC, et al. Antibiotic prophylaxis in Wertheim-Meigs surgery. A single dose vs three doses. Eur J Gynaecol Oncol 1994;XV:14–18.

80. KOBAMATSU Y, MAKINODA S, YAMADA T, et al. Evaluation of the improvement of cephems on the prophylaxis of pelvic infection after radical hysterectomy. Gynecol Obstet Invest 1991;32: 102–106.

81. GRAHAM JE JR. Infectious morbidity in gynecologic oncology. J Reprod Med 1990;35:348–352.

82. MORRIS WT. Prophylaxis against sepsis in patients undergoing major surgery. World J Surg 1993;17:178–183.

83. McDONALD PJ, O'LOUGHLIN JA. Prophylactic antibiotics and prevention of surgical sepsis. Baillieres Clin Obstet Gynaecol 1993;7:219–236.

84. SHERIDAN RL, TOMPKINS RG, BURKE JF. Prophylactic antibiotics and their role in the prevention of surgical wound infection. Adv Surg 1994;27:43–65.

85. GORBACH SL. SESSION II: Clinical uses of prophylaxis. Antimicrobial prophylaxis for appendectomy and colorectal surgery. Rev Infect Dis 1991;13:S815–S820.

86. MENAKER GJ. The use of antibiotics in surgical treatment of the colon. Surg Gynecol Obstet 1987;164:581–586.

87. BECK DE, HARFORD FJ, DiPALMA JA. Comparison of cleansing methods in preparation for colonic surgery. Dis Colon Rectum 1985;28:491–495.

88. WOLFF BG, BEART RW JR, DOXOIS RR, et al. A new bowel preparation for elective colon and rectal surgery: a prospective, randomized clinical trial. Arch Surg 1988;123:895–900.

89. KAISER AB, HERRINGTON JL JR, HERRINGTON JL JR, et al. Cefoxitin versus erythromycin, neomycin and cefazolin in colorectal operations: importance of the duration of the surgical procedure. Ann Surg 1983;198:525–530.

90. NICHOLS RL. Effects of preoperative neomycin erythromycin intestinal preparation on the incidence of infectious complications following colon surgery. Ann Surg 1973;178:453–462.

91. CLARKE JS, CONDON RE, BARTLETT JG, et al. Preoperative oral antibiotics reduce septic complications of colon operations: results of prospective randomized, double-blind clinical study. Ann Surg 1977;186:251–259.

92. STELLATO TA, DANZIGER LH, GORDON N, et al. Antibiotics in elective colon surgery. A randomized trial of oral, systemic, and oral/systemic antibiotics for prophylaxis. Am Surg 1990;56: 251–254.

93. WEAVER M, BURDON DW, YOUNGS DJ, et al. Oral neomycin and erythromycin compared with single-dose systemic metronidazole and ceftriaxone prophylaxis in elective colorectal surgery. Am J Surg 1986;151:437–442.

94. COPPA GF, ENG K. Factors involved in antibiotic selection in elective colon and rectal surgery. Surgery 1990;104:383–386.

95. SCHOETZ DJ JR, ROBERTS PL, MURRAY JJ, et al. Addition of parenteral cefoxitin to regimen of oral antibiotics for elective colorectal operations. A randomized prospective surgery. Ann Surg 1990;212:209–212.

96. PORTNOY J, KAGAN E, GORDON P, et al. Prophylactic antibiotics in elective colorectal surgery. Dis Colon Rectum 1983;26:310–313.

97. MORRIS DL, WILSON SR, PAIN J, et al. A comparison of aztreonam/metronidazole and cefotaxime/metronidazole in elective colorectal surgery: antimicrobial prophylaxis must include gram-positive cover. J Antimicrob Chemother 1990;25:673–678.

98. DAJANI AS, BISNO AL, CHUNG KJ, et al. Prevention of bacterial endocarditis: recommendations by the American Heart Association. JAMA 1990;264:2919–2922.

99. OFFENBARTL K, BENGMARK S. Intraabdominal infections and gut origin sepsis. World J Surg 1990;14:191–195.

100. STOUTENBEEK CHP, VAN SACNE HKF, MIRANDA DR, et al. The effect of selective decontamination of the digestive tract on colonization and infection rate in multiple trauma patients. Intensive Care Med 1984;10:185–192.

101. KERVER AJH, ROMMES JH, MEVISSEN-VERHAGE EAE, et al. Colonization and infection in surgical intensive care patients—a prospective study. Intensive Care Med 1987;13:347–351.

102. KERVER AJH, ROMMES JH, MEVISSEN-VIRHAGE EAE, et al. Prevention of colonization and infection in critically ill patients: a prospective randomized study. Crit Care Med 1988;16:1087–1093.

103. DESAI MH, RUTAN RL, HEGGERS JP, et al. Candida infection with and without nystatin prophylaxis: an 11-year experience with patients with burn injury. Arch Surg 1992;127:159–162.

104. KLASTERSKY J, GLAUSER MP, SCHIMPFF C, et al. Prospective randomized comparison of three antibiotic regimens for empirical therapy for suspected bacteremic infection in febrile granulocytopenic patients. Antimicrob Agents Chemother 1986;29:263–270.

105. DEITCH EA, WINTERTON J, BERG R. The gut as a portal of entry for bacteremia: role of protein malnutrition. Ann Surg 1987;205:681–691.

106. DEITCH EA, WINTERTON J, BERG R. Effect of starvation, malnutrition, and trauma on the gastrointestinal tract flora and bacterial translocation. Arch Surg 1987;122:1019–1024.

107. CERRA FB. Hypermetabolism, organ failure, and metabolic support. Surgery 1987;101:1–13.

108. GALLUP DG, NOLAN TE. The gynecologist and multiple organ failure syndrome (MOFS). Gynecol Oncol 1993;48:293–300.

109. CIRISANO FD, GREENSPOON JS, STENSON R, et al. The etiology and management of diarrhea in the gynecologic oncology patient. Gynecol Oncol 1993;50:45–48.

110. REINKE CM, MESSICK CR. Update on Clostridium difficile-induced colitis, part 1. Am J Hosp Pharm 1994;51:1771–1781.

111. REINKE CM, MESSICK CR. Update on Clostridium difficile-induced colitis, part 2. Am J Hosp Pharm 1994;51:1892–1901.

112. GERDING DN, JOHNSON S, PETERSON LR, et al. Clostridium difficile-associated diarrhea and colitis. Infect Control Hosp Epidemiol 1995;16:459–477.

113. ANAND A, GLATT AE. Glostridium difficile infection associated with antineoplastic chemotherapy: a review. Clin Infect Dis 1993;17:109–113.

114. WALTERS BAJ, ROBERTS RK, SENEVIRATNE E. Contamination and cross infection with Clostridium difficile in an intensive care unit. Aust N Z J Med 1982;12:255–258.

115. TRUDEL JL, DESCHENES M, MAYRAND S, et al. Toxic megacolon complicating pseudomembranous enterocolitis. Dis Colon Rectum 1995;38(10) 1033–1038.

116. KELLY CP, POTHOULAKIS C, LAMONT JT. Clostridium difficile colitis (Review Article). N Engl J Med 1994;330:257–262.

117. BONNAR J. Venous thromboembolism and gynecologic surgery. Clin Obstet Gynecol 1985;28(2):432–446.

118. WEINMANN EE, SALZMAN EW. Deep-vein thrombosis. N Engl J Med 1994;24:1630–1640.

119. CLARKE-PEARSON DL, DELONG ER, SYNAN IS, et al. Variables associated with postoperative deep venous thrombosis: a prospective study of 411 gynecology patients and creation of a prognostic model. Obstet Gynecol 1987;69:146–150.

120. GENTON E, TURPIE AGG. Venous thromboembolism associated with gynecologic surgery. Clin Obstet Gynecol 1980;23(1):209–241.

121. WALSH JJ, BONNAR J, WRIGHT FW. A study of pulmonary embolism and deep vein thrombosis after major gynecological surgery using labeled fibrinogen, phlebography and lung scanning. J Obstet Gynecol Br Commonw 1974;81:311–316.

122. NICOLAIDES A, KAKKAR V, FIELD ES, et al. The origin of deep vein thrombosis: a venographic study. Br J Radiol 1971;44:653–663.

123. KAKKAR VV, HOWE CT, FLANG C, et al. Natural history of postoperative deep-venous thrombosis. Lancet 1969;2:230–232.

124. BALLARD RM, BRADLEY-WATSON PJ, JOHNSTONE FD, et al. Low doses of subcutaneous heparin in the prevention of deep vein thrombosis after gynaecological surgery. J Obstet Gynaecol Br Commonw 1973;80:469–663.

125. CLAYTON JK, ANDERSON JA, McNICOL GP. Effect of cigarette smoking on subsequent postoperative thromboembolic disease in gynaecological patients. Br Med J 1978;2(6134):402.
126. KAKKAR VV. Prevention of fatal pulmonary embolism. Haemostasis 1993;23S:42–50.
127. KAKKAR VV. An international multicenter trial: Prevention of fatal postoperative pulmonary embolism by low doses of heparin. Lancet 1975;2:45–51.
128. GINSBERG JS. Management of venous thromboembolism (Review). N Engl J Med 1996;335:1816–1828.
129. CARTER CJ, KELTON JG, JIRSH J, et al. The relationship between the hemorrhagic and antithrombotic properties of low molecular weight heparin in rabbits. Blood 1982;59:1239–1245.
130. SALZMAN EW, ROSENBERG RD, SMITH MH, et al. Effect of heparin and heparin fractions on platelet aggregation. J Clin Invest 1980;65:64–73.
131. KAKKAR VV, COHEN AT, EDMONSON RA, et al. Low molecular weight versus standard heparin for prevention of venous thromboembolism after major abdominal surgery. Lancet 1993;341: 259–265.
132. WEITZ JI. Low-molecular-weight heparins (Review). N Engl J Med 1997;337(10):688–698.
133. Multicenter Trial Committee. Dihydroergotamine-heparin prophylaxis of postoperative deep vein thrombosis: a multicenter trial. JAMA 1984;251:2960–2966.
134. POLLER L, McKERNAN A, THOMSON JM, et al. Fixed minidose warfarin: a new approach to prophylaxis against venous thrombosis after major surgery. Br Med J 1987;295:1309–1312.
135. TURNER GM, COLE SE, BROOKS JH. The efficacy of graduated compression stockings in the prevention of deep vein thrombosis after major gynaecological surgery. Br J Obstet Gynaecol 1984;91:588–591.
136. CLARKE-PEARSON DL, SYNAN IS, HINSHAW WM, et al. Prevention of postoperative venous thromboembolism by external pneumatic calf compression in patients with gynecologic malignancy. Obstet Gynecol 1984;63:92–98.
137. CLARKE-PEARSON DL, SYNAN IS, DODGE R, et al. A randomized trial of low-dose heparin and intermittent pneumatic calf compression for the prevention of deep venous thrombosis after gynecologic oncology surgery. Am J Obstet Gynecol 1993;168:1146–1154.
138. Consensus Conference. Prevention of venous thrombosis and pulmonary embolism. JAMA 1986;256(6):744–749.
139. CLARKE-PEARSON DL, DeLONG E, SYNAN IS, et al. A controlled trial of two low-dose heparin regimens for the prevention of postoperative deep vein thrombosis. Obstet Gynecol 1990;75:684–689.
140. WILLE-JORGENSEN P, LAUSEN I, JORGENSEN LN. Is there a need for long-term thromboprophylaxis following general surgery? Haemostasis 1993;23(S1):10–14.
141. VANOOIJEN B. Subcutaneous heparin and postoperative wound hematomas. Arch Surg 1986;121:937–940.
142. OSTER G, TUDEN RL, COLDITZ GA. Prevention of venous thromboembolism after general surgery: cost-effectiveness analysis of alternative approaches to prophylaxis. Am J Med 1987;82: 889–899.
143. SAMAMA M, BERNARD P, BONNARDOT JP, et al. Low molecular weight heparin compared with unfractionated heparin in prevention of postoperative thrombosis. Br J Surg 1988;75:128–131.
144. SASAHARA AA, KOPPENHAGEN, HARING R, et al. Low molecular weight heparin plus dihydroergotamine for prophylaxis of postoperative deep vein thrombosis. Br J Surg 1986;73(9):697–700.
145. ABRAMOWICZ M. Dihydroergotamine-heparin to prevent postoperative deep vein thrombosis. Med Lett Drugs Ther 1985;27(688):45–46.
146. SALVIAN AJ, BAKER JD. Effects of intermittent pneumatic calf compression in normal and postphlebitic Legs. J Cardiovasc Surg 1988;29:37–41.
147. SCHWARZ RE, MARRERO AM, CONLON KC, et al. Inferior vena cava fiters in cancer patients: introduction and outcome. J Clin Oncol 1996;14(2):652–657.
148. ZINNER MJ, ZUIDEMA GD, SMITH PL, et al. The prevention of upper gastrointestinal tract bleeding in patients in an intensive care unit. Surg Gynecol Obstet 1981;153:214–220.
149. PRIEBE HJ, SKILLMAN JJ, BUSHNESS LS, et al. Antacid versus cimetidine in preventing acute gastrointestinal bleeding: a randomized trial in 75 critically ill patients. N Engl J Med 1980;302:426–430.

150. RUDDELL WSJ, AXON ATR, FINDALY JM, et al. Effect of cimetidine on the gastric bacterial flora. Lancet 1980;1:672–674.
151. DONOWITZ LG, PAGE MC, MILEUT BL, et al. Alteration of normal gastric flora in critical care patients receiving antacid and cimetidine therapy. Infect Control 1986;7:23–26.
152. HORAN TC, WHITE JW, JARVIS WR, et al. Nosocomial infection surveillance, 1984. Mor Mortal Wkly Rep CDC Surveill Summ 1986;35(1):17SS–29SS.
153. SAMLOFF IM, O'DELL C. Inhibition of peptic activity by sucralfate. Am J Med 1985;79S(2C): 15–18.
154. DRIKS MR, CRAVEN DE, CELLI BR, et al. Nosocomial pneumonia in intubated patients given sucralfate as compared with antacids or histamine type 2 blockers. N Engl J Med 1987;317:1376–1382.
155. AXELROD L. Glucocorticoid therapy. Medicine 1976;55:39–65.
156. GRABER AL, NEY RL, NICHOLSON WE, et al. Natural history of pituitary-adrenal recovery following long-term suppression with corticosteroids. J Clin Endocrinol Metab 1965;25:11–16.
157. KEHLET H, BINDER C. Value of ACTH test in assessing HPA function in glucocorticoid-treated patients. Br Med J 1973;1:147–149.
158. SALEM M, TAINSH RE, BROMBERG J, et al. Perioperative glucocorticoid coverage: a reassessment 42 years after emergence of a problem. Ann Surg 1994;219(4):416–425.
159. GOLDMANN DR. Perioperative endocrinologic problems. In: MERLI GJ, WEITZ HH, editors. Medical Management of the Surgical Patient. Philadelphia, PA: WB Saunders Company; 1992. p 227–245.
160. SONNENDECKER EWW, GUIDOSSI F, MARGOLIUS KA. Splenectomy during primary maximal cytoreductive surgery for epithelial ovarian cancer. Gynecol Oncol 1989;35:301–306.
161. MORRIS M, GERSHENSON DM, BURKE TW, et al. Splenectomy in gynecologic oncology: indications, complications, and technique. Gynecol Oncol 1991;43:118–122.
162. FEROE DD, AUGUSTINE SD. Hypothermia in the PACU. Crit Care Nurs Clin North Am 1991;3(1):135–144.
163. ORR JW JR, HOLLOWAY RW, ORR PF. Postoperative care of the gynecologic patient. In: COPELAND LJ, JARRELL JF, MCGREGOR JA, editors. Textbook of Gynecology. Philadelphia, PA: WB Saunders Company; 1992. p 670–694.
164. KRUSE JA, CARLSON RW. Rapid correction of hypokalemia using concentrated intravenous potassium chloride infusions. Arch Intern Med 1990;150:613–617.
165. KUNIS CL, LOWENSTEIN J. The emergency treatment of hyperkalemia. Med Clin North Am 1981;65:165–175.
166. ALLON M, COPKNEY C. Albuterol and insulin for treatment of hyperkalemia in hemodialysis patients. Kidney Int 1990;38:869–872.
167. LILLEMOE KD, ROMOLO JL, HAMILTON SR, et al. Intestinal necrosis due to sodium polystyrene (Kayexalate) in sorbitol enemas: clinical and experimental support for the hypothesis. Surgery 1987;101:267–272.
168. MULLEN JL, BUZBY GP, MATTHEWS DC, et al. Reduction of operative morbidity and mortality by combined preoperative and postoperative nutritional support. Ann Surg 1980;192:604–613.
169. MASSAD LS, VOGLER G, HERZOG TJ, et al. Correlates of length of stay in gynecologic oncology patients undergoing inpatient surgery. Gynecol Oncol 1993;51:214–218.
170. CAMPOS ACL, MEGUID MM. A critical appraisal of the usefulness of perioperative nutritional support. Am J Clin Nutr 1992;55:117–130.
171. The Veterans Affairs Total Parenteral Nutrition Cooperative Study Group. Perioperative total parenteral nutrition in surgical patients. N Engl J Med 1991;325:525–532.
172. GRANT JP, editor. Handbook of Total Parenteral Nutrition. 2nd ed. Philadelphia, PA: WB Saunders Company; 1992. p 15–47.
173. BAUE AE. Nutrition and metabolism in sepsis and multisystem organ failure. Surg Clin North Am 1991;71:549–565.
174. VINNARS E, HAMMARQVIST F, VON DER DECKEN A, et al. Role of glutamine and its analogs in posttraumatic muscle protein and amino acid metabolism. JPEN J Parenter Enteral Nutr 1990;14:125S–129S.
175. KEMPER M, WEISSMAN C, HYMAN AI. Caloric requirements and supply in critically ill surgical patients. Crit Care Med 1992;20:344–348.

176. Schlichtig R, Ayres SM. Nutritional assessment of the critically ill. In: Nutritional Support of the Critically Ill. Chicago: Year Book Medical Publishers; 1988. p 75–95.

177. Willatts SM. Nutrition. Br J Anaesth 1986;58:201–222.

178. AMA Department of Foods and Nutrition. Guidelines for essential trace element preparations for parenteral use. JAMA 1979;241:2051–2054.

179. Bozzetti F, Terno G, Camerini E, et al. Pathogenesis and predictability of central venous catheter sepsis. Surgery 1982;91:383–389.

180. Bjornson HS, Colley R, Bower RH, et al. Association between microorganism growth at the catheter insertion site and colonization of the catheter in patients receiving total parenteral nutrition. Surgery 1982;92:720–727.

181. Pemberton B, Lyman B, Lander V, et al. Sepsis from triple- vs single-lumen catheters during total parenteral nutrition in surgical or critically ill patients. Arch Surg 1986;121:591–594.

182. Padberg FT, Ruggiero J, Blackburn GL, et al. Central venous catheterization for parenteral nutrition. Ann Surg 1981;193:264–270.

183. Haire WD, Lieberman RP. Defining the risks of subclavian-vein catheterization. N Engl J Med 1994;331:1769–1770.

184. Bern MM, Lokich JJ, Wallach SR, et al. Very low doses of warfarin can prevent thrombosis in central venous catheters. Ann Intern Med 1990;112:423–428.

185. Tschirhart JM, Rao MK. Mechanism and management of persistent withdrawal occlusion. Am Surg 1988;54:326–328.

186. Haire WD, Lieberman RP, Lund GB, et al. Obstructed central venous catheters: restoring function with a 12-hour infusion with low-dose urokinase. Cancer 1990;66:2279–2285.

187. Edwards TW. Optimizing opioid treatment of postoperative pain. J Pain Symptom Manage 1990;5:S24.

188. Donovan M, Dillon P, McGuire L. Incidence and characteristics of pain in a sample of medical-surgical inpatients. Pain 1987;30:69–78.

189. Hopf HW, Weitz S. Postoperative pain management. Arch Surg 1994;129:128–132.

190. Lutz LJ, Lamer TJ. Management of postoperative pain: review of current techniques and methods. Mayo Clin Proc 1990;65:584–596.

191. Rose PG, Piver MS, Batista E, et al. Patient-controlled analgesia in gynecologic oncology. J Reprod Med 1989;34:651–654.

192. Lange MP, Dahn MS, Jacobs LA. Patient-controlled analgesia versus intermittent analgesia dosing. Heart Lung 1988;17:495–498.

193. Moss G, Regal ME, Lichtig L. Reducing postoperative pain, narcotics, and length of hospitalization. Surgery 1986;99:206–210.

194. Dahl JB, Daugaard JJ, Larsen HV, et al. Patient-controlled analgesia: a controlled trial. Acta Anaesthesiol Scand 1987;31:744–747.

195. Rybro L, Schurizek BA, Petersen TK, et al. Postoperative analgesia and lung function: a comparison of intramuscular with epidural morphine. Acta Anaesthesiol Scand 1982;26:514–518.

196. Hjortso NC, Neumann P, Frosig F, et al. A controlled study on the effect of epidural analgesia with local anaesthetics and morphine on morbidity after abdominal surgery. Acta Anaesthesiol Scand 1985;29:790–796.

197. Drummond GB, Littlewood DG. Respiratory effects of extradural analgesia after lower abdominal surgery. Br J Anaesth 1977;49:999–1004.

198. Cuschieri RJ, Morran CG, Howie JC, et al. Postoperative pain and pulmonary complications: comparison of three analgesic regimens. Br J Surg 1985;72:495–498.

199. Cullen ML, Staren ED, El-Ganzouri A, et al. Continuous epidural infusion for analgesia after major abdominal operations: a randomized, prospective, double-blind study. Surgery 1985;98:718–728.

200. Lysak SZ, Anderson PT, Carithers RA, et al. Postoperative effects of fentanyl, ketorolac, and piroxicam as analgesics for outpatient laparoscopic procedures. Obstet Gynecol 1994;83:270–275.

201. Stouten EM, Armbruster S, Houmes RJ, et al. Comparison of ketorolac and morphine for postoperative pain after major surgery. Acta Anaesthesiol Scand 1992;36:716–721.

202. PARKER RK, HOLTMANN BH, SMITH I, et al. Use of ketorolac after lower abdominal surgery. Anesthesiology 1994;80:6–12.

203. BRADFORD TH, ROBERTSON K, NORMAN PF, et al. Reduction of pain and nausea after laparoscopic sterilization with bupivacaine, metoclopramide, scopolamine, ketorolac, and gastric suctioning. Obstet Gynecol 9115;85:687–691.

204. WONG HY, CARPENTER RL, KOPACZ DJ, et al. A randomized, double-blind evaluation of ketorolac tromethamine for postoperative analgesia in ambulatory surgery patients. Anesthesiology 1993;78:6–14.

205. ROGERS JEG, FLEMING BG, MAGINTOSH KC, et al. Effect of timing of ketorolac administration on patient-controlled opioid use. Br J Anaesth 1995;75:15–18.

206. JOSLYN AF. Ondansetron, clinical development for postoperative nausea and vomiting: current studies and future directions. Anaesthesia 1994;49S:34–37.

207. KENNY GNC. Risk factors for postoperative nausea and vomiting. Anaesthesia 1994;49S:6–10.

208. NAYLOR RJ, INALL FC. The physiology and pharmacology of postoperative nausea and vomiting. Anaesthesia 1994;49S:2–5.

209. WATCHA MF, WHITE PF. Postoperative nausea and vomiting: its etiology, treatment, and prevention. Anesthesiology 1992;77:162–164.

210. ALON E, HIMMELSEHER S. Ondansetron in the treatment of postoperative vomiting: a randomized double-blind comparison with droperidol and metoclopramide. Anesth Analg 1992;75:561–565.

211. ANDERSON R, KROHG K. Pain as a major cause of postoperative nausea. Can Anaesth Soc J 1976;23:366–369.

212. ABRAMSON DJ. Charles Penrose and the Penrose drain. Surg Gynecol Obstet 1973;136:285–286.

213. SARR MG, PARIKH KJ, MINKEN SL, et al. Closed-suction versus Penrose drainage after cholecystectomy. Am J Surg 1987;153:394–398.

214. SOMERS RG, JABLON LK, KAPLAN MJ, et al. The use of closed suction drainage after lumpectomy and axillary node dissection for breast cancer: a prospective randomized trial. Ann Surg 1992;215:146–149.

215. JENSEN JK, LUCCI JA III, DISAIA PJ, et al. To drain or not to drain: a retrospective study of closed-suction drainage following radical hysterectomy with pelvic lymphadenectomy. Gynecol Oncol 1993;51:46–49.

216. PETRU E, TAMUSSINO K, LAHOUSEN M, et al. Pelvic and paraaortic lymphocysts after radical surgery because of cervical and ovarian cancer. Am J Obstet Gynecol 1989;161:937–941.

217. CHOO YC, WONG LC, WONG KP, et al. The management of intractable lymphocyst following radical hysterectomy. Gynecol Oncol 1986;24:309–316.

218. GALANDUIK S, FAZIO VW. Postoperative irrigation-suction drainage after pelvic colonic surgery. Dis Colon Rectum 1991;34:223–228.

219. ORR JW JR, BARTER JF, KILGORE LC, et al. Closed suction pelvic drainage after radical pelvic surgical procedures. Am J Obstet Gynecol 1986;155:867–871.

220. COHAN RH, SAEED M, SCHWAB SJ, et al. Povidone-iodine sclerosis of pelvic lymphoceles: a prospective study. Urol Radiol 1988;10:203–206.

221. BARTZEN PJ, HAFFERTY FW. Pelvic laparotomy without an indwelling catheter: a retrospective review of 949 cases. Am J Obstet Gynecol 1987;156:1426–1432.

222. KINGDOM JCP, KITCHENER HC, MACLEAN AB. Postoperative urinary tract infection in gynecology: implications for an antibiotic prophylaxis policy. Obstet Gynecol 1990;76:636–638.

223. IRELAND D, TACCHI D, BINT AJ. Effect of single-dose prophylactic co-trimoxazole on the incidence of gynaecological postoperative urinary tract infection. Br J Obstet Gynaecol 1982;89:578–580.

224. BURG R, GEIGLE CF, FASO JM, et al. Omission of routine gastric decompression. Dis Colon Rectum 1978;21:98–100.

225. COLVIN DB, LEE W, EISENSTAT TE, et al. The role of nasointestinal intubation in elective colonic surgery. Dis Colon Rectum 1986;29(5):295–213.

226. CHEADLE WG, VITALE GC, MACKIE CR, et al. Prophylactic postoperative nasogastric decompression: a prospective study of its requirement and the influence of cimetidine in 200 patients. Ann Surg 1985;202:361–366.

227. MOSS G. Discharge within 24 hours of elective cholecystectomy. Arch Surg 1986;121:1159–1161.

228. MACRAE HM, FISCHER JD, YAKIMETS WW. Routine omission of nasogastric intubation after gastrointestinal surgery. Can J Surg 1992;35:625–628.

229. BAUER JJ, GELERNT IM, SALKY BA, et al. Is routine postoperative nasogastric decompression really necessary? Ann Surg 1985;202:233–236.

230. SCHIPPERS E, HOLSCHER AH, BOLLSCHWEILER E, et al. Return of interdigestive motor complex after abdominal surgery: end of postoperative ileus? Dig Dis Sci 1991;36:621–626.

231. FRANKEL AM, HOROWITZ GD. Nasoduodenal tubes in short-stay cholecystectomy. Surg Obstet Gynecol 1989;168:433–436.

232. MOSS G, REGAL ME, LICHTIG LK: Reducing postoperative pain narcotics and length of hospitalization. Surgery 1986;90:206–210.

233. BICKEL A, SHTAMLER B, MIZRAHI S. Early oral feeding following removal of nasogastric tube in gastrointestinal operations: a randomized prospective study. Arch Surg 1992;127:287–289.

234. HORAN TC, GAYNES RP, MARTONE WJ, et al. CDC definitions of nosocomial surgical site infections, 1992: a modification of CDC definitions of surgical wound infections. Am J Infect Control 1992;20:271–274.

235. SUDARSKY LA, LASCHINGER JC, COPPA GF, et al. Improved results from a standardized approach in threatening patients with necrotizing fascitis. Ann Surg 1987;206:661–665.

236. FRY DE, CLEVENGER FW. Reoperation for intra-abdominal abscess. Surg Clin North Am 1991;71:159–174.

237. BOYD ME. Postoperative gynecologic infections. Can J Surg 1987;30:7–9.

238. HOUANG ET. Antibiotic prophylaxis in hysterectomy and induced abortion: a review of the evidence. Drugs 1991;41:19–37.

239. CROMBLEHOLME WR, OHM-SMITH M, ROBBIE MO, et al. Ampicillin/sulbactam versus metronidazole-gentamicin in the treatment of soft tissue pelvic infections. Am J Obstet Gynecol 1987;156:507–512.

240. CRUSE PJE. The epidemiology of surgical infection: a 10-year prospective study of 62,939 wounds. Surg Clin North Am 1980;60:27–40.

241. SAWYER RG, PRUETT TL. Wound infections. Surg Clin North Am 1994;74:519–536.

242. BROWN SE, ALLEN HH, ROBINS RN. The use of delayed primary wound closure in preventing wound infections. Am J Obstet Gynecol 1977;127:713–717.

243. WOOLSEY RM, MCGARRY JD. The cause, prevention and treatment of pressure sores. Neurol Clin 1991;9(3):797–808.

244. ALVAREZ OM, JARCZYNSKI E. Pressure ulcers: physical, supportive, and local aspects of management. Clin Podiatr Med Surg 1991;8(4):869–890.

245. JESTER J, WEAVER V. A report of clinical investigation of various tissue support surfaces used for the prevention, early intervention and management of pressure ulcers. Ostomy Wound Manage 1990;19:39–45.

246. LINDAN O, GIRBENWAY RM, PIAZZA JM. Pressure distribution on the human body. I. Evaluation of lying and sitting positions using a "bed of springs and nails." Arch Phys Med Rehabil 1965;45:378–385.

247. LANDIS EM. Microinjection studies of capillary blood pressure in human skin. Heart 1930;15:209–228.

248. KOSIAK M. Etiology and pathology of ischemic ulcers. Arch Phys Med Rehabil 1959;40:62–69.

249. TAYLOR TV, RIMMER S, DAY B, et al. Ascorbic acid supplementation in the treatment of pressure sores. Lancet 1974;2(7880):544–546.

250. HALLBOOK T, LANNER E. Serum zinc and healing of venous leg ulcers. Lancet 1972;2(7781):780–782.

251. FALYONS J. Monitoring practice. Nurs Times 1994;90(16):69–78.

252. MEECHAN M. Multisite pressure ulcer prevalence survey. Decubitus 1990;3:14–17.

253. ROBNETT MK. The incidence of skin breakdown in a surgical intensive care unit. J Nurs Qual Assur 1986;1:77–81.

254. National Pressure Ulcer Advisory Panel. Pressure ulcers prevalence, cost and risk assessment: consensus development conference statement. Decubitus 1989;2:24–28.

255. HOFMAN A, GEELKERKEN RH, WILLE J, et al. Pressure sores and pressure-decreasing mattresses: controlled clinical trial. Lancet 1994;343:568–571.

256. BRYAN CS, DEW CE, REYNOLDS KL. Bacteremia associated with decubitus ulcers. Arch Intern Med 1983;143:2093–2095.

257. MUSTOE TA, CUTLER NR, ALLMAND RM, et al. A phase II study to evaluate recombinant platelet-derived growth factor-BB in the treatment of stage 3 and 4 pressure ulcers. Arch Surg 1994;129:213–219.

258. RUBIN SC, BENJAMIN I, HOSKINS WJ, et al. Intestinal surgery in gynecologic oncology. Gynecol Oncol 1989;34:30–33.

259. HOFFMAN MS, BARTON DP, GATES J, et al. Complications of colostomy performed on gynecologic cancer patients. Gynecol Oncol 1992;44:231–234.

260. PEARL RK, PRASAD L, ORSAY CP, et al. Early local complications from intestinal stomas. Arch Surg 1985;120:1145–1147.

261. HAMPTON BG. Peristomal and stomal complications.In: HAMPTON BG, BRYANT RA, editors. Ostomies and Continent Diversions: Nursing Management. St. Louis: Mosby-Year Book Inc; 1992. p 105–128.

262. ALLEN-MERSH TG, THOMSON JPS. Surgical treatment of colostomy complications. Br J Surg 1988;75:416–418.

263. ORR JW JR. Introduction to pelvic surgery—pre- and post-operative care. In: GUSBERG SB, SHINGLETON HM, DEPPE G, editors. Female Genital Cancer. New York: Churchill Livingstone; 1988. p 497–534.

264. STGEHLING L. Preoperative blood ordering. Int Anesthesiol Clin 1982;20:45–57.

265. Blood component therapy. ACOG Technical Bulletin Number 199. November 1994.

266. SAZAMA K. Reports of 355 transfusion-associated deaths: 1976 through 1985. Transfusion 1990;30:583–590.

267. GOLDBERG GL, GIBBON DG, SMITH HO, et al. Clinical impact of chemotherapy-induced thrombocytopenia in patients with gynecologic cancer. J Clin Oncol 1994;12:2317–2320.

268. National Institutes of Health Consensus Conference. Fresh-frozen plasma: indications and risks. JAMA 1985;253:551–557.

269. NESS PM, PERKINS HA. Cryoprecipitate as a reliable source of fibrinogen replacement. JAMA 1979;241:1690–1691.

270. KREBS HB. Intestinal injury in gynecologic surgery: a ten-year experience. Am J Obstet Gynecol 1986;155:509–514.

271. ALVAREZ RD. Gastrointestinal complications in gynecologic surgery: a review for the general gynecologist. Obstet Gynecol 1988;72:533–540.

272. KREBS HB, GOPERUD DR. Mechanical intestinal obstruction in patients with gynecologic disease: a review of 368 patients. Am J Obstet Gynecol 1987;157:467–471.

273. HOLDER WD JR. Intestinal obstruction. Gastroenterol Clin North Am 1988;17(2):317–340.

274. FABRI PJ, ROSEMURGY A. Reoperation for small intestinal obstruction. Surg Clin North Am 1991;71:131–146.

275. MONK BJ, BERMAN ML, MONTZ FJ. Adhesions after extensive gynecologic surgery: clinical significance, etiology, and prevention. Am J Obstet Gynecol 1994;170:1936–1403.

276. BROLIN R, CRASNA M, MAST B. Use of tubes and radiographs in the management of small bowel obstruction. Ann Surg 1987;206:26–133.

277. BUTTS DE. Perioperative care of the patient with diabetes mellitus. Plast Surg Nurs 1990;10:7–31.

278. ORLAND MJ. Diabetes mellitus. In: WOODLY M, WHELAN A, editors. Manual of Medical Therapeutics. 27th ed. Boston: Little, Brown and Company; 1992. p 375–399.

279. UNGER RH, FOSTER DW. Diabetes mellitus. In: WILSON JD, FOSTOR DW, editors. Williams Textbook of Endocrinology. 8th ed. Philadelphia, PA: WB Saunders Company; 1992. p 1255–1333.

280. VINICO F. Atherosclerosis and diabetes mellitus. Diabetes Spect 1988;1:319–324.
281. GAVIN LA. Perioperative management of the diabetic patient. Endocrinol Metab Clin North Am 1992;21:457–473.
282. NESTO RW, PHILLIPS RT, KETT KG, et al. Angina and exertional myocardial ischemia in diabetic and nondiabetic patients: assessment by exercise thallium scintigraphy. Ann Intern Med 1988;108:170–175.
283. SEKI S, YOSHIDA H, MONOKI Y, et al. Impaired pulmonary oxygenation of diabetic origin in patients undergoing coronary artery bypass grafting. Cardiovasc Surg 1993;1:72–78.
284. HJORTRUP A, SORENSEN C, DYREMOSE E, et al. Influence of diabetes mellitus on operative risk. Br J Surg 1985;72:783–785.
285. SCHUMANN D. Postoperative hypoglycemia: clinical benefits of insulin therapy. Heart Lung 1990;19:165–173.
286. KAUKINEN S, SALMI J, MARTTINEN A, et al. Postoperative hyperglycaemia—are the patients diabetic? Exp Clin Endocrinol 1992;100:85–89.
287. BRANDI LS, FREDIANI M, OLEGGINI M, et al. Insulin resistance after surgery: normalization by insulin treatment. Clin Sci 1990;79:443–450.
288. HOOGWERF BJ. Perioperative management of diabetes mellitus: striving for metabolic balance. Cleve Clin J Med 1992;59(5):447–449.
289. MCMURRAY JF JR. Wound healing with diabetes mellitus: better glucose control for better wound healing in diabetes. Surg Clin North Am 1984;64:769–778.
290. WHEAT LJ. Infection and diabetes mellitus. Diabetes Care 1980;3:187–197.
291. DAVI G, CATALANO I, AVERNA M, et al. Thromboxane biosynthesis and platelet function in type II diabetes mellitus. N Engl J Med 1990;322:1796–1794.
292. GOLDSTEIN DE, PARKER KM, ENGLAND JD, et al. Clinical application of glycosylated hemoglobin measurements. Diabetes 1982;31(Suppl. 3):70–78.
293. WALTS LF, MILLER J, DAVIDSON MB, et al. Perioperative management of diabetes mellitus. Anaesthiology 1981;55:104–109.
294. LJUNGVIST O, THORELL A, GUTNIAK M, et al. Glucose infusion instead of preoperative fasting reduces postoperative insulin resistance. J Am Coll Surg 1994;178:329–336.
295. Adams III JE, SIGARD GA, ALLEN BT, et al. Diagnosis of perioperative myocardial infarction with measurement of cardiac troponin I. N Engl J Med 1994;330:670–674.
296. GRAEBER GM. Creatine kinase (CK): its use in the evaluation of perioperative myocardial infarction. Surg Clin North Am 1985;65:539–551.
297. VAL PG, PELLETIER LC, HERNANDEZ MG, et al. Diagnostic criteria and prognosis of preoperative myocardial infarction following coronary bypass. J Thorac Cardiovasc Surg 1983;86: 878–886.
298. ACC/AHA Task Force Report. Guidelines for the early management of patients with acute myocardial infarction. JACC 1990;16(2):249–292.
299. CHARLSON ME, MACKENZIE CR, GOLD JP, et al. Risk for post-operative congestive heart failure. Surg Gynecol Obstet 1991;172(2):95–104.
300. EICKHOFF TC. Pulmonary infections in surgical patients. Surg Clin North Am 1980;60:175–183.
301. RODRIGUEZ JL, GIBOONS KJ, BITZER LG, et al. Pneumonia: incidence, risk factors, and outcome in injured patients. J Trauma 1991;31:907–912.
302. MARTIN LF, ASHER EF, CASEY JM, et al. Postoperative pneumonia: determinants of mortality. Arch Surg 1984;119:379–383.
303. Centers for Disease Control. Nosocomial infection surveillance, 1984. CDC Surveill Summ 1986;35:17S–29S.
304. DUNN DL. Gram-negative bacterial sepsis and sepsis syndrome. Surg Clin North Am 1994;74:621–635.
305. FRY DE. Postoperative pneumonia in the intensive care unit. Surg Gynecol Obstet 1993;177:41S–49S.
306. MILLEDGE JS, NUNN JF. Criteria of fitness for anaesthesia in patients with chronic obstructive lung disease. Br Med J 1975;3:670–673.
307. FLENLEY DC. Chronic obstructive pulmonary disease. Dis Mon 1988;34:543–599.

308. BOSSER SA, ROCK P. Asthma and chronic obstructive lung disease. In: BRESLOW MJ, MILLER CJ, ROGERS MC, editors. Perioperative management. St. Louis: CV Mosby Company; 1990. p 259–280.

309. ZIBRAK JD, O'DONNELL CR, MARTON K. Indications for pulmonary function testing. Ann Intern Med 1990;112:763–771.

310. MEYERS JR, LEMBECK L, O'KANE H, et al. Changes in functional residual capacity of the lung after operation. Arch Surg 1975;110:576–583.

311. BARNES PJ. A new approach to the treatment of asthma. N Engl J Med 1989;321:1517–1527.

312. EASTON PA, JADUE C, DHINGRA S, et al. A comparison of the bronchodilating effects if a beta-2 adrenergic agent (albuterol) and an anticholinergic agent (ipratropium bromide) given by aerosol alone or in sequence. N Engl J Med 1986;315:735–739.

313. HOU SH, BUSHINSKY DA, WISH JB, et al. Hospital-acquired renal insufficiency: a prospective study. Am J Med 1983;74:243–248.

314. SMITHIES NM, CAMERON JS. Can we predict outcome in acute renal failure? Nephron 1989;51:297–300.

315. KELLERMAN PS. Perioperative care of the renal patient. Arch Intern Med 1994;154:1674–1688.

316. SCHUSTERMAN N, STROM BL, MURRAY TG, et al. Risk factors and outcome of hospital-acquired acute renal failure. Am J Med 1987;83:75–71.

317. CHARLSON ME, MACKENZIE R, GOLD JP, et al. Postoperative renal dysfunction can be predicted. Surg Gynecol Obstet 1989;169:303–309.

318. WILKES BM, MAILLOUX LU. Acute renal failure: pathogenesis and prevention. Am J Med 1986;80:1129–1136.

319. MEYER RD. Risk factors and comparisons of clinical nephrotoxicity of aminoglycosides. Am J Med 1986;80:119S–125S.

320. ALLEN GC. Malignant hyperthermia and associated disorders. Curr Opin Rheumatol 1993; 719–724.

321. PINSON CW, SCHUMAN ES, GROSS GF, et al. Surgery in long-term dialysis patients: experience with more than 300 cases. Am J Surg 1986;151:567–571.

322. BLUMBERG A, WIEDMANN P, SHAW S, et al. Effect of various therapeutic approaches on plasma potassium and major regulating factors in terminal renal failure. Am J Med 1988;85:507–512.

323. ESCHBACK JW, EGRIE JC, DOWNING MR, et al. Correction of the anemia of end-stage renal disease with recombinant human erythropoietin: results of a combined phase I and II clinical trial. N Engl J Med 1987;316:73–78.

324. LIVIO M, MANNUCCI PM, VIGANO G, et al. Conjugated estrogens for the management of bleeding associated with renal failure. N Engl J Med 1986;315:731–735.

325. LEWIS SL, van EPPS DE. Neutrophil and monocyte alterations in chronic dialysis patients. Am J Kidney Dis 1987;9:381–395.

326. FRIEDMAN LS, MADDREY WC. Surgery in the patient with liver disease. Med Clin North Am 1987;71:453–476.

327. HARVILLE DD, SUMMERSKILL WHJ. Surgery in acute hepatitis. JAMA 1963;184:257–261.

328. MARTINEZ J, PALESCAK JE. Hemostatic alterations in liver disease. In: ZAKIM D, BOYER TD, editors. Hepatology: A Textbook of Liver Disease. Philadelphia, PA: WB Saunders Company; 1992. p 546–580.

329. ROBERTS HR, CEDERBAUM AI. The liver and blood coagulation: physiology and pathology. Gastroenterology 1979;63:297–320.

330. CHILD CG, TURCOTTE JC. Surgery and portal hypertension. In: CHILD CG, editor. The Liver and Portal Hypertension. Philadelphia, PA: WB Saunders Company; 1994. p 1–85.

331. PUGH RNH, MURRAY-LYON IM, DAWSON JL, et al. Transection of the oesophagus for bleeding oesophageal varices. Br J Surg 1973;60:646–649.

332. STONE HH. Preoperative and postoperative care. Surg Clin North Am 1977;57:409–419.

333. GOLDMANN, DR. Surgery in patients with endocrine dysfunction. Med Clin North Am 1987;71(3):499–509.

334. SEMENKOVICH CF. Endocrine diseases. In: WOODLEY M, WHELAN A, editors. Manual of Medical Therapeutics. Boston: Little, Brown and Company; 1993. p 400–405.

335. DANIELS GH, MARTIN JB. Neuroendocrine regulation and diseases of the anterior pituitary and hypothalamus. In: ISSELBACHER KJ, BRAUNWALD E, WILSON JD, MARTIN JB, FAUCI AS, KASPER DL, editors. Harrison's Principles of Internal Medicine. New York: McGraw-Hill; 1994. p 1911–1913.

336. CLUTTER WE. Mineral and metabolic bone disease. In: WOODLEY M, WHELAN A, editors. Manual of Medical Therapeutics. Boston: Little, Brown and Company; 1993. p 427–433.

337. MAZZE RI, KALLEN B. Reproductive outcome after anesthesia and operation during pregnancy: a registry study of 5405 cases. Am J Obstet Gynecol 1989;161:1178–1185.

338. BRODSKY JB, COHEN EN, BROWN BW, et al. Surgery during pregnancy and fetal outcome. Am J Obstet Gynecol 1980;138:1165–1167.

339. LEVINSON G, SHNIDER SM. Anesthesia for surgery during pregnancy. In: SHNIDER SM, LEVINSON G, editors. Anesthesia for Obstetrics. Baltimore: Williams and Wilkins; 1994. p 188–277.

340. VINCENT RD. Anesthesia for the pregnant patient. Clin Obstet Gynecol 1994;37(2):256–273.

341. MOISE KJ. Effect of advancing gestational age on the frequency of fetal ductal constriction in association with maternal indomethacin use. Am J Obstet Gynecol 1993;168:1350–1353.

342. HILL LM, JOHNSON CE, LEE RA. Cholecystectomy in pregnancy. Obstet Gynecol 1975;46:291–293.

343. SPEROFF L, GLASS RH, KASE NG. The endocrinology of pregnancy. In: Clinical Gynecologic Endocrinology and Infertility. Baltimore: Williams and Wilkins; 1989. p 251–289.

344. DILTS PV, BRINKMAN CR, KIRSCHBAUM TH, et al. Uterine and systemic hemodynamic relationships and their response to hypoxia. Am J Obstet Gynecol 1965;103:138–157.

345. US Bureau of the Census, Statistical Abstract of the United States: 1993 (113th edition). Washington, DC, 1993.

346. YANCIK R. Frame of reference: old age as the context for prevention and treatment of cancer. In: YANCIK R, editor. Perspectives on Prevention and Treatment of Cancer in the Elderly. New York: Raven Press; 1993. p 5.

347. GOODWIN JS, SAMET JM, KEY CR, et al. Stage at diagnosis of cancer varies with the age of the patient. J Am Geriatr Soc 1986;34:20–26.

348. GROVER SA, COOK EF, ADAM J, et al. Delayed diagnosis of gynecologic tumors in elderly women: relation to national medical practice patterns. Am J Med 1989;86:151–157.

349. WHEAT ME, MANDELBLATT JS, KUNITZ G. Pap smear screening in women 65 and older. J Am Geriatr Soc 1988;36:827–830.

350. SAMET J, HUNT WC, KEY C, et al. Choice of cancer therapy varies with age of patient. JAMA 1986;255:3385–3390.

351. KENNEDY AW, FLAGG JS, WEBSTER KD. Gynecologic cancer in the very elderly. Gynecol Oncol 1989;32:49–54.

352. GRANT PT, KEFFREY JF, FRASER RC, et al. Pelvic radiation therapy for gynecologic malignancy in geriatric patients. Gynecol Oncol 1989;33:185–188.

353. KIRSHNER CV, DESERTO TM, ISAACS JH. Surgical treatment of the elderly patient with gynecologic cancer. Surg Gynecol Obstet 1990;170:379–384.

354. LAWTON FG, HACKER NF. Surgery for invasive gynecologic cancer in the elderly female population. Obstet Gynecol 1990;76:287–289.

355. WARNER MA, HOSKING MP, LOBDELL CM, et al. Effects of referral bias on surgical outcomes: a population-based study of surgical patients 90 years of age or older. Mayo Clin Proc 1990;65:1185–1191.

356. LICHTINGER M, AVERETTE H, PENALVAER M, et al. Major surgical procedures for gynecologic malignancy in elderly women. South Med J 1986;79:1506–1510.

357. FUCHTNER C, MANETTA A, WALKER JL, et al. Radical hysterectomy in the elderly patient: analysis of morbidity. Am J Obstet Gynecol 1992;166:593–597.

358. MATTHEWS CM, MORRIS M, BURKE TW, et al. Pelvic exenteration in the elderly patient. Obstet Gynecol 1992;79:773–777.

359. ALTARAS MM, BEN-BARUCH G, AVIRAM R, et al. Treatment results for ovarian cancer in women older than 70 years (Abstract). Gynecol Oncol 1993;50: 270.

360. LAU HC, GRANICK MS, AISNER AM, et al. Wound care in the elderly patient. Surg Clin North Am 1994;74:441–463.

361. WATTERS JM, CLANCEY SM, MOULTON SB, et al. Impaired recovery of strength in older patients after major abdominal surgery. Ann Surg 1993;218:380–393.

362. HARPER CM, LYLES YM. Physiology and complications of bedrest. J Am Geriatr Soc 1988;36:1047–1054.

363. BRATZLER D, HOUCK PM. Antimicrobial prophylaxis for surgery: an advisory statement from the National Surgical Infection Prevention Project. Clin Infect Dis 2004;38:1706–1715.

364. FORSE RA, KARAM B, MACLEAN LD, CHRISTOU NV. Antibiotic prophylaxis for surgery in morbidly obese patients. Surgery 1989;106:750–756.

365. SESSLER DI. Non-pharmacologic prevention of surgical wound infection. Anesthesiol Clin 2006;24(2):279–297.

366. KURZ A, SESSLER DI, LENHARDT RA. Perioperative normothermia to reduce the incidence of surgical-wound infection and shorten hospitalization. N Engl J Med 1996;334:1209–1215.

367. GREIF R, AKÇA O, HORN E-P, et al. Supplemental perioperative oxygen to reduce the incidence of surgical wound infection. N Engl J Med 2000;342:161–167.

368. HOPF HW, HUNT TK, WEST JM, et al. Wound tissue oxygen tension predicts the risk of wound infection in surgical patients. Arch Surg 1997;132:997–1005.

369. HEMSELL DL, JOHNSON ER, HEMSELL PG, et al. Cefazolin is inferior to cefotetan as single-dose prophylaxis for women undergoing elective total abdominal hysterectomy. Clin Infect Dis 1995;20:677–684.

370. Antibiotic prophylaxis for gynecologic procedures. ACOG Practice Bulletin No. 104. May 2009.

371. SOPER DE, BUMP RC, HURT WG. Bacterial vaginosis and trichomoniasis vaginitis are risk factors for postoperative cuff cellulitis after abdominal hysterectomy. Am J Obstet Gynecol 1990;163:1016–1021.

372. LARSSON PG, CARLSSON B. Does pre- and postoperative metronidazole treatment lower vaginal cuff infection rate after abdominal hysterectomy among women with bacterial vaginosis? Infect Dis Obstet Gynecol 2002;10:133–140.

373. KOCAK I, USTÜN C, EMRE B, UZEL A, et al. Antibiotics prophylaxis in laparoscopy. Ceska Gynekol 2005;70:269–272.

374. HUGHES ES. Asepsis in large-bowel surgery. Ann R Coll Surg Engl 1972 Dec;51(6):347–356

375. IRVING AD, SCRIMGEOUR D. Mechanical bowel preparation for colonic resection and anastomosis. Br J Surg. 1987 Jul;74(7):580–581.

376. SLIM K, FLAMEIN R, BRUGERE C. Preoperative bowel preparation–is it useful? J Chir (Paris). 2004 Sep;141(5):285–289.

377. BUCHER P, GERVAZ P, SORAVIA C, MERMILLOD B, ERNE M, MOREL P. Randomized clinical trial of mechanical bowel preparation versus no preparation before elective left-sided colorectal surgery. Br J Surg. 2005 Apr;92(4):409-14. Erratum in: Br J Surg. 2005 Aug;92(8):1051.

378. GUENAGA KK, MATOS D, WILLE-JØRGENSEN P, et al. Mechanical bowel preparation for elective colorectal surgery. Cochrane Database Syst Rev 2008; (1):CD001544.

379. GUENAGA KK, MATOS D, WILLE-JØRGENSEN P. Mechanical bowel preparation for elective colorectal surgery. Cochrane Database Syst Rev 2009 Jan 21;(1):CD001544.

380. SLIM K, VICAUT E, LAUNAY-SAVARY MV, et al. Updated systematic review and meta-analysis of randomized clinical trials on the role of mechanical bowel preparation before colorectal surgery. Ann Surg 2009;249(2):203–209.

381. RUSSMANN S, LAMERATO L, MOTSKO SP, et al. Risk of further decline in renal function after the use of oral sodium phosphate or polyethylene glycol in patients with a preexisting glomerular filtration rate below 60 ml/min. Am J Gastroenterol 2008;103:2707–2716.

382. KHURANA A, MCLEAN L, ATKINSON S, FOULKS CJ. The effect of oral sodium phosphate drug products on renal function in adults undergoing bowel endoscopy. Arch Intern Med 2008;168(6): 593–597.

383. WILSON W, TAUBERT KA, GEWITZ M, et al. AHA guideline: "Prevention of infective endocarditis." Circulation 2007;116:1736–1754.

384. CAPRINI. VTE risk assessment tools and guideline-based thromboprophylaxis strategies for surgical cancer patients. First Report: Late Breaking Clinical Developments—Princeton CME 2008; 10–19.

385. HEIT JA, SILVERSTEIN MD, MOHR DN, et al. Risk factors for deep vein thrombosis and pulmonary embolism: a population-based case-control study. Arch Intern Med 2000;160(6):809–815.

386. LYMAN GH, KHORANA AA, FALANGA A, et al. American Society of Clinical Oncology guideline: recommendations for venous thromboembolism prophylaxis and treatment in patients with cancer. J Clin Oncol 2007;25(34):5490–5505.

387. KHORANA AA, FRANCIS CW, CULAKOVA E, et al. Thromboembolism in hospitalized neutropenic cancer patients. J Clin Oncol 2006;24:484–490.

388. KOBBERVIG CE, HEIT JA, JAMES AH, et al. The effect of patient age on the incidence of idiopathic vs. secondary venous thromboembolism: a population-based cohort study (Abstract 3516). Blood 2004;104: 957a.

389. AGNELLI G, BOLIS G, CAPUSSOTTI L, et al. A clinical outcome-based prospective study of venous thromboembolism after cancer surgery. The RISTOS project. Ann Surg 2006;243:89–95.

390. CHEW HK, WUN T, HARVEY D, et al. Incidence of venous thromboembolism and its effect on survival among patients with common cancers. Arch Intern Med 2006;166:458–464.

391. KRÖGER K, WEILAND D, OSE C, et al. Risk factors for venous thromboembolic events in cancer patients. Ann Oncol 2006;17(2):297–303.

392. SOUTO JC, ALMASY L, BORRELL M, et al Genetic susceptibility to thrombosis and its relationship to physiologic risk factors: the GAIT study. Am J Hum Genet 2000;67:1452–1459.

393. SANSON BJ, SIMIONI P, TORMENE D, et al. The incidence of venous thromboembolism in asymptomatic carriers of a deficiency of antithrombin, protein C, protein S: a prospective cohort study. Blood 1999;94:3702–3706.

394. KENNEDY M, ANDREESCU AC, GREENBLATT MS, et al Factor V Leiden, prothrombin 20210 A and the risk of venous thromboembolism among cancer patients. Br J Haematol 2005;128:386–388.

395. BLOM JW, DOGGEN CJ, OSANTO S, ROSENDAAL FR Malignancies, prothrombic mutations, and the risk of venous thrombosis. JAMA 2005;293:715–722.

396. KHORANA AA, FRANCIS CW, CULAKOVA E, LYMAN GH Risk factors for chemotherapy-associated venous thromboembolism in a prospective observational study. Cancer 2005;104:2822–2829.

397. BOHLIUS J, WILSON J, SEIDENFELD J, et al. Recombinant human erythropoietins and cancer patients: updated meta-analysis of 57 studies including 9353 patients. J Natl Cancer Inst 2006;98: 708–714.

398. ZANGARI M, ANAISSIE E, BARLOGIE B, et al. Increased risk of deep-vein thrombosis in patients with multiple myeloma receiving thalidomide and chemotherapy. Blood 2001;98:1614–1615.

399. ZANGARI M, BARLOGIE B, ANAISSIE E, et al. Deep vein thrombosis in patients with multiple myeloma treated with thalidomide and chemotherapy: effects of prophylactic and therapeutic anticoagulation. Br J Haematol 2004;126:715–721.

400. KABBINAVAR F, HURWITZ HI, FEHRENBACHER L. Phase II, randomized trial comparing bevacizumab plus fluorouracil (FU)/leucovorin (LV) with FU/LV alone in patients with metastatic colorectal cancer. J Clin Oncol 2003;21:60–65.

401. NALLURI SR, CHU D, KERESZTES R, et al. Risk of venous thromboembolism with the angiogenesis inhibitor bevacizumab in cancer patients: a meta-analysis. JAMA 2008;300:2277–2285.

402. HERNANDEZ RK, SØRENSEN HT, PEDERSEN L, et al. Tamoxifen treatment and risk of deep venous thrombosis and pulmonary embolism: a Danish population-based cohort study. Cancer 2009;115(19):4442–4449.

403. GALLUS AS. Prevention of post-operative deep leg vein thrombosis in patients with cancer. Thromb Haemost 1997;78:126–132.

404. PRANDONI P, TRUJILLO-SANTOS J, SURICO T, et al. Recurrent thromboembolism and major bleeding during oral anticoagulant therapy in patients with solid cancer: findings from the RIETE registry. Haematologica 2008;93(9):1432–1434.

405. SØRENSEN HT, MELLEMKJAER L, OLSEN JH, BARON JA. Prognosis of cancers associated with venous thromboembolism. N Engl J Med 2000;343(25):1846–1850.

406. CLARKE-PEARSON DL, SYNAN IS, HINSHAW WM, et al. Prevention of postoperative venous thromboembolism by external pneumatic calf compression in patients with gynecologic malignancy. Obstet Gynecol 1984;63:92–98.

407. MAXWELL GL, SYNAN I, DODGE R, et al. Pneumatic compression versus low molecular weight heparin in gynecologic oncology surgery: a randomized trial. Obstet Gynecol 2001;98(6):989–995.

408. CLARKE-PEARSON DL, SYNAN IS, DODGE R, et al. A randomized trial of low-dose heparin and intermittent pneumatic calf compression for the prevention of deep venous thrombosis following gynecologic oncology surgery. Am J Obstet Gynecol 1993;168:1146–1153.

409. CLARKE-PEARSON DL. Prevention of venous thromboembolism in gynecologic surgery patients. Curr Opin Obstet Gynecol 1993;5(1):73–79.

410. CLARKE-PEARSON DL, DODGE RK, SYNAN I, et al. Venous thromboembolism prophylaxis: patients at high risk to fail intermittent pneumatic compression. Obstet Gynecol 2003;101(1):157–163.

411. MARTINO MA, BORGES E, WILLIAMSON E, et al. Pulmonary embolism after major abdominal surgery in gynecologic oncology. Obstet Gynecol 2006;107(3):666–671.

412. WILLE-JØRGENSEN P, RASMUSSEN MS, ANDERSEN BR, BORLY L. Heparins and mechanical methods for thromboprophylaxis in colorectal surgery. Cochrane Database Syst Rev 2003; (4):CD001217.

413. KHORANA A. The NCCN clinical practice guidelines on venous thromboembolic disease: strategies for imprving VTE prophylaxis in hospitalized cancer patients. Oncologist 2007;12:1361–1370.

414. Prevention of fatal postoperative pulmonary embolism by low doses of heparin: an international multicentre trial. Lancet 1975;2:45–51.

415. CLAGETT GP, REISCH JS. Prevention of venous thromboembolism in general surgical patients: results of meta-analysis. Ann Surg 1988;208:227–240.

416. Efficacy and safety of enoxaparin versus unfractionated heparin for prevention of deep vein thrombosis in elective cancer surgery: a double-blind randomized multicentre trial with venographic assessment. ENOXACAN Study Group. Br J Surg 1997;84(8):1099–1103.

417. COHEN AT, DAVIDSON BL, GALLUS AS, et al. Efficacy and safety of fondaparinux for the prevention of venous thromboembolism in older acute medical patients: randomised placebo controlled trial. BMJ 2006;332(7537):325–329.

418. BERGQVIST D, AGNELLI G, COHEN AT, et al. Duration of prophylaxis against venous thromboembolism with enoxaparin after surgery for cancer. N Engl J Med 2002;346(13):975–980.

419. RASMUSSEN MS, JORGENSEN LN, WILLE-JØRGENSEN P, et al. Prolonged prophylaxis with dalteparin to prevent late thromboembolic complications in patients undergoing major abdominal surgery: a mulitcenter randomized open-label study. J Thromb Haemost 2006;4:2384–2390.

420. EINSTEIN MH, KUSHNER DM, CONNOR JP, et al. A protocol of dual prophylaxis for venous thromboembolism prevention in gynecologic cancer patients. Obstet Gynecol 2008;112(5):1091–1097.

Chapter 7

Perioperative Infections: Prevention and Therapeutic Options

Amy Stenson, MD, MPH

POSTOPERATIVE FEVER

Postoperative fever is common in the first few days after surgery; however, it is most often noninfectious in etiology and is self-limited.[1,2] Although most postoperative fevers will resolve spontaneously, they may also be a manifestation of a serious surgical complication. The differential diagnosis should be broad and include both infectious and noninfectious etiologies such as nosocomial pneumonia, urinary tract infections, drug-related or neoplastic fevers, and deep pelvic thrombosis. The possibility of a serious surgical site infection (SSI) must always be kept in mind. Atelectasis is no longer thought to be a significant cause of postoperative fever, though both occur commonly after surgery.[3] The most common cause of postoperative fever is operative site inflammation due to the release of fever-associated cytokines (IL-1, IL-6, TNF-alpha, and IFN-gamma) stimulated by tissue trauma during surgery.[4,5] The extent of tissue trauma sustained during a given surgery correlates with the development of postoperative fever, e.g., a laparoscopic procedure is less likely to result in fever than the same procedure done through a laparotomy.[6–8]

The evaluation of a patient with postoperative fever should begin with a thorough history and physical exam. It is usually unnecessary to order a battery of expensive tests; laboratory and radiologic testing should be guided by the findings of the evaluation and the patient's overall status.[9,10] Frequent clinical reevaluation of the patient

Gynecologic Oncology: Evidence-Based Perioperative and Supportive Care, Second Edition.
Edited by Scott E. Lentz, Allison E. Axtell and Steven A. Vasilev.
© 2011 John Wiley & Sons, Inc. Published 2011 by John Wiley & Sons, Inc.

can help distinguish patients with mild self-limited symptoms from a patient with a more serious infectious process developing.

In distinguishing between infectious and noninfectious fevers, it is important to note that infectious fevers typically occur later (2.7 days vs. 1.6 days) and last longer (5.4 days vs. 3.4 days) than noninfectious fevers.[2] In the immediate postoperative period, fever is most likely due to medications or blood products administered perioperatively, trauma prior to or during surgery, or an infectious process present before the start of the surgery. Malignant hyperthermia normally presents within 30 minutes of receiving anesthesia, but can sometimes be delayed several hours.[11] Although SSIs typically present later, there are several organisms in particular that can present emergently in the immediate postoperative period: group A *Streptococcus*, MRSA, and *Clostridium perfringens* among others can lead to fulminant, necrotizing infections of the skin and fascia.[12–14]

In the first few weeks following surgery, there can be many causes of fever, including nosocomial infections. SSIs, catheter infections, pneumonia, and urinary tract infections are the most likely etiologies. Patients receiving ventilation are at high risk for ventilator-associated pneumonia.[15] Aspiration pneumonia should be considered, particularly in patients with diminished mental status or gag reflex. Catheter site infections and urinary tract infections should be ruled out. Noninfectious etiologies include pancreatitis, myocardial infarction, pulmonary embolism, thrombophlebitis, acute gout, alcohol withdrawal, and medication-related fevers.

A patient presenting more than 4 weeks from surgery with a fever will likely be found to have an infection. Consideration should be given to indolent SSIs, particularly if graft material has been used. If a patient has been given blood products, they may present with a related infection such as cytomegalovirus, hepatitis, HIV, or a parasitic infection resulting from blood transfusion.[16] Infective endocarditis from perioperative bacteremia typically presents during this time period.

SURGICAL INFECTION GENESIS

The most common etiology of SSI is thought to be direct inoculation of the surgical site by the patient's own flora during surgery. Contamination by endogenous bacteria may occur at the time of gynecologic operations despite vigorous preoperative skin and vaginal cleansing. The most common pathogens in a clean case are the staphylococcal species. If the surgery involves a viscus being opened, the pathogens resulting in SSI are generally a reflection of the endogenous flora of that organ and are usually polymicrobial. The species of microorganisms causing SSI have not changed dramatically in recent years, but the incidence of antibiotic resistance has markedly increased.[17] Contamination can also occur from exogenous sources from the operating room environment or staff. For example, group A streptococci carriage by OR personnel has resulted in several outbreaks of SSIs.

The vagina contains both aerobic and anaerobic organisms (anaerobes > aerobes). Pelvic infections may occur as a consequence of the introduction of pathogenic exogenous organisms and/or by the presence of normal vaginal flora in an abnormal location (e.g., in the endometrium, oviducts, or peritoneal cavity) in sufficient numbers to overwhelm the host defense system. Bacterial vaginosis is a complex alteration of vaginal flora that results in an increased concentration of potentially pathogenic anaerobic bacteria, and is associated with an increased risk of posthysterectomy cuff cellulitis.[18]

When an inoculation of mixed (aerobic and anaerobic) organisms derived from bowel flora is introduced into an abnormal location (e.g., peritoneal cavity), a biphasic infection pattern may ensue.[19] Initially, peritonitis secondary to the effects of aerobic gram-negative organisms such as *Escherichia coli* precedes abscess formation composed largely of anaerobic organisms, predominantly of the bacteroides group. Approximately 40% of laboratory animals infected in this manner but not treated with antibiotics die of peritonitis while nearly 100% of surviving animals develop abscess.[19]

A small number of *E. coli* or *Bacteroides fragilis* colony forming units introduced into a wound is not sufficient to produce a wound infection. Large numbers of *E. coli* alone or combined with *B. fragilis* can induce a wound infection, and even greater numbers of *B. fragilis* by itself can be harmless.[20] However, once a threshold is exceeded for either, a wound infection develops. Thus, a sufficient inoculum of single or multiple organisms that can overwhelm the host-defense mechanism appears to be necessary to cause disease.[20]

RISK FACTORS FOR INFECTION

Many factors influence the likelihood of developing an infection. Important patient factors to consider include age, nutritional status, diabetes, smoking, obesity, immune status, colonization with microorganisms, coexistent infections, cancer, history of irradiation, and length of preoperative stay.[21,22] Modifiable patient characteristics should be addressed prior to surgery, if possible. Operative characteristics associated with infection include the duration of the surgery, type of surgery performed, preoperative skin preparation, surgeon preparation, antimicrobial prophylaxis, sterilization of equipment, use of foreign bodies (grafts, drains), and operative technique.[23] Meticulous attention to preoperative preparation of the patient, operating environment, and surgeon as well as to intraoperative factors including anesthetic considerations and operative technique can substantially impact infection rates.

SURGICAL PROCEDURE CLASSIFICATION

The national Academy of Sciences and the National Research Counsel developed a wound classification scheme more than 35 years ago based on the degree of expected microbial contamination during surgery.

Wound Type	Definitions	% Infection
Clean	Uninfected Minimal inflammation Wound closed primarily No visus involvement	1.3%–2.9%
Clean–contaminated	Clean wound with entry of viscus No unusual contamination	2.4%–7.7%
Contaminated	Open, fresh accidental wound Major break in sterile technique Gross spillage from viscus Acute purulent inflammation	6.4%–15.2%
Dirty	Old traumatic wounds Devitalized tissue Foreign bodies Fecal contamination Perforated viscus prior to surgery	7.1%–40%

Although this classification system has been widely used, it has not been validated as a good predictor of infection. In 1990, the National Nosocomial Infections Surveillance System (NNIS) was developed to stratify patients undergoing surgery into four risk groups.[24] The system assigns one point for the presence of each of three risk factors:

1. American Society of Anesthesiology (ASA) preoperative score of 3–5.
2. A surgical wound classified as contaminated or dirty.
3. An operation lasting over a certain length of time defined by type of surgery.

NNSI Index	Points	Risk of Infection
1	Zero	1.5%
2	One	2.9%
3	Two	6.8%
4	Three	13%

This system has been validated for many types of surgery and has been found to perform better than the simpler wound classification alone.[25–27]

SURGICAL SITE INFECTIONS

The Center for Disease Control and Prevention define SSIs based on the location and extent of the infection.[28] SSIs are defined as occurring within 30 days of the surgery if there is no implant or within one year if an implant has been left in place. Superficial incisional SSIs are defined as an infection that involves only skin or subcutaneous tissue at the site of the incision. The diagnosis can be made by observing purulent drainage from the incision, isolating organisms from the fluid or tissue involved, or by identifying pain, swelling, erythema, or heat near the incision. Deep incisional SSIs involve the deep soft tissues and can be diagnosed by identifying purulent drainage from the deep part of the incision, an abscess, or a wound dehiscence. An organ space infection involves any part of the anatomy (organs or spaces) other than the incision, that was opened or manipulated during the surgery. It is associated with purulent discharge, abscess formation or organisms isolated from the involved anatomy. Any of these SSIs can also be diagnosed at the discretion of the attending physician/surgeon.[28]

Prevention of SSIs

For patients undergoing a surgical procedure, SSIs are the most common nosocomial infection, developing in 2%–5% of patients undergoing surgery.[26] This largely preventable complication of surgery leads to increased patient morbidity, need for treatment, and length of hospital stay, which results in rapidly escalating health-care costs.[29,30] One study demonstrated an increase in 8-week postdischarge costs of $5155 versus $1773 for patients with and without a SSI respectively.[31]

Many traditional infection control practices and policies have not been shown to be effective in clinical studies. The most important factors in preventing SSI include the general health of the patient, operative technique, and timely administration of appropriate preoperative antibiotics.

Smoking Cessation

Cigarette smokers are known to be at higher risk for both cardiopulmonary and infectious complications at the time of surgery. Smoking cessation, if completed at least 8 weeks before surgery has been shown to decrease wound infections. A randomized blinded clinical trial in Denmark showed that the overall complication rate was significantly different 18% versus 52% in the smoking intervention group and controls, respectively, and for wound-related complications (5% vs. 31%).[32] However, abstinence from smoking immediately prior to surgery does not improve outcomes and may increase the risk of pulmonary complications.[33]

Management of Diabetes

Diabetes is a common chronic disease that affects approximately 7% of the population and about 20% of patients undergoing surgery. These patients are at increased risk for cardiovascular disease, perioperative infection, and postoperative cardiovascular complications.[22] It is important to optimize glycemic control perioperatively in order to minimize complications. This is often difficult as there is a complex interplay between surgery, anesthesia, and the postoperative course leading to labile blood glucose levels.[34] Studies have shown that a preoperative blood glucose level of more than 200 mg/dL increases the odds ratio for SSI to 10.2 in cardiothoracic surgery.[35]

Another cohort study showed that for each 50 mg/dL increase in blood glucose, the odds ratio for infection increased 1.23.[36] Maintaining normoglycemia perioperatively is thus considered important to decreasing infection rates, in addition to minimizing the risks of cardiopulmonary complications and overall mortality.

Preoperative Cleansing

There is no benefit to preoperative showering or bathing with an antiseptic preparation.[37] Similarly, vaginal douching has been shown to be ineffective at preventing SSI and may even be harmful by selecting for pathogenic organisms.[38]. It is best not to alter the normal flora of the skin or vagina prior to surgery. Patients should be advised to simply bathe or shower normally the night prior to surgery to remove debris from the skin surface.

Hair Removal

Many surgeons prefer to have hair removed prior to surgery to provide a clean field and to prevent hair from entering the operative space. Clinical trials have failed to show a difference in infection rates when comparing patients who have had hair removed prior to surgery compared with those who have not.[41] A recent meta-analysis compared shaving with clipping and found that there were statistically significantly more SSIs when people were shaved rather than clipped (RR 2.02, 95% CI 1.21–3.36).[41] There seems to be no difference in SSIs when patients' hair are clipped 1 day prior to surgery or on the day of surgery. If hair needs to be removed, it should be clipped, not shaved.

Use of Barrier Devices

The use of barrier devices such as masks, caps, gowns, drapes, and shoe covers does not appear to significantly reduce SSIs in clinical trials.[42–44] However, the use of these barrier agents is recommended by the Occupational Health and Safety Administration primarily to protect the operating room staff from exposure to infectious agents through body fluids. Double gloving in particular has been shown to decrease glove failure rates from 51% to 7%.[45] Some advocate the use of glove liners or triple gloving to further reduce the risk of glove failure.[44]

Bowel Preparation

Bowel preparation has been an accepted practice for many years; however, recent data calls this into question. Mechanical bowel preparation has been shown to increase the likelihood of bowel content spillage in colorectal surgery.[46] A recent meta-analysis found that bowel preparation does not decrease SSIs, may increase anastomotic leaks at the time of bowel reanastomosis and may increase overall complication rates.[47,48] It has been shown that mechanical bowel preparation alters the intestinal mucosa, leading to loss of superficial mucus, epithelial cells, and increased inflammation, which are known risk factors for anastomotic leakage.[49] Bowel preparation may be helpful for improved bowel handling, but should not be considered to decrease infectious complications.[50] The utility of bowel preparation for gynecologic laparoscopy was evaluated in a randomized, blinded clinical trial and found no difference in surgical difficulty, operating times or postoperative complications between intervention and control.[51] Patients undergoing bowel preparation reported significantly increased preoperative discomfort.[51]

Temperature Regulation

Perioperative hypothermia is thought to promote SSIs. Even mild decreases in temperature may lead to vasoconstriction and decreased oxygen tension in tissues. This has been confirmed by several studies that have shown that hypothermia predisposes patients to infection (19% vs. 6%) and that preoperative warming results in lower infection rates compared with no warming (5% vs. 14%).[52,53]

Surgical Hand Hygiene

Surgeons' hands are colonized by coagulase negative staphylococci and coryneform bacteria as well as any pathogens picked up from patient contact.[54] They are therefore a source of considerable potential contamination in the perioperative care of patients if appropriate hygiene is not maintained.

Artificial nails are a risk factor for carriage of gram-negative organisms that can contribute to SSIs and are discouraged.[55] Long nails have also been associated with outbreaks of unusual pathogens such as *Pseudomonas aeruginosa* in intensive care units.[56] Operating room personnel and other health-care workers are encouraged to keep short (<1/4 inch), natural nails clean and to use nail cleaners and brushes to remove debris prior to surgical antiseptic scrub/rub.[57]

Although clinical trials are lacking to confirm a reduction in SSI rates with preoperative scrubbing, this is an accepted and recommended practice.[57] The duration and technique required for adequate surgical scrub has changed over time and is a matter debate. The traditional 10-minute surgical scrub with iodine and a brush have been largely replaced with faster techniques that are more tolerable for the surgical team. Most recently, hand rubbing with an aqueous alcoholic solution has been recommended as an alternative to the traditional scrub with antimicrobial soap.

Chlorhexidine achieved significantly greater reductions in adjusted mean log10 bacterial count than did povidone–iodine and chloroxylenol immediately after scrubbing and for up to 6 hours. This difference persisted with repeated scrubbing over multiple days.[58]

A cluster randomized trial compared a 75% aqueous alcoholic solution containing propanol-1, propanol-2, and mecetronium etilsufate with a hand-scrubbing protocol using either 4% povidone–iodine or 4% chlorhexidine gluconate. There was no difference in the rates of SSI (2.44% with hand rubbine vs. 2.48% with hand scrubbing.) However, the adherence to protocol and the acceptability of the method to the surgical teams was better with the hand-rubbing protocol. It is recommended that a nonantiseptic hand washing be performed for 1 minute at the start of the day and again if hands are soiled.[59] Hand-rubbing with liquid aqueous alcoholic solution can thus be safely used as an alternative to traditional surgical hand-scrubbing.[57,59,60]

Bacterial Vaginosis

Bacterial vaginosis is a risk factor for SSI, particularly cuff cellulitis after hysterectomy. Preoperative and postoperative treatment with metronidazole for patients diagnosed with bacterial vaginosis should be carried out for at least 4 days beginning just before surgery. The practice significantly reduces vaginal cuff infection.[18]

Antimicrobial Prophylaxis

Antibiotic prophylaxis is one of the mainstays of preventing SSI. It works by eradicating or retarding the growth of endogenous microorganisms. The timing of antibiotic prophylaxis is very important. Clinical trials have demonstrated that the optimal time for dosing a patient with preoperative antibiotics is between 30 minutes and 2 hours prior to surgery. For most antibiotics, a 60-minute window prior to anesthesia is ideal; however, for vancomycin or fluoroquinolones dosing within 60–120 minutes ensures adequate drug levels and prevents antibiotic drug reactions at the time of anesthesia.[61] Antibiotics given sooner, or later are not as effective.[62]

Time of Administration with Respect to Incision Time	Percent with SSI	Odds Ratio (95% CI)
Early (2–24 hours prior)	3.8	4.3 (1.8–10.4)
Preoperative (0–2 hours prior)	0.6	1.0
Perioperative (within 3 hours after)	1.4	2.1 (0.4–7.4)
Postoperative (more than 3 hours after)	3.3	5.8 (2.4–13.8)

Adapted from Reference 62.

For cases that are longer, antibiotics should be re-dosed in intervals of one or two times the half-life of the drug, which maintains adequate levels throughout the operation.[63] For cefazolin, this suggests the need for a second dose after 3 hours. A second dose may be appropriate in surgical cases with an increased blood loss (greater than 1500 mL). Antibiotic doses should be increased for morbidly obese patients with a BMI over 35 or weight greater than 100 kg.[64] The standard dose of cefazolin should be increased from 1 to 2 g in these patients.

Not all surgery requires prophylaxis with antibiotics. Clean surgery generally does not require prophylaxis unless there is a high-risk indication. Contaminated and dirty cases generally require therapeutic courses of broad-spectrum antibiotics. Cases that are most important to ensure adequate prophylaxis is given are clean-contaminated cases, which represent a relatively high proportion of gynecologic surgery. Some advocate prophylaxis for procedures involving placement of prosthetic materials, such as synthetic mesh.

Recently, a prospective cohort study verified the low incidences of complications in benign laparoscopic surgery, where no cases of SSI were noted in 300 women, half of whom had received antibiotics.[65] Gynecologic surgery where prophylaxis is not indicated include clean laparoscopy and laparotomy where the vagina is not entered, hysteroscopy, hysterosalpingogram or chromotubation (unless there is a history of pelvic inflammatory disease or dilated fallopian tubes), IUD insertion, endometrial biopsy, and urodynamics.[66]

The selection of antibiotics varies by perceived risk of exposure to various pathogens. There are minor differences in published guidelines.[61,66] Here we will present some of the options. An example of common prophylaxis for different surgeries is given in the following table.

Surgery	Common Pathogens	Recommended Antibiotics	Dosage (adults)
Hysterectomy or gynecologic procedures involving mesh	Enteric gram-negatives Anaerobes Group B *Streptococcus* Enterococci	Cefazolin, Cefotetan, or Cefoxitin Ampicillin–sulbactam Clindamycin or Metronidazole plus Gentamicin or Quinolone or Aztreonam	1–2 g IV 3 g IV 600 mg IV 500 mg IV 1.5 mg/kg IV 400 mg IV 1 g IV
Abortion	Same as for hysterectomy	Doxycycline	300 mg po (100 mg 1 hour prior and 200 mg po after procedure)
Colorectal	Enteric gram-negatives Anaerobes Enterococci	Oral: Neomycin plus Metronidazole or Erythromycin Cefotetan, Cefoxitin or Cefazolin plus Metronidazole Ampicillin–sulbactam Ertapenem	1 g 2 g 1 g 1–2 g IV 500 mg IV 3 g IV 1 g IV

Adapted from References 61 and 66.

First-generation cephalosporins such as Cefazolin exhibit activity against most gram-positive organism such as staphylococci and streptococci, which comprise the normal skin flora. The broader spectrum gram-positive and gram-negative coverage of second-generation cephalosporins such as cefoxitin or cefotetan provide improved coverage for bowel flora. There is some resistance among gram-negative aerobes, and adding metronidazole or substituting therapy with ampicillin/sulbactam can increase the spectrum of coverage.

There is evidence from the colorectal literature that ertapenem is more effective than cefotetan in preventing SSI, with lower SSI infection rates (17 vs. 26%), though the incidence of *Clostridium difficile* infection was higher (1.7% vs 0.6%).[67,68] Ertapenem has also been found to be more cost effective with per hospitalization cost savings of $2181.[69] However, there is concern that prophylactic use of this agent could lead to resistance and diminish the ability to effectively treat more serious infections.

Generally, penicillin allergic patients can still be treated with cephalosporins, since cross-reactivity is uncommon unless the patient has a history of severe IgE-mediated reactions. If the patient has history suggestive of this type of allergy, an alternative such as clindamycin (600–900 mg IV) or vancomycin (1 g IV) should be considered. If coverage for gram-negative organisms is desired, then an additional antibiotic can be added such as levofloxacin, ciprofloxacin, gentamicin, or aztreonam.

The possibility of antimicrobial resistance should be considered for patients who are at high risk for colonization with resistant organisms, such as patients with long preoperative hospitalization. In these patients, consideration can be given to prophylaxis with vancomycin.[61]

Despite the recognized utility of antibiotic prophylaxis, there are significant inconsistencies in its use. A sample of Medicare patients in 2001 found that only 93% of patients received prophylaxis, only 56% were given within 1 hour before incision, and only 41% were discontinued within 24 hours of surgery.[70] Efforts to improve these numbers resulted in significant improvement in rates to 95% of patients receiving appropriately timed prophylaxis and 85% having appropriate discontinuation of antibiotics within 1 hour of surgery.[71]

Surgical Technique

There is no substitute for meticulous surgical technique to minimize blood loss, tissue ischemia and tissue damage in preventing SSIs. Excessive use of electrosurgical cautery and/or dissection may increase tissue damage, increase dead space, and predispose the wound to infection. Laparoscopy as compared to laparotomy decreases infection rates.[27] The use of prosthetics or mesh increases infection rates. Longer surgical times are also associated with increased risk of infection; good operative technique can minimize operating times and therefore further reduce the risks of infection. In general, the number of personnel in the operating environment during surgery should be kept to a minimum to avoid inadvertent contamination.

Wound Closure

Peritoneal closure is not recommended as it has been shown in studies to promote adhesions, infection, and inflammation both in animal studies and in surgery.[72,73] Peritoneal nonclosure is thought to be equally effective, faster, associated with lower postoperative morbidity and is cost-saving in the range of $330 per case. Closure of Camper's fascia has been shown to decrease hematomas and seromas, particularly in patients with >2 cm subcutaneous tissue. Skin staples may be preferable to subcuticular closure, as the risk of infection is thought to be lower, and staples are less likely to mask wound drainage and impending separation.[74,75] In general, skin closure is left to the discretion of the surgeon.

Drains

The use of drains is sometimes necessary to prevent the development of fluid collections or infection at the end of surgery. This should be based on the likelihood of significant postoperative fluid build-up and remains largely the discretion of the surgeon. A drain may also be used to irrigate the wound with antibiotic or debridement solution, which has the potential to decrease wound infection.[76] Complications from drains may include infection, hemorrhage, kinking, and hernia. Drainage of subcutaneous tissue has not been shown to improve outcomes, may actually increase the risk of infection in contaminated incisions, and should not be part of standard practice.[76] If a drain is used, a closed system with negative pressure is preferred.

Foley Catheters

Foreign objects, whether catheters or other prosthetics, are rapidly enveloped by a bio-film, consisting of thrombin, fibrin, fibronectin, and microbial production of an organic polymer matrix.[77,78] If human cells attach to the artificial material ahead of bacteria, the likelihood of an infection is less likely. Microbial adherence depends upon the material of the prosthetic, with Teflon or silicon being more resistant to adherence than polyvinylchloride. The microbes may not initially derive sufficient nutrients to replicate and to produce disease. However, when the devices are exposed to the outside environment (e.g., Foley catheter into the bladder through a highly colonized distal urethra), the replicating bacteria can serve as a nidus of infection and continued seeding requiring antibiotic therapy with removal and/or replacement.[79] Bacteriuria develops in up to 30% of patients with catheters in place for less than 1 month and in almost all patients with prolonged catheterization.[79] Pyelonephritis and systemic sepsis can complicate both short- and long-term catheterization.

Although suggested by some, prophylactic antibiotics do not have a clear role for prevention of urinary tract infections in patients with indwelling catheter.[80] They may be effective in the immediate postoperative period, for patients with catheters in place for 1–3 days.[81] In the absence of clear data, such a strategy should be individualized relative to risk factors. Prolonged catheterization should be avoided whenever possible.

Central Venous Catheters

Short-term catheters are associated with a higher rate of bacteremia and infection than long-term insertions, with a rate as high as 15%.[77] They should be kept in place for the minimal amount of time possible to decrease infectious morbidity. The use of antiseptic impregnated or antimicrobial-impregnated catheters decreases infection rates significantly.[82-84] Upper extremity placement of peripheral and subclavian placement for central catheters is preferred to minimize infection. The most common organisms involved are coagulase negative staph, *S. aureus* and *Candida* species. Skin site contamination, at the time of insertion or subsequent care, is the most common cause of infection and reflects skin flora migrating up along the external surface of the catheter from the skin exit site.[78] Seeding from distant infections represents the least frequent mechanism, although *Candida* species infections are likely related to hematogenous seeding from the gastrointestinal tract.

Subcutaneous reservoir port catheters are associated with low infectious complication rates.[78] As noted above, this depends upon minimal contamination at insertion. The definition of catheter infection is not clearly outlined in many reports and includes exit site infections as well as catheter related bacteremia. Signs of localized exit site infection, in the absence of positive blood cultures, can be treated with local care and intravenous antibiotics. Removal of the catheter should be considered if there is no response to these measure or if tunnel infection/cellulitis is present.[77]

Catheter-related bacteremia due to coagulase-negative staphylococci needs to be confirmed by more than one blood culture due to the high prevalence of contamination by this organism.[77] If confirmed, it should be noted that more than half of these organisms are resistant to anti-staphylococcal penicillins and cephalosporins. Vancomycin therapy for 5–7 days is indicated. If no rapid response is evident, removal of the catheter should be considered and antibiotic therapy administered for 7–10 days if uncomplicated. In the event of sepsis despite removal, a prolonged 4-week course is required. Uncomplicated systemic catheter-related infection can be cured with antibiotics administered through the catheter 85% of the time. An absolute indication for removal is persistence of fevers and positive blood cultures despite antibiotic therapy. If signs of infection persist despite antibiotic therapy and catheter removal, endocarditis or septic thrombophlebitis should be ruled out.[77] Candidemia induced by a central venous catheter should be treated with a short course of Amphotericin (2 weeks at 0.5 mg/kg), and evaluation for systemic candidiasis. If infection persists beyond 48 hours, a longer treatment course will be required and the catheter should be removed.[77]

SSI MANAGEMENT

Superficial and Deep Incisional

Wound Infection

Wound infections or superficial SSIs are diagnosed clinically and are typically associated with fever, localized erythema, induration and pain at the site of the incision. Separation of the wound may occur. Most wound infections can be treated with wound drainage, irrigation, debridement, packing, and oral antibiotics. Irrigation and debridement should be performed with normal saline and gauze and not Dakins solution or Iodophor, as these agents lead to decreased wound macrophage and fibroblast function and thus retarding the healing process. After 3 or 4 days, if the wound looks healthy, it can be reapproximated. Closure by secondary intention generally takes many weeks to months and frequently leads to a less satisfactory cosmetic result. If the wound is associated with cellulitis, antibiotic therapy may be necessary. Early wound infection with red-striae may suggest group A or B, hemolytic streptococci, requiring therapy with penicillin and clindamycin or cephalosporins, which have activity against these organisms. For complex wounds, a wound-vacuum may be used to assist with wound closure, but this should be used after adequate debridement has taken place and the wound is granulating.

Necrotizing Fasciitis

Should the wound not bleed or if the patient cannot feel the surgical manipulations, one has to consider the diagnosis of necrotizing fasciitis that may be associated with aerobic and anaerobic organisms, especially *Streptococcus*, group A, C, or G and *Clostridia* species. Findings may include unexplained, progressive pain, rapidly spreading erythema, and subcutaneous crepitus. The patient may also present with fever, malaise, myalgia, diarrhea, and anorexia. Early recognition is critical as the rapid progression of this disease may result in extensive tissue destruction, limb loss, systemic toxicity, and death.[85] Treatment should consist of ampicillin–sulbactam and clindamycin or metronidazole with urgent, aggressive surgical resection of diseased tissue to margins that bleed.[86] This surgical course may be required multiple times daily because this disease may pursue a fulminant course with rapid development of multiorgan dysfunction if allowed to spread. If broader coverage is desired, ticarcillin–clavulanate or piperacillin–tazobactam can be substituted for ampicillin or an additional antibiotic can be added (fluoroquinolone, aminoglycoside, cephalosporin, or carbapenems.) Mortality rates remain high (14%–34%), even with appropriate therapy.[85,87–89]

Intra-Abdominal/Pelvic Infections

Gynecologic Ascending Infections As noted, the vagina normally harbors bacteria and bacterial vaginosis has been linked to the development of upper genital tract infections, especially at midcycle when the cervical mucus is thin and penetrable or at menses when it is absent. Sexually transmitted disease pathogens such as *Gonorrhea* and *Chlamydia* as well as enteric flora are thought to damage surface epithelium in an ascending fashion from the endocervix, endometrium, and fallopian tube. The female genital tract is susceptible to infection by organisms whenever there is instrumentation or surgery performed with contact with the endometrium or endocervix. These are impossible to sterilize prophylactically with topical agents. If infection occurs, coverage should include a third-/fourth-generation cephalosporin and doxycycline to cover gram-negative organisms and atypicals. Complications of this type of infection include sterility, tuboovarian abscess formation, and the development of chronic pelvic pain.

Bowel Related If peritonitis develops postoperatively without evidence of intra-abdominal gas, but with elevated WBC and temperature, then expectant management with aggressive antibiotic therapy should be instituted immediately and continued until the patient improves. However, if peritonitis with evidence of a perforated viscus is noted, surgical intervention is mandatory.

Recognized injury of the unprepared large bowel is associated with both aerobic and anaerobic organism contamination. As described above, a biphasic infection pattern may develop. Peritonitis leading to mortality may occur unless appropriate operative management (i.e., repair of injury with or without colostomy) and prophylactic or therapeutic antibiotic therapy is promptly instituted, depending on the degree of contamination.

Small bowel contents have a very low concentration of potentially pathogenic organisms, depending upon the site and presence or absence of obstruction. In general, recognized injury is treated surgically without antibiotic therapy/prophylaxis. In the presence of bowel obstruction, feculent overgrowth can occur, particularly of anaerobes, and production of endo- and exotoxins can lead to septic shock and death. Although newer techniques have dramatically improved diagnostic accuracy, there is no absolutely reliable way to distinguish simple from strangulated obstruction, especially in the presence of carcinomatosis[90] Many would suggest that in the presence of any of the following classical findings, surgery is indicated: (1) fever, (2) tachycardia, (3) localized tenderness, and (4) leukocytosis.[91] Also, in cases of carcinomatosis-induced obstruction, conservative management may be futile and the obstruction is often amenable to surgical relief.[90] However, morbidity and cost data suggest that conservative management should be pursued when possible.[92] Chemotherapy may be considered as an alternative to surgical intervention and may be associated with less morbidity, particularly in patients with platinum sensitive tumors.[93] Decisions have to be individualized depending upon localization of the malignant process, probability of successful bypass/resection, and life expectancy. The use of perioperative antibiotics in simple adhesive small bowel obstruction depends on the likelihood of contamination and is generally used. For more complicated cases, prophylaxis is recommended. If employed, coverage should include skin and bowel flora.

Clinically, significant translocation of bacteria occurs under conditions of mucosal injury.[94] This may include mesenteric ischemia and strangulation due to small bowel obstruction but may also be due to radiation or other therapeutic insults. In the presence of ischemia or longer standing obstruction, the feculent environment predisposes to anaerobic predominance.[95] Antibiotic selection should bear these factors in mind and in general have broad-spectrum coverage, including for skin, bowel, and anaerobic organisms.

Abscesses The second phase of the bi-phasic infection pattern, especially if the antibiotic choice was insufficient in its spectrum or activity, is abscess formation. Although there is evidence that these may respond to antibiotic therapy alone, there are a variety of intervention strategies available. It is possible to adequately drain some abscesses with sonographic or radiologic assistance. Ultrasound or CT-assisted aspiration (with or without irrigation) may be performed in patients failing antibiotic therapy, especially in postoperative patients in whom reoperative surgery may be hazardous. This therapeutic option should be restricted to those individuals in whom there is no evidence of perforation. If there is evidence of perforation such as with ruptured appendicitis or bowel anastomosis leakage, surgical intervention and correction of the defect is necessary. Exploratory laparotomy with or without extirpation of genital tract structures may be necessary if the patients are unresponsive to antibiotic therapy and if their clinical condition warrants it. On a separate note, a tubo-ovarian abscess presenting in a postmenopausal woman with no clear etiology should be investigated for possible malignancy, as this is likely in about half of cases.[96]

Lymphocyst Infection   Lymphocyst formation is a rare occurrence after pelvic lymphadenectomy. Collections can occasionally become infected as a result of direct inoculation from the gut flora or from hematogenous spread. Thus, they are apt to represent mixed infections and should be treated with antibiotics and drainage. Prophylactic drains have been proven ineffective in preventing lymphocyst occurrence and infection after radical pelvic surgery.[97–99]

Treatment of Intra-Abdominal Infections

Intravenous Antibiotic Choices   In order to provide antibiotic coverage for aerobes and anaerobes, a variety of therapeutic options can be considered. It has been customary to use an aminoglycoside-based regimen that includes an antianaerobic agent. This combination was successful in 86% (range 70%–100%) of cases included in a large meta-analysis of 28 studies comparing these agents to newer regimens.[100] Using once-daily dosing of an aminoglycoside has been shown to increase adherence, improve efficacy, and possibly decrease toxicity compared to multiple daily dosing.[101] *Enterococcus* coverage is not necessary for routine coverage of intra-abdominal infections, but if indicated, the extended coverage penicillin/beta-lactamase agents such as piperacillin/tazobactam or ampicillin/sulbactam can be used.

Third-generation cephalosporins provide a simple alternative and are very effective as monotherapy in treating intra-abdominal infections. Cefoxitin alone is successful in 85% (range 78%–97%) of cases, while cefotetan alone resulted in 95% (range 90%–98%) success. Cefuroxime (a second-generation cephalosporin) can be combined with metronidazole as an alternative resulting in 87% success. Increased success can be obtained by combining a third-/fourth-generation cephalosporin with an anti-anaerobic agent, which resulted in 92% (75%–100%) of cases successfully treated. Monbactams such as aztreonam combined with anti-anaerobic coverage are successful in 84% of cases (range 71%–100%). Carbapenems can be very effective as monotherapy; rates of cure were 87% (range 69%–100%) for imipenem/cilastatin and 87% in one study of ertapenem, while the cure rate for meropenem were even higher at 95% (91%–100%). These agents have the additional advantage of covering *Enterococcus*, which may be desired for certain patients. Fluoroquinolones coupled with antianaerobic agents can successfully treat intra-abdominal infections in 82% (range 74%–97%) of cases and have the advantage of excellent oral bioavailability. Clindamycin and metronidazole remain the accepted antimicrobials for anti-anaerobic coverage.[100]

Oral Antibiotics: Primary or Completion Traditionally, the oral antibiotic following parenteral therapy did not provide the same spectrum of activity. However, exceptions to this general rule include some of the fluoroquinolones and metronidazole.[102] Upon resolution of the peritonitis or upon ability to tolerate enteral medications, oral therapy can be instituted with identical circulating and tissue concentrations as with the intravenous therapy. Completion therapy for intra-abdominal infection with oral antibiotics has been shown to be effective and is recommended when patients are able to tolerate oral intake.[103] Also, in selected cases the oral form may be administered primarily. There is insufficient data to provide guidelines for duration of total therapy.[100] Convention has dictated that for infections without abscesses, a 5- to 7-day course of therapy be administered while for those with abscesses, a 10- to 14-day course be administered. Randomized controlled trials are lacking and are indicated.

Extra-Abdominal Infection Sites

Pneumonia Nosocomial pneumonia is defined as occurring more than 48 hours after hospital admission and is the most common cause of nosocomial infection-induced mortality.[104, 105] Clinically, it is diagnosed in the presence of fever, purulent sputum, leukocytosis, and a decline in oxygenation.

The most common isolates are aerobic gram-negative rods (*E. coli, Klebsiella pneumoniae, Enterobacter, Pseudomonas*) and gram-positive cocci (*S. aureus,* MRSA, *Streptococcus*) aspirated from the oropharynx.[106] More rarely, nosocomial pneumonia can be due to viruses or fungi.

Mechanical ventilation is often complicated by nosocomial pneumonia, having a relative risk of 7–10 times that seen in nonventilated patients.[107] Each hospital and intensive care facility monitors the pathogens associated with these infections. Selective pressures from antibiotic usage leading to resistant organisms responsible for these infections have been routinely reported and may explain the high death rate despite the availability of potent antibiotics. Additionally, breakdowns in standard protocols for ventilator management may lead to infections. Contamination of the condensate forming in the tubing is frequent. If this condensate is not drained frequently and the tubing not changed every 24–48 hours (CDC recommendation is 24 hours), it may be inoculated into the tracheobronchial tree during patient positioning. Personnel may be responsible for horizontal infection spread (e.g., lack of hand washing or gloving). While ventilator-associated pneumonia may be due to aspiration of refluxed pathogens colonizing the stomach and duodenum, studies involving selective enteral antibiotic decontamination of the digestive tract as prophylaxis have had mixed results. Regular oral care with antiseptic reduces the risk of ventilator-associated pneumonia and should be employed in ventilated patients.[108] Prevention of aspiration through positioning in the semirecumbent position and subglottic drainage are also helpful to reduce VAP. Silver coated endotracheal tubes are beneficial in reducing VAP (4.8% vs. 7.5%) particularly in patients ventilated for more than 24 hours.[109]

Empiric treatment should be based on clinical findings and Gram's stain results from an uncontaminated sputum specimen or tracheal aspirate. The patient's recent exposure to antibiotic therapy, the resident hospital flora, and the presence of underlying disease should guide therapy until specific culture data is available. Diagnosis should be made by chest radiograph and culture of the lower respiratory tract if possible.[110] Although bronchoalveolar lavage or protected specimen brushing may be more sensitive or specific, the cost-effectiveness is not clear.

Empiric therapy is generally with ceftriaxone 2 g IV qd, ampicillin–sulbactam 3 g IV q6h, piperacillin–tazobactam 4.5 g IV q6h, levofloxacin 750 mg IV qd, or ertapenem 1 gm IV qd. If the patient has risk factors for a drug-resistant organism, then coverage should be expanded to a three-drug regimen. These patients should receive combination therapy with a beta-lactam (or aztreonam if beta-lactam allergic), an antipseudomonal fluoroquinolone (ciprofloxacin or levofloxacin) and an aminoglycoside (gentamicin or tobramycin). In critically ill patients with nosocomial pneumonia due to *Pseudomonas* or other gram-negative rods, combination regimens should be used and guided by sensitivity of the culture. Monotherapy may be considered in less critically ill patients. Vancomycin or linezolid should be initiated for MRSA.[111] Treatment modifications are based on clinical response and sensitivity patterns.

Urinary Tract Infection   Diagnosis of cystitis is established based on symptomatology and urinalysis and confirmed by urine culture. Empiric therapy for uncomplicated lower tract infections should be based on local hospital infection surveillance susceptibility patterns, Gram stain and patient issues such as allergies, age, and renal function. Treatment options include beta-lactams, trimethoprim/sulfamethoxazole, nitrofurantoin, and fluoroquinolone among others and can be given as a short course (3 days) in most cases.[112]

Pyelonephritis normally progresses from a lower urinary tract infection that is asymptomatic or undertreated. If untreated, it can progress and result in significant renal damage. Diagnosis is made by history and the findings of costovertebral angle (CVA) tenderness and high fevers. Laboratory studies include CBC to look for elevated WBC, urinalysis to evaluate for pyuria and white cell casts as well as culture with sensitivity. Generally, urinary tract infections are caused by enteric organisms, such as *E. coli* or *Klebsiella*. More unusual organisms such as *Staphylococcus saprophyticus* are associated with abnormalities such as stones. Patients may be initially treated with oral agents if tolerated. In uncomplicated cases, fluoroquinolones such as ciprofloxacin should be used. Trimethoprim–sulfamethoxazole is an alternative, but resistance rates are higher. For patients not able to tolerate oral intake or with more complicated infections, ceftriaxone, or fluoroquinolone IV monotherapy can be used initially. Ampicillin and gentamicin can also be used, as they provide coverage for the often-encountered gram-negative bacilli and enterococci. In the event of progressive systemic sepsis, multiagent regimens targeting gram-negative rods and enterococci should be selected. Modifications should be based on clinical response and culture and sensitivity profiles. Patients who do not coalesce should be evaluated radiologically for obstruction, abscess, or other complications.

Clostridium Difficile Colitis   Pseudomembranous antibiotic-induced colitis is a common complication of prolonged broad-spectrum antibiotic therapy.[113] Colonization of the intestinal tract occurs by the fecal–oral route and overgrowth occurs as a result of antimicrobial therapy disrupting the normal bowel flora. Clinical symptoms include significant diarrhea for at least 1–2 days. Flexible sigmoidoscopy can quickly identify pseudomembranes in most cases; however, it is not generally necessary. Testing for stool cytotoxin presence is more sensitive and is highly specific. Treatment is cessation of the inciting antibiotic and the institution of oral metronidazole for mild to moderate cases.[114] For severe cases, vancomycin continues to be the agent of choice. Patients in whom *C. difficile* is not found, but who have symptoms of enteric infection, can be treated with oral quinolones. In the presence of associated bacteremia, a third-generation cephalosporin is effective against the most common offending pathogens: *Campylobacter*, *Salmonella*, *Shigella*, and *E. coli.*

Systemic Sepsis   The definitions of systemic inflammatory response syndrome and sepsis are presented elsewhere. When sepsis has been diagnosed, antibiotic therapy should be instituted immediately after obtaining cultures. Empiric antibiotic selection guidelines for sepsis are as follows: The initial treatment should consist of vancomycin plus one of the following: a third-/fourth-generation cephalosporin, piperacillin-tazobactam, ticarcillin–clavulanate or carbapenems.

If *Pseudomonas* is a possible pathogen then vancomycin should be combined with two of the following: (1) ceftazidime or cefepime, (2) imipenem or meropenem, (3) piperacillin–tazobactam or ticarcillin–clavulanate, (4) ciprofloxacin, (5) gentamicin or amikacin, or (6) aztreonam.

Once culture results have come back, a single agent with documented sensitivity is recommended as this is associated with less morbidity than a continued multiagent regimen.[115] Patients should be observed closely for clinical response, side effects, and the development of complications such as nosocomial superinfection. Therapy is normally continued for 7–10 days, though longer courses are indicated for patients with a slow clinical response or in certain populations, e.g., neutropenic patients.[116]

Fungal Infection   *Candida* species accounts for approximately 9% of nosocomial bloodstream infections.[117] The increase in fungemia is thought to reflect the use of total parenteral nutrition, central venous catheterization, and broad-spectrum antibiotics. *Candida albicans* accounts for about half of all cases, with *Candida glabrata* responsible for 26%, *Candida parapsilosis* 16%, *Candida tropicalis* 8%, and *Candida krusei* 3%.[118] It may be important to differentiate between these types as antifungal susceptibility varies among species. Risk factors for candidemia include immunocompromised patient, location in an intensive care unit, presence of a central venous catheter, urinary catheter, and use of systemic antibiotics.[119] Meticulous aseptic technique when inserting and managing indwelling catheters and shortening inpatient systemic antibiotic usage, if possible, should reduce the risk of fungemia. The gold standard method to diagnosis candidemia is positive blood cultures, but these are not always sensitive and treatment may be instituted based on clinical suspicion. Treatment will be based on the local prevalence of resistant *Candida* species, prior treatment history, and immune status. Treatment options include polyenes such as amphotericin B, azoles such as fluconazole and echinocandins such as caspofungin.[120] For nonneutropenic patients, fluconazole may be started initially.

PHARMACOECONOMICS

A description of the various forms of economic analysis is provided elsewhere, in Evidence-Based Medicine and Decision Support. Use of pharmacoeconomics in formulary decision making provides a better alternative to purchasing the "cheapest" agent as measured by unit cost. Incorporating outcomes analysis and proper attention to total relevant cost data gathering allows equitable comparison of agents and results in optimized care rather than simple cost cutting.

Economic assessment of antibiotic usage should generally be based on comparison of the marginal or incremental benefits versus the marginal costs of administration. This holds true for prophylaxis as well as therapeutic use. As noted previously, the actual definition of "costs," and accurate assigning thereof, significantly influences the outcome analysis. Opportunity costs and human suffering/morbidity cost should not be lost in favor of pure economics. However, wasteful infection control measures, such as use of prophylactic antibiotics for greater than 24 hours, compromises patient care, and is a reflection of poor scarce resources utilization.

With respect to direct costs, evaluating excess costs of infection per operation takes into account (1) the costs of infection care, (2) the infection rate, and (3) the number of surgical procedures performed per year.[121] On an excess cost per case basis, clean operations may not rank very highly due to the low expected rate of infection. However, due to the volume of cases, excess cost per year may total more than the clean contaminated to dirty cases on a sheer volume basis. These factors should be considered in determining the effectiveness of infection control measures, including use of prophylactic antibiotics and the duration of their administration.[122]

Formulary decisions and antibiotic usage may be made based upon the following types of analyses, depending upon the question being posed:

Cost minimization: Do the products have the same patient outcomes but differing vendor prices?

Cost effectiveness: What is the total cost of therapy versus the outcomes gained if the agents are dissimilar in patient outcomes?

Cost utility: Use of which antibiotic results in patient outcomes that are optimal when adjusted for patient preferences (e.g., side effects, duration and route of therapy, inpatient/outpatient)?

Cost–benefit: Which program area (e.g., antibiotics) of the formulary requires greatest attention and more benefit per dollar due to higher ascribed value of outcomes than another program (e.g., antihypertensives)?

CLINICAL REALITIES

Prior to economic evaluation, there must be clinical effectiveness clearly demonstrated. Failure of antibiotic therapy requiring surgery with extirpation of organs or prolonged intensive care is very costly, no matter how costs are defined and suffering may be extreme. Unfortunately, in many areas there are insufficient definitive studies suggesting that one antibiotic or one combination of antibiotics is superior to another. We are left with having to examine the outcomes of various therapies for the treatment of specific conditions. In the case of treatment of presumed tuboovarian abscesses, therapy with a cephalosporin with doxycycline or gentamicin with clindamycin may fail up to 25% of the time, leading to the need for more costly interventions such as surgery.[123] Additionally, approximately one third of those who initially responded required surgery with extirpation of some pelvic structures before being cured of their infection. With such a high failure rate when employing standard therapies, alternate therapies should be considered and further research encouraged, even when these agents are significantly more costly when prices are compared directly.

Each intravenous administration is costly, thus the administrative cost of dosing a drug multiple times daily may be far more costly than the direct unit cost of the drug alone, sometimes overshadowing the inflated costs of new agents. Even if the efficacy of a new single daily dose agent is not superior to conventional therapies, there may be a favorable cost-effectiveness ratio to the use of single daily dosing. While clinical and economic evaluation of antibiotic usage is very complex and currently imprecise, treatment patterns ought not be based on the best drug detailer pitch or personal anecdotal experience alone. Audit programs, incorporating infection control surveillance and outcomes analysis, have been proposed as effective means of eliminating wasteful practices while optimizing care.[124]

SSI SURVEILLANCE AND INFECTION CONTROL PROGRAM

Active surveillance of SSIs and organized programs to prevent and control this common complication are essential to good perioperative care.[125, 126] Active reporting of SSI rates to individual surgeons and chiefs of staff is an important component of minimizing infection.[127] The report should be presented as surgeon-specific, service-specific, and organized by surgical risk index scores; however, confidentiality must be maintained. For outpatient procedures, SSI tracking may be more difficult, and some use questionnaires or automated health plan and pharmacy data to identify patients with a SSI.

There has been clear demonstration that hospitals that participate in comprehensive infection control programs such as the National Surgical Infection Prevention Collaborative or the Surgical Infection Prevention and Surgical Care Improvement Projects can significantly decrease SSI rates and improve patient outcomes.[71, 128]

REFERENCES

1. GARIBALDI RA, BRODINE S, MATSUMIYA S, et al. Evidence for the non-infectious etiology of early postoperative fever. Infect Control 1985;6(7):273–277.

2. GALICIER C, RICHET H. A prospective study of postoperative fever in a general surgery department. Infect Control 1985;6(12):487–490.

3. ENGOREN M. Lack of association between atelectasis and fever. Chest 1995;107(1):81–84.

4. BLATTEIS CM, SEHIC E, LI S. Pyrogen sensing and signaling: old views and new concepts. Clin Infect Dis 2000;31(suppl 5):S168– S177.

5. CONTI B, TABAREAN I, ANDREI C, et al. Cytokines and fever. Front Biosci 2004;9:1433–449.

6. DAULEH MI, RAHMAN S, TOWNELL NH. Open versus laparoscopic cholecystectomy: a comparison of postoperative temperature. J R Coll Surg Edinb 1995;40(2):116–118.

7. MUZII L, BASILE S, ZUPI E, et al. Laparoscopic-assisted vaginal hysterectomy versus minila-parotomy hysterectomy: a prospective, randomized, multicenter study. J Minim Invasive Gynecol 2007;14(5):610–615.

8. MEDEIROS LR, ROSA DD, BOZZETTI MC, et al. Laparoscopy versus laparotomy for benign ovarian tumour. Cochrane Database Syst Rev 2009 (2):CD004751.

9. SCHEY D, SALOM EM, PAPADIA A, et al. Extensive fever workup produces low yield in determining infectious etiology. Am J Obstet Gynecol 2005;192(5):1729–1734.

10. SCHWANDT A, ANDREWS SJ, FANNING J. Prospective analysis of a fever evaluation algorithm after major gynecologic surgery. Am J Obstet Gynecol 2001;184(6):1066–1067.

11. SCHULTE-SASSE U, HESS W, EBERLEIN HJ. Postoperative malignant hyperthermia and dantrolene therapy. Can Anaesth Soc J 1983;30(6):635–640.

12. MILLER LG, PERDREAU-REMINGTON F, RIEG G, et al. Necrotizing fasciitis caused by community-associated methicillin-resistant *Staphylococcus aureus* in Los Angeles. N Engl J Med 2005;352(14):1445–1453.

13. NOLAN TE, KING LA, SMITH RP, et al. Necrotizing surgical infection and necrotizing fasciitis in obstetric and gynecologic patients. South Med J 1993;86(12):1363–1367.

14. BROOK I, FRAZIER EH. Clinical and microbiological features of necrotizing fasciitis. J Clin Microbiol 1995;33(9):2382–2387.

15. HORAN TC, CULVER DH, GAYNES RP, et al. Nosocomial infections in surgical patients in the United States, January 1986-June 1992. National Nosocomial Infections Surveillance (NNIS) System. Infect Control Hosp Epidemiol 1993;14(2):73–80.

16. DODD RY. Transmission of parasites by blood transfusion. Vox Sang 1998;74(suppl 2):161–163.

17. SCHABERG DR, CULVER DH, GAYNES RP. Major trends in the microbial etiology of nosocomial infection. Am J Med 1991;91(3B):72S-75S.

18. LARSSON PG, CARLSSON B. Does pre- and postoperative metronidazole treatment lower vaginal cuff infection rate after abdominal hysterectomy among women with bacterial vaginosis? Infect Dis Obstet Gynecol 2002;10(3):133–140.

19. WEINSTEIN WM, ONDERDONK AB, BARTLETT JG, et al. Experimental intra-abdominal abscesses in rats: development of an experimental model. Infect Immun 1974;10(6):1250–1255.

20. KELLY MJ. The quantitative and histological demonstration of pathogenic synergy between *Escherichia coli* and *Bacteroides fragilis* in guinea-pig wounds. J Med Microbiol 1978;11(4): 513–523.

21. GUINAN JL, MCGUCKIN M, NOWELL PC. Management of health-care–associated infections in the oncology patient. Oncology (Williston Park). 2003;17(3):415–420; discussion 23–26.

22. MALONE DL, GENUIT T, TRACY JK, et al. Surgical site infections: reanalysis of risk factors. J Surg Res 2002;103(1):89–95.

23. National Nosocomial Infections Surveillance (NNIS) System report, data summary from October 1986-April 1998, issued June 1998. Am J Infect Control 1998;26(5):522–533.

24. CULVER DH, HORAN TC, GAYNES RP, et al. Surgical wound infection rates by wound class, operative procedure, and patient risk index. National Nosocomial Infections Surveillance System. Am J Med 1991;91(3B):152S-157S.

25. FRIEDMAN ND, BULL AL, RUSSO PL, et al. Performance of the national nosocomial infections surveillance risk index in predicting surgical site infection in australia. Infect Control Hosp Epidemiol 2007;28(1):55–59.

26. The Society for Hospital Epidemiology of America; The Association for Practitioners in Infection Control; The Centers for Disease Control; The Surgical Infection Society. Consensus paper on the surveillance of surgical wound infections. Infect Control Hosp Epidemiol 1992;13(10): 599–605.

27. GAYNES RP, CULVER DH, HORAN TC, et al. Surgical site infection (SSI) rates in the United States, 1992–1998: the National Nosocomial Infections Surveillance System basic SSI risk index. Clin Infect Dis 2001;33(suppl 2):S69–S77.

28. MANGRAM AJ, HORAN TC, PEARSON ML, et al. Guideline for prevention of surgical site infection, 1999. Hospital Infection Control Practices Advisory Committee. Infect Control Hosp Epidemiol 1999;20(4):250–278; quiz 79–80.

29. VEGAS AA, JODRA VM, GARCIA ML. Nosocomial infection in surgery wards: a controlled study of increased duration of hospital stays and direct cost of hospitalization. Eur J Epidemiol 1993;9(5):504–510.

30. POULSEN KB, BREMMELGAARD A, SORENSEN AI, et al. Estimated costs of postoperative wound infections. A case-control study of marginal hospital and social security costs. Epidemiol Infect 1994;113(2):283–295.

31. PERENCEVICH EN, SANDS KE, COSGROVE SE, et al. Health and economic impact of surgical site infections diagnosed after hospital discharge. Emerg Infect Dis 2003;9(2):196–203.

32. MOLLER AM, VILLEBRO N, PEDERSEN T, et al. Effect of preoperative smoking intervention on postoperative complications: a randomised clinical trial. Lancet. 2002 12; 359(9301):114–117.

33. MOORE S, MILLS BB, MOORE RD, et al. Perisurgical smoking cessation and reduction of postoperative complications. Am J Obstet Gynecol 2005;192(5):1718–1721.

34. JACOBER SJ, SOWERS JR. An update on perioperative management of diabetes. Arch Intern Med 1999;159(20):2405–2411.

35. TRICK WE, SCHECKLER WE, TOKARS JI, et al. Modifiable risk factors associated with deep sternal site infection after coronary artery bypass grafting. J Thorac Cardiovasc Surg 2000;119(1):108–114.

36. ESTRADA CA, YOUNG JA, NIFONG LW, et al. Outcomes and perioperative hyperglycemia in patients with or without diabetes mellitus undergoing coronary artery bypass grafting. Ann Thorac Surg 2003;75(5):1392–1399.

37. WEBSTER J, OSBORNE S. Preoperative bathing or showering with skin antiseptics to prevent surgical site infection. Cochrane Database Syst Rev 2006 (2):CD004985.

38. AMSTEY MS, JONES AP. Preparation of the vagina for surgery. A comparison of povidone-iodine and saline solution. JAMA 1981;245(8):839–841.

39. BLACKMORE MA, TURNER GM, ADAMS MR, et al. The effect of pre-operative povidone iodine vaginal pessaries on vault infections after hysterectomy. Br J Obstet Gynaecol 1981;88(3):308–313.

40. KJOLHEDE P, HALILI S, LOFGREN M. The influence of preoperative vaginal cleansing on postoperative infectious morbidity in abdominal total hysterectomy for benign indications. Acta Obstet Gynecol Scand 2009;88(4):408–416.

41. TANNER J, WOODINGS D, MONCASTER K. Preoperative hair removal to reduce surgical site infection. Cochrane Database Syst Rev 2006 (2):CD004122.

42. TUNEVALL TG. Postoperative wound infections and surgical face masks: a controlled study. World J Surg 1991;15(3):383–387; discussion 7–8.

43. LIPP A, EDWARDS P. Disposable surgical face masks: a systematic review. Can Oper Room Nurs J 2005;23(3):20–21, 4–5, 33–38.

44. TANNER J, PARKINSON H. Double gloving to reduce surgical cross-infection. Cochrane Database Syst Rev 2006;3:CD003087.

45. QUEBBEMAN EJ, TELFORD GL, WADSWORTH K, et al. Double gloving. Protecting surgeons from blood contamination in the operating room. Arch Surg 1992;127(2):213–216; discussion 6–7.

46. MAHAJNA A, KRAUSZ M, ROSIN D, et al. Bowel preparation is associated with spillage of bowel contents in colorectal surgery. Dis Colon Rectum 2005;48(8):1626–1631.

47. ZHU QD, ZHANG QY, ZENG QQ, et al. Efficacy of mechanical bowel preparation with polyethylene glycol in prevention of postoperative complications in elective colorectal surgery: a meta-analysis. Int J Colorectal Dis 2010;25(2):267–275.

48. WILLE-JORGENSEN P, GUENAGA KF, MATOS D, et al. Pre-operative mechanical bowel cleansing or not? An updated meta-analysis. Colorectal Dis 2005;7(4):304–310.

49. BUCHER P, GERVAZ P, EGGER JF, et al. Morphologic alterations associated with mechanical bowel preparation before elective colorectal surgery: a randomized trial. Dis Colon Rectum 2006;49(1):109–112.

50. ROVERA F, DIONIGI G, BONI L, et al. Mechanical bowel preparation for colorectal surgery. Surg Infect (Larchmt) 2006;7(suppl 2):S61–S63.

51. MUZII L, BELLATI F, ZULLO MA, et al. Mechanical bowel preparation before gynecologic laparoscopy: a randomized, single-blind, controlled trial. Fertil Steril 2006;85(3):689–693.

52. KURZ A, SESSLER DI, LENHARDT R. Perioperative normothermia to reduce the incidence of surgical-wound infection and shorten hospitalization. Study of Wound Infection and Temperature Group. N Engl J Med 1996;334(19):1209–1215.

53. MELLING AC, ALI B, SCOTT EM, et al. Effects of preoperative warming on the incidence of wound infection after clean surgery: a randomised controlled trial. Lancet 2001;358(9285):876–880.

54. ROTH RR, JAMES WD. Microbial ecology of the skin. Annu Rev Microbiol 1988;42:441–464.

55. POTTINGER J, BURNS S, MANSKE C. Bacterial carriage by artificial versus natural nails. Am J Infect Control. 1989;17(6):340–344.

56. MOOLENAAR RL, CRUTCHER JM, SAN JOAQUIN VH, et al. A prolonged outbreak of *Pseudomonas aeruginosa* in a neonatal intensive care unit: did staff fingernails play a role in disease transmission? Infect Control Hosp Epidemiol 2000;21(2):80–85.

57. BOYCE JM, PITTET D. Guideline for Hand Hygiene in Health-Care Settings: recommendations of the Healthcare Infection Control Practices Advisory Committee and the HICPAC/SHEA/APIC/IDSA Hand Hygiene Task Force. Infect Control Hosp Epidemiol 2002;23(suppl 12):S3–S40.

58. ALY R, MAIBACH HI. Comparative antibacterial efficacy of a 2-minute surgical scrub with chlorhexidine gluconate, povidone-iodine, and chloroxylenol sponge-brushes. Am J Infect Control 1988;16(4):173–177.

59. PARIENTI JJ, THIBON P, HELLER R, et al. Hand-rubbing with an aqueous alcoholic solution vs traditional surgical hand-scrubbing and 30-day surgical site infection rates: a randomized equivalence study. JAMA. 2002;288(6):722–727.

60. TANNER J, SWARBROOK S, STUART J. Surgical hand antisepsis to reduce surgical site infection. Cochrane Database Syst Rev 2008 (1):CD004288.

61. Antimicrobial prophylaxis for surgery. Treat Guidel Med Lett 2009;7(82):47–52.

62. CLASSEN DC, EVANS RS, PESTOTNIK SL, et al. The timing of prophylactic administration of antibiotics and the risk of surgical-wound infection. N Engl J Med 1992;326(5):281–216.

63. DELLINGER EP, GROSS PA, BARRETT TL, et al. Quality standard for antimicrobial prophylaxis in surgical procedures. Infectious Diseases Society of America. Clin Infect Dis 1994;18(3): 422–427.

64. FORSE RA, KARAM B, MACLEAN LD, et al. Antibiotic prophylaxis for surgery in morbidly obese patients. Surgery 1989;106(4):750–756; discussion 6–7.

65. LITTA P, SACCO G, TSIROGLOU D, et al. Is antibiotic prophylaxis necessary in elective laparoscopic surgery for benign gynecologic conditions? Gynecol Obstet Invest 2009;69(2):136–139.

66. ACOG practice bulletin No. 104: antibiotic prophylaxis for gynecologic procedures. Obstet Gynecol 2009;113(5):1180–1189.

67. ITANI KM, WILSON SE, AWAD SS, et al. Ertapenem versus cefotetan prophylaxis in elective colorectal surgery. N Engl J Med 2006;355(25):2640–2651.

68. ITANI KM, JENSEN EH, FINN TS, et al. Effect of body mass index and ertapenem versus cefotetan prophylaxis on surgical site infection in elective colorectal surgery. Surg Infect (Larchmt) 2008;9(2):131–137.

69. WILSON SE, TURPIN RS, KUMAR RN, et al. Comparative costs of ertapenem and cefotetan as prophylaxis for elective colorectal surgery. Surg Infect (Larchmt) 2008;9(3):349–356.

70. BRATZLER DW, HOUCK PM, RICHARDS C, et al. Use of antimicrobial prophylaxis for major surgery: baseline results from the National Surgical Infection Prevention Project. Arch Surg 2005;140(2):174–182.

71. DELLINGER EP, HAUSMANN SM, BRATZLER DW, et al. Hospitals collaborate to decrease surgical site infections. Am J Surg 2005;190(1):9–15.

72. KOMOTO Y, SHIMOYA K, SHIMIZU T, et al. Prospective study of non-closure or closure of the peritoneum at cesarean delivery in 124 women: Impact of prior peritoneal closure at primary cesarean on the interval time between first cesarean section and the next pregnancy and significant adhesion at second cesarean. J Obstet Gynaecol Res 2006;32(4):396–402.

73. TULANDI T, AL-JAROUDI D. Nonclosure of peritoneum: a reappraisal. Am J Obstet Gynecol 2003;189(2):609–612.

74. BOESCH CE, UMEK W. Effects of wound closure on wound healing in gynecologic surgery: a systematic literature review. J Reprod Med 2009;54(3):139–144.

75. EDLICH RF, BECKER DG, THACKER JG, et al. Scientific basis for selecting staple and tape skin closures. Clin Plast Surg 1990;17(3):571–578.

76. FARNELL MB, WORTHINGTON-SELF S, MUCHA P JR, et al. Closure of abdominal incisions with subcutaneous catheters. A prospective randomized trial. Arch Surg 1986;121(6):641–648.

77. RAAD, II, BODEY GP. Infectious complications of indwelling vascular catheters. Clin Infect Dis 1992;15(2):197–208.

78. GOLDMANN DA, PIER GB. Pathogenesis of infections related to intravascular catheterization. Clin Microbiol Rev 1993;6(2):176–192.

79. GARIBALDI RA, BURKE JP, DICKMAN ML, et al. Factors predisposing to bacteriuria during indwelling urethral catheterization. N Engl J Med 1974;291(5):215–219.

80. WARREN JW. Catheter-associated urinary tract infections. Int J Antimicrob Agents 2001;17(4):299–303.

81. NIEL-WEISE BS, VAN DEN BROEK PJ. Antibiotic policies for short-term catheter bladder drainage in adults. Cochrane Database Syst Rev 2005 (3):CD005428.

82. RAAD I, DAROUICHE R, DUPUIS J, et al. Central venous catheters coated with minocycline and rifampin for the prevention of catheter-related colonization and bloodstream infections. A randomized, double-blind trial. The Texas Medical Center Catheter Study Group. Ann Intern Med 1997;127(4):267–274.

83. HANNA H, BENJAMIN R, CHATZINIKOLAOU I, et al. Long-term silicone central venous catheters impregnated with minocycline and rifampin decrease rates of catheter-related bloodstream infection in cancer patients: a prospective randomized clinical trial. J Clin Oncol 2004;22(15):3163–3171.

84. VEENSTRA DL, SAINT S, SAHA S, et al. Efficacy of antiseptic-impregnated central venous catheters in preventing catheter-related bloodstream infection: a meta-analysis. JAMA 1999;281(3):261–267.

85. WONG CH, CHANG HC, PASUPATHY S, et al. Necrotizing fasciitis: clinical presentation, microbiology, and determinants of mortality. J Bone Joint Surg Am 2003;85-A(8):1454–1460.

86. SUDARSKY LA, LASCHINGER JC, COPPA GF, et al. Improved results from a standardized approach in treating patients with necrotizing fasciitis. Ann Surg 1987;206(5):661–665.

87. DARENBERG J, LUCA-HARARI B, JASIR A, et al. Molecular and clinical characteristics of invasive group A streptococcal infection in Sweden. Clin Infect Dis 2007;45(4):450–458.

88. KAUL R, MCGEER A, LOW DE, et al. Population-based surveillance for group A streptococcal necrotizing fasciitis: Clinical features, prognostic indicators, and microbiologic analysis of seventy-seven cases. Ontario Group A Streptococcal Study. Am J Med 1997;103(1):18–24.

89. STEVENS DL, TANNER MH, WINSHIP J, et al. Severe group A streptococcal infections associated with a toxic shock-like syndrome and scarlet fever toxin A. N Engl J Med 1989;321(1):1–7.

90. TANG E, DAVIS J, SILBERMAN H. Bowel obstruction in cancer patients. Arch Surg 1995;130(8):832–836; discussion 6–7.

91. STEWARDSON RH, BOMBECK CT, NYHUS LM. Critical operative management of small bowel obstruction. Ann Surg 1978;187(2):189–193.

92. KREBS HB, HELMKAMP BF. Management of intestinal obstruction in ovarian cancer. Oncology (Williston Park) 1989;3(5):25–31; discussion 2, 5–6.

93. BRYAN DN, RADBOD R, BEREK JS. An analysis of surgical versus chemotherapeutic intervention for the management of intestinal obstruction in advanced ovarian cancer. Int J Gynecol Cancer 2006;16(1):125–134.

94. ANTEQUERA R, BRETANA A, CIRAC A, et al. Disruption of the intestinal barrier and bacterial translocation in an experimental model of intestinal obstruction. Acta Cient Venez 2000;51(1):18–26.

95. BENNION RS, WILSON SE, SEROTA AI, et al. The role of gastrointestinal microflora in the pathogenesis of complications of mesenteric ischemia. Rev Infect Dis 1984;(suppl 1):S132–S138.

96. PROTOPAPAS AG, DIAKOMANOLIS ES, MILINGOS SD, et al. Tubo-ovarian abscesses in postmenopausal women: gynecological malignancy until proven otherwise? Eur J Obstet Gynecol Reprod Biol 2004;114(2):203–209.

97. SRISOMBOON J, PHONGNARISORN C, SUPRASERT P, et al. A prospective randomized study comparing retroperitoneal drainage with no drainage and no peritonization following radical hysterectomy and pelvic lymphadenectomy for invasive cervical cancer. J Obstet Gynaecol Res 2002;28(3): 149–153.

98. JENSEN JK, LUCCI JA 3rd, DISAIA PJ, et al. To drain or not to drain: a retrospective study of closed-suction drainage following radical hysterectomy with pelvic lymphadenectomy. Gynecol Oncol 1993;51(1):46–49.

99. LOPES AD, HALL JR, MONAGHAN JM. Drainage following radical hysterectomy and pelvic lymphadenectomy: dogma or need? Obstet Gynecol 1995;86(6):960–963.

100. MAZUSKI JE, SAWYER RG, NATHENS AB, et al. The Surgical Infection Society guidelines on antimicrobial therapy for intra-abdominal infections: evidence for the recommendations. Surg Infect (Larchmt). 2002;3(3):175–233.

101. HATALA R, DINH T, COOK DJ. Once-daily aminoglycoside dosing in immunocompetent adults: a meta-analysis. Ann Intern Med 1996;124(8):717–725.

102. SOLOMKIN JS, REINHART HH, DELLINGER EP, et al. Results of a randomized trial comparing sequential intravenous/oral treatment with ciprofloxacin plus metronidazole to imipenem/cilastatin for intra-abdominal infections. The Intra-Abdominal Infection Study Group. Ann Surg 1996;223(3):303–315.

103. SOLOMKIN JS, DELLINGER EP, BOHNEN JM, et al. The role of oral antimicrobials for the management of intra-abdominal infections. New Horiz 1998;6(suppl 2):S46–S52.

104. Guideline for prevention of nosocomial pneumonia. Centers for Disease Control and Prevention. Respir Care 1994;39(12):1191–1236.

105. CRAVEN DE, PALLADINO R, MCQUILLEN DP. Healthcare-associated pneumonia in adults: management principles to improve outcomes. Infect Dis Clin North Am 2004;18(4):939–962.

106. WEBER DJ, RUTALA WA, SICKBERT-BENNETT EE, et al. Microbiology of ventilator-associated pneumonia compared with that of hospital-acquired pneumonia. Infect Control Hosp Epidemiol 2007;28(7):825–831.

107. RELLO J, QUINTANA E, AUSINA V, et al. Incidence, etiology, and outcome of nosocomial pneumonia in mechanically ventilated patients. Chest 1991;100(2):439–444.

108. CHAN EY, RUEST A, MEADE MO, et al. Oral decontamination for prevention of pneumonia in mechanically ventilated adults: systematic review and meta-analysis. BMJ 2007;334(7599):889.

109. KOLLEF MH, AFESSA B, ANZUETO A, et al. Silver-coated endotracheal tubes and incidence of ventilator-associated pneumonia: the NASCENT randomized trial. JAMA 2008;300(7):805–813.

110. Guidelines for the management of adults with hospital-acquired, ventilator-associated, and healthcare-associated pneumonia. Am J Respir Crit Care Med 2005;171(4):388–416.

111. WUNDERINK RG, CAMMARATA SK, OLIPHANT TH, et al. Continuation of a randomized, double-blind, multicenter study of linezolid versus vancomycin in the treatment of patients with nosocomial pneumonia. Clin Ther 2003;25(3):980–992.

112. KATCHMAN EA, MILO G, PAUL M, et al. Three-day vs longer duration of antibiotic treatment for cystitis in women: systematic review and meta-analysis. Am J Med 2005;118(11):1196–1207.

113. BARTLETT JG. Narrative review: the new epidemic of *Clostridium difficile*-associated enteric disease. Ann Intern Med 2006;145(10):758–764.

114. LEFFLER DA, LAMONT JT. Treatment of *Clostridium difficile*-associated disease. Gastroenterology 2009;136(6):1899–1912.

115. PAUL M, BENURI-SILBIGER I, SOARES-WEISER K, et al. Beta lactam monotherapy versus beta lactam-aminoglycoside combination therapy for sepsis in immunocompetent patients: systematic review and meta-analysis of randomised trials. BMJ 2004;328(7441):668.

116. DELLINGER RP, LEVY MM, CARLET JM, et al. Surviving Sepsis Campaign: international guidelines for management of severe sepsis and septic shock: 2008. Crit Care Med 2008;36(1):296–327.

117. WISPLINGHOFF H, BISCHOFF T, TALLENT SM, et al. Nosocomial bloodstream infections in US hospitals: analysis of 24,179 cases from a prospective nationwide surveillance study. Clin Infect Dis 2004;39(3):309–317.

118. HORN DL, NEOFYTOS D, ANAISSIE EJ, et al. Epidemiology and outcomes of candidemia in 2019 patients: data from the prospective antifungal therapy alliance registry. Clin Infect Dis 2009;48(12):1695–1703.

119. PUZNIAK L, TEUTSCH S, POWDERLY W, et al. Has the epidemiology of nosocomial candidemia changed? Infect Control Hosp Epidemiol 2004;25(8):628–633.

120. PAPPAS PG, KAUFFMAN CA, ANDES D, et al. Clinical practice guidelines for the management of candidiasis: 2009 update by the Infectious Diseases Society of America. Clin Infect Dis 2009;48(5):503–535.

121. LYNCH W, MALEK M, DAVEY PG, et al. Costing wound infection in a Scottish hospital. Pharmacoeconomics 1992;2(2):163–170.

122. KAISER AB, ROACH AC, MULHERIN JL Jr, et al. The cost effectiveness of antimicrobial prophylaxis in clean vascular surgery. J Infect Dis 1983;147(6):1103.

123. REED SD, LANDERS DV, SWEET RL. Antibiotic treatment of tuboovarian abscess: comparison of broad-spectrum beta-lactam agents versus clindamycin-containing regimens. Am J Obstet Gynecol 1991;164(6 Pt 1):1556–1561; discussion 61–62.

124. DAVEY PG ND. What is the value of preventing postoperative infections? New Horizons 1998;6(2 sup):S64–S69.

125. HALEY RW, CULVER DH, WHITE JW, et al. The efficacy of infection surveillance and control programs in preventing nosocomial infections in US hospitals. Am J Epidemiol 1985;121(2):182–205.

126. HALEY RW, QUADE D, FREEMAN HE, et al. The SENIC Project. Study on the efficacy of nosocomial infection control (SENIC Project). Summary of study design. Am J Epidemiol. 1980;111(5):472–485.

127. CONDON RE, SCHULTE WJ, MALANGONI MA, et al. Effectiveness of a surgical wound surveillance program. Arch Surg 1983;118(3):303–307.

128. BRATZLER DW, HUNT DR. The surgical infection prevention and surgical care improvement projects: national initiatives to improve outcomes for patients having surgery. Clin Infect Dis 2006;43(3):322–330.

Chapter 8

Intraoperative and Perioperative Considerations in Laparoscopy

Steven A. Vasilev and Scott E. Lentz

INTRODUCTION

Ott and Kelling developed laparoscopy at the turn of the century[1,2] and Jacobaeus' soon thereafter reported his extensive experience.[3] However, it wasn't until the 1990s that operative laparoscopy finally came of age, largely due to vastly improved technology. Laparoscopic procedures have become the standard in many cases, and have been widely adopted by nearly all surgical disciplines. Although these procedures have decreased morbidity and cost under some circumstances, they are associated with specific perioperative complications and considerations. This chapter reviews fundamental intra- and perioperative physiology related to pneumoperitoneum, medical management, and morbidity associated with advanced laparoscopic surgical procedures, including prevention and care of complications. Most evidence is Level II-3 to III. Areas achieving Level I support are especially noted.

PHYSIOLOGY OF PNEUMOPERITONEUM

Until the 1990s, laparoscopy was largely used in short diagnostic or finite therapeutic interventions, such as tubal ligation in younger women. When first introduced, these short procedures were well tolerated despite intra-abdominal pressures as high as 40 mm Hg commonly used at the time. Therefore, little attention was paid to understanding the physiology of prolonged pneumoperitoneum. Although the physiologic alterations discussed in this chapter and summarized in Table 8.1 are generally well tolerated, they can cause significant challenges in elderly or obese patients with

Gynecologic Oncology: Evidence-Based Perioperative and Supportive Care, Second Edition.
Edited by Scott E. Lentz, Allison E. Axtell and Steven A. Vasilev.
© 2011 John Wiley & Sons, Inc. Published 2011 by John Wiley & Sons, Inc.

Table 8.1 Physiologic Changes/Complications During Laparoscopy

---

Pneumoperitoneum
- Circulatory changes: venous return and filling pressures/cardiac contractility/afterload
- Respiration/ventilation changes: minute ventilation/airway pressure/lung volumes/gas exchange

Trendelenburg and reverse position
- Circulatory changes: heart rate/stroke volume /systemic vascular resistance
- Respiration/ventilation changes: minute ventilation/work of breathing/lung volumes/gas exchange

Carbon dioxide insufflation
- Circulatory changes: arrhythmias/cardiac contractility/venous gas embolization

Respiration/ventilation changes: dead space ventilation/hypercarbia–acidemia

---

cardiopulmonary compromise. There is an urgent need for further research pertaining to pneumoperitoneum in the critically ill or compromised patient.[4] In these cases, gasless laparoscopy may be a viable alternative to laparotomy for some of the more limited procedures that these patients could tolerate[5–7] **Level I.**

Carbon Dioxide

Normal cellular oxidative metabolism produces CO_2.[8] Blood flow to tissues, local tissue perfusion, ventilatory capacity, and buffering systems all contribute to homeostasis and determine plasma CO_2 concentrations (discussed in Chapter 4). During laparoscopy, exogenous CO_2 contributes an additional volume and exposure length–related stress on intracellular and plasma homeostatic mechanisms, acting as an irritant and potential local cellular immune depressant within the peritoneum. Copious intraoperative irrigation may lessen the former effect[9, 10] **Level I.**

Carbon dioxide is the preferred laparoscopic insufflation gas due to noncombustibility and a high diffusion coefficient, which reduces, but does not eliminate, the potential for gas embolism. However, this diffusibility also leads to rapid systemic absorption, causing an increase in arterial pco_2 and decreased pH, which may be arrhythmogenic.[11, 12, 14] Particular care is theoretically warranted in patients with sickle cell disease who may be in danger of crisis precipitated by alterations in pH and pco_2, although small series have documented laparoscopy to be safe in this setting.[15]

Controlling mechanical ventilation minute volume (V_T = rate $\times$ tidal volume) allows maintenance of a normal pco_2 and pH in most otherwise healthy patients. A twofold increase in minute ventilation results in a pco_2 adjustment of 5 mm Hg. Thus, ventilation is a highly effective method of clearing volatile acid. However, diaphragmatic elevation due to pneumoperitoneum decreases lung volumes. In order to compensate, peak airway pressures must increase in order to deliver constant tidal volumes for CO_2 homeostasis.[16] The consequences of this are discussed below. By and large, homeostatic disturbances lead to clinically significant findings only in patients with abnormal cardiopulmonary function and limited homeostatic reserves.[17]

These reserves may be limited by increased ventilatory dead space as seen in chronic obstructive pulmonary disease, impaired tissue perfusion, or poor cardiac output due to cardiovascular disease.

While it is imperative that all patients be closely monitored with end-tidal CO_2 readings, it is especially critical in patients with chronic lung or cardiac disease in whom radial artery cannulation may be indicated.[17] End tidal CO_2 (Etco$_2$) is the most common intraoperative noninvasive method for assessing adequacy of ventilation and accurately reflects changes in pco$_2$ in normal patients. However, it may differ significantly, and possibly in divergent direction, from Paco$_2$ in the presence of significant ventilation/perfusion (V/Q) mismatch.[18–20] Thus, blood gas monitoring should be considered in patients with known cardiorespiratory disease or those who develop intraoperative hypoxemia or high airway pressures.[17]

Alternate Gases

Argon

Argon is an inert gas with a poor solubility index relative to CO_2. Although not ordinarily used as a substitute gas for creation of a pneumoperitoneum, through use of the argon beam coagulator (ABC), argon gas can contribute significantly to the gas mix achieved intraoperatively. Animal studies suggest lesser effects on most hemodynamic indices and pulmonary gas exchange than CO_2. However, systemic vascular resistance index (SVRI) and stroke volume (SV) depression by 30% has been reported.[21] Additionally, deleterious effects of an accidental embolism may be more severe due to the solubility characteristics of argon.[22] At the very least, argon gas is more likely to be retained in the abdomen and is associated with greater pain at 72 hours due to decreased solubility and absorption[23] **Level I.** Therefore, when using the ABC, the abdomen should be continuously vented and argon flow rate limited to 4–6 LPM. One, or preferably two, high flow CO_2 insufflator(s) will maintain adequate pneumoperitoneum with continuous venting.

Nitrous Oxide

The relatively low blood solubility of nitrous oxide (N_2O) increases the risk for gas embolism, and its potential support of combustion generally restricts intraperitoneal use to diagnostic procedures. Additionally, the considerably lower solubility, compared with nitrogen and methane, results in nitrous oxide diffusing into the intestinal lumen faster than the latter gases diffuse out. With inspired nitrous oxide anesthesia, the intestine may expand, obstructing view or the ability to retract intestine, especially during laparoscopic procedures exceeding 4 hours.[24, 25] If intestinal perforation is sustained intraoperatively, an explosion hazard exists due to nitrogen/methane mix.[26] On balance, there is little to support use of N_2O for insufflation in operative laparoscopy. However, for shorter diagnostic procedures it may cause less pain than CO_2, possibly due to lack of hydrogen ion mediated peritoneal irritation.[27, 28] Inhalational N_2O use should be limited to shorter cases to prevent bowel distention.[25, 29]

Lung Volumes, Compliance, and Ventilation

Changes in lung volumes accompany laparoscopy as a result of increased abdominal pressures displacing the diaphragm cephalad, and steep Trendelenburg position common to pelvic procedures. Total lung compliance and functional residual capacity may be reduced, producing areas of ventilation-perfusion (V/Q) mismatch.[30] Although mechanical ventilation may overcome some of these problems, increased peak airway pressures can become prohibitive, risking barotrauma even in patients with normal lungs. A special challenge occurs in the obese patient in whom high peak airway pressures are necessary just to overcome chest wall resistance and decreased lung volumes.[12, 16]

Another risk of steep Trendelenburg is inadvertent intraoperative right mainstem bronchial intubation with resulting hypoxemia. The proposed mechanism involves a tethered endotracheal tube at the mandible while the diaphragm displaces the lung and carina cephalad.[31, 32] Keeping intra-abdominal pressures in the 10–15 mm Hg range and Trendelenburg position at a minimum will help minimize these problems. Limited Trendelenburg position is potentially prohibitive when performing some advanced laparoscopic procedures, and the anesthetists should pay constant careful attention to the possibility of inadvertent right mainstem intubation.

Postoperative spirometry demonstrates a significant difference between lower abdominal and upper abdominal surgery effect on lung volumes. Minor pelvic surgery produces no significant changes beyond the day of surgery. In contradistinction, forced vital capacity (FVC), forced expiratory volume at one second (FEV-1), and peak expiratory flow rate are significantly reduced beyond the day of surgery following laparoscopic cholecystectomy.[33]

Oxygenation

The effect of pneumoperitoneum on oxygenation is minimal in healthy patients (American Society of Anesthesiologists (ASA) Class 1 patients) who are mechanically ventilated during laparoscopy.[12] The possible causes of hypoxemia are listed in Table 8.2. ASA Class 2 and 3 patients are at higher risk on several parameters as listed.[12]

Intraoperative monitoring via pulse oximetry is usually adequate, correlating well with arterial blood gas measurements. However, if laser, argon beam coagulation, or cautery-induced smoke is allowed to accumulate, carboxyhemoglobin levels can become significantly elevated, producing inaccurate pulse oximetry readings[13] **Level II-2.**

Cardiovascular Changes

Changes in central venous return, and hence cardiac output, depend upon the degree of intra-abdominal pressure and position of the patient.[34, 35] While both may decrease if pressures exceed 20 mm Hg, return and output may increase if pressures are

Table 8.2   Hypoxemia Risk Factors and Etiologies

Preexisting conditions
- Cardiopulmonary dysfunction
- Morbid obesity

Hypoventilation
- Patient position
- Pneumoperitoneum
- Endotracheal tube obstruction
- Inadequate/dead space ventilation

V/Q mismatch
- Atelectasis and reduced FRC
- Endobronchial intubation
- Pneumothorax

Reduced cardiac output
- Pneumomediastinum/pneumopericardium
- Arrhythmias
- Myocardial depression: anesthesia/sepsis/acidosis
- Gas embolism
- Reduced filling pressures/vena cava compression

Technical failure
- Hypoxic gas mixture delivery
- Ventilator dysfunction

kept between 10 and 15 mm Hg due to a shift of circulating blood volume from the abdominal mesentery and vena cava into the chest. Trendelenburg position *may* increase return, while a reverse Trendelenburg position decreases return in euvolemic patients. However, in the hypovolemic patient, Trendelenburg position can decrease filling pressures and increase systemic vascular resistance, resulting in a decreased cardiac output.[36, 37] Additionally, higher mean airway pressures during mechanical ventilation may contribute to decreased cardiac output.

Elderly patients with limited cardiovascular reserves do not readily compensate for the above changes and thus more commonly evidence significant hemodynamic alterations with increased abdominal pressures and steep positions. For this reason, right heart catheterization and close monitoring may be indicated for prolonged procedures in the compromised or elderly patient.

Neuroendocrine Hormonal Response

Primarily elicited by afferent neural input, levels of stress hormones are typically increased during and after laparotomy, and mediate widespread physiologic effects

Table 8.3 Perioperative Neuroendocrine Response to Surgery and Stress Effects

System/Organ		Effect Alteration	Lap	LSC
Pituitary	Increased ACTH	Impaired free water excretion	++	+
	Increased TSH	Hyponatremia	+	+
	Increased growth hormone		+	+
	Increased vasopressin (ADH)		+	+++
Autonomic nervous system	Increased plasma nor-epi	Sodium retention	+	+
		Hypokalemia		
		Glucose intolerance	-	
		Lipolysis		
		Protein catabolism		
Adrenal	Increased catecholamines	Arrhythmogenic	+	++
		Tachycardia	+	+
	Increased cortisol	Tachypnea	+	+
	Increased aldosterone	Widened pulse pressure		
		Glucose intolerance		
		Lipolysis		
		Protein catabolism		
Pancreas	Increased glucagon	Hyperglycemia	+	+
	Dec/Inc insulin	Lipolysis	+	+
		Protein catabolism		
Thyroid	Variable T4 and T3 effect		+	+

in proportion to the degree of insult. Cardiovascular changes in heart rate, blood pressure, and myocardial performance are mediated primarily by the catecholamines. Additionally, accelerated fat and protein metabolism combined with impaired glucose utilization contribute to a catabolic state. Overall these major alterations can be poorly tolerated by compromised patients and can be persistent. After a laparotomy, plasma vasopressin (ADH) can remain elevated for 5–7 days, reducing the ability to excrete free water, whereas during laparoscopy, available data suggests a more rapid ADH normalization despite higher intraoperative levels, ostensibly due to greater peritoneal stretch/pressure receptor activation[38] **Level I.**

A key question surrounds whether or not laparoscopy favorably blunts some of these stress response effects at clinically significant levels. Table 8.3 summarizes the relative alterations found in laparotomy vs. laparoscopy. The physiologic effects tend to be complex, variable, time dependent, and synergistic such that this summary by no means reflects all situations at any given point in time. Although preliminary animal data seems promising, limited clinical data, primarily comparing open vs. laparoscopic cholecystectomy, fails to substantiate a major difference in any stress response parameters, with most differences in response being of short duration[39–43] **Level I.** In addition, there are significant questions regarding the overall impact of immunomodulation/inflammatory response seen with laparoscopy. Even though the beneficial effects are apparent, reflected by reduced pain and fevers, the immunosuppression may alter infection response cascades in a negative fashion.[44]

Renal Perfusion

Pneumoperitoneum reduces urine output by several mechanisms similar to that which occur in other abdominal compartment syndromes such as malignant tense ascites. Firstly, a 15 mm Hg intra-abdominal pressure translates into a 15 mm Hg decrease in blood perfusion and a 60% reduction in renal cortical perfusion.[45] This in turn leads to a 50% reduction in urine output. If only one kidney is compressed, as may occur in a laparoscopic retroperitoneal para-aortic node dissection with unilateral retroperitoneal insufflation, a 25% reduction in urine output may be evident.[45, 46] Additionally antidiuretic hormone (ADH) and aldosterone elevation due to increased intraperitoneal pressures further mediates decreased urine output, which may persist into the immediate postoperative period.[47] Maintaining the intra-abdominal pressures between 10 and 15 mm Hg may improve renal perfusion and lessens the probability of decreased urine output, thereby lessening the hazard of inadvertent iatrogenic fluid overload.[45, 47, 48]

Splanchnic and Hepatic Perfusion

Animal data suggests intraperitoneal pressure increase results in mechanical compression of the splanchnic capillary beds, increasing systemic vascular resistance. To limit this effect and its role in reduced cardiac output, maintaining pressures at 10–15 mm Hg is recommended.[49, 50] Hepatic blood flow is also affected, but to a much lesser extent.[49, 50]

Gastrointestinal Distention

Spinal and epidural blockade above T5 interrupts sympathetic nervous system innervation to the gastrointestinal tract, with the epidural approach achieving a more controlled, slower onset of blockade. The resulting unopposed parasympathetic activity leads to relaxed sphincters and contracted intestines, facilitating positioning and retraction of bowel for upper retroperitoneal dissection.

Inhalational anesthesia with nitrous oxide increases sympathetic tone and possibly directly influences gaseous intestinal dilatation, making it a less desirable agent when optimal intestinal contraction is desired in longer complicated cases.[25, 29, 52]

COMPLICATIONS

In a 1991 survey by the American Association of Gynecologic Laparoscopists (AAGL), a mortality rate of 1.8 per 100,000 procedures was reported.[53] Although possible underreporting limits interpretation of available data, it appears that operative laparoscopy is still associated with low mortality, despite the fact that an increase in more complex surgeries has led to higher complication rates.[54] A large prospective clinical series (25,764 cases) reported an operative laparoscopy complication rate of 17.9 per 1000, as opposed to 2.7 per 1000 for diagnostic laparoscopy and 4.5 per 1000 for sterilization procedures.[55] This correlation of complexity and morbidity was confirmed by a large French study comprising 29,966 operations. The same series reported a statistically significant correlation between surgeon's current experience and rate of complications.[56]

Cardiovascular Collapse and Cardiac Arrest

Acute cardiovascular collapse during or immediately following laparoscopy is a rare but life-threatening complication, occurring at a rate of less than 0.5%. Causes for cardiovascular collapse are numerous, most commonly metabolic abnormalities, gas embolism, pneumothorax, pneumomediastinum, myocardial ischemia, hemorrhage, and cardiac arrhythmia.

Metabolic Abnormalities

Clinically significant metabolic abnormalities leading to significant cardiac dysfunction occur at a rate of less than 5 per 10,000 laparoscopic cases.[53] The most frequently occurring changes of hypercarbia, hypoxemia, and acidemia can cause hypertension and cardiac brady- or tachyarrhythmias in compromised patients.

These metabolic abnormalities can be minimized by limiting peritoneal CO_2 exposure as much as possible (i.e., by expeditiously completing the operative procedure) and keeping intraperitoneal pressures between 10 and 15 mm Hg.[57] Pulse oximetry evaluation should be continuous and adequate ventilation of the patient must be maintained as reflected by end tidal CO_2 or arterial measurements. Volume cycled mechanical ventilation must be adjusted to compensate for the excess CO_2 absorbed via the peritoneal surface and Trendelenburg position limited in order to minimize pressure against the intra-abdominal diaphragmatic surface. If significant changes in oxygenation are noted or cardiac arrhythmias occur, the pneumoperitoneum must be immediately evacuated, Trendelenburg position reversed, and efforts focused on acutely decreasing pCO_2 while increasing pO_2 and pH.

Gas Embolism

This is an extremely rare but potentially fatal complication, occurring in the range of 15 per 100,000 laparoscopies.[58] CO_2 is used preferentially during laparoscopy partly because of its solubility relative to air and N_2O, minimizing the chances of fatal embolization. Since CO_2 is rapidly absorbed, small amounts can be injected into the venous circulation without clinical consequence.[59] Etiology of clinically significant embolism may be multifactorial, including direct vessel insufflation via the Verres needle or through a significant rent in a low pressure venous vessel. However, with high intraperitoneal pressures, gas embolism can theoretically occur following extensive tissue dissection without a major vessel injury.

If a large gas embolus lodges in a significant venous channel or right atrium or ventricle, an obstruction to blood flow can result. Clinical sequelae may include cardiovascular collapse, acute pulmonary hypertension and right heart failure, or cerebrovascular accident. Embolism risk can be minimized by limiting intraperitoneal pressures, especially when alternative gases such as argon are used (ABC), closure of open vessels, and the conservative use of Trendelenburg position.

Intraoperative findings may include sudden onset hypoxemia, hypotension, asystole or ventricular fibrillation associated with basilar rales, and a pathognomonic but often fleeting "mill wheel" murmur. One of the earliest signs may be a transient and sudden increase in $Etco_2$.[60] Postoperatively, there may be associated signs such as seizures, motor/sensory deficits, or bronchoconstriction and noncardiogenic pulmonary edema.[61,62]

Intraoperative therapy includes immediate termination of the procedure with decompression of the pneumoperitoneum, adequate ventilation with 100% O_2, and aggressive cardiovascular support. Cardiac arrest may occur if large volume air/gas is acutely infused ($>$100 cc). The patient should be placed in Trendelenburg position and a left lateral decubitus position to minimize embolized gas entering the pulmonary circulation, although this traditional maneuver has limited effect on outcome. An attempt may be made to extract larger gas volumes via a right heart catheter. Once the patient is stable, hyperbaric oxygen unit therapy has been suggested for treatment of clinically significant emboli. Proposed therapy is 30 minutes of hyperbaric oxygen at 3 atmospheres.[63] Finally, the use of corticosteroids in order to reduce lung injury remains controversial.[64]

Pneumothorax

Clinically recognized pneumothorax occurs at a rate of less than 0.08%. CO_2 can either enter the pleural space across congenital defects in the diaphragm, at the time of alveolar bleb rupture, via the transdiaphragmatic lymphatics, or pneumoretroperitoneal dissection of gas through the aortic and esophageal diaphragmatic hiatus.[65] Some of these mechanisms are potentiated by excessive intraperitoneal pressures and the length of time that these pressures are maintained. Alveolar blebs in particular are more likely to rupture at the higher peak inspiratory pressures and volumes that are necessary to counteract the effects of increased intra-abdominal pressure on the diaphragm.

N_2O has a blood:gas partition coefficient (0.47) that is 34 times that of nitrogen (0.014). This differential solubility allows N_2O to enter an air filled cavity from blood 34 times faster than nitrogen can leave the cavity. Therefore, in the presence of an intraoperatively diagnosed closed pneumothorax, N_2O is contraindicated because it can cause the volume of the pneumothorax to double rapidly. In fact, in the presence of subcutaneous emphysema appearing during laparoscopy associated with decreasing pulmonary compliance should raise the possibility of unrecognized pneumothorax and N_2O use discontinued.

Therapy of pneumothorax includes early recognition initially based on a significant decrease or loss of breath sounds on the affected side. Subcutaneous emphysema of the chest wall and neck should alert the anesthesiologist to the possibility of associated pneumothorax and a chest film ordered. If pneumothorax is the result of congenital defects in the diaphragm, decompression of the pneumoperitoneum and hyperexpansion of the lungs may suffice. Should the postoperative chest radiograph(s) demonstrate a persistent, large (greater than 30%), or expanding pneumothorax, a small bore tube thoracostomy with the tip placed at the apex is mandated. The chest tube should be connected to water seal, not to wall suction, as the latter may prolong bronchopleural leak. Simple pneumothorax usually requires the chest tube to be in place for 24 hours following resolution of an air leak. If there is clinical perioperative evidence of a tension pneumothorax, emergency chest tube thoracostomy is indicated and should not be delayed by a radiographic workup.

Pneumomediastinum

Occurring at a rate of less than 0.01%, this complication is most likely due to dissection of CO_2 along the aortic or esophageal hiatus or passage of CO_2 through congenital defects in the mediastinum.[65] It may also follow inappropriate placement of the Verres needle into the falciform ligament or dorsal retroperitoneum with the CO_2 dissecting cephalad.

Prevention focuses on appropriate Verres needle placement, minimization of retroperitoneal dissection, and maintenance of low intraperitoneal pressures and degree of Trendelenburg position. Diagnosis is usually based on loss, or distancing, of heart sounds with associated hypotension. Pneumomediastinal decompression may be performed using a transcutaneous large bore spinal needle, and the pneumoperitoneum evacuated.

Pneumopericardium

There are only a few reported cases of pneumopericardium that is usually associated with pneumomediastinum.[66, 67] Causation, prevention, and management are the same as for pneumomediastinum. Surgical decompression is imperative if a significant decrease in cardiac output occurs.

Myocardial Ischemia

Patients predisposed to myocardial ischemia are ill-equipped to tolerate increased afterload. In ASA III or IV patients, an intraperitoneal pressure of 15 mm Hg leads to elevation in mean arterial pressure, peripheral vascular resistance, and central venous pressure, with a significant reduction in cardiac output. Additionally, mixed venous oxygen saturation (sVO_2) drops in half of these patients. The fall in cardiac output is likely due to inadequate ventricular reserve in these patients, emphasizing the need for very close monitoring in the presence of cardiac compromise history.[68]

Hemorrhage

Hemorrhage may occur as a result of either arterial or venous injury. While arterial injury is readily evidenced by brisk bleeding, pressure equalization between the venous and intraperitoneal compartments may hide or minimize a significant venous injury. Intraoperative surgical management of vascular injury is discussed below. To avoid postoperative cardiovascular collapse from an unrecognized major venous injury, hemostasis should be ascertained at the end of the procedure, as the intraperitoneal pressures are slowly decreased during pneumoperitoneum evacuation. If ongoing hemorrhage is suspected in the postoperative period, laparotomy may be indicated to arrest the bleeding and evacuate any hematomas that may compromise organ function by direct pressure via a compartment syndrome in an enclosed retroperitoneal space.

Cardiac Arrhythmia

Acidemia, hypoxemia, and hypercarbia contribute to various arrhythmias, which commonly occur intraoperatively.[14] Most are ventricular in origin. Tachyarrhythmias can be precipitated by surgical stress response increases in catecholamine levels, and may be further potentiated by Halothane anesthesia.[14, 69] In addition to the metabolic etiologies, vagal stimulation via peritoneal distention may result in bradyarrhythmias or asystole.[69–73] Increasing intraperitoneal pressure quickly can lead to a sudden decrease in venous return and bradycardia via the Bainbridge reflex. Additionally, Mobitz type I block has been reported with propofol, fentanyl, and vecuronium, possibly preventable with an anticholinergic premedication.[74] In general, bradycardia may occur more frequently when anticholinergic and nonvagolytic neuromuscular blockers are not used.

Other Causes of Cardiovascular Collapse

Excessive compression of the vena cava and vasovagal response have both been proposed as causes of cardiovascular collapse.[72] The former can be minimized by keeping intraperitoneal pressures between 10 and 15 mm Hg and limiting the degree of Trendelenburg position. The latter may be prevented by atropine sulfate premedication. Additionally, the possibility of an adverse drug reaction should be entertained in the absence of any of the above.

Subcutaneous Emphysema

Subcutaneous emphysema occurs in up to 50% of patients undergoing laparoscopic lymph node dissections.[75] In the absence of a retroperitoneal dissection, rates are much lower, approximating 2%. The majority of the subcutaneous emphysema cases are due to improper Verres needle placement and insufflation superficial to the rectus fascia or due to prolonged cases with improperly sealed sleeves. Genital emphysema is probably due to CO_2 dissection through the inguinal ring and a patent Canal of Nuck. Emphysema of the neck and face may be associated with anterior thoracoabdominal wall emphysema and may accompany a pneumomediastinum/pneumothorax.

Management of subcutaneous emphysema includes adequate analgesics to control the pain associated with cutaneous distension. Pressure dressings can be applied in an attempt to facilitate CO_2 absorption. In rare cases of extensive emphysema, a patient's ability to clear the absorbed CO_2 may be overcome, requiring extended mechanical ventilation.

Extraperitoneal Insufflation

Extraperitoneal insufflation follows either improper placement of a Verres needle or the insertion of an operative sleeve superficial to the peritoneum. Prevention includes open laparoscopy or direct placement of the first sleeve into the peritoneal cavity prior to establishing a pneumoperitoneum. These techniques are described below under the section discussing gastrointestinal injuries. Extraperitoneal insufflation at the time of Verres or sleeve placement can be minimized by using a continuous motion through an adequate skin incision. The sleeve should be placed at a 45–60 degree angle to the peritoneum, which is usually tightly adherent to the anterior abdominal wall fascia. Unfortunately, preperitoneal insufflation is usually not recognized until the laparoscope is placed and it is noted that the peritoneum has been displaced by the insufflating gas. At this time the gas tubing should be disconnected from the sleeve, the stop cock left open, the laparoscope removed, and the diaphragm of the sleeve held open. The anesthesiologist should be asked to Valsalva the patient in an attempt to increase the intraperitoneal pressure and expel the extraperitoneal CO_2 through the open trocar. One should not attempt to blindly penetrate the distended peritoneum with a trocar in the sleeve as such a maneuver has a significant risk of injuring an intraperitoneal structure. After the extraperitoneal insufflation has been maximally decompressed, the Verres needle should be reintroduced via an alternative site such as the left upper quadrant. A low intercostal, subcostal, or cul-de-sac approach can also be used.

Anesthetic Complications

Anesthesia complications, independent of laparoscopy are rare, occurring at most in 1.4 of every 1,000 cases.[76] The majority of anesthesia related deaths are due to hypoventilation. This can be caused by failed or esophageal intubation, but may also follow inadvertent endobronchial intubation. The former can be prevented in the difficult case by using newer techniques of intubation such as flexible endoscopic direction. Appropriate monitoring via pulse oximetry allows early recognition of hypoxemia. Initial endobronchial intubation can be avoided by using appropriate length (i.e., shorter) endotracheal tubes. However, the possibility of intraoperative migration of the ET tube with steep Trendelenburg position must be kept in mind.[31,32]

Laryngeal mask airway (LMA) may be a safe alternative for shorter cases. During a 2-year survey study period, a subset of 2222 patients underwent an abdominal procedure under general anesthesia via LMA of whom 44% were subjected to positive pressure ventilation. On 579 occasions, the procedures lasted for 2 hours. There were 18 critical incidents involving the airway, none of which involved intensive care management.[77]

Higher intra-abdominal pressures and steep Trendelenburg position increase the risk of regurgitation of gastric contents and subsequent aspiration pneumonitis. This risk can be minimized by assuring that the patient has been NPO for 8 hours prior to surgery and by the use of cuffed endotracheal tubes, the pressure of which requires monitoring in longer cases. Although intraoperative oral-gastric tube suction may not decrease an already low aspiration pneumonitis rate (<0.1%), it may improve surgical field exposure and may decrease risk of instrument injury.[78]

Hypothermia

Decrease in core body temperature may be minimized in laparoscopic procedures due to less extensive visceral exposure to ambient temperatures and irrigation fluid. However, at least one randomized controlled trial demonstrates that core body temperature can still be lowered during laparoscopy and is a function of the length of anesthesia rather than the irrigant temperature. Use of ambient temperature, or lower, irrigant poses the greatest risk and can lower the core temperature by 1.7 (+/− 0.2) degrees[79] **Level I**. Depending on starting temperatures, this decrease may approach clinical significance and may intraoperatively affect platelet function among other variables. Use of preconditioned CO_2 (heated and hydrated) reduces hypothermia, shortens recovery room stay and reduces postoperative pain due to the favorable effect of humidification on reducing peritoneal irritation[80] **Level I.**

Deep Venous Thrombosis

Pneumoperitoneum causes pelvic venous compression, which leads to venous stasis in the lower extremities. For those gynecologic procedures that require Trendelenburg position, this venous stasis is lessened, thus potentially lowering the incidence of venous thromboembolism (VTE). The incidence of VTE during laparoscopy appears to be low, but may be underreported. In a large population based registry study of laparoscopic cholecystectomy (105,850 cases), the rates of symptomatic VTE measured within 3 months of the procedure were lower for laparoscopy than for open procedures (0.2% vs. 0.5%).[210] Two randomized trials have compared routine postoperative Doppler sonography, each comparing graduated compression stockings (GCS) versus GCS with low molecular weight heparin (LMWH). Among the 927 patients between the two trials, only 3 patients were found to have VTE and there were no significant differences between the two groups. The very low rate of VTE in laparoscopic

Table 8.4   Risk Factors for VTE

Surgery
Trauma (major trauma or lower-extremity injury)
Immobility, lower extremity paresis
Cancer (active or occult)
Cancer therapy (hormonal, chemotherapy, angiogenesis inhibitors, radiotherapy)
Venous compression (tumor, hematoma, arterial abnormality)
Previous VTE
Increasing age
Pregnancy and the postpartum period
Estrogen-containing oral contraceptives or hormone replacement therapy
Selective estrogen receptor modulators
Erythropoesis-stimulating agents
Acute medical illness
Inflammatory bowel disease
Nephrotic syndrome
Myeloproliferative disorders
Paroxysmal nocturnal hemoglobinuria
Obesity
Central venous catheterization
Inherited or acquired thrombophilia

patients makes it unlikely that a prospective, randomized trial of sufficient power will resolve the dispute concerning the most optimal form of thromboprophylaxis[211,212] **Level I**. Current recommendations by the American College of Chest Physicians for patients undergoing entirely laparoscopic procedures in the absence of risk factors for VTE other than surgery are limited to frequent and early ambulation. In those patients with other risk factors for VTE (Table 8.4), prophylaxis is recommended using one or more of graduated compression stockings, intermittent pneumatic compression stockings, unfractionated, or low molecular weight heparin[213] **Level II-2** (Chapter 6).

Operative Injuries

Specific organ system injuries are discussed individually later, but special attention to trocar placement is warranted. Trocar insertion represents the point of a laparoscopic procedure where injuries are most likely to occur, particularly because there is a blind element to this step in any procedure. Trocar placement caused a certain amount of trepidation when laparoscopy was initially introduced as it ran contrary to usual surgical principles of adequate exposure to limit risk of injury.

Trocar insertion during laparoscopy has evolved along with the procedures and technology associated with this surgical discipline. Originally performed in a stepwise manner, using the Veress needle followed by trocar insertion into a distended abdomen, many practitioners today prefer a direct entry technique using the desired trocar. Laparoscopic trocars have also evolved to include bladed or bladeless tips, with or without direct visibility by inserting the laparoscope into the trocar itself. Preferred entry methods for laparoscopy continue to be driven in large part by the training of a particular surgeon, with little regard for evidence in choosing or maintaining a specific method. That said, there are a number of prospective, randomized trials in laparoscopy which can guide decision making. It is worth noting that the most significant limitation to the published trials in laparoscopy is the tendency to specifically exclude patients who have undergone prior surgery as well as a variable limitation on the acceptable maximum body mass index (BMI). Also notable is the finding that there are unusually high complication rates among obese patients who undergo laparoscopy, an important issue as the BMI of the general population increases.

No single entry technique has proven to be superior to any other in terms of preventing surgical complications. Whether choosing a stepwise entry (insufflation followed by trocar insertion) or a direct entry technique (using any available trocar system), there was no difference in solid organ injury **Level I**. What has been demonstrated to be different are the rates of failed peritoneal entry and the rate of extraperitoneal insufflation. Compared to a needle entry method, the direct trocar insertion reduces entry failures (OR 0.22, 0.08–0.56) and reduces extraperitoneal insufflation (OR 0.06, 0.02–0.23) **Level I**. There are no trials that compare direct vision entry to the needle approach, nor are there direct head-head comparisons of direct vision versus blind trocar insertions.[197–202]

Radially expanding trocar systems are designed to allow insertion of a laparoscopic trocar through an expanding sleeve that is initially inserted using a 2-mm needle. The presumed advantages of this method are reduced insertion injury since the incising instrument is much smaller than the trocar itself and a smaller fascial defect relative to the size of the trocar, with a presumed lower rate of incisional herniation. Prospective randomized trials comparing this system to standard trocar insertion show no differences in injury rates but a reduction in trocar site bleeding events (OR 0.06, 95% CI: 0.01, 0.46)[203] **Level I**.

Vascular Injury

Vascular injuries are among the most frequent laparoscopic surgery–related complications. Unfortunately, not all injuries are recognized intraoperatively.

Minor Vascular Injury

The superficial and deep inferior epigastric vessels are frequently injured with an incidence approaching 2.5%.[85, 86] If not appreciated intraoperatively, a hemoperitoneum may develop or an anterior abdominal wall extraperitoneal hematoma may form. This may be heralded by a progressively decreasing hemoglobin/hematocrit, changes in vital signs, a palpable lateral abdominal wall mass, or simply by pain and bleeding from the incision(s).

Management of a significant or expanding hematoma may include wound exploration, hematoma evacuation, and vessel ligation under general anesthesia. In the unstable patient, selective and rapid angiographic embolization may be an option. However, inferior to superior deep epigastric artery arborization and anastomosis is variable, such that embolization may not provide enough decrease in pulse pressure to ensure hemostasis.[87]

Major Vascular Injury

Major vessel injury occurs with a frequency of approximately 0.1%, most often at the aortic bifurcation,[88,89] usually during Verres needle or umbilical sleeve placement. Mortality rates of 10%–40% have been reported with major vessel injury as well as significant morbidity and high transfusion rates.[89–91] Injury risk can be minimized by angling the Verres needle or trocar toward the pelvis below the bifurcation of the aorta, which is usually deep to the umbilicus in the nonobese patient.

Injury to major pelvic vessels after the laparoscope has been placed is less common due to the ability to visualize accessory trocar placement. Such injuries can still occur unless the surgeon is very familiar with the retroperitoneal course of the common and external iliac vessels. Injury can also occur due to the misuse or inappropriate settings of a given instrument such as the ABC whose power may be set too high and/or directed at one area for too long. Large veins can appear flat and blend into the adjacent anatomy in the presence of pneumoperitoneum and Trendelenburg position. Thus injury may go undetected until the venturi effect of CO_2 suction into the vessel is appreciated.

Arterial injury due to placement of a Verres needle will be appreciated immediately, while an injury to a major venous vessel may initially go unrecognized. If bleeding is encountered through the Verres needle, the stopcock should be closed and the needle left in place. This functionally tamponades the bleeding and leads the surgeon to the site of injury. When the site of injury is identified via laparotomy, a 4-0 vascular Prolene® figure of eight suture can be placed around the defect and secured while the Verres needle is removed.

Major vascular injuries due to initial trocar insertion are usually appreciated after the laparoscope is introduced. In the presence of brisk intraperitoneal bleeding or expanding hematoma, it may be prudent to perform a midline laparotomy. A posterior parietal peritoneal incision should be made lateral to the injury and a complete and thorough retroperitoneal exploration performed, including evaluation for concomitant ureteral injury.

Many vascular injuries can be repaired using endoscopic techniques. Laparoscopic vascular clips can be used as the first-line effort to obtain hemostasis. Additionally, as a preemptive measure, placement of a surgical mini-laparotomy sponge in the peritoneal cavity for immediate availability may help stem hemorrhage should an injury occur. If laparoscopic repair is not immediately successful, immediate exploratory laparotomy is important. If the patient is in steep Trendelenburg position, blood can drain into the upper abdomen where it can pool and remain hidden from view, despite extensive hemorrhage. If an extensive major vessel laceration has occurred, especially of an artery, intraoperative vascular surgery consultation should be obtained. Perioperative sequelae can be minimized by employing vascular techniques that ensure that the vessel lumen is not narrowed and that a thrombus has not formed.

Mesenteric Vascular Injury

The incidence of mesenteric vessel injury is unknown. These injuries may occur at the time of Verres needle or initial trocar placement and often are not appreciated until the laparoscope is placed. Because of extensive anastomoses, most small vessel injuries can be repaired via laparoscopy using clips and electrocautery. If multiple ligations are required, care must be taken to ensure that blood supply to the nearby bowel segment has not been interrupted to the point of causing ischemia. In addition to visual inspection, options include laparoscopic Doppler examination at the mesenteric border, intravenous fluorescein facilitated bowel segment evaluation, or a planned second look laparoscopy within 24–48 hours.[92] A technique that may facilitate this involves leaving a flexible drain in one or two sleeve sites, through which a 5-mm scope and accessory sleeve can be re-placed in 24–48 hours with minimal risk of trocar reinsertion bowel injury.[93] Injuries to the superior mesenteric artery require revascularization. However, if the injury involves the inferior mesenteric artery, ligation may be safely accomplished in the majority of patients due to excellent collateral blood supply.[92]

Gastrointestinal Tract Injury and Dysfunction

The incidence of intestinal injury during laparoscopy is apparently 0.002%–0.2%.[94–96] The majority of these injuries occur at the time of Verres needle or primary trocar placement. Prior abdominal surgery increases the risk and at one time was considered a strong relative contraindication to laparoscopy.

Open laparoscopy techniques carry the advantage of peritoneal cavity entry under direct visualization. Unfortunately, this does not completely avoid bowel injury, maintenance of pneumoperitoneum may be difficult, and risk of subcutaneous emphysema increased if the Hasson sleeve sutures do not provide a tight seal. In spite of the perceived safety of open laparoscopy, there appear to be no improvements in the rates of vascular or visceral injury when comparing the open approach to either needle entry[207, 208] or direct trocar entry[198] **Level I.**

An alternative is to place the initial trocar at another site, away from the umbilicus or prior abdominal incisions. Some have described a low intercostal or subcostal Verres needle placement, while others have demonstrated the efficacy of direct 2- or 5-mm trocar introduction in the left upper quadrant, just lateral to the midclavicular line[100–102] **Level II-1.** If the left upper quadrant entry is chosen, a nasogastric tube should be preemptively placed to ensure stomach decompression. Once the anatomy and adhesion location is appreciated, additional ports can be safely introduced under direct visualization.

Electrosurgical bowel injury usually occurs with the use of unipolar current and direct injury or conduction to the intestine via insulation failure or capacitive coupling.[103] Prevention rests with reusable instrument insulation testing on a regularly scheduled basis. Disposable instruments should never be reused. The uninsulated end of the electrosurgical instrument should be fully visible and in contact with whatever structure is to be cut or coagulated prior to activating current. Unfortunately, due to insulation failure, this does not always prevent electrothermal bowel injury.

Newer instrumentation has led to the development of the bipolar vessel sealing instruments, a purported advance from the original bipolar instrumentation. These instruments employ an amperage sensor, which is able to modulate the current applied for tissue desiccation. By controlling the delivered current, the potential for capacitive coupling is reduced thereby limiting unintended thermal injury. A third agent of tissue dissection is the ultrasonic coagulating shears (Harmonic Scaplel^{TM}). This device performs by ultrasonically vibrating one of the two blades on a dissecting instrument creating sufficient heat during hydrolysis to cause protein denaturation and coagulation. The advantage of this device is the absence of any electrical current and elimination of possible cautery injury. However, compared to the electrosurgical instruments this unit retains heat at the device tip for a markedly longer period and can result in delayed thermal injury if used for immediate tissue division and blunt dissection.

No direct comparison of the three technologies exists in the gynecologic oncology literature. Complication rates are comparable according to the various manufacturers of the devices. In one of the few comparative reviews of the three methods, a randomized allotment of 61 consecutive colorectal laparoscopic procedures were collected. Monopolar endoscopic scissors were found to be inferior to the other modalities with respect to dissection time and need for endoscopic clip usage for bleeding control. A cost analysis of the same instruments found that both the bipolar vessel sealing and the ultrasonic coagulating shears were more cost-effective than monopolar instrumentation, assuming that a center performed more than 200 laparoscopic procedures per year[207] **Level I.**

The ABC is a useful innovation based on gas-mediated electrosurgical dissection, especially in the retroperitoneum.[104] While embolism remains a theoretical risk, the superficial electrical current penetration (0.3–0.9 mm) at lower wattage settings is a predictable and welcome characteristic. In comparison, unipolar cautery is associated with a variable depth of tissue injury, up to 3 mm even with brief exposure. Additionally, the ABC insulation is constructed in such a fashion that capacitive coupling risk is minimized.

Verres needle simple puncture injury to the small intestine, signaled by the return of enteric contents, is often managed by removing the needle and attempting placement elsewhere. There are no large series to either support or refute this practice and management rests with the surgeon's experience and specific findings in this situation. Large bowel injury management in a similar fashion has been reported.[106] This assumes extensive manipulation has not occurred, which may have caused a significant laceration.[107] Simple Verres puncture is analogous to the same event occurring at time of paracentesis with a large bore needle, which is probably a relatively common occurrence. There is no evidence to support use of prophylactic antibiotics should a simple puncture occur, in the absence of prolonged small bowel obstruction with feculent bowel contents or extensive injury to the large bowel.

Bowel injuries larger than a Verres needle puncture must be surgically closed. This can be performed via laparoscopy if the surgeon has mastered the necessary skills or via a minilaparotomy and exteriorization of the injured bowel segment. If an electrosurgical injury appears to be greater than 0.5 cm, it may be prudent to resect the injured area with closure or anastomosis, depending on the size and configuration of the defect. Although it is difficult to gauge the extent of electrosurgical damage, small injuries can be over sewn. If a large enterotomy occurs involving over half of the antimesenteric circumference, or the bowel has been devascularized, a bowel resection is indicated via laparoscopy or laparotomy. Management of all of the above injuries will vary with surgeon's experience, specific findings and other contributing factors, such as a history of radiation therapy.

A thorough mechanical and antibiotic bowel prep has previously been advocated for any patient scheduled for operative laparoscopy who has had prior abdominal surgery. The role of bowel prep has evolved in response to several Level I publications detailing its role in contemporary surgery (Chapter 6). Most researchers agree that there is little role for antibiotic bowel preparation in modern surgical practice (open or laparoscopic). This is elegantly detailed in a comprehensive analysis by the Cochrane Collaborative Group.[209] The role of mechanical prep is less well accepted. In the literature specific to gynecologic surgery, there is only one publication to address the issue of mechanical bowel prep. As shown in Figure 8.1, all patient perceived

Use of bowel preparation in laparoscopy

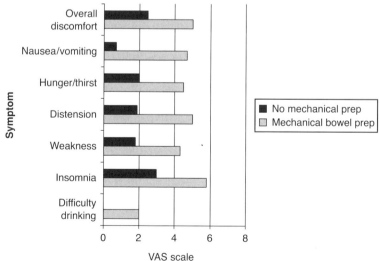

Modified from Muzii et al. *Fert Ster,* 2006:85(3) 689-693

Figure 8.1 Use of bowel preparation in laparoscopy. Modified from Reference 204.

symptoms are reduced in patients who do not receive preoperative bowel prep, but these differences were not statistically significant. Additionally, there were no differences in surgical factors (quality of exposure, difficulty of procedure, need for conversion to laparotomy) between the two groups[204] **Level I.**

Even in cases of minimal but grossly evident fecal intraoperative contamination, colostomy is indicated only if there has been significant delay in diagnosis, extensive tissue necrosis, gross intraperitoneal infection, or cardiovascular compromise and hypoxemia.[105, 108] Copious isotonic peritoneal lavage should be considered when large bowel injury occurs and antibiotic therapy initiated with broad spectrum agents covering mixed GI flora.[109, 110]

A potentially lethal complication is the unrecognized intraoperative bowel injury. This may be due to unappreciated electrosurgical damage or direct operative injury. About 40%–70% of bowel injuries are not recognized during surgery and often become evident only after the patient has been discharged.[95, 96] Delay in diagnosis is usually due to a low index of suspicion. These situations are associated with severe sepsis and death.[95, 96] Thus, initial therapy includes aggressive fluid resuscitation and antibiotic therapy. After effective resuscitation, or if the patient fails to rapidly stabilize, exploratory laparotomy with appropriate drainage, repair and/or diversion should be performed. In a stable patient with a localized process, percutaneous CT guided drainage is becoming the preferred alternative.[111] After the inflammation subsides, the patient can be returned to the operating room and definitive surgery performed.

Postoperative ileus is common in patients who have undergone either long or extensive operative laparoscopic procedures. This is due to the additive effect of prolonged anesthetic agent exposure, direct bowel manipulation, and possibly chemical peritonitis secondary to carbon dioxide byproducts.[4, 9] The potential for ileus can be minimized by reducing operative time. However, the physiologic events affecting bowel function during laparoscopy are probably more complex than suggested by the above discussion. Animal data indicates that gut inflammatory response, as reflected by blunted serum and gut mucosal IL-6 (interleukin), is minimized by laparoscopy.[97]

Should the symptoms of ileus fail to abate within 72 hours of bowel rest, a bowel obstruction must be suspected and appropriate radiographic studies performed.

Urinary Tract Injury

Bladder Injury

Injury to the bladder during gynecologic operative laparoscopy occurs at a rate of 0.02%–8.3%.[98] Laparoscopically assisted hysterectomy is associated with the highest reported rates. Injuries are more common when the bladder is incompletely drained, when the anatomy is distorted due to prior surgery, when inflammatory states or carcinomatosis are present, or when advanced operative procedures are performed. For example, with radical laparoscopic hysterectomy, injury rates approaching 30% have been reported.[112] Subsequent reports have not substantiated such high rates of injury, reflecting the dynamics of a lengthy learning curve, volume/outcomes relationship and ever improving technology in such surgery.[104]

During laparoscopic-assisted vaginal hysterectomy, at time of vesicouterine reflection development, low posterior bladder wall injuries can occur. These can be minimized by sharp dissection and attention to detail in dissecting distorted tissue planes that may be the result of prior surgery or inflammatory states.

Risk of Verres needle/trocar injury is reduced by adequate and/or continuous bladder drainage. For longer procedures, a Foley catheter should be introduced and removed at the completion of the procedure. As has been described above, appropriate caution and attention to technique must be taken at time of placement of the Verres needle and umbilical sleeve. Injury at the time of suprapubic sleeve placement is almost always preventable since placement can be done under direct visualization.

Fortunately, intraoperatively recognized bladder dome injuries are easily managed. Small defects, especially if extraperitoneal, such as those caused by a Verres needle or 5-mm trocar can be managed solely with 5–10 days of bladder drainage. Larger injury repair may be effected laparoscopically, closing the bladder in one or two layers, depending upon the extent of injury and the presence or absence of electrosurgical injury.[113] The bladder should be placed at rest and drained completely for approximately 5 days, a point at which 50% of tensile strength has been regained.[114] In patients who have received pelvic radiation, drainage should empirically be continued for a longer period of time. No data exists as to the appropriate length of time for similar healing. However, since the bladder is one of the most rapidly healing tissues in the body, in the absence of such cofactors, prolonged drainage is unwarranted.

Bladder injury unrecognized intraoperatively can cause major postoperative morbidity and usually leads to reoperation.[99] Approximately half of patients with bladder injuries will not present for many days postoperatively, particularly if an extensive thermal injury was sustained, which can cause a delayed rather than immediate cystotomy.[98] Peritonitis, fevers, ileus, or urine leaking from an incision site may be observed. Intravenous urography and/or cystography will usually confirm an injury and its location. Management may be affected by inflammation and scarring, which may mandate repair via laparotomy.

Urachal and Vesicourachal Diverticulum

This extremely rare injury is caused by placing a trocar through the diverticular cyst or patent urachus.[115] The injury can be avoided by recognizing the urachus, assuming it is patent, and angling the suprapubic trocar lateral in such a way as to avoid the structure. Preoperative assessment has been described using ultrasound and contract studies.[116] If recognized at the time of surgery, the urachus should be ligated above and below the site of injury. The patient may present postoperatively with urine draining from her umbilical incision. The diagnosis can be confirmed with a cystogram. Treatment may simply entail continuous bladder drainage, confirming closure of the urachus with repeat cystogram prior to catheter removal.

Ureteral Injuries

Although these injuries are rare (less than 0.01%–0.2%), there may be a relative increase in occurrence as more complex surgical procedures are performed.[117] The ureter may be injured at the pelvic brim during division of the ovarian vessels, in the broad ligament during lysis of adhesions or ablation of endometriosis/carcinomatosis, or at the level of the uterine artery as could occur during cardinal ligament division. All of these injuries are preventable by identifying the ureter throughout its retroperitoneal course and dissecting it free from the site of surgery.

Injuries that are intraoperatively identified are associated with the best outcomes. However, these injuries are usually recognized postoperatively, at which time the morbidity increases.[118] Ureteral injury should be suspected postoperatively in the presence of fever, leukocytosis, peritonitis, flank pain/tenderness, a urinoma/pelvic mass, or hematuria.[111] Radiographic studies such as intravenous pyelogram or CT urogram should be employed to determine the presence and site of injury. Traditional therapy involves exploratory surgery with primary repair, reimplantation, and interposition techniques. However, selected patients may be successfully managed with ureteroscopy, stent placement, and percutaneous drainage.[119, 120] These include patients with minor leaks or partial obstruction due to a kink caused by adjacent absorbable suture placement.

Nerve Injuries

Nerve injuries are extremely rare in gynecologic laparoscopy.[121] Most commonly these are due to stretching or pressure injury (neurapraxia). Rarely, transection of a nerve (neurotmesis) can occur.

Brachial palsy can be due to prolonged steep Trendelenburg position combined with a shoulder brace or hyperabducted arms strapped to an armboard. These injuries can be avoided by placing the arms at the patient's side, avoiding the use of shoulder braces, and ensuring that no undue pressure from equipment occurs. The latter is ensured with extensive padding and avoiding encroachment on the arm. Physical therapy usually results in good outcomes.

Femoral, sciatic, and peroneal nerve injuries can be due to positioning, hip hyperflexion, and direct pressure. Allen stirrups, which support the knee and foot, in combination with proper positioning limit such injury. If nerve injury is suspected postoperatively due to foot drop or gait disturbance, neurologic evaluation should be sought. Electromyographic and nerve conduction studies can help isolate the defect. Physical therapy should then be initiated with expected full recovery. However, complete recovery may require several months.

Neurotmesis, or transection of the nerve, is potentially more serious. However, the nerves at risk for this are the genitofemoral nerve branches bordering the psoas muscle lateral to the external iliac artery and the obturator nerve, which lies deep in the obturator space. Only radical laparoscopic surgery, including pelvic lymph node dissection, exposes these nerves to such injury. The genitofemoral nerve is composed of several branches, all or some of which may be transected during pelvic lymph node dissection, and are not repaired. Although bothersome medial thigh dysesthesia may result, this can resolve over time. If the obturator nerve is transected, it should be repaired using microsurgical technique. Despite dual motor innervation, adductor function of the leg may be impaired. With epineurial repair and/or postoperative physiotherapy, recovery is complete in most instances.[121]

Incisional Complications

Wound Infections

Laparoscopy is usually a clean or clean contaminated operation, depending upon the intraperitoneal procedure performed. Therefore, infections are uncommon (0.1%–3.0%)[53, 82, 83, 122–126] **Level I**. The umbilicus, where the Verres needle and principal sleeve is placed, should be thoroughly cleansed.[82, 124] In an effort to minimize the risk of infection, all attempts should be made to maintain aseptic technique. Antibiotics are not used routinely in laparoscopy and are only recommended for prophylaxis as dictated by open procedure indications as discussed in Chapter 7.

Incision site infection management includes opening the skin for debridement and administration of appropriate antibiotics in the event of cellulitis. Initial coverage, which should be modified when culture results become available, should include activity against staph species and hemolytic streptococci. Finally, although necrotizing fasciitis is rare after laparoscopy, it may occur and can be difficult to assess due to the small incision size.[81, 127] The index of suspicion must remain low in order to initiate timely, aggressive, and effective therapy.

Wound Dehiscence and Incisional Hernias

The incidence of these complications is probably underreported but is likely between 0.2% and 0.02%.[128, 129] The cause of these wound complications is inadequate closure of a fascial incision. As would be expected, the larger the size of the sleeve used, the more likely that a hernia will occur. The vast majority (86.3%) occur at 10 mm or greater size sleeve sites and three quarters of hernias develop at the umbilical site.[129] Prevention centers on adequate primary closure of the incisional defect. Adequacy of closure is key since primary fascial closure is completed in 18%–60% of patients who subsequently develop a hernia at 10- to 12-mm sleeve sites.[128, 129] Adequate closure can be ensured by placing the sutures under direct laparoscopic visualization at all 10 mm or greater sleeve sites. Also, placing the trocars via a "Z" technique (i.e., offsetting the skin incision and peritoneal entry site) may help reduce the risk of a hernia tract by relying on natural staggered tissue apposition.

In the event of a hernia or wound dehiscence, management should include conventional techniques of surgical evaluation for bowel involvement and hernia repair. Up to 17% of laparoscopic hernias present with evidence of small or large intestine morbidity.[129]

Postoperative Pain

Although definitive studies have not been performed, the degree of pain that follows a laparoscopic procedure is often not fully appreciated and is multifactorial. Incisional pain may be decreased, but operative site pain will depend on the degree of tissue inflammation, ischemia, and trauma related to the procedure performed. Also, pain may be due to carbon dioxide mediated peritoneal irritation.[28] For this reason, consideration may be given to small dose hypobaric lidocaine-fentanyl spinal anesthesia for short-duration laparoscopic procedures[130, 131] **Level I.** Postural spinal headache may occur, but patient acceptance was shown to be high.

Various series report that 35%–65% of patients experience shoulder pain.[132, 135] Thorough attempts at deflating the pneumoperitoneum at procedure conclusion must be undertaken, including Valsalva provided by the anesthesiologist. Evaluated in a small case study, with the patient in the Trendelenburg position, five positive pressure ventilations for 5 second each were employed at the conclusion of the procedure. This resulted in a reduction of shoulder discomfort in 57% of cases[205] **Level III.** No prospective randomized trials of this method have been conducted. Patients undergoing gasless laparoscopy have similar pain location and duration patterns.[137] Shoulder tip pain may be reduced by bupivacaine irrigation (10 cc of 0.5% bupivacaine in 500 cc normal saline) to both hemidiaphragms at the end of surgery.[138–140]

Even though CO_2 is rapidly absorbed, free gas can be demonstrated under the diaphragm for up to 3 days postoperatively, although it is uncommon after 24 hours.[132–134] A large volume of gas under the diaphragm on an upright chest film more than 24 hours postoperatively should signal the strong possibility of viscus perforation.[134] Placing a drain into the peritoneal cavity for 6 hours after surgery, especially in a suprahepatic location, may significantly decrease pain severity.[145]

Postoperative analgesic requirements may be reduced but are not eliminated due to the lack of a laparotomy incision. Incisional pain may be reduced if subcutaneous lidocaine or bupivacaine are used at closure.[139, 140] However, conflicting Level I data exists, supporting preemptive injection as being more effective[141] **Level I.** In general, pain is easier to manage if analgesic therapy is instituted preemptively in the postoperative period. A common regimen may include parenteral nonsteroidal anti-inflammatory drugs, with a narcotic analgesic added as needed. Postoperative administration of Tramadol (3 mg/kg) was shown in one study to reduce postanesthetic shivering and additional analgesic use, thus reducing postanesthesia recovery time[142] **Level I.** However, administration of narcotics or injectable nonsteroidal agents earlier, at or immediately preceding induction, fails to impact postoperative consumption of analgesics[143, 144] **Level I.** A more detailed discussion regarding pain management is offered in Chapter 15.

The patient should be reassured that the pain will subside and that it does not represent an unexpected complication or a failure of the procedure, but rather a physiologic sequelae to surgical trauma and pneumoperitoneum.

Postoperative Nausea

Postoperative nausea, dizziness, and emesis are common after laparoscopy, are related to the total amount of CO_2 used, often prolong length of stay, and increase costs.[52, 146] These effects can persist for 24 hours or more in up to 25% of patients.[147] Risk factors for nausea and emesis include female gender, anxiety, obesity, history of motion sickness, and performance of the procedure during menses.[148–151] Emesis rates seem to be lowest during the third and fourth weeks of the menstrual cycle.[150]

The emetogenic potential of anesthetic and analgesic agents is variable. Nitrous oxide may contribute to nausea in longer procedures via intestinal dilatation and autonomic effects,[29,334,152,153] but this has not been confirmed by all investigators. Recently, nitrous oxide has been directly implicated in nausea during laparoscopic surgery. The role of nitrous oxide in laparoscopic surgery has become the stuff of legend. A great deal of myth and fable have led to very fixed opinions on the appropriateness (or lack thereof) when considering N_2O in patients undergoing laparoscopic surgery. A full discourse on N_2O is outside the scope of this book, but some background is necessary when considering the role of N_2O in laparoscopy. While nitrous oxide is both analgesic and sedating, it also contributes to postoperative nausea and vomiting (PONV). Several mechanisms are proposed to explain the effect on PONV: (1) increased middle ear pressure, (2) activation of the chemoreceptor trigger zone through the dopamine system, (3) direct interaction with opioid receptors, and (4) bowel distension. The effects of distension on PONV are disputed, but one meta-analysis showed that each additional hour of anesthesia using N_2O doubled the risk of bowel distension when compared to air/oxygen (OR 2.09, 95% CI: 1.27–3.59).

In a randomized trial of women undergoing laparoscopy for gynecologic surgery, three different concentrations of N_2O were tested to determine the effect on PONV. Using the widely validated VAS scale for nausea, varying the concentration of nitrous oxide during laparoscopic surgery did not lessen the degree of postoperative nausea. In fact, in the absence of prophylactic antiemetic therapy, the absence of all nitrous oxide led to the lowest incidence of nausea **Level I**.[196] This result is limited only in the fact that the researchers specifically excluded patients with BMI > 33, which limits its broad applicability. Otherwise, the commonly used inhalational agents seem to be equivalent in emetogenic potential.[52] Epidural anesthesia may be superior to general anesthesia in reducing emesis, but this advantage may be decreased depending upon which systemic agents are used.[154] For example, Propofol as a systemic agent is associated with very low rates of emesis.[155] In contrast, narcotic analgesics contribute significantly to nausea and emesis.[156] Several investigators have reported reduction in postoperative nausea and emesis following parenteral ketorolac administered prior to conclusion of laparoscopy.[157,158] Other intraoperatively administered agents that may prophylactically reduce postoperative nausea by acting centrally are intravenous metoclopramide (0.1–0.2 mg/kg), IV droperidol (10–20 mcg/kg), and dexamethasone (0.17 mg/kg),[52,159–161] although metoclopramide has higher potential for side effects. Ondansetron, a serotonin antagonist, may be superior to the above agents with minimal side effects[162–164] **Level I**. However, this benefit may be marginal with a higher marginal cost and in the face of evidence that demonstrates that the serotonin metabolite 5-HT3 (5-hydroxytryptamine) is not elevated after gynecologic laparoscopy.[165,166] Finally, transdermal scopolamine applied preoperatively has been reported to be effective.[167] Since the genesis of nausea and emesis is multifactorial, each patient has to be preoperatively evaluated individually and in some cases multiple agent regimens applied.

LAPAROSCOPIC PROCEDURES DURING PREGNANCY

Surgical procedures performed during pregnancy by any route carry a risk of fetal loss and theoretical first trimester anesthetic exposure related teratogenesis. Although pelvic and abdominal laparoscopic surgery has become widely accepted in nonpregnant patients, pregnancy has been considered a relative contraindication mostly due to potential for direct trauma, theoretical physiologic concerns, and animal data.

Potential physiologic advantages of an operative laparoscopic approach during pregnancy include decreased postoperative narcotic requirements, diminished postoperative maternal hypoventilation, and more rapid bowel function return.[168] However, risks include direct trauma from blind trocar and Verres needle introduction, physiologic sequelae due to increased intra-abdominal pressure and/or direct CO_2 effects.[168-177] The latter two effects may lead to reduced uterine blood flow and/or uterine contractions. This in turn may lead to premature labor and/or fetal acidosis. Clinically, significant reduction in uterine blood as a direct result of pneumoperitoneum is unproven. In an animal model, fetal acidosis, decreased uterine blood flow and increased intrauterine pressure has been reported during CO_2 pneumoperitoneum. Maternal respiratory alkalosis compensated to a degree and most importantly, all ewes delivered normal lambs at term gestation.[178,179] Gasless laparoscopy utilizing mechanical methods for abdominal wall elevation has been proposed as an alternative to pneumoperitoneum to eliminate such concerns.[180,181] However, further research into the physiologic effects of laparoscopy during pregnancy is required in order to determine optimal management.

Multiple case reports, small series, and reviews suggest that operative laparoscopy during pregnancy is safe during first, second, and possibly third trimesters, depending upon the procedure(s) performed.[169,182-192] However, limited clinical data, reports of complications, and animal model–based physiologic concerns mandate caution until prospective trials prove safety.[179,193]

In the absence of strong Level I data, the Society of American Gastrointestinal Endoscopic Surgeons (SAGES) offers the following consensus guidelines for operative laparoscopy during pregnancy[194]:

1. When possible, operative intervention should be deferred until the second trimester, when fetal risk is lowest.

2. Since pneumoperitoneum enhances lower extremity venous stasis, already present in the gravid patient, and since pregnancy induces a hypercoagulable state, pneumatic compression devices must be utilized.

3. Fetal and uterine status, as well as maternal end tidal CO_2 and arterial blood gases, should be monitored.

4. The uterus should be protected with a lead shield if intraoperative cholangiography is a possibility. Fluoroscopy should be utilized selectively.

5. Given the enlarged gravid uterus, abdominal access should be attained using an open technique.

6. Dependent positioning should be utilized to shift the uterus off of the inferior vena cava.

7. Pneumoperitoneum pressures should be minimized to 8–12 mm Hg and not allowed to exceed 15 mmHg.

8. Obstetrical consultation should be obtained preoperatively.

SIMULATION TRAINING

As laparoscopic procedures have become more complex, training methods have evolved to accommodate these changes. The old "apprentice-style" model is no longer sufficient to provide education in procedures that are often lengthy, intricate, and highly specialized. This also coincides with a broad shift in the overall model of medical education that allows for less "on-the-job" training than has been previously tolerated.

As a result, many teaching programs employ various styles of simulation training. This style of education has been the standard in the aviation industry and is well known as the method of choice in areas where direct experience is very rare or exceedingly dangerous, such as NASA. It is this same level of preparatory exactitude that teaching programs have sought in order to maximize exposure of the trainees while simultaneously limiting complication rates and improving patient safety. Simulation training is commonly performed in one of three ways. Live animal or cadaver training provides the closest simulation to "real life," but is very expensive, requires large amounts of support personnel, and is highly regulated to ensure safety of the subjects and appropriate handling of the living material. Video trainers (VT) are most likely the commonest form of simulators, consisting of a box trainer attached to a video system that requires the trainee to perform a series of actions that mimic surgical steps. These systems are inexpensive and highly reproducible, but they lack applicability to specific surgical procedures. Virtual reality (VR) trainers have evolved in concert with improvements in graphic technology and computer processing speeds. VR trainers fill the gap between live surgical training on animal models or cadavers and the abstract nature of VT systems. These trainers are generally more expensive than VT systems, but can graphically mimic real life procedures and simulations without patient risk or harm. Incorporation of VT into surgical residency training has resulted in improved global performance during laparoscopic procedures compared to traditional surgical training.[206](**Level I**)

The role of VR trainers has been controversial, as the costs of the systems must be weighed against the costs of increased operative times and complication rates. No publications in gynecologic oncology have looked specifically at the impact of VR trainers in laparoscopic surgery, but a comprehensive review prepared according to the Cochrane methodology was performed in the general surgery literature. This review is strengthened by the fact that results were stratified based on the prior laparoscopic experience of the subjects. As the authors noted, the available literature on the subject is heavily biased, but a handful of conclusions could be drawn. In trainees with no prior laparoscopic experience, there was no difference in job speed or time to complete a task when comparing VR versus VT. Additionally, as was previously seen with VT, the VR training improved the time to perform a job when compared to no simulation training at all. VR did offer improved operative scores (performed by observers evaluating tissue trauma and ability to keep instruments in sight) among trainees with limited prior laparoscopic experience when compared with the VT group. Simulation training has proven to provide important presurgical training in the residency experience, but the method of choice remains a source of dispute. **Level I**

REFERENCES

1. OTT D. Die Direkte Beleuchtung der Bauchhole, der Haranblase, des Dichdarams und des Uterus zu Diagnostichen Zwecken. Rev Med Tcheque 1909;2:27–30.
2. KELLING G. Zur Coelioskopie. Arch Klin Chir 1923;126:226–229.
3. JACOBAEUS HC. Uber die Moglichkeit die Zystoskopie bei Untersuchung seroser Hohlungen anzumenden. Munch Med Wochenschr 1911;58:2017–2019.
4. HOLTHAUSEN UH, NAGELSCHMIDT M, TROIDL H. CO_2 pneumoperitoneum: what we know and what we need to know. World J Surg 1999;23:794–800.
5. KOIVUSALO AM, KELLOKUMPU I, LINDGREN L. Postoperative drowsiness and emetic sequelae correlate to total amount of carbon dioxide used during laparoscopic cholecystectomy. Surg Endosc 1997;11:42–44.
6. CASATI A, VALENTINI G, FERRARI S, et al. Cardioerspiratory changes during gynaecological laparoscopy by abdominal wall elevation: comparison with carbon dioxide pneumoperitoneum. Br J Anaesth 1997;78:51–54.
7. Goldberg Jm, MAURER WG. A randomized comparison of gasless laparoscopy and CO_2 pneumoperitoneum. Obstet Gynecol 1997;90:416–420.
8. NUNN JF. Nunn's Applied Respiratory Physiology. 4th ed. Stoneham, MA: Butterworth; 1993: 219–246.
9. TASKIN O, BUHUR A, BIRINCIOGLU M, et al. The effects of duration of CO_2 insufflation and irrigation on peritoneal microcirculation assessed by free radical scavengers and total glutathione levels during operative laparoscopy. J Am Assoc Gynecol Laparosc 1998;5:129–133.
10. KOPERNIK G, AVINOACH E, GROSSMAN Y, et al. The effect of a high partial pressure of carbon dioxide environment on metabolism and immune functions of human peritoneal cells: relevance to carbon dioxide pneumoperitoneum. Am J Obstet Gynecol 1998;179:1503–1510.
11. ALEXANDER GD, BROWN EM. Physiologic alterations during pelvic laparoscopy. Am J Obstet Gynecol 1969;105:1078–1081.
12. PURI GD, SINGH H. Ventilatory effects of laparoscopy under general anesthesia. Br J Anaesth 1992;68:211–213.
13. OTT DE. Carboxyhemoglobinemia due to peritoneal smoke absorption from laser tissue combustion at laparoscopy. J Clin Laser Med Surg 1998;16:309–315.
14. SCOTT DB, JULIAN DG. Observations on cardiac arrhythmias during laparascopy. Br J Med 1972;1:411–413.
15. WARE RE, KINNEY TR, CASEY JR, et al. Laparoscopic cholecystectomy in young patients with sickle hemoglobinopathies. J Pediatr 1992;120:58–61.
16. SEED TF, SHAKESPEARE TF, MULDOON MJ. Carbon dioxide homeostasis during anaesthesia for laparoscopy. Anaesthesia 1970;25:223–231.
17. WITTGEN CM, ANDRUS CH, FITZGERALD SD, et al. Analysis of the hemodynamic and ventilatory effects of laparoscopic cholecystectomy. Arch Surg 1991;126:997–1001.
18. KALHAN SB, REANEY JA, COLLINS RL. Pneumomediastinum and subcutaneous emphysema during laparoscopy. Cleve Clin J Med 1990;57:639–642.

19. LIU SY, LEIGHTON T, DAVIS I, et al. Prospective analysis of cardiopulmonary responses to laparoscopic cholecystectomy. J Laparoendosc Surg 1991;1:241–244.

20. McKINSTRY LJ, PERVERSEFF RA, YIP RW. Arterial and end-tidal carbon dioxide in patients undergoing laparoscopic cholecytectomy. Anethesiology 1992;77(A):108–112.

21. EISEHNAUER DM, SAUNDERS CJ, HO HS, et al. Hemodynamic effects of argon pneumoperitoneum. Surg Endosc 1994;8:315–321.

22. MANN C, BOCCARA G, GREVY V, et al. Argon pneumoperitoneum is more dangerous than CO2 pneumoperitoneum during venous gas embolism. Anesth Analg 1997;85(6):1367–1371.

23. REICHERT JA. Argon as distending medium in laparoscopy compared with carbon dioxide and nitrous oxide. J Am Assoc Gynecol Laparosc 1996;3:S41.

24. EGER EI, SAIDMAN LJ. Hazards of nitrous oxide anesthesia in bowel obstruction and pneumothorax. Anesthesiology 1965;26:61–66.

25. TAYLOR E, FEINSTEIN R, WHITE RF, et al. Anesthesia for laparoscopic cholecystectomy. Is nitrous oxide contraindicated? Anesthesiology 1992;76:541–543.

26. NEUMAN GG, SIDEBOTHAM G, NEGOIANU E, et al. Laparoscopy explosion hazards with nitrous oxide. Anesthesiology 1993;78:857–859.

27. SHARP JR, PIERSON WP, BRADY CE. Comparison of CO_2 and N_2O induced discomfort during peritoneoscopy under local anesthesia. Gatroenterology 1982;82:453–456.

28. MINOLI G, TERRUZZI V, SPIZZI GC, et al. The influence of carbon dioxide and nitrous oxide on pain during laparoscopy: a double blind, controlled trial. Gastrointest Endosc 1982;28:173–175.

29. LONIE DS, HARPER NJN. Nitrous oxide anesthesia and vomiting: the effect of nitrous oxide anaesthesia on the incidence of vomiting following gynaecological laparoscopy. Anaesthesia 1986;41:703–708.

30. VERSICHELEN L, SERREYN R, ROLLY G, et al. Physiopathologic changes during anesthesia administration during gynecological laparoscopy. J Reprod Med 1984;29:697–700.

31. WILCOX S, VANDAM LD. Alas, poor Trendelenburg and his position! A critique of its uses and effectiveness. Anesth Analg 1988;67:574–577.

32. BURTON A, STEINBROOK RA. Precipitous decrease in oxygen saturation during laparoscopic surgery. Anesth Analg 1993;76:1177.

33. JORIS J, KABA A, LAMY M. Postoperative spirometry with laparoscopy for lower abdominal or upper abdominal surgical procedures. Br J Anaesth 1997;79:422–426.

34. MOTEW M, IVANKOVICH AD, BIENIARZ J, et al. Cardiovascular effects and acid base and blood gas changes during laparoscopy. Am J Obstet Gynecol 1973;115:1002–1012.

35. HODGSON C, McCLELLAND RMA, NEWTON JR. Some effects of peritoneal insufflation of carbon dioxide at laparoscopy. Anaesthesia 1970;25:382–390.

36. SIBBALD WJ, PATERSON NAM, HOLLIDAY RL, et al. The Trendelenburg position: hemodynamic effects in hypotensive and normotensive patients. Crit Care Med 1979;7:218–224.

37. SING R, O'HARA D, SAWYER MAJ, et al. Trendelenburg position and oxygen transport in hypovolemic adults. Ann Emerg Med 1994;23:564–568.

38. ORTEGA AE, PETERS JH, INCARBONE R, et al. A randomized prospective comparison of the metabolic and stress hormonal responses of laparoscopic and open cholecystectomy. J Amer Coll Surg 1996;183:249–256.

39. AKTAN A, BUYUKGEBIZ O, YEGEN C, et al. How minimally invasive is laparoscopic cholecystectomy? Surg Laparosc Endosc 1994;4:18–21.

40. MEALY K, GALLAGHER H, BARRY M, et al. Physiological and metabolic response to open and laparoscopic cholecystectomy. Br J Surg 1992;79:1061–1064.

41. McMAHON AJ, O'DWYER PJ, CRUISHANK AM, et al. Comparison of metabolic responses to laparoscopic and minilaparotomy cholecystectomy. Br J Surg 1993;80:1255–1258.

42. KEHLET H. Surgical stress response: does endoscopic surgery confer an advantage? World J Surg 1999;23:801–807.

43. BOUVY ND, MARQUET RL, TSENG LN, et al. Laparoscopic vs. conventional bowel resection in the rat. Earlier restoration of serum insulin-like growth factor 1 levels. Surg Endosc 1998;12:412–415.

44. HACKAM DJ, ROTSTEIN OD. Host response to laparoscopic surgery: mechanisms and clinical correlates. Can J Surg 1998;41:103–111.

45. CHIU AW, CHANG LS, BIRKETT DH, et al. The impact of pneumoperitoneum, pneumoretroperi-
toneum and gasless laparoscopy on the systemic and renal hemodynamics. J Amer Coll Surg
1995;181:397–406.

46. VASILEV SA, MCGONIGLE KF. Extraperitoneal laparoscopic paraaortic lymph node dissection. Gynecol Oncol 1996;61:315–320.

47. MANSOUR MA, STIEGMANN GV, YAMAMOTO M, et al. Neuroendocrine stress response after minimally invasive surgery. Surg Endosc 1992;6:294–297.

48. PUNNONEN R, VIINAMAKI O. Vasopressin release during laparoscopy: Role of increased intra-
abdominal pressure. Lancet 1982;16:175–176.

49. ISHIZAKI Y, BANDAI Y, SHIMOMURA K, et al. Changes in splanchnic blood flow and cardiovascular
effects following peritoneal insufflation of carbon dioxide. Surg Endosc 1993;7:420–423.

50. WINDBERGER UB, AUER R, KEPLINGER F, et al. The role of intra-abdominal pressure on splanchnic
and pulmonary hemodynamic and metabolic changes during carbon dioxide pneumoperitoneum.
Gastrointest Endosc 1999;49:84–91.

51. JUNGHANS T, BOHM B, GRUNDEL K, et al. Does pneumoperitoneum with different gases,
body positions, and intraperitoneal pressures influence renal and hepatic blood flow? Surgery
1997;121:206–211.

52. WATCHA MF, WHITE PF. Postoperative nausea and vomiting. Anesthesiology 1992;77:162–184.

53. HULKA JF, PETERSON HB, PHILLIPS JM, et al. American Association of Gynecologic Laproscopist'
1991 membership survey on operative laparoscopy. J Reprod Med 1993;38:569–571.

54. HULKA JF, PETERSON HB, PHILLIPS JM, et al. American Association of Gynecologic Laproscopist'
1993 membership survey. J Am Assoc Gynecol Laparosc 1995;2:133–136.

55. JANSEN FW, KAPITEYN K, TRIMBOS-KEMPER T, et al. Complications of laparoscopy: a prospective
multicentre observational study. Br J Obstet Gynaecol 1997;104:595–600.

56. CHAPRON C, QUERLEU D, BRUHAT MA, et al. Surgical complications of diagnostic and operative
gynaecological laparoscopy: a series of 29,966 cases. Hum Reprod 1998;13:867–872.

57. TOUB DB, SEDLACEK TV, CAMPION MJ. Acidemia associated with the use of high-flow insufflators
during laparoscopy. Am J Obstet Gynecol 1994;170:959–960.

58. OSTMAN PL, PAUTLE-FISHER FH, FAURE EA, et al. Circulatory collapse during laparoscopy. J Clin
Anesth 1990;2:129–132.

59. GAFF TD, ARBGAST NR, PHILLIPS OC, et al. Gas embolism: a comparative study of air and carbon
dioxide as embolic agents in the systemic vascular system. Am J Obstet Gynecol 1959;78:259–265.

60. SHULMAN D, ARONSON HB. Capnography in the early diagnosis of carbon dioxide embolism. Can
Anaesth Soc J 1984;31:455–459.

61. ALBERTINE KH. Lung injury and neutrophil density during air embolization in sheep after leukocyte
depletion with Nitorgen mustard. Am Rev Respir Dis 1988;138:1444–1447.

62. SLOAN TB, KIMOVEC MA. Detection of venous air embolism by airway pressure monitoring. Anesthesiology 1986;64:645–648.

63. WINTER PH, ALVIS HJ, GAG M. Hyperbaric treatment of cerebral air embolism during cardiopulmonary bypass. JAMA 1971;21(5):1786–1788.

64. BERNARD GR, ARTIGAS A, BRIGHAM KL, et al. The American-European Consensus Conference on
ARDS: definitions, mechanisms, relevant outcomes and clinical trial coordination. Am Rev Respir
Crit Care Med 1994;149:818–824.

65. SHAH P, RMAKANTAN R. Pneumoperitoneum and pneumomediastinum: Unusual complications of
laparoscopy. J Post Grad Med 1990;36:31–32.

66. PASCUAL JB, BARANDA MM, TARRERO MT, et al. Subcutaneous emphysema, pseudomediastinum,
bilateral pneumothorax and pneumopericardium after laparoscopy. Endoscopy 1990;22:59–61.

67. KNOS GB, SUNG, YF, TOLEDO A. Pneumopericardium associated with laparoscopy. J Clin Anesth
1991;3:56–59.

68. SAFRAN D, SGAMBATI S, ORLANDO R 3rd. Laparoscopic surgery in high risk cardiac patients. Surg
Gynecol Obstet 1993;176:548–554.

69. HARRIS MNE, PLANTEVIN OM, CROWTHER A. Cardiac arrhythmias during anaesthesia for laparoscopy. Br J Anaesth 1984;56:1213–1216.

70. MYLES PS. Bradyarrhythmias and laparoscopy: a prospective study of heart rate changes during laparoscopy. Aust N Z J Obstet Gynaecol 1991;31:171–173.

71. CARMICHAEL DE. Laparoscopy—Cardiac considerations. Fertil Steril 1971;22:69–70.

72. DOYLE DJ, MARK PWS. Laparoscopy and vagal arrest. Anaesthesia 1989;44:448.

73. SHIFREN JL, ADLESTEIN L, FINKLER NJ. Asystolic Cardiac Arrest: a rare complication of laparoscopy. Obstet Gynecol 1992;79:840–841.

74. GANANSIA MF, FRANCOIS TP, ORMEZZANO X, et al. Atrioventricular Mobitz I block during propofol anesthesia for laparoscopic tubal ligation. Anesth Analg 1989;69:524–525.

75. NORD HJ. Complications of Laparoscopy. Endoscopy 1992:24;693–700.

76. HULKA JF, SOCERSTROM RM, CORSON SL, et al. Complications Committee of the American Association of Gynecologic Laparoscopist: First Annual Report. J Reprod Med 1975;10:301–306.

77. VERGHESE C, BRIMACOMBE JR. Survey of laryngeal mask airway usage in 11,910 patients: safety and efficacy for conventional and nonconventional usage. Anesth Analg 1996;82:129–133.

78. SCOTT DB. Regurgitation during laparoscopy. Br J Anaesth 1980;52:559–561.

79. MOORE SS, GREEN CR, WANG FL. The role of irrigation in the development of hypothermia during laparoscopic surgery. Am J Obstet Gynecol 1997;176(3):598–602.

80. OTT DE, REICH H, LOVE B, et al. Reduction of laparoscopic induced hypothermia, postoperative pain and recovery room length of stay by pre-conditioning gas with the Insuflow device: a prospective randomized controlled multi-center trial. J Soc Laparoendsc Surg 1998;2:321–329.

81. DEZIEL DJ, MILLIKAN KW, ECONOMOU SG, et al. Complications of laparoscopic cholecystectomy: Results of a national survey of 4,292 hospitals and analysis of 77,604 cases. Am J Surg 1993;165:9–14.

82. LARSON GM, VITALE GC, CASEY J, et al. Multipractice analysis of laparoscopic cholecystectomy in 1,983 patients. Am J Surg 1992;163:221–226.

83. The Southern Surgeons Club. A prospective analysis of 1518 laparoscopic cholecystectomies. N Engl J Med 1991;324:1073–1078.

84. SCHWENK W, BOHM B, JUNGHANS T, et al. Intermittent sequential compression of the lower limbs prevents venous stasis in laparoscopic and conventional colorectal surgery. Dis Colon Rectum 1997;40(9):1056–1062.

85. PRING DW. Inferior epigastric hemorrhage, an avoidable complication of laparoscopic clip sterilization. Br J Obstet Gynaecol 1983;90:480–482.

86. HULKA JF, LEVY BS, PARKER WH, et al. Laparoscopic assisted vaginal hysterectomy: American Association of Gynecologic Laparsocopists' 1995 membership survey. J Am Assoc Gynecolo Laparosc 1997;4:167–171.

87. GOTTLIEB ME, CHANDRASEKHAR B, TERZ JJ, et al. Clinical applications of the extended deep inferior epigastric flap. Plastic Recon Surg 1986;78:788–792.

88. BAADSGAARD SE, BILE S, EGEBLAD K. Major vascular injury during gynecologic laparoscopy. Acta Obstet Gynecol Scand 1989;68:283–285.

89. SAVILLE LE, WOODS MS. Laparoscopy and major retroperitoneal vascular injuries (MVRI). Surg Endosc 1995;9:1096–1100.

90. CHAPRON CM, PIERRE F, LACROIX S, et al. Major vascular injuries during gynecologic laparoscopy. J Am Coll Surg 1997;185:461–465.

91. LAM A, ROSEN DMB. Laparoscopic bowel and vascular complications: should the Verres needle and cannula be replaced? J Am Assoc Gynecol Laparosc 1996;3:S24.

92. SHACKFORD SR, SISE MJ. Renal and mesenteric vascular trauma. In: BONGARD FS, WILSON SE, PERRY MO, editors. Vascular Injuries in Surgical Practice. Norwalk, CT: Appleton and Lange, 1991: 179–181.

93. NASSAR AH, HTWE T, HEFNY H, et al. The abdominal drain: a convenient port for second look laparoscopy. Surg Endosc 1996;10:1114–1115.

94. ALVAREZ RD. Gastrointestinal complications in gynecologic surgery: a review for the general gynecologist. Obstet Gynecol 1988;72:533–540.

95. BISHOFF JT, ALLAF ME, KIRKELS W, et al. Laparoscopic bowel injury: incidence and clincal presentation. J Urol 1999;161:887–890.

96. SCHRENK P, WOISETSCHLAGER R, RIEGER R, et al. Mechanism, management, and prevention of laparoscopic bowel injuries. Gastrointest Endosc 1996;43:572–574.

97. TUNG PH, WANG Q, OGLE CK, et al. Minimal increase in gut-mucosal interleukin-6 during laparoscopy. Surg Endosc 1998;12:409–411.

98. OSTRZENSKI A, OSTRZENSKA KM. Bladder injury during laparoscopic surgery. Obstet Gynecol Surv 1998;53:175–180.

99. SAIDA MH, SADLER RK, VANCAILLIE TG, et al. Diagnosis and management of serious urinary complications after major operative laparoscopy. Obstet Gynecol 1996;87:272–276.

100. CHILDERS JM, BRZECHFFA PR, SURWIT EA. Laparoscopy using the left upper quadrant as the primary trocar site. Gynecol Oncol 1993;50:221–225.

101. LEE PI, CHI YS, CHANG YK, et al. Minilaparoscopy to reduce complications from cannula insertion in patients with previous pelvic or abdominal surgery. J Am Assoc Gynecol Laparosc 1999;6:91–95.

102. BRUHAT MA, GOLDCHMIT R. Minilaparoscopy in gynecology. Eur J Obstet Gynecol Reprod Biol 1998;76:207–210.

103. GROSSKINSKY CM, RYDER RM, PENDERGRASS HM, et al. Laparoscopic capacitance: a mystery measured. Am J Obstet Gynecol 1993;169:1632–1635.

104. SPIRTOS NM, SCHLAERTH JB, KIMBALL RE, et al. Laparoscopic radical hysterectomy with aortic and pelvic lymphadenectomy. Am J Obstet Gynecol 1996;174:1763–1768.

105. FLINT LM, VITALE GC, RICHARDSON JD, et al. The injured colon: relationships of management to complications. Ann Surg 1981;619–623.

106. BERRY MA, RANGRAJ M. Conservative treatment of recognized laparoscopic colonic injury. J Soc Laparoendosc Surg 1998;2:195–196.

107. BIRNS MT. Inadvertent instrumental perforation of the colon during laparoscopy: non surgical repair. Gastrointest Endosc 1989;35:54–55.

108. RIDGEWAY CA, FRAME SB, RICE JC, et al. Primary repair vs. colostomy for treatment of penetrating colon injuries. Dis Colon Rectum 1989;32:1046–1049.

109. HESELTINE PNR, BERNE TV, YELLIN AE. The efficacy of cefoxitin vs. clindamycin/gentamycin in surgically treated stab wounds of the bowel. J Trauma 1986;26:241–244.

110. ROWLANDS BJ, ERICSSON CH, FISCHER RP. Penetrating abdominal trauma: the use of operative findings to determine length of antibiotic therapy. J Trauma 1987;27:250–255.

111. GAZELLE GS, MUELLER PR. Abdominal abscess: imaging and intervention. Radiol Clin North Am32:5 913–932 1994.

112. SEDLACEK TV. Laparoscopic radical hysterectomy: the next evolutionary step in the treatment of invasive cervical cancer. J Gynecol Tech 1995;1:223–230.

113. REICH H, McGLYNN F. Laparoscopic repair of bladder injury. Obstet Gynecol 1990;76:909.

114. DEGNER DA, WALSHAW R. Healing responses of the lower urinary tract. Vet Clin North Am Small Anim Pract 1996;26(2):197–206.

115. McLUCAS B, MARCH C. Urachal sinus perforation during laparoscopy: a case report. J Reprod Med. 1990;75:573–574.

116. OSTRZENSKI A, OSBORNE NG, OSTRZENSKA K, et al. Peroperative contrast ultrasonographic diagnosis of patent urachal sinus. Int Urogynecol J Pelvic Floor Dysfunct 1998;9:52–54.

117. WOODLAND MB. Ureteral injury during laparoscopy-assisted vaginal hysterectomy with the endoscopic linear stapler. Am J Obstet Gynecol 1992;167:756–757.

118. GRAINGER DA, SODERSTROM RM, SCHIFF SF, et al. Ureteral injuries at laparoscopy: insights into diagnosis, management, and prevention. Obstet Gynecol 1990;75:839–843.

119. KOONINGS PP, HUFFMAN JL, SCHLAERTH JB. Uerteroscopy: a new asset in the management of postoperative ureterovaginal fistulas. Obstet Gynecol 1992;80(3):548–549.

120. SELZMAN AA, SPIRNAK JP, KURSH ED. The changing management of ureterovaginal fistulas. J Urol 1995;153(3Pt 1):626–628.

121. VASILEV SA. Obturator nerve injury: a review of management options. Gynecol Oncol 1994;53:152–155.

122. ATWOOD SEA, HILL ADK, MURPHY PG, et al. A prospective randomized trial of laparoscopic versus open appendectomy. Surgery 1992;112:457–501.

123. PETERS JH, GIBBONS GD, INNES JT, et al. Complications of laparoscopic cholecytectomy. Surgery 1991;110:769–778.

124. PIER A, GOTZ F, BACHER C. Laparoscopic appendectomy in 625 cases: from innovation to routine. Surg Laparosc Endosc 1991;1(1):8–13.

125. SCHULTZ L, GRABER J, PIETRAFITTA J, et al. Laser laparoscopic herniorrhaphy: a clinical trial preliminary results. J Laparoendosc Surg 1990;1:41–45.

126. SCOTT-CONNER CEH, HALL TJ, ANGLIN BL, et al. Laparoscopic appendectomy: initial experience in a teaching program. Ann Surg 1992;215:660–668.

127. SOTREL G, HIRSCH E, EDELIN KC. Necrotizing fasciitis following diagnostic laparoscopy. Obstet Gynecol 1983;62S:67S–69S.

128. KADAR N, REICH H, LUI CY, et al. Incisional hernias after major laparoscopic gynecologic procedures. Am J Obstet Gynecol 1993;168:4193–4195.

129. MONTZ FJ, HOLSCHNEIDER CH, MUNRO MG. Incisional hernia following laparoscopy: a survey of the American Association of Gynecologic Laparoscopists. Obstet Gynecol 1994;84(5):881–884.

130. VAGHADIA H, MCLEOD DH, MITCHELL GW, et al. Small dose hypobaric lidocaine-fentanyl spinal anesthesia for short duration outpatient laparoscopy. I.A randomized comparison with conventional dose hyperbaric lidocaine. Anesth Analg 1997;84:59–64.

131. CHILVERS CR, VAGHADIA H, MITCHELL GW, et al. Small dose hypobaric lidocaine-fentanyl spinal anesthesia for short duration outpatient laparoscopy. II. Optimal fentanyl dose. Anesth Analg 1997;84:65–70.

132. DOBBS FF, KUMAR V, ALEXANDER JL, et al. Pain after laparoscopy related to posture and ring versus clip sterilization. Br J Obstet Gynaecol 1987;94:262–266.

133. SCHAUER PR, PAGE CP, GHIATAS AA, et al. Incidence and significance of subdiaphragmatic air following laparoscopic cholecystectomy. Am Surg 1997;63:132–136.

134. TOUB DB, ZUBERNIS J, CAMPION MJ, et al. Resolution of free intraperitoneal air after laparoscopy: utility of abdominal radiography in the diagnosis of bowel injury. J Am Assoc Gynecol Laparosc 1994;1: S37.

135. KENEFICK JP, LEADER A, MALTBY JR, et al. Laparoscopy: blood gas values and minor sequelae associated with three techniques based on Isoflurane. Br J Anaesth 1987;59:189–194.

136. CHAMBERLAIN G. The recovery of gases insufflated at laparoscopy. Br J Obstet Gynaecol 1984;91:367–370.

137. GUIDO RS, BROOKS K, MCKENZIE R, et al. A randomized, prospective comparison of pain after gasless laparoscopy and traditional laparoscopy. J Am Assoc Gynecol Laparosc 1998;5:149–153.

138. CUNNIFFE MG, MCANENA OJ, DAR MA, et al. A prospective randomized trial of intraoperative bupivicaine irrigation for management of shoulder tip pain following laparoscopy. Am J Surg 1998;176:258–261.

139. ZULLO F, PELLICANO M, CAPPIELLO F, et al. Pain control after microlaparoscopy. J Am Assoc Gynecol Laparosc 1998;5:161–163.

140. ABDOLHOSSEINZADEH M, ASGARIEH S, HAJIAN H. Postoperative pain after lidocaine injection intraperitoneally and subcutaneously for laparoscopic surgery. J Am Assoc Gynecol Laparosc 1995;2: S1.

141. KE RW, PORTERA SG, BAGOUS W, et al. A randomized double blinded trial of pre-emptive analgesia in laparoscopy. Obstet Gynecol 1998;92:972–975.

142. DE WITTE J, RIETMAN GW, VANDENBROUCKE G, et al. Postoerative effects of tramadol administered at wound closure. Eur J Anaesthesiol 1998;15:190–195.

143. WINDSOR A, MCDONALD P, MUMTAZ T, et al. The analgesic efficacy of tenoxicam versus placebo in day case laparoscopy: a randomised parallel double blind trial. Anaesthesia 1996;51:1066–1069.

144. RASANAYAGAM R, HARRISON G. Preoperative oral administration of morphine in day-case gynaecological laparoscopy. Anaesthesia 1996;51:1179–1181.

145. ALEXANDER JI, HULL MGR. Abdominal pain after laparoscopy: the value of a gas drain. Br J Obstet Gynaecol 1987;94:267–269.

146. METTER SE, KITZ DS, YOUNG ML, et al. Nausea and vomiting after outpatient laparoscopy: Incidence, impact on recovery room stay and cost. Anesth Analg 1987;66:S116.

147. CHUNG F, UN V, SU J. Postoperative symptoms 24 hours after ambulatory anaesthesia. Can J Anesth 1996;43:1121–1127.

148. PALAZZO MGA, STRUNIN L. Anaesthesia and emesis: etiology. Can Anaesth Soc J 1984;31:178–187.

149. BOULTON TB, CHIR B. Oral chlorpromazine hydrochloride. Anaesthesia 1955;10:233–246.

150. BEATTIE WS, LINDBLAD T, BUCKLEY DN, et al. The incidence of postoperative nausea and vomiting in women undergoing laparoscopy is influenced by the day of menstrual cycle. Can J Anaesth 1991;38:298–302.

151. BELLVILLE JW. Postanesthetic nausea and vomiting. Anesthesiology 1961;22:773–780.

152. HOVORKA J, KORTILLA K, ERKOLA O. Nitrous oxide does not increase nausea and vomiting following gynaecological laparoscopy. Can J Anesth 1989;36:145–148.

153. SENGUPTA P, PLANTEVIN OM. Nitrous oxide and day case laparoscopy: effects on nausea, vomiting, and return to normal activity. Br J Anaesth 1988;60:570–573.

154. BRIDENBAUGH LD. Regional anaesthesia for outpatient surgery—a summary of 12 years experience. Can Anaesth Soc J 1983;30:548–552.

155. GUNAWARDENE RD, WHITE DC. Propofol and emesis. Anaesthesia 1988;43:65–67.

156. RISING S, DODGSON MS, STEEN PA. Isoflurane v fentanyl for outpatient laparoscopy. Acta Anaesth Scand 1985;29:251–255.

157. OH S, FABRICK J, PAGUALAYAN G. Evaluation of toradol for pain control after laparoscopic cholecystectomy. Anesthesiology 1992;77:440–443.

158. CALHOUN B, VIANI B, LARUE D. The effect of ketorolac on patients undergoing laparoscopic cholecystectomy. Anesthesiology 1992;77:48–52.

159. PARRIS WC, LEE EM. Anaesthesia for laparoscopic cholecystectomy. Anaesthesia 1991;46:997.

160. PANDIT SK, KOTHARY SP, PANDIT UA, et al. Dose-response study of droperidol and metoclopramide as antiemetics for outpatient anesthesia. Anesth Analg 1989;68:798–802.

161. ROTHENBERG DM, MCCARTHY RJ, PENG CC, et al. Nausea and vomiting after dexamethasone versus droperidol following outpatient laparoscopy with a propofol based general anesthetic. Acta Anaesthesiol Scand 1998;42:637–642.

162. ALON E, HIMMELSEHER S. Ondansetron in the treatment of postoperative vomiting: a randomized double blind comparison with droperidol and metoclopramide. Anesth Analg 1992;75:561–565.

163. WETCHLER BV, SUNG YF, DUNCALF D, et al. Ondansetron decreases emetic symptoms following outpatient laparoscopy. Anesthesiology 1990;73:A35.

164. POLATI E, VERLATO G, FINCO G, et al. Ondasteron versus metaclopramide in the treatment of postoperative nausea and vomiting. Anesth Analg 1997;85:395–399.

165. BORGEAT A, HASLER P, FAHTI M. Gynecologic laparoscopic surgery is not associated with an increase of serotonin metabolites excretion. Anesth Analg 1998;87:1104–1108.

166. SNIADACH MS, ALBERTS MS. A comparison of the prophylactic antiemetic effect of ondasteron and droperidol on patients undergoing gynecologic laparoscopy. Anesth Analg 1997;85:797–800.

167. BAILY PL, STREISAND JB, PACE NL, et al. Transdermal scopolamine reduces nausea and vomiting after outpatient laparoscopy. Anesthesiology 1990;72:977–980.

168. CURET MJ, ALLEN D, JOSLOFF RK, et al. Laparoscopy in pregnancy. Arch Surg 1996;131:546–551.

169. REEDY MB, GALAN HL, RICHARDS WE, et al. Laparoscopy during pregnancy. A survey of laparoendosocopic surgeons. J Reprod Med 1997;42:33–38.

170. ARVIDSSON D, GERDIN E. Laparoscopic cholecystectomy during pregnancy. Surg Laparoscopy Endosc 1991;1:193–194.

171. PUCCI RO, SEED RW. Case report of laparoscopic cholecystectomy in the third trimester of pregnancy. Am J Obstet Gynecol 1991;165:401–402.

172. MORRELL DG, MULLINS JR, HARRISON PB. Laparoscopic cholecystectomy during pregnancy in symptomatic patients. Surgery 1992;112:856–859.

173. SOPER NJ, HUNTER JG, PETRIE RH. Laparoscopic cholecystectomy during pregnancy. Surg Endosc 1992;6:115–117.

174. CONSTANTINO GN, VINCENT GJ, MUKALIAN CG, et al. Laparoscopic cholecystectomy in pregnancy. J Laparoendosc Surg 1994;4:161–164.

175. POSTA CG. Laparoscopic surgery in pregnancy: Report on two cases. J Laparoendosc Surg 1995;4:161–164.

176. WILLIAMS JK, ROSEMURGY AS, ALBRINK MH, et al. Laparoscopic cholecystectomy in pregnancy: a case report. J Reprod Surg 1995;40:243–244.

177. MARTIN IG, DEXTER SP, McMAHON MJ. Laparoscopic cholecystectomy in pregnancy. A safe option during the second trimester. Surg Endosc 1996;10:508–510.

178. CURET MJ, VOGT DA, SCHOB O, et al. Effects of CO_2 pneumoperitoneum in pregnant ewes. J Surg Res 1996;63:339–344.

179. HUNTER JG, SWANSTROM L, THORNBURG K. Carbon dioxide pneumoperitoneum induces fetal acidosis in a pregnant ewe model. Surg Endosc 1995;9:272–279.

180. IAFRATI MD, YARNELL R, SCHWAITZBERG SD. Gasless laparoscopic cholecystectomy in pregnancy. J Laparoendosc Surg 1995;5:127–130.

181. AKIRA S, YAMANAKA A, ISHIHARA T, et al. Gasless laparoscopic ovarian cystectomy during pregnancy: comparison with laparotomy. Am J Obstet Gynecol 1999;180:554–557.

182. LUXMAN D, COHEN JR, DAVID MP. Laparoscopic myomectomy in pregnancy. J Am Assoc Gynecol Laparosc 1995;2:S28.

183. DUFUOR P, DELEBECQ T, VINATIER D, et al. Appendicitis in pregnancy. Seven case reports. J Gynecol Obstet Biol Reprod (Paris) 1996;25:411–415.

184. BARONE JE, BEARS S, CHEN S, et al. Outcome study of cholecystectomy in pregnancy. Am J Surg 1999;177:232–236.

185. GEISLER JP, ROSE SL, MERNITZ CS, et al. Non-gynecologic laparoscopy in the second and third trimester pregnancy: obstetric implications. J Soc Laparoendosc Surg 1998;2:235–238.

186. GURBUZ AT, PEETZ ME. The acute abdomen in the pregnant patient. Is there a role for laparoscopy? Surg Endosc 1997;11:98–102.

187. REEDY MB, KALLEN B, KUEHL TJ. Laparoscopy during pregnancy: a study of five fetal outcome parameters with use of the Swedish Health Registry. Am J Obstet Gynecol 1997;177:673–679.

188. NEZHAT FR, TAZUKE S, NEZHAT CH, et al. Laparoscopy during pregnancy: a literature review. J Soc Laparoendosc Surg 1997;1:17–27.

189. MORICE P, LOUIS-SYLVESTRE C, CHAPRON C, et al. Laparoscopy for adnexal torsion in pregnant women. J Reprod Med 1997;42:435–439.

190. YUVAL Y, SORIANO D, GOLDENBERG M, et al. Is operative laparoscopy contraindicated in the first trimester of pregnancy? J Am Assoc Gynecol Laparosc 1995;2:S61–S62.

191. CONRON RW Jr, ABBRUZZI K, COCHRANE SO, et al. Laparoscopic procedures in pregnancy. Am Surg 1999;65:259–263.

192. SORIANO D, YEFET Y, SEIDMAN DS, et al. Laparoscopy versus laparotomy in the management of adnexal masses during pregnancy. Fertil Steril 1999;71:955–960.

193. AMOS JD, SCHORR SJ, NORMAN PF, et al. Laparoscopic surgery during pregnancy. Am J Surg 1996;171:435–437.

194. Guidelines for laparoscopic surgery during pregnancy. Society of American Gastrointestinal Endoscopic Surgeons. Surg Endosc 1998;12:189–190.

195. GURUSAMY K, AGGARWAL R, PALANIVELU L, et al. Systematic review of randomized controlled trials on the effectiveness of virtual reality training for laparoscopic surgery Br J Surg 2008;95:1088–1097.

196. MRAOVIC B, IMURINA T, SONICKI Z, et al. The dose–response of nitrous oxide in postoperative nausea in patients undergoing gynecologic laparoscopic surgery: a preliminary study. Int Anes Res Soc 2008;107(3):818–823.

197. AGRESTA F, DeSIMONE P, CIARDO LF, et al. Direct trocar insertion versus Veress needle in nonobese patients undergoing laparoscopic procedures. Surg Endosc 2004;18:1778–1781.

198. BEMELMAN WA, DUNKER MS, BUSCH ORC, et al. Efficacy of establishment of pneumoperitoneum with the Veress needle, Hasson trocar, and modified blunt trocar (TrocDoc): a randomized study. J Laparoendosc Adv Surg Tech 2000;10(6):325–330.

199. BORGATTA L, GRUSS L, BARAD D, et al. Direct trocar Insertion vs. Verres Needle use for laparoscopic sterilization. J Reprod Med 1990;35(9):891–894.

200. BYRON JW, MARKENSON G, MIYAZAWA K. A randomized comparison of Verres needle and direct trocar insertion for laparoscopy. Surgery 1993;177:259–262.

201. GUNEC MZ, YESILDAGLAR N, BINGOL B, et al. The safety and efficacy of direct trocar insertion with elevation of the rectus sheath instead of the skin for pneumoperitoneum. Surg Laparosc Endosc Percutan Tech 2005;15(2):80–81.

202. TANSATIT T, WISAWASUKMONGCHOL W, BUNYAVEJCHEVIN S. A randomized, prospective study comparing the use of the missile trocar and the pyramidal trocar for laparoscopy access. J Med Assoc Thai 2006;89(7):941–947.

203. FESTE JR, BOJAHR B, TURNER DJ. Randomized trial comparing a radially expandable needle system with cutting trocars. JSLS 2000;4:11–15.

204. MUZII L, BELLATI F, ZULLO MA, et al. Mechanical Bowel preparation before gynecologic laparoscopy: a randomized, single blind, controlled trial. Fert Ster 2006:85(3):689–693.

205. PHELPS P, CAKMAKKAYA OS, APFEL CC, et al. A simple clinical maneuver to reduce laparoscopy-induced shoulder pain: a randomized controlled trial. Obstet Gynecol 2008;111:1155–1160.

206. SCOTT DJ, BERGEN PC, REGE RV, et al. Laparoscopic training on bench models: better and more cost effective than operating room experience? J Am Coll Surg 2000;191:272–283.

207. HUBNER M, DEMARTINES N, MULLER S, et al. Prospective randomized study of monopolar scissors, bipolar vessel sealer and ultrasonic shears in laparoscopic colorectal surgery Br J Surg 2008;95:1098–1104.

208. COGLIANDOLO A, MANGANARO T, SAITTA FP, et al. Blind versus open approach to laparoscopic cholecystectomy. Surg Laparosc Endosc 1998;8(5):353–355.

209. GUENAGA KKFG, ATALLAH ÁN, CASTRO AA, et al. Mechanical bowel preparation for elective colorectal surgery. Cochrane Database Syst Rev 2005;1:CD001544. DOI: 10.1002/14651858.CD001544.pub2.

210. WHITE RH, ZHOU H, ROMANO PS. Incidence of symptomatic venous thromboembolism after different elective or surgical procedures. Thromb Haemost 2003;90:446–455.

211. TINCANI E, PICCOLI M, TURRINI F, et al. Video LAPAROSCOPIC surgery: is out-of-hospital thromboprophylaxis necessary? J Thromb Maemost 2005;3:216–220.

212. BACA I, SCHNEIDER B, KOHLER T, et al. Prevention of venous thromboembolism in patients undergoing minimally invasive surgery with a short-term hospital stay: results of a multicentric, prospective, randomised, controlled trial with a low-molecular weight heparin. Chirurg 1997;68:1275–1280.

213. GEERTS WH, BERGQVIST D, PINEO GF, et al. Prevention of venous thromboembolism: American College of Chest Physicians Evidence-Based Clinical Practice Guidelines (8th edition). Chest 2008;133(6 Suppl):381S–453S.

Part Three

Oncologic Perioperative Decision Making

Chapter 9

Cervical Carcinoma

Fidel A. Valea, MD

INTRODUCTION

Cervical cancer is the second most common malignancy in women worldwide, with an estimated 555,100 new cases and 309,800 deaths attributable to this disease.[1,2] The American Cancer Society estimates that in 2008 there will be approximately 11,070 cases of cervical cancer and 3870 deaths in the United States.[3] The median age at diagnosis in North America is 47 years with nearly half the cases diagnosed before the age of 35. Women over the age of 55 have a disproportionately higher mortality from this disease as they present with more advanced disease.[4] Although the incidence and mortality rates have been decreasing in many developed countries due to mass screening and early detection, these rates remain high in underdeveloped countries that do not have effective screening programs. In the United States the relative 5-year survival rate for cervical cancer patients diagnosed with localized disease is 92% and 70% for all stages respectively.

The incidence of cervical carcinoma in the United States is substantially higher among minority women as well as women of lower socioeconomic status, predominantly because these individuals have not had good access to health care and cervical cancer screening programs. They also lack screening for common illness such as diabetes, hypertension, and cardiovascular disease[5]. Therefore, careful attention to nongynecologic symptoms as well as a high index of suspicion of other medical illnesses is critical when treating patients with cervical cancer. Furthermore, HIV seropositivity has been identified as a risk factor for cervical cancer, and in patients with HIV, cervical cancer is considered an AIDS-defining illness. Other risk factors for cervical cancer include early age of first intercourse, history of multiple sexual partners, smoking, and a large number of pregnancies, but the single most important risk factor is a persistent infection with one of the high risk HPV types.[6]

Gynecologic Oncology: Evidence-Based Perioperative and Supportive Care, Second Edition.
Edited by Scott E. Lentz, Allison E. Axtell and Steven A. Vasilev.
© 2011 John Wiley & Sons, Inc. Published 2011 by John Wiley & Sons, Inc.

THE SURGICAL TREATMENT OF CERVICAL CANCER

The treatment of cervical cancer depends on the stage at presentation. Although a combination of chemotherapy and radiation is superior to surgical treatment for advanced disease, it is comparable to surgical treatment for early stage disease (stage IIa or less). The surgical treatment of invasive cervical cancer can be grouped into categories based on extent and status of disease.[5]

Microinvasive Cervix Cancer

Microinvasive cervical cancer is a term that was first introduced in 1947 by Mestwerdt.[7] It was meant to identify patients that were at such low risk of metastatic disease that they did not require radical treatment. Although stromal invasion can be seen in a small biopsy, the diagnosis of microinvasive cervical cancer can only be made in a conization or hysterectomy specimen.[8] More recently, cervical conization and large loop excision of the transformation zone (LLETZ) are considered equally efficacious when the latter is performed by experienced operators who limit thermal artifact and properly orient the specimen, thus simplifying histologic analysis[9-11] (**Levels II-1, II-3**). Patients with squamous lesions, which are occult, invade to less than 3 mm below the basement membrane, and no confluent lesion is wider than 7 mm (FIGO stage Ia1), can be treated with extrafascial hysterectomy alone, with cure rates approaching 100% because the risk of parametrial and/or lymphatic spread is 1% or less. Disease extent can only be accurately assessed after an excisional procedure has been performed and negative surgical margins obtained. The decision to perform an extrafascial hysterectomy based on frozen section evaluation of a cone or LLETZ specimens has been associated with inaccuracies when compared to standard histologic review and may lead to inappropriate surgical management[12] (**Level II-3**).

In a woman who desires future fertility, an excisional procedure, such as conization or LLETZ, is considered adequate therapy for a stage Ia1 microinvasive cervical cancer, assuming that the margins of excision are negative and the postexcision endocervical curettage (ECC) is also negative[13] (**Level II-3**). Residual invasion has been detected in 13% of patients in cases where either the internal margin of excision or the ECC revealed dysplasia or 33% when both revealed dysplasia.[14] A repeat excisional procedure is recommended prior to definitive treatment with hysterectomy to rule out more extensive invasive disease. A woman who does not desire any further childbearing and has negative margins of excision should consider definitive treatment with a simple extrafascial hysterectomy. The presence of lymphovascular space invasion (LVSI) is controversial in an Ia1 cervix cancer and should not be considered in the treatment plan unless it is extensive.[13]

Another group of patients with occult, microinvasive cancers and 3–5 mm of invasion and no more than 7 mm of lateral spread, stage Ia2 cervix cancer deserve special consideration. Unfortunately, there is limited data on patients with this stage of cervical cancer. Because of the very low incidence of lymph node metastases (2%–3%), conservative treatments have been investigated with mixed results.[5,13] In one review, patients who met these criteria were associated with more treatment failures, and multivariate analysis demonstrated that both simple hysterectomy and omission of lymphadenectomy were associated with higher recurrence rates.[15] The current recommendations are to treat these patients with radical surgery or chemoradiation with comparable results.

Microinvasive Adenocarcinoma

When the International Federation of Gynecologists and Obstetricians (FIGO) last revised the staging of cervical cancer in 1994, the microstaging of occult cervical cancer, stage Ia disease, applied to squamous lesions and did not include adenocarcinomas. The term "microinvasive adenocarcinoma" has gained more popularity in the literature as the definitions of microinvasive disease have been applied to adenocarcinomas.

The most recent and extensive review of the topic identified more than 1500 cases of microinvasive adenocarcinoma of the cervix.[16] Of the patients that had ≤3 mm of invasion and had a lymph node dissection, 3/261 had positive lymph nodes (1.1%). Patients with 3.1–5.0 mm of invasion who underwent a lymph node dissection were found to have metastases to the lymph nodes in 2/264 cases (0.8%). Unfortunately, the lack of uniformity in treatment as well as in reporting hinders the interpretation of these results. The presence of LVSI was not a prognostic indicator in this review. In a separate review, Ostör identified 436 cases of microinvasive adenocarcinoma of the cervix, of which 219 had pelvic lymph node dissection and 5 (2%) had metastases, supporting the notion that microinvasion in glandular lesions may be comparable to squamous lesions.[17] Finally, in a recent population-based study from the Surveillance, Epidemiology and End Results (SEER) database, 131 cases of stage Ia1 and 170 cases of stage Ia2 adenocarcinomas were treated between 1988 and 1997.[18] The censored survival was 99.2% and 98.2%, respectively, with a mean follow-up of 46.5 months. Although, there is no true consensus, it seems reasonable to treat the entity: "microinvasive adenocarcinoma of the cervix" in a manner similar to its squamous counterpart, provided one understands the difficulty in following glandular lesions that are treated conservatively.

Stage IB1 up to Early Stage IIa Cervical Cancer

Patients with cervical cancer confined to the cervix or have early vaginal involvement (stage IIa) are usually considered ideal surgical candidates, but can be treated with either radical hysterectomy and bilateral pelvic lymphadenectomy or chemoradiation therapy combining whole pelvic teletherapy with local brachytherapy and weekly chemotherapy. These treatment modalities are recognized as having equal cure rates in a randomized series.[19] Surgery is often preferred to radiotherapy in younger women because ovarian function is preserved and sexual function is not compromised following radiation. In addition, the late complications of radiation are avoided when patients are treated with surgery alone. As such, radiation is usually reserved for the medically unfit patient.[13] Age alone should not be used as the deciding factor as older women have comparable morbidity to their younger counterparts.[20] However, women with early cervical cancer treated with radical surgery may occasionally benefit from a combined approach including adjuvant radiation if surgical margins are compromised, if regional lymphatic spread is present, or if other high risk features are present.[21–23] In a landmark Gynecologic Oncology Group (GOG) trial, Scdlis and colleagues identified three high risk features: deep stromal invasion (>1/3), LVSI, and large tumor diameter (>4 cm). If two of these risk factors were present, the addition of postoperative radiation therapy improved the recurrence-free rate at 2 years from 79% to 88%[22] (**Level I**).

Surgical Treatment of Advanced Cervical Cancer (Stage IIB and Greater)

Although radiation can be used to treat all stages of cervical cancer, it is the predominant treatment for advanced, stage IIB or greater, cervical cancer. Yet, it wasn't until 1999 when three separate randomized clinical trials established chemoradiation with cisplatin as the best treatment for advanced cervical cancer[24–26] (**Level I**).

In the first study, the GOG randomized patients into one of three treatment arms. Each had the same radiation but one also received weekly cisplatin, another received hydroxyurea, cisplatin, and 5-fluorouracil, and the last received hydroxyurea alone. The progression-free survival favored the cisplatin-containing regimens, 70% vs. 67% vs. 50%, respectively.[24] In the second trial, the Radiation Therapy Oncology Group (RTOG) randomized 403 patients to either pelvic and para-aortic radiation or pelvic radiation with concurrent cisplatin and 5-fluorouracil. The 5-year actuarial survival favored the group that received chemotherapy, 73% vs. 58% with a median follow-up of 43 months.[25] In the final trial, the GOG and Southwest Oncology Group (SWOG) randomized 388 patients with surgically staged negative para-aortic nodes to receive standard pelvic radiation in addition to either hydroxyurea or cisplatin and 5-fluorouracil. The overall survival favored the group receiving the cisplatin-containing regimen.[26]

Each of the above trials included patients who had disease confined to the pelvis with negative para-aortic nodes. Historically, clinical staging of para-aortic nodes has failed to consistently recognize para-aortic node metastases, missing anywhere from 7% to 29% of the cases.[13] Until recently, the role of surgery in this group of patients was limited to evaluating the presence of metastases to the para-aortic lymph nodes without any proof of survival advantage if the patients were surgically staged. However, a recent GOG study compared patients who had negative surgically staged para-aortic nodes to patients who had para-aortic lymph node status determined radiographically (GOG 85 and 120 vs. GOG 165).[27] In this trial, the surgically staged patients had a better 4-year progression-free survival (48.9% vs. 36.3%) and a better overall survival (54.3% vs. 40%) compared to patients who had radiographic evaluation of their para-aortic nodes, thus emphasizing the importance of surgical para-aortic lymph node staging in advanced cervical cancer.

The role of positron emission tomography (PET) and PET/CT continues to be evaluated but reported sensitivities are not consistent enough to be helpful, ranging from 38% to 86%.[28, 29] This is an area that still needs to be explored further if surgical staging is to be replaced.

The management of grossly enlarged para-aortic nodes is also quite controversial as there is evidence that resecting these nodes through an extraperitoneal approach converts their prognosis to that of patients with micrometastases.[30–32] Opponents of this cite the high likelihood that patients with bulky para-aortic nodes have disseminated disease and are probably incurable.

Advanced and Recurrent Cervix Cancer

Total pelvic exenteration (TPE), with en bloc removal of the pelvic organs including bladder, rectum, and vagina, continues to be the only curative option for patients with centrally recurrent cancer of the cervix with no evidence of sidewall or distant involvement after definitive radiation. In very select cases the procedure could be limited to a posterior exenteration with preservation of the bladder or an anterior exenteration with preservation of the rectum. Opponents of these limited procedures voice concerns over the potential for incomplete excisions. Hence, they should only be done in very limited circumstances. TPE can also be used to treat the occasional patient who presents with stage IVB disease and fistula to either the rectum or bladder if no disseminated disease is noted on imaging of the chest, abdomen, and pelvis.

The operation was first described by Brunschwig in 1948.[33] Since then, several modifications have occurred that have increased the acceptance of this procedure. The most notable of these was the creation of a urinary conduit and subsequently a continent urinary pouch.[34–36] Other modifications include vaginal reconstruction and low rectal anastamosis.

Patient selection is very important when considering TPE for recurrent cervical cancer. Patients with weight loss, hydronephrosis, leg edema, and hip pain rarely benefit from the procedure.[37] Preoperative evaluation should include imaging of the chest, abdomen, and pelvis, looking for evidence of metastatic disease. Although this is usually performed utilizing CT or MRI scans, more recently the role of PET scanning is expanding to include the evaluation of metastatic disease.[38] In addition, an extensive medical and psychological assessment is done to ensure the patient's ability to withstand the operative procedure and the prolonged morbidity and body changes that result from this operation. A preoperative consultation with an enterostomal therapist is helpful for patient education and proper positioning/marking of possible stomas. Absolute contraindications to curative TPE include any metastatic disease outside of the pelvis detected either preoperatively or intraoperatively. Not every patient who is explored for an exenteration actually goes through with it. In one large series from M.D. Anderson, procedure for approximately 28% of the patients who were explored for exenteration was aborted.[39] Reasons for aborting the procedure included the presence of intraperitoneal disease in 44%,

Table 9.1   Mortality and Survival Data for Patients with Cervical Cancer (Data Abstracted from Original Article When Possible) Undergoing Pelvic Exenteration

Author and Year	No. of Patients	Operative Mortality	5-Year Survival Rate
Douglas et al., 1957[40]	23	1 (4.3%)	5 (21.7%)
Parsons et al., 1964[41]	112	24 (21.4%)	24 (21.4%)
Brunschwig, 1965[42]	535	86 (16.1%)	108 (20.2%)
Kiselow et al., 1967[43]	207	16 (7.7%)	68 (32.9%)
Krieger et al., 1969[44]	35	4 (11.4%)	13 (37.1%)
Ketcham et al., 1970[45]	162	12 (7.4%)	62 (38.3%)
Symmonds et al., 1975[46]	198	16 (8.1%)	64 (32.3%)
Rutledge et al., 1977[37]	296	40 (13.5%)	99 (33.4%)
Averette et al., 1984[47]	92	23 (25%)	34 (37%)
Morley et al., 1989[48]	66	2 (3%)	44 (66.7%)
Lawhead et al., 1989[49]	65	6 (9.2%)	15 (23.1%)
[a]Soper et al., 1989[50]	69	5 (7.2%)	28 (40.5%)
Shingleton et al., 1989[51]	143	9 (6.3%)	71 (49.7%)
[a]Sharma et al., 2005[52]	48	2 (4.2%)	16 (33.3%)
Goldberg et al., 2006[53]	95	1 (1.1%)	46 (48.4%)
Total	**2146**	**246 (11.6%)**	**697 (32.5%)**

[a]Included a small number of patients with other pelvic malignancies.

nodal disease in 40%, parametrial fixation in 13%, and hepatic or bowel involvement in the rest. Peritoneal cytology was only predictive of disease in patients with adenocarcinomas.

Operative mortality has decreased over the years with most centers averaging less than 10% in the more recent series (Table 9.1). The 5-year cumulative survival rate after TPE is also quite variable but averages about 32%. Unfortunately, TPE for cervical cancer carries a high degree of morbidity that cannot be compared to TPE for other conditions, as most of the latter patients have not been radiated. Enteric complications including bowel obstruction and fistulas are the most serious, with particularly high mortality rates with surgical correction. In one series from the University of Miami, 22.5% of the patients were reexplored for gastrointestinal complications, with a mortality rate of 53.3%.[54] Similarly, Orr and his colleagues reported that gastrointestinal complications accounted for 60% of all nonmalignant indications for reoperation after exenteration and 15% of patients after exenteration developed gastrointestinal tract fistulas.[55] The avoidance of irradiated small bowel to small bowel anastamoses seems to decrease the fistula rate. Hence, enterocolostomy is the recommended anastamosis if possible. The use of any sort of "mesh" or foreign graft material to cover the denuded pelvis is also associated with a very high rate of complications and should be avoided.[53] Given the high complication and mortality rates with TPE, it is imperative that the clinician select patients very carefully for this procedure.

TECHNIQUES OF RADICAL HYSTERECTOMY

Although initially described by Meigs in 1944, this is the most common operation for the treatment of early stage cervical cancer.[56] Its 5-year survival rate is comparable to radiotherapy (83% vs. 74%) in a large randomized trial for stage Ib–IIa cervix cancer.[19] Although many modifications of the operation have been described, there is no randomized data as to the utility and safety of the modifications. In 1974, Piver et al. described the following five classes of extended hysterectomies.[57]

Type I: Extrafascial hysterectomy. This is the traditional, simple hysterectomy used for noninvasive disease and even suitable for stage Ia1 microinvasive cervical cancer.

Type II, Modified Radical Hysterectomy. This is the extended hysterectomy that was initially described by Wertheim in 1912.[58] It involved the removal of the medial half of the cardinal and uterosacral ligaments, the upper one-third of the vagina and division of the uterine artery where it crossed the ureter. As described, the pelvic lymph nodes were only selectively removed. Although there is no randomized data, many use this operation to treat stage Ia2 cervical cancer.[13] There is some retrospective data that the type II hysterectomy is appropriate for this population of patients. In one recent small series, none of the patients with negative margins at the time of either a cone biopsy or LLETZ procedure had residual disease at the time of radical hysterectomy; suggesting that less aggressive treatments could be considered.[59] In a much larger series of these patients (lesion size ≤ 2 cm, lymph nodes negative, and depth of invasion ≤ 10 mm), the incidence of parametrial involvement was only 0.6% in patients, also suggesting the potential for less radical surgery, but acknowledging the importance of pelvic lymphadenectomy.[60]

Type III: Radical hysterectomy. This is the traditional operation for early stage, invasive cervical cancer (stage Ib–IIa) where the uterine artery is divided at its origin, and the ureter is dissected free from the parametrial tissue surrounding it in the "tunnel" between the crossing of the uterine artery and its entrance into the bladder. This allows for removal of the entire cardinal and uterosacral ligaments, the parametria, and the upper one third of the vagina. It also includes a complete pelvic lymphadenectomy.

Type IV: Extended radical hysterectomy. This operation differs from the type III in that the superior vesicle artery is sacrificed, the ureter is completely dissected from all its attachments in the pelvis, and the upper three fourths of the vagina is excised. Only on rare occasions is this operation necessary for primary treatment of cervical cancer or even selective small central recurrences.

Type V: Partial exenteration. This operation is also rarely used in modern practice as it involves removal of the distal ureters and part of the bladder with reimplantation of both ureters. Although described for cancer encasing the distal ureter, most of these patients are best treated with chemoradiation.

Preoperative Evaluation

The goal of a preoperative evaluation is to assess surgical risk and formulate a risk/benefit ratio of surgical management. In addition, careful preoperative assessment of the patient enables preventive measures to be taken, which decrease surgical risk and morbidity. Preoperative care begins with a careful history including the current illness, medical history, surgical history, gynecologic history, family history, social history, and documentation of medications, allergies to medications, and habits. Inherent in this screening evaluation is a complete physical examination with particular attention to the cardiovascular, respiratory, renal/urinary, gastrointestinal, immune, and nervous systems. Furthermore, nutritional status is evaluated as well as infectious, thromboembolic, and bleeding risks.

Prognostic risk stratification to identify perioperative and long-term cardiac risk in selected patients undergoing gynecologic surgery is part of good clinical practice.[61] Noninvasive cardiac testing may be used selectively in patients undergoing noncardiac surgery to provide useful estimates of short- and long-term risk of cardiac events. Results from noninvasive testing and the magnitude of abnormality should then be used to formulate decisions regarding the need for therapy, even surgical intervention, prior to the planned elective gynecologic operation. Controversy exists regarding the guidelines for ordering noninvasive studies including the preoperative electrocardiogram (ECG).[61,62] Exercise variables have been proposed as criteria to screen patients who may benefit from other noninvasive cardiac studies beyond the ECG. Marked exercise-induced ST segment shift or angina at low workloads as well as an inability to increase or actually decrease systolic blood pressure with progressive exercise may then be indications for further testing. The predictive value for a perioperative event, i.e., death or myocardial infarction, ranges from 5% to 25% for a positive exercise ECG test and from 90% to 95% for a negative test. When an exercise ECG is not feasible (approximately 30%–50% of patients), pharmacological stress imaging should be used in patients who require further perioperative noninvasive risk stratification. In one recent meta-analysis of noninvasive cardiac tests, dobutamine stress echocardiography was the best predictor of perioperative cardiac death and nonfatal myocardial infarction compared to dipyridamole myocardial scintigraphy or dipyridamole stress echocardiography.[63] Prior to this, the reported sensitivity and specificity of dobutamine-induced echocardiographic wall motion abnormalities in patients with peripheral vascular disease were similar to those of myocardial perfusion scintigraphy[64] (**Level II-2**).

For most gynecologic procedures, a chest radiograph is not routinely recommended unless the patient is over 60 years of age, since the yield in asymptomatic nonsmokers without preexisting pulmonary disease is low and, therefore, not supported by evidence.[65,66] However, when performing surgery for an invasive gynecologic malignancy, it is important to exclude lung metastasis although this is also an unusual occurrence and the cost effectiveness of chest radiographs in asymptomatic women with early gynecologic cancers is not well established.[67]

Crossmatching of packed red blood cell units is also not part of the routine evaluation for gynecologic surgery, although some consider it because of the potential for vascular injury and rapid blood loss during lymph node dissections and/or radical hysterectomy. Even the routine performance of urinalysis, complete blood count, and blood chemistries is not supported by the literature and should be done only for particular indications or when abiding by the local hospital guidelines.[62]

There are some tests that should be done for staging purposes. The chest X-ray was mentioned above but also some evaluation of the urinary system needs to be done to rule out hydronephrosis. Although the cost effectiveness of this practice for very early stage disease is not proven, it should at least be performed for stage Ib or greater cervical cancers. Some substitute CT or MRI with contrast as reasonable alternatives that also give potential information on lymph node status. In patients with more advanced disease, an exam under anesthesia with possible proctoscopy and cystoscopy can be performed to evaluate for rectal and bladder involvement respectively but these patients are usually best treated with radiation. Recent publications have supported the use of sonography to detect the presence of bladder invasion with a high degree of accuracy.[68]

Preoperative Preparation

Once the patient has been clinically staged, the various treatment options discussed, informed consent obtained, and the patient deemed medically fit for surgery, she needs to undergo preoperative preparation.

Preoperative fasting. Although the standard practice has always been to restrict anything by mouth from midnight before surgery, recent trials have found that drinking clear fluids up to a few hours before surgery did not increase the risk of regurgitation during or after the surgery.[69]

Preoperative hair removal. The practice of preoperative hair removal from the surgical site is common practice. However, there does not appear to be any difference in surgical site infections (SSIs) between patients who have had their hair removed prior to surgery and those who have not. If hair removal is deemed necessary, clipping or depilatory creams result in fewer SSIs than using a razor[70] (**Level I**).

Skin preparation. In a recent Cochrane Systematic Review, there was insufficient evidence from randomized trials to support or refute the use of one antiseptic over another as long as one is being utilized. In addition, there was no definitive evidence to show that iodophor-impregnated drapes had any effects on wound infection rates when compared to using no incise drape at all.[71]

Preoperative antibiotics. The use of prophylactic antibiotics to prevent SSIs has been common practice for many years. The long duration of surgery and significant amount of blood loss associated with this procedure is probably a good reason alone to administer prophylactic antibiotics. The type of antibiotic used has been a source of many trials, with no convincing evidence that one antibiotic is better than the next. Most agree that a single dose of an antibiotic is all that is required to diminish SSIs. Most commonly used are the first- and second-generation cephalosporins, ampicillin, and even doxycycline.[72,73] Prolonged operative time leads to increased operative site infection presumably due to a decrease in tissue perfusion secondary to transient hypothermia.[74]

Bowel preparation. Although there are no prospective trials evaluating the utility of bowel preparation prior to radical hysterectomy, there are numerous studies in the colorectal surgery literature that conclude that mechanical preparation is not necessary prior to elective colorectal surgery.[75] Whether this applies to elective radical hysterectomy is unproven. Opponents to this practice cite visualization as a problem in the unprepared bowel. Unfortunately, there is no data to support this notion.

Thromboembolic prophylaxis. The incidence of venous thrombosis in a large series of 397 radical hysterectomies was only 2.7%.[76] In an older series, encompassing both endometrial and cervical cancer operations, the incidence of significant thromboemboli was 7.8%.[77] Although the precise incidence of venous thromboembolic (VTE) complications after radical hysterectomy is not known, it ranges between 11% and 18% in gynecologic cancer surgeries, and it is common practice to use VTE prophylaxis to reduce the morbidity and mortality associated with these events.[78] In a recent survey of the Society of Gynecologic Oncologists, 42% of the members who replied preferred the use of double prophylaxis (anticoagulant and sequential compression devices), while 41% used sequential compression devices alone for the prevention of VTE in women undergoing major gynecologic cancer surgery.[79] Although most agree that prophylaxis is important, there is no randomized data in the radical hysterectomy patient.

Intraoperative Considerations

Careful intraoperative management simplifies postoperative care and reduces complications. Every effort possible should be made to accomplish a safe and expeditious surgical procedure.

Patient positioning and incision selection. Generally, patients undergoing abdominal radical hysterectomy with lymph node dissection for cervical cancer are positioned in the supine position. Alternatively, a low lithotomy positioning can also be used, but care must be exercised to avoid peroneal nerve injury. This nerve injury occurs commonly after improper patient positioning when the peroneal nerve becomes entrapped between the head of the fibula and the stirrup.[80] Moreover, femoral and/or obturator nerve injuries can be prevented by avoiding hip hyperextension and hip overabduction, respectively.[81,82]

Although on occasions, adequate operative exposure can be obtained through a Pfannenstiel incision, a low transverse muscle dividing Maylard or Cherney incision is more commonly used as they both provide excellent exposure of the pelvic sidewalls. Alternatively, a low vertical incision can also be used with the advantage that it would provide better exposure of the para-aortic nodes, which is rarely necessary in early stage disease.[13, 83]

Intraoperative blood loss. Compared to less radical therapy such as extrafascial hysterectomy, patients treated with radical hysterectomy experience increased blood loss and more frequently require transfusions. The estimated average blood loss associated with radical hysterectomy varies with operator experience, patient body habitus and anatomy, as well as lesion size. Averages ranging from 800 to 1500 mL are reported.[13, 84] Hence, it is appropriate to at least order a type and screen prior to surgery in the event that blood is needed intraoperatively.

Drainage after lymph node dissection. After pelvic lymphadenectomy it has been common practice to leave closed-suction drains in the bed of dissection to prevent lymphocyst formation. Recently, with the use of prophylactic antibiotics and leaving the retroperitoneal space open, the need for drains has come into question as they may be associated with more morbidity.[85] Hence, drains are used less and less after pelvic lymphadenectomy.

Bladder drainage. Bladder dysfunction is very common after radical hysterectomy. As such, prolonged bladder drainage was common either with a suprapubic or a transurethral foley catheter.[86] There is some older evidence that the incidence of lower urinary tract infection can be reduced with suprapubic as opposed to transurethral catheterization.[87] More recently, the duration of prolonged bladder drainage has been challenged and 69% of the patients were able to void with low postvoid residual (PVR) volumes of less than 75 cc within 6–9 days of surgery.[88] The remaining 31% of patients were managed with intermittent self-catheterization until their PVR volumes were less than 75 cc. Because of this shorter need for catheterization, many are using a foley catheter in lieu of suprapubic drainage with removal at 1 week postoperation.

Surgical adhesion prevention. Adhesion formation after gynecologic surgery is the second leading cause of adhesive small bowel obstruction. In one large population-based series, 31.9% of patients who underwent surgery on their reproductive tract in 1986 had at least one admission during the ensuing 10 years that was attributable to adhesion formation.[89] In a 2006 Cochrane database systematic review of pharmacological agents for adhesion prevention, there was some evidence that hyaluronic acid agents may decrease the proportion of adhesions and prevent the deterioration of preexisting adhesions. There was insufficient evidence for the use of steroids, icodextrin 4%, polyethylene glycol derivatives, and dextran.[90] When comparing barrier agents, a separate Cochrane review identified an oxidized regenerated cellulose adhesion barrier, Interceed, as reducing the incidence of adhesions following abdominal surgery, but meticulous hemostasis was paramount. Gore-Tex was superior to Interceed in preventing adhesions, but its usefulness was limited by the need to subsequently remove it.[91] In the only published report addressing specifically radical hysterectomies, a cost-effective analysis tree was created demonstrating that routine use of a hyaluronate–carboxymethylcellulose barrier, Seprafilm, was cost-effective in preventing subsequent adhesion-related expenses.[92]

ROUTINE POSTOPERATIVE ASSESSMENT AND MANAGEMENT

The specific details of postoperative assessment and management depend on the extent, duration, and type of operative procedure, as well as the existence of preoperative comorbidities. The surgeon must also focus on problems unique to the patient's medical condition relative to the radicality of the operation.

Postoperative Laboratory Tests

Postoperative laboratory evaluation should be tailored to the extent of surgery, specific fluid and electrolyte concerns, and the patient's preoperative condition. A blood hemoglobin concentration and hematocrit should be obtained within the immediate 24-hour postoperative period for any patient with an estimated intraoperative blood loss greater than 250 cc or an expected postoperative hemoglobin concentration or hematocrit of below 10 gm/dL or 30%, respectively. No other routine blood work is necessary unless a complication develops.

Decisions regarding the postoperative evaluation and monitoring of serum chemistries should be made based on the clinical situation in combination with the preexisting medical comorbid conditions. Patients with postoperative ileus and emesis with nasogastric tube decompression should be monitored for serum electrolyte abnormalities as they can lead to other complications such as cardiac arrythmias in patients with low potassium. A serum calcium concentration should be obtained on patients transfused with more than 2 units of packed red blood cells because the preservatives in banked blood chelate ionized calcium.

Activity

Venous stasis, atelectasis, and ileus are common morbidities following surgery for cervical cancer. Rapid postoperative recovery and the prevention of complications from these conditions rest on early and progressive ambulation of the patient. Early ambulation, beginning within the first 24-hour postoperative period, is recommended and should be steadily increased daily until discharge. In general, when patients are at bed rest, they should be positioned with the head of the bed elevated to avoid aspiration of secretions and gastric contents and with pneumatic sequential compression stockings in place.

Intake and Output

The frequency of postoperative intake and output monitoring and reporting depend on the surgery performed and the postoperative condition of the patient. It should be closely monitored for the first 24 hours or at least until the patient is consistently having a urine output of 0.5–1.0 cc/hour/kg. An output below this amount may be a sign of renal hypoperfusion and hypovolemia, which may lead to other complications.

Diet and Nutrition

Most patients undergoing a radical hysterectomy for cervical cancer or even TPE for recurrent disease are usually nutritionally replete and anabolic at the time of surgery. Therefore, the majority of patients will not require hyperalimentation. In general, oral intake can safely begin on the first postoperative day, once sensorium has normalized, even after retroperitoneal node dissections or anastomosis of the colon and small intestine[93] (**Level I**). A more conservative approach is recommended for patients who have previously been treated with pelvic and/or abdominal radiotherapy, especially in the presence of an intestinal anastomosis.

Pulmonary Care

Patients undergoing radical abdominal hysterectomy for cervical cancer have numerous risk factors for pneumonia. Some of these risk factors include poor respiratory effort due to pain from abdominal incision, anesthesia with endotracheal intubation, decreased clearance of endobronchial secretions, impaired sensorium from analgesics and sedative-hypnotics, immobility, and occasionally obesity. Although incentive spirometry has not been found to alter pulmonary volumes and arterial gas values in prospective studies, it has been found to reduce postoperative pulmonary complications such as atelectasis and pneumonia. This protective effect appears to be significant only for moderate and high risk patients (e.g., those with history of chronic obstructive pulmonary disease, reactive airway disease, general anesthesia time greater than 120 minutes)[94, 95] (**Level I**). However, deep breathing alone may be as effective as incentive spirometry in preventing postoperative pulmonary complications among patients at low risk for pulmonary complications, such as those less than 60 years of age with an ASA (American Society of Anesthesia) score equal to 1[95] (**Level I**).

Wound Care

Wound infections are more common in obese patients with a subcutaneous tissue depth of greater than or equal to 3 cm.[96] Such patients may benefit from a subcutaneous closed drainage system. One prospective, randomized study on 197 obese patients undergoing gynecologic surgery showed that overall wound complication rates decreased from 31% to 20% when drains were placed[97] (**Level I**). Drains are generally left in place for 72 hours until drainage is less than 50 cc in 24 hours.

Some surgeons recommend abdominal binders to improve support of the abdominal wall in obese patients. However, this practice is unstudied and of questionable benefit for pain control or hernia prevention. Primarily, closed incisions should be kept clean and dry. Showers or sponge baths beginning on the second postoperative day can facilitate hygiene by clearing peri-incisional debris, which may contain a high bacterial inoculum, as reepithelialization occurs within the first 24 hours after surgery. Although exact data is lacking, skin staples/skin sutures are generally removed 3–10 days after surgery. Some surgeons prefer delayed staple/skin suture removal (10–14 days after surgery) in patients at increased risk of superficial skin separation such as those who are obese, radiated, malnourished, immunosupressed, or diabetic.

Follow-Up

After hysterectomy, patients are generally seen in an outpatient setting 1–2 weeks after surgery. Staples or skin staples are removed if still in place, intestinal function assessed, signs and symptoms of infection investigated, and, finally, results of surgical and pathological findings reviewed. Patients who require wound or drain care (including suprapubic catheters) should be seen weekly until wound or drain care is discontinued. Six weeks after surgery, the vaginal cuff is examined and patients are generally released to return to work unless complications have occurred.

SURGICAL COMPLICATIONS

Complications following radical hysterectomy are not uncommon, the most frequent of which is a urinary tract infection, short-term, occurring approximately 8% of the time, probably because of the need for an indwelling urinary catheter.[13] However, the most common long-term complication following radical hysterectomy is bladder dysfunction with a wide incidence (8%–80%) depending on how thoroughly it is assessed.[98] Fortunately, the incidence of the major complications of radical hysterectomy are decreasing, including hemorrhage, infections, lymphocysts, and ureteral fistulas.[5]

> *Postoperative bladder dysfunction.* The pathophysiology of this occurrence is believed to be due to the partial interruption of the autonomic fibers that innervate the bladder and other pelvic organs during a radical pelvic dissection. It occurs more commonly with the more radical dissections. In one small series, long-term bladder abnormalities were discovered in 76% of patients after a type IV radical hysterectomy although only 29% of them reported any symptoms.[98] Interestingly, in 210 patients who had urodynamic studies prior to radical hysterectomy for cervical cancer in a separate series, only 17% had normal findings. Forty-five percent of the patients had bladder storage

dysfunction and 51% had urinary incontinence.[99] Two types of dysfunctional abnormalities can be seen after radical hysterectomy: a hypertonic bladder with elevated urethral pressure and, less commonly, a hypotonic bladder that carries a much worse prognosis with a higher need for self-catheterization.[100] In the immediate postoperative period, voiding dysfunctions are common and the bladder should be drained for at least a week, as 69% of patients are able to void by that time.[88] Urodynamic evaluations are helpful in the early diagnosis and management of patients with bladder dysfunction after radical hysterectomy. In one series, 46 women who underwent radical hysterectomy had both pre- and postoperative urodynamic evaluations. Decreased bladder compliance and detrusor function are commonly found in these patients.[101] The patient usually complains of the loss of sensation to void and difficulty emptying the bladder. Although the majority of bladder dysfunctions resolve on their own, usually within 3 weeks, as patients compensate for their sensory and motor loss, some do not, and the patients require either prolonged bladder drainage or preferably self-catheterization. Once PVR (<75 mL) and voiding (150–400 mL) volumes are normal, bladder catheterization or drainage can be discontinued.

Medications have been used to try and diminish the magnitude of bladder dysfunction. In a randomized, double-blind, placebo-controlled study of 79 cervical cancer patients after radical hysterectomy, Madeiro et al. showed that there was significant improvement in a variety of parameters including higher maximum flow rates and lower PVR volumes in patients who received bethanacol and cisapride compared to a placebo[102] (**Level I**). In a separate study of 64 patients receiving early rehabilitative treatment with kinesitherapy and/or pharmacological therapy after bladder catheter removal, 91% of 50 symptomatic patients had satisfactory functional recovery of the bladder activity.[103] Whether rehabilitative techniques such as kinesitherapy and pharmacological therapy are beneficial still needs further investigation.

Sexual function after radical hysterectomy. This continues to be an area of great controversy. Radical surgery with subsequent damage to the hypogastric plexus of nerves may be associated with changes in vaginal function and anatomy that lead to sexual dysfunction. In one large Swedish case-controlled study, women treated for early-stage cervical reported more problems with insufficient vaginal lubrication, elasticity, and vaginal shortening, as well as more dyspareunia than controls who did not have cancer.[104] Interestingly, the frequency of orgasm was similar in the two groups. This is in contrast to other small series that did not show any major changes.[105] The incidence and extent of these complications have been thought to correlate directly with patient age, primary tumor size, extent of surgery, and possibly the use of adjuvant postoperative radiotherapy, although these claims have not been substantiated.

In an attempt to decrease some of the complications associated with radical hysterectomy, some authors have described a nerve-sparing radical hysterectomy that preserves the function of the hypogastric nerve.[106, 107] The hypogastric nerve was identified and preserved below the ureter and lateral to the uterosacral ligament. The nerve plexus was retracted laterally to allow dissection of the parametrium and it was again avoided with careful dissection of the posterior vesicouterine ligament. There are many modifications of this technique; the survival results of one large series are comparable to the traditional radical hysterectomy results with less morbidity.[108] Although the procedure is feasible, it is more difficult in obese patients or in those with bulky tumors. Despite the many small series showing efficacy and less morbidity, more data is needed to substantiate its role in the treatment of cervical cancer. Other issues and potential approaches are discussed further in Chapter 18.

Other urologic complications. Patients undergoing radical hysterectomy are also at increased risk of urinary tract fistula formation; although, the exact incidence is not known as most cases are not reported. Vesicovaginal fistulas occur in about 1% and ureterovaginal fistulas occur in about 2% of patients after radical hysterectomy.[5] In a recent large series of 536 women who underwent radical hysterectomy, the incidence of intraoperative injury to the ureter and the bladder were 1.3% and 1.5%, respectively. Postoperative ureterovaginal and vesicovaginal fistulas were reported in 2.4% and 2.6%, respectively.[109] Factors associated with these complications included obesity, diabetes, postoperative surgical infections, and stage of disease.

When bladder injuries are recognized and immediately repaired, the potential for long-term sequelae is low. Unfortunately, early recognition is not always feasible. Late recognition of bladder damage usually is associated with a vesicovaginal fistula that appears 3–12 days postoperatively, with urine leaking through the vagina. Bladder damage can be avoided during radical hysterectomy with careful dissection of the bladder from the uterine cervix and upper vagina, and safe retraction of the bladder during vaginal closure. Once a vesicovaginal fistula is suspected, the diagnosis can often be readily made by filling the bladder with a dilute solution of blue fluid (methylene blue in saline) and inspecting the vaginal wall and cuff for leakage. Cystoscopy may also be helpful in determining the site and anatomic location of the fistula. In addition, cystoscopy is important because foreign material, such as sutures in the bladder, can be removed during this procedure, perhaps accelerating spontaneous healing. When a fistula is not immediately obvious, a tampon may be placed in the vagina after methylene blue solution has been instilled into the bladder. After allowing the patient to walk for 10–15 minutes, staining of the upper portion of the tampon is highly suggestive of a vesicovaginal fistula. If the tampon is not stained blue, but the patient remains wet, a ureterovaginal fistula is suspected. A ureterovaginal fistula may also be diagnosed in the office by having the patient take oral phenazopyridine, which stains the urine orange and can be detected on the upper portion of a tampon. It can also be diagnosed with an intravenous pyelogram (IVP) or by retrograde pyelography.

The timing of fistula repair is an area of great controversy. In the past, many recommended delayed repair of a vesicovaginal fistula for a few months after discovery to allow maturation of the fistulous tract. Cure rates are approximately 90% with delayed repair.[110] In addition, delayed surgical closure permits a trial of spontaneous healing with the use of continuous bladder drainage. This has been shown to be successful in select patients with small fistulas. When surgical repair is necessary, repair may be accomplished using either a vaginal or an abdominal approach, although vaginal is the preferred in 90% of cases, and either an open or endourologic approach with similar results.[110, 111] The type of repair, whether immediate or delayed, has comparable results as well, 87% vs. 90%, respectively.[111] However, the authors did caution that patients with fistulas after radical hysterectomies were more likely to have poor outcomes than fistulas after other gynecologic procedures.

Of all injuries to the urinary tract, those involving the ureter are the most difficult to recognize and produce the most serious complications. Ureteral injuries generally occur at four locations during gynecologic surgery: (1) at or above the infundibulo-pelvic ligament and near the pelvic brim (this can occur during infundibulo-pelvic ligament ligation or during an aortic lymphadenectomy); (2) in the base of the broad ligament where the ureter passes beneath the uterine vessels (this site of ureteral injury is more common when the ureter is dissected out of the cardinal ligament during a radical hysterectomy); (3) along the lateral pelvic sidewall just above the uterosacral ligaments (this site of ureteral injury is most common when a pelvic lymphadenectomy is performed or when the rectovaginal septum is developed during a radical hysterectomy); and (4) the site where the ureter leaves the cardinal ligament and enters the bladder (this site of injury can occur with both an extrafascial and radical hysterectomy). Ureteral injuries can occur for a variety of reasons (Table 9.2).

The displacement of the ureter by cervical or intraligamentous tumors, inflammatory exudates in the base of the broad ligament, previous pelvic irradiation, endometriosis, postoperative adhesions, and retroperitoneal masses all predispose to ureteral injury.[112]

Ureteral injuries are almost always avoided during extrafascial hysterectomy when dissection is accomplished immediately adjacent to the cervix medial to the ureter. A radical hysterectomy requires complete dissection of the terminal ureter potentially compromising the ureteral blood supply that leads to ischemia and necrosis. Even though meticulous dissection is essential, it does not completely protect against this injury. As in bladder injuries, intraoperative recognition and immediate repair are critical to fistula prevention. If the ureteral sheath is traumatized during radical hysterectomy, placement of a semipermanent ureteral catheter for a

Table 9.2   Types of Ureteral Injuries in Pelvic Surgery

A crushing injury from misapplication of surgical clamps
Ligation with suture
Thermal injury from surgical energy devices
Ischemia with stripping of the ureteral adventitia and devascularization
Transection (either partial or complete)
Angulation with secondary, partial, or complete obstruction
Resection of a segment of ureter as part of radical pelvic surgery for cancer

few weeks should be considered while revascularization of the ureter takes place. Perioperative, retroperitoneal, closed suction drains can be used when ureteral damage is suspected, not only to identify but also to prevent urinoma formation. When the ureter has been partially or completely divided or is so devitalized by suture or clamping that necrosis is likely to occur, more aggressive management is indicated. The appropriate repair for a severely injured ureter depends on the level of the ureteral injury in the pelvis, the length of the segment traumatized or removed, the mobility of the ureter and bladder, the quality of the pelvic tissues, the condition for which the operation is being performed, and the general condition and anticipated lifetime of the patient. When possible, direct reimplantation of the ureter, a ureteroneocystostomy, is the preferred method. When injury to the pelvic ureter is so extensive that the proximal ureter cannot be brought to the bladder without tension, several techniques are available to reduce the ureteral-vesical gap. These include the Boari bladder flap tube technique and the psoas muscle hitch. If the ureter is transected above the pelvic brim, the preferred method is either a ureteroureterostomy or the interposition of an intestinal segment between the injured ureter and the bladder[112].

When a ureteral injury is not recognized at the time of operation, it can usually be demonstrated using an IVP, computerized tomography with contrast, or retrograde radiographic studies. Once identified, the initial step in management of a ureteral injury is urinary diversion, preferably with a ureteral stent. Retrograde urography allows more accurate delineation of the precise anatomy and can be performed in combination with retrograde ureteral stent placement. If a stent can be successfully placed, the ureter will generally heal spontaneously in the absence of previous radiation. The catheter should be left in place for 14–28 days to allow the ureter to heal without stricture formation. After stent removal, a follow-up urogram or ultrasound should be performed at 4- to 6-week intervals to rule out hydronephrosis and stricture. If a ureteral catheter does not pass the obstruction during cystoscopy, ureteroscopy may be considered in an attempt to save an open operative procedure.[113] Otherwise, either immediate ureteral repair or percutaneous nephrostomy should be performed to preserve remaining renal function. When percutaneous nephrostomy is successful, definite surgery may be deferred for 6–12 weeks as many ureteral injuries will resolve with percutaneous nephrostomy alone. Moreover, antegrade ureteral stent placement through the percutaneous nephrostomy may promote spontaneous healing.[114]

Controversy exists as to the management of ureteral obstruction secondary to ureteral ligation discovered in the immediate postoperative period. Early (48–72 hours after surgery) repair (usually ureteroneocystostomy) is favored by many clinicians as this may be accomplished before inflammation and scarring occur. Certainly, surgery should be delayed in the patient with significant pelvic infection or in any patient whose medical status is compromised and in whom surgery for ureteral obstruction might pose a significant threat.

Lymphedema and lymphocysts. Lymphedema is a late and quite disabling complication of radical hysterectomy specifically related to the pelvic lymphadenectomy. It has been reported to occur in up to 25% of patients.[115] In another series of 233 patients having a pelvic lymphadenectomy, 20.2% developed lymphedema.[116] The onset of swelling was 53% by 3 months, 71% by

6 months, and 84% by 1 year. Just as in other studies, the addition of radiation postoperatively also increased the risk of lymphedema. Lymphocysts are also a common occurrence after pelvic lymphadenectomy occurring 44% of the time in one series.[117] Fortunately, the majority (81%) resolve on their own within 1 year.

Pulmonary embolism. Although the incidence of pulmonary embolism is only 1% after radical hysterectomy, it is the most common cause of perioperative mortality.[5] The presence of cancer, pelvic surgery, and even advanced age make the gynecologic oncology patient high risk for VTE complications. A recent systematic review enforced that all gynecologic oncology surgical patients should receive VTE prophylaxis.[78] They did not see any difference between heparin, low molecular weight heparin, and sequential compression devices. They are all effective and no method was superior to the other.

LESS INVASIVE THERAPIES FOR EARLY STAGE CERVICAL CANCER

Sentinel Node Identification

The concept of sentinel node identification for cervical cancer was introduced by Dargent in 2000.[118] Since then, several have been successful in identifying a sentinel node using a combination of a radiolabeled colloid (technetium-99m) and blue dye injected into the cervix preoperatively.[119, 120] The accuracy of the sentinel node predicting lymph node status was 94% in one series.[120] A recent review identified 831 women who had lymphatic mapping as part of their treatment for cervical cancer. A sentinel node was identified 90% of the time with a false negative rate of 8% and a negative predictive value over 97%.[121] The results of large randomized trials in this area will soon shed light on the future of this technology in cervical cancer.

Laparoscopic Lymph Node Staging

Until recently, the whole concept that surgical staging of cervical cancer improved survival was unproven. However, patients with surgically proven negative nodes had a better survival than patients with negative nodes evaluated radiographically.[27] The surgically staged patients had a better 4-year progression-free survival (48.9% vs. 36.3%) and a better overall survival (54.3% vs. 40%) compared to patients who had radiographic evaluation of their para-aortic nodes. Although several have proposed laparoscopic staging in cervical cancer, the theoretical advantages of this procedure have not been proven.[122]

Radical Vaginal Hysterectomy

The traditional radical vaginal hysterectomy described by Shauta was compared to the radical abdominal hysterectomy by Roy et al.[123] They described less febrile morbidity and comparable outcomes. With the rising use of laparoscopic surgery, the operation has been replaced by the laparoscopic assisted radical vaginal hysterectomy that has the added advantage of lymph node dissection. Although shorter hospital stays and less blood loss have been reported, without compromising survival, more data is required to truly assess the utility of this procedure.[124, 125]

Total Laparoscopic Radical Hysterectomy

Because of the advances in equipment and surgical technique, the traditional type III radical hysterectomy can now be done completely laparoscopically.[126] The authors report less morbidity, blood loss, and shorter hospital stays with comparable outcomes to the more traditional operation after a short follow-up. In a case-controlled fashion, the same institution compared total laparoscopic hysterectomy with radical abdominal hysterectomy and also noted reduced operative blood loss, postoperative infectious morbidity, and postoperative length of stay without sacrificing the size of radical hysterectomy specimen margins; however, total laparoscopic radical hysterectomy was associated with increased operative time.[127]

Robotic Radical Hysterectomy

The first robot-assisted radical hysterectomy was described in 2003.[128] Since then, a recent report comparing robotic, laparoscopic, and abdominal radical hysterectomies in a matched fashion confirmed the decrease in blood loss and length of hospital stay associated with both robotic and laparoscopic radical hysterectomies compared to abdominal radical hysterectomy.[129] The number of lymph nodes and recurrence rates were similar between the three groups but robotic surgery was associated with a shorter operative time compared to laparoscopy. In a separate series from the University of North Carolina, a case-controlled design was used to compare 51 robotic radical hysterectomies to 49 abdominal radical hysterectomies.[130] In this series operative blood loss, operative time, hospital stay, and lymph node counts all favored the robotic approach. Although the advantages of robotic surgery, which include three-dimensional vision, 7 degrees of intra-abdominal articulation, motion scaling, and tremor reduction, make it a popular alternative, more data is required to define its role in the treatment of early stage cervical cancer.

Fertility-Preserving Surgery in Early Stage Cervical Cancer

One surgical alternative for the early stage patient with desires for future fertility is the radical trachelectomy. Over 900 cases have been reported in the worldwide literature, with most of them accomplished vaginally (RVT), usually with a laparoscopic pelvic lymphadenectomy, and the rest abdominally.[131] There have been over 300 pregnancies reported with 196 live births and a 10% prematurity rate before 32 weeks.

Recurrences have been reported in 4% of patients. In a single institution series from Toronto, 90 patients who underwent RVT and laparoscopic pelvic lymphadenectomy were compared to a matched series of radical abdominal hysterectomies (RAH) with similar characteristics. The mean operating time was the same between the two groups although the RVT group experienced more intraoperative complications (13% vs. 2%, $p < 0.01$).[132] As expected, blood loss and hospital stay also favored the RVT group. The 5-year recurrence-free survival rates were comparable between the two groups, 95% vs. 100% for RVT vs. RAH, respectively. These authors use a conservative limit of less than 2 cm lesion size as their cutoff. In a separate series by Dargent, 82 patients underwent RVT and there were three recurrences all in the 21 patients with lesions greater than 2 cm.[133] As such, most consider lesion size greater than 2 cm associated with a higher risk of recurrence. Because the radical trachelectomy allows for preservation of the uterus and the potential for reproduction, the RVT is a viable alternative for the young woman with early stage cancer who still wants to preserve fertility.

MANAGEMENT OF COEXISTING PREGNANCY AND CERVICAL CANCER

Carcinoma of the cervix is the most frequently diagnosed malignancy during pregnancy with approximately 1% of all cervical cancers diagnosed in pregnant women.[134] In a large series from the University of Southern California it complicated an estimated 1.2 cases per 10,000 pregnancies, representing 27 cases of cervical cancer during pregnancy at a single institution with a predominant Latina population; 24 out of 27 were Latinas.[135] When deciding on therapy for these malignant neoplasms, one must consider the extent of the disease, the patient's attitude toward pregnancy termination, and the gestational age of the fetus. The preponderance of the existing evidence suggests that pregnancy does not have a detrimental effect on prognosis from accelerated tumor growth.[134–136]

Vaginal bleeding is the most common symptom seen in carcinoma of the cervix in both the pregnant as well as the nonpregnant woman. Unfortunately, this symptom usually appears only among those with advanced disease. Because most cervical cancers in pregnancy are early stage lesions, 20%–30% of the pregnant patients with invasive cervical carcinoma are asymptomatic at the time of diagnosis.[13,137] The methods for screening, diagnosis, and treatment of dysplasia and cervical cancer in the pregnant or postpartum woman are the same as in the nonpregnant patient. Frequently, a careful physical examination including visual inspection and cervical biopsy are sufficient to diagnose this malignancy.

Fortunately, the Pap smear is as sensitive and accurate in detecting cervical neoplasia during pregnancy as in the nonpregnant state as half of cervical cancers in asymptomatic pregnant patients will be detected through Pap smear screening.[137] All Pap smears in pregnancy suggesting a high grade abnormality should be investigated with physical examination and colposcopy. If invasion is suspected, a colposcopically directed biopsy should be performed. Cervical biopsies are safe during pregnancy and have not been associated with an increased incidence of pregnancy loss. An

ECC, however, should be avoided. If the cytologic and colposcopic impression only suggest intraepithelial neoplasia (CIN), the pregnancy should be allowed to continue anticipating a vaginal delivery if indicated. Further evaluation can be postponed until 6 weeks postpartum when the affects of pregnancy on the cervix have resolved. Occasionally, a Pap smear and/or colposcopic examination will only suggest CIN but the entire transformation zone will not be visualized. This examination is unsatisfactory and frequently occurs in the first trimester. Repeat colposcopy in the second trimester generally allows eversion of the endocervix making colposcopy more satisfactory and allowing complete visualization of the transformation zone and cervical lesion.

Only lesions suggestive of invasion require biopsy in pregnancy. Similarly, cone biopsy can generally be avoided in pregnancy and should be performed only if invasive disease is suspected or the extent of an early microinvasive lesion requires further evaluation for treatment planning. When performed, a "coin" rather than a cone biopsy can usually be performed safely without interrupting the pregnancy.[5]

Once the diagnosis of cervical cancer has been established in pregnancy, treatment planning is similar to the nonpregnant patient as described above. However, a delay in treatment may be considered until fetal viability in selected cases. Such a delay, may, in theory, allow cancer progression and worsen prognosis, but this has not been substantiated by the limited case series[134–138] (**Level II-2**). Strong consideration to a short delay in therapy should be given if the diagnosis of cancer is made after 24 weeks but before fetal viability and lung maturity (approximately 33–36 weeks gestation) in an attempt to avoid neonatal morbidity associated with premature delivery. Using this approach, the maximum delay in treatment would only be 12 weeks (24–36 weeks) and would generally be expected to be much shorter. Nevertheless, any decision to delay treatment should be thoroughly discussed with the patient and partner focusing on risks to the mother and the fetus.[13]

The treatment of a stage Ia1 cervical cancer diagnosed by cervical conization with negative margins is fairly straightforward. The pregnancy can be allowed to progress and anticipate a vaginal delivery once the cone bed has healed. Cases of patients with more advanced disease and less than 20 weeks gestation are more complex but they should be encouraged to proceed with treatment for the cancer without delay, as delay at this point in the pregnancy can be prolonged. Patients at 28 weeks gestation or greater should be encouraged to wait for fetal lung maturity prior to delivery and then treat their cancer.[13] The cases of patients between 20 and 28 weeks of gestation with greater than Ia1 cervical cancers are more complicated. Although there is no proven change in prognosis with delay, each case needs to be individualized and all factors taken into consideration.[135–139] If the patient's cancer is amenable to radical hysterectomy, it should be performed with pelvic lymphadenectomy after a planned classical cesarean delivery or with the fetus *in situ* prior to viability.

Radiation therapy is equally efficacious to surgery in treating patients with early stage cervical cancer in pregnancy and the treatment of choice in more advanced stages. It should be performed before fetal viability as it will usually induce abortion. If abortion does not occur, surgical evacuation of the uterus with hysterotomy must be performed prior to proceeding on with brachytherapy. This at least allows for the surgical evaluation of lymph nodes. If an advanced cancer is detected in the later stages of pregnancy and/or a radical hysterectomy with pelvic lymphadenectomy is not performed at the time of cesarean section, whole-pelvic irradiation my begin immediately after the cesarean incision has healed and intracavitary irradiation can follow completion of the whole-pelvic irradiation.

URETERAL OBSTRUCTION

The patient with bilateral ureteral obstruction and uremia secondary to the extension of cervical cancer presents a serious dilemma for the clinician. Management should be divided into two subsets of patients: those who have not received prior radiation therapy and those who have recurrent disease after pelvic irradiation.

The patient with bilateral ureteral obstruction from untreated cancer or from recurrent pelvic disease after surgical therapy should consider some form of urinary diversion followed by appropriate radiation therapy. Because the salvage rate in this clinical situation is low, supportive care alone allowing progressive uremia and demise should also be considered as an alternative to more aggressive therapy in certain cases. If aggressive management is selected, the patients will live longer but require placement of retrograde ureteral stents using cystoscopy if possible. If not, a percutaneous nephrostomy followed by antegrade stent placement is a reasonable alternative.[140–142] Another option is surgical urinary diversion such as a urinary conduit, connecting both ureters into an isolated loop of ileum (Bricker procedure) or creating a continent pouch from a segment of bowel.[143]

The case of a patient with bilateral ureteral obstruction following a full dose of pelvic radiation therapy is a more complicated problem. Less than 5% of these patients will have obstruction caused by radiation fibrosis, and often this group is difficult to identify.[144] In order to identify patients whose obstruction is a result of recurrent disease, an examination under anesthesia, cystoscopy, and proctoscopy with multiple biopsies is recommended. When recurrent cancer is absent, simple diversion of the urinary stream can be lifesaving, and therefore all patients must be considered as possibly belonging to this category until recurrent malignancy is found.

When the presence of recurrent disease has been unequivocally established as the cause of bilateral ureteral obstruction, the decision process becomes somewhat philosophical. Numerous studies suggest that "useful life" is not achieved by urinary diversion in this subset of patients.[143,145,146] One series reported on 47 cases (5 with cervical cancer) with ureteral obstruction secondary to advanced pelvic malignancy. The average survival time was 5.3 months, with only 50% of the patients alive at 3 months and only 22.7% alive at 6 months. After the diversion, 63.8% of the survival time was spent in the hospital.[145] A separate study reported on a group of patients with recurrent pelvic cancer and renal failure who underwent urinary conduit diversion with no increase in survival time.[143] Some suggest that these patients should not undergo urinary diversion, as a more preferable terminal course (i.e., uremia) is thereby eliminated from the patient's options. Obviously, these decisions should be made in consultation with the family and with the patient if possible. When urinary diversion is performed, other clinical manifestations of recurrent pelvic cancer (i.e., severe pelvic pain, repeated infections, and hemorrhage) are frequently encountered leading to increased suffering. Pain control and progressive cachexia are major management problems. Episodes of massive pelvic hemorrhage are associated with difficult decisions for transfusion as well. An extension of the inpatient hospital stay is inevitable, and the financial impact on the patient and her family can be considerable.

REFERENCES

1. WAGGONER SE. Cervical cancer. Lancet 2003;361:2217–2225.
2. American Cancer Society. Global Cancer Facts & Figures 2007.
3. JEMAL A, SIEGEL R, WARD E, et al. Cancer statistics, 2008. CA Cancer J Clin 2008;58:71–96.
4. SUNG H, KEARNEY KA, MILLER M, et al. Papanicolau smear history and diagnosis of invasive cervical carcinoma among members of a large prepaid health plan. Cancer 2000;88:2283–2289.
5. DISAIA PJ, CREASMAN WT. Invasive cervical cancer. In: DISAIA PJ, CREASMAN WT, editors. Clinical Gynecologic Oncology. St. Louis: Mosby; 2007.
6. WRIGHT TC, SCHIFFMAN M. Adding a test for human papillomavirus DNA to cervical-cancer screening. NEJM 2003;348:489–490.
7. MESTWERDT G. Die Fruhdiagnose des Kollumkarzinoms. Zentralbl Gynakol 1947;69:198–202.
8. OSTÖR AG. Studies on 200 cases of early squamous cell carcinoma of the cervix. Int J Gynecol Pathol 1993;12:193–207.
9. PRENDIVILLE W. Large loop excision of the transformation zone. Clin Obstet Gynecol 1995;38:622–639.
10. BENNETT BB, STONE IK, ANDERSON CD, et al. Deep loop excision for prehysterectomy endocervical evaluation. Am J Obstet Gynecol 1997;176:82–86.
11. HOFFMAN MS, COLLINS E, ROBERTS WS, et al. Cervical conization with frozen section before planned hysterectomy. Obstet Gynecol 1993;82:394–398.
12. WOODFORD HD, POSTON W, ELKINS TE. Reliability of the frozen section in sharp knife cone biopsy of the cervix. J Reprod Med 1986;31:951–953.
13. BEREK JS, HACKER NF. Cervical cancer. In: BEREK JS, HACKER NF, editors. Practical Gynecologic Oncology. Philadelphia, PA: Lippincott, Williams & Wilkins; 2005.
14. ROMAN LD, FELIX JC, MUDERSPACH LI, et al. Risk of residual invasive disease in women with microinvasive squamous cancer in a conization specimen. Obstet Gynecol 1997;90:759–764.
15. ELLIOTT P, COPPLESON M, RUSSELL P, et al. Early invasive (FIGO stage IA) carcinoma of the cervix: a clinico-pathologic study of 476 cases. Int J Gynecol Cancer 2000;10:42–52.
16. BISSELING KC, BEKKERS RL, ROME RM, et al. Treatment of microinvasive adenocarcinoma of the uterine cervix: a retrospective study and review of the literature. Gynecol Oncol 2007;107:424–430.
17. OSTÖR AG. Early invasive adenocarcinoma of the uterine cervix. Int J Gynecol Pathol 2000;19:29–38.
18. WEBB JC, KEY CR, QUALLS CR, et al. Population-based study of microinvasive adenocarcinoma of the uterine cervix. Obstet Gynecol 2001;97:701–706.
19. LANDONI F, MANEO A, COLOMBO A, et al. Randomised study of radical surgery versus radiotherapy for stage Ib–IIa cervical cancer. Lancet 1997;350:535–540.
20. LAWTON FG, HACKER NF. Surgery for invasive gynecologic cancer in the elderly female population. Obstet Gynecol 1990;76:287–291.
21. PETERS WA III, LIU PY, BARRETT RJ II, et al. Concurrent chemotherapy and pelvic radiation therapy compared with pelvic radiation therapy alone as adjuvant therapy after radical surgery in high-risk early-stage cancer of the cervix. J Clin Oncol 2000;18:1606–1613.
22. SEDLIS A, BUNDY BN, ROTMAN MZ, et al. A randomized trial of pelvic radiation therapy versus no further therapy in selected patients with stage IB carcinoma of the cervix after radical hysterectomy and pelvic lymphadenectomy: a Gynecologic Oncology Group study. Gynecol Oncol 1999;73:177–183.

23. KRIDELKA FJ, BERG DO, NEUMAN M, et al. Adjuvant small field pelvic radiation for patients with high risk, stage IB lymph node negative cervix carcinoma after radical hysterectomy and pelvic lymph node dissection. A pilot study. Cancer 1999;86:2059–2065.

24. ROSE PG, BUNDY BN, WATKINS EB, et al. Concurrent cisplatin-based radiotherapy and chemotherapy for locally advanced cervical cancer. N Engl J Med 1999;340:1144–1153.

25. MORRIS M, EIFEL PJ, LU J, et al. Pelvic radiation with concurrent chemotherapy compared with pelvic and para-aortic radiation for high-risk cervical cancer. N Engl J Med 1999;340: 1137–1143.

26. WHITNEY CW, SAUSE W, BUNDY BN, et al. Randomized comparison of fluorouracil plus cisplatin versus hydroxyurea as an adjunct to radiation therapy in stage IIB–IVA carcinoma of the cervix with negative para-aortic nodes: a Gynecologic Oncology Group and Southwest Oncology Group study. J Clin Oncol 1999;17:1339–1348.

27. GOLD MA, TIAN C, WHITNEY CW, et al. Surgical versus radiographic determination of para-aortic lymph node metastases before chemoradiation for locally advanced cervical carcinoma: a Gynecologic Oncology Group study. Cancer 2008;112:1954–1963.

28. ROH JW, SEO SS, LEE S, et al. Role of positron emission tomography in pretreatment lymph node staging of uterine cervical cancer: a prospective surgicopathologic correlation study. Eur J Cancer 2006;41:2086–2092.

29. MOTA F, De OLIVEIRA C. Patients with locally advanced cervical cancer should not undergo routine pretreatment surgical staging. Eur J Gynaecol Oncol 2006;27:109–114.

30. COSIN JA, FOWLER JM, CHEN MD, et al. Pretreatment surgical staging of patients with cervical carcinoma: the case for lymph node debulking. Cancer 1998;82:2241–2248.

31. HACKER NF, WAIN GV, NICKLIN JL. Resection of bulky positive lymph nodes in patients with cervical cancer. Int J Gynecol Cancer 1995;5:250–256.

32. KIM PY, MONK BJ, CHABRA S, et al. Cervical cancer with paraaortic metastases: significance of residual paraaortic disease after surgical staging. Gynecol Oncol 1998;69:243–247.

33. BRUNSCHWIG A, PIERCE VK. Necropsy findings in patients with carcinoma of the cervix: implications for treatment. Am J Obstet Gynecol 1948;56:1134–1137.

34. BRICKER EM. Bladder substitution after pelvic evisceration. Surg Clin North Am 1950;30:1511–1521.

35. ROWLAND RG, MITCHELL ME, BIHRLE R, et al. Indiana continent urinary reservoir. J Urol 1987;137:1136–1139.

36. LOCKHART JL. Remodeled right colon: an alternative urinary reservoir. J Urol 1987;138:730–734.

37. RUTLEDGE FN, SMITH JP, WHARTON JT, et al. Pelvic exenteration: analysis of 296 patients. Am J Obstet Gynecol 1977;129:881–892.

38. HAVRILESKY LJ, WONG TZ, SECORD AA, et al. The role of PET scanning in the detection of recurrent cervical cancer. Gynecol Oncol 2003;90:186–190.

39. MILLER B, MORRIS M, RUTLEDGE F, et al. Aborted exenterative procedures in recurrent cervical cancer. Gynecol Oncol 1993;50:94–99.

40. DOUGLAS RG, SWEENEY WJ. Exenteration operations in the treatment of advanced pelvic cancer. Am J Obstet Gynecol 1957;73:1169–1182.

41. PARSONS L, FRIEDELL GH. Radical surgical treatment of cancer of the cervix. Proc Natl Cancer Conf 1964;5:241–246.

42. BRUNSCHWIG A. What are the indications and results of pelvic exenteration? JAMA 1965;194:274.

43. KISELOW M, BUTCHER HR, BRICKER EM. Results of the radical surgical treatment of advanced pelvic cancer: a fifteen-year study. Ann Surg 1967;166:428–436.

44. KRIEGER JS, EMBREE HK. Pelvic exenteration. Cleve Clin Q 1969;36:1–8.

45. KETCHAM AS, DECKERS PJ, SUGARBACKER EV, et al. Pelvic exenteration for carcinoma of the uterine cervix: a 15-year experience. Cancer 1970;26:513–521.

46. SYMMONDS RE, PRATT JH, WEBB MJ. Exenterative operations: experience with 198 patients. Am J Obstet Gynecol 1975;121:907–918.

47. AVERETTE HE, LICHTINGER M, SEVIN BU, et al. Pelvic exenteration: a 15-year experience in a general metropolitan hospital. Am J Obstet Gynecol 1984;150:179–184.

48. MORLEY GW, HOPKINS MP, LINDENAUER SM, et al. Pelvic exenteration, University of Michigan: 100 patients at 5 years. Obstet Gynecol 1989;74:934–943.

49. LAWHEAD RA Jr, CLARK DG, SMITH DH, et al. Pelvic exenteration for recurrent or persistent gynecologic malignancies: a 10-year review of the Memorial Sloan-Kettering Cancer Center experience (1972–1981). Gynecol Oncol 1989;33:279–282.

50. SOPER JT, BERCHUCK A, CREASMAN WT, et al. Pelvic exenteration: factors associated with major surgical morbidity. Gynecol Oncol 1989;35:93–98.

51. SHINGLETON HM, SOONG SJ, GELDER MS, et al. Clinical and histopathologic factors predicting recurrence and survival after pelvic exenteration for cancer of the cervix. Obstet Gynecol 1989;73:1027–1034.

52. SHARMA S, ODUNSI K, DRISCOLL D, et al. Pelvic exenteration for gynecological malignancies: twenty-year experience at Roswell Park Cancer Institute. Int J Gynecol Cancer 2005;15: 475–482.

53. GOLDBERG GL, SUKUMVANICH P, EINSTEIN MH, et al. Total pelvic exenteration: the Albert Einstein College of Medicine/Montefiore Medical Center experience (1987 to 2003). Gynecol Oncol 2006;101:261–268.

54. LICHTINGER M, AVERETTE H, GIRTANNER R, et al. Small bowel complications after supravesical urinary diversion in pelvic exenteration. Gynecol Oncol 1986;24:137–142.

55. ORR JW Jr, SHINGLETON HM, HATCH KD, et al. Gastrointestinal complications associated with pelvic exenteration. Am J Obstet Gynecol 1983;145:325–332.

56. MEIGS J. Carcinoma of the cervix: the Wertheim operation. Surg Gynecol Obstet 1944;78:195–199.

57. PIVER MS, RUTLEDGE F, SMITH JP. Five classes of extended hysterectomy for women with cervical cancer. Obstet Gynecol 1974;44:265–272.

58. Wertheim E. The extended abdominal operation for carcinoma uteri (based on 500 operative cases). Am J Obstet 1912;66:169–174.

59. SURI A, FRUMOVITZ M, MILAM MR, et al. Preoperative pathologic findings associated with residual disease at radical hysterectomy in women with stage IA2 cervical cancer. Gynecol Oncol 2009;112:110–113.

60. COVENS A, ROSEN B, MURPHY J, et al. How important is removal of the parametrium at surgery for carcinoma of the cervix? Gynecol Oncol 2002;84:145–149.

61. FLEISHER LA, BECKMAN JA, BROWN KA, et al. ACA/AHA 2007 guidelines on preoperative cardiovascular evaluation and care for noncardiac surgery: a report of the American College of Cardiology/American Heart Association Task Force on Practice Guidelines. J Am Coll Cardiol 2007;50:e159–e242.

62. Task Force on Preanesthesia Evaluation. Practice advisory for preanesthesia evaluation: a report by the American Society of Anesthesiologists Task Force on preanesthesia evaluation. Anesthesiology 2002;96:485–496.

63. KERTAI MD, BOERSMA E, BAX JJ, et al. A meta-analysis comparing the prognostic accuracy of six diagnostic tests for predicting perioperative cardiac risk in patients undergoing major vascular surgery. Heart 2003;89:1327–1334.

64. CHAITMAN BR, MILLER DD. Perioperative cardiac evaluation for noncardiac surgery noninvasive cardiac testing. Prog Cardiovasc Dis 1998;40:405–418.

65. ISHAQ M, KAMAL RS, AQIL M. Value of routine pre-operative chest X-ray in patients over the age of 40 years. JPMA J Pak Med Assoc 1997;47:279–281.

66. RITZ JP, GERMER CT, BUHR HJ. Preoperative routine chest x-ray: expensive and of little value. Langenbecks Arch Chir Suppl Kongressbd 1997;114:1051–1053.

67. LIM EHL, LIU EHC. The usefulness of routine preoperative chest x-rays and ECGs: a prospective audit. Singapore Med J 2003;44:340–343.

68. HUANG WC, YANG JM, YANG YC, et al. Ultrasonographic characteristics and cystoscopic correlates of bladder wall invasion by endophytic cervical cancer. Ultrasound Obstet Gynecol 2006;27: 680–687.

69. BRADY M, KINN S, STUART P. Preoperative fasting for adults to prevent perioperative complications. Cochrane Database Syst Rev 2003;(4):CD004423.

70. TANNER J, WOODINGS D, MONCASTER K. Preoperative hair removal to reduce surgical site infection. Cochrane Database Syst Rev 2006;(3):CD004122.

71. EDWARDS P, LIPP A, HOLMES A. Preoperative skin antiseptics for preventing surgical wound infections after clean surgery (Review). Cochrane Database Syst Rev 2004;(3):CD003949.

72. ROSENSHEIN NB, RUTH JC, VILLAR J, et al. A prospective randomized study of doxycycline as a prophylactic antibiotic in patients undergoing radical hysterectomy. Gynecol Oncol 1983;15: 201–206.

73. ORR JW Jr, SISSON PF, PATSNER B, et al. Single-dose antibiotic prophylaxis for patients undergoing extended pelvic surgery for gynecologic malignancy. Am J Obstet Gynecol 1990;162:718–712.

74. KURZ A, SESSLER DI, LENHARDT R. Perioperative normothermia to reduce the incidence of surgical-wound infection and shorten hospitalization. Study of Wound Infection and Temperature Group [see comments]. N Engl J Med 1996;334:1209–1215.

75. GUENAGA KKFG, ATALLAH ÁN, CASTRO AA, et al. Mechanical bowel preparation for elective colorectal surgery. Cochrane Database Syst Rev 2005;(1):CD001544.

76. SIVANESARATNAM V, SEN DK, JAYALAKSHMI P, et al. Radical hysterectomy and pelvic lymphadenectomy for early invasive cancer of the cervix—14-year experience. Int J Gynecol Cancer 1993;3:231–238.

77. CLARKE-PEARSON DL, JELOVSEK FR, CREASMAN WT. Thromboembolism complicating surgery for cervical and uterine malignancy: incidence, risk factors, and prophylaxis. Obstet Gynecol 1983;61:87–94.

78. EINSTEIN MH, PRITTS EA, HARTENBACH EM. Venous thromboembolism prevention in gynecologic cancer surgery: a systematic review. Gynecol Oncol 2007;105:813–819.

79. MARINO MA, WILLIAMSON E, RAJARAM L, et al. Defining practice patterns in gynecologic oncology to prevent pulmonary embolism and deep venous thrombosis. Gynecol Oncol 2007;106:439–445.

80. JACOBS D, AZAGRA JS, DELAUWER M, et al. Unusual complication after pelvic surgery: unilateral lower limb crush syndrome and bilateral common peroneal nerve paralysis. Acta Anaesthesiol Belg 1992;43:139–143.

81. GOMBAR KK, GOMBAR S, SINGH B, et al. Femoral neuropathy: a complication of the lithotomy position. Reg Anesth 1992;17:306–308.

82. VASILEV SA. Obturator nerve injury: a review of management options. Gynecol Oncol 1994;53:152–155.

83. HELMKAMP BF, KREBS HB, CORBETT SL, et al. Radical hysterectomy: current management guidelines. Am J Obstet Gynecol 1997;177:372–374.

84. LERNER HM, JONES HW III, HILL EC. Radical surgery for the treatment of early invasive cervical carcinoma (stage IB): review of 5 years' experience. Obstet Gynecol 1980;56:413–418.

85. JENSEN JK, LUCCI JA, DI SAIA PJ, et al. To drain or not to drain: a retrospective study of closed-suction drainage following radical hysterectomy with pelvic lymphadenectomy. Gynecol Oncol 1993;51:46–49.

86. BANDY LC, CLARKE-PEARSON DL, SOPER JT, et al. Long-term effects on bladder function following radical hysterectomy with and without postoperative radiation. Gynecol Oncol 1987;26:160–168.

87. HAYASAKI M. Studies on the causes and prophylaxis of urinary tract infection following radical hysterectomy for cervical cancer. Nippon Sanka Fujinka Gakkai Zasshi 1982;34:2185–2194.

88. CHAMBERLAIN DH, HOPKINS MP, ROBERTS JA, et al. The effects of early removal of indwelling urinary catheter after radical hysterectomy. Gynecol Oncol 1991;43:98–102.

89. ELLIS H, MORAN BJ, THOMPSON JN, et al. Adhesion-related hospital readmissions after abdominal and pelvic surgery: a retrospective cohort study. Lancet 1999;353:1476–1480.

90. METWALLY M, WATSON A, LILFORD R, et al. Fluid and pharmacological agents for adhesion prevention after gynaecological surgery. Cochrane Database Syst Rev 2006;(2):CD001298.

91. AHMAD G, DUFFY JMN, FARQUHAR C, et al. Barrier agents for adhesion prevention after gynaecological surgery. Cochrane Database Syst Rev 2008;(2):CD000475.

92. BRISTOW RE, SANTILLAN A, DIAZ-MONTES TP, et al. Prevention of adhesion formation after radical hysterectomy using a sodium hyaluronate–carboxymethylcellulose (HA–CMC) barrier: a cost-effective analysis. Gynecol Oncol 2007;104:739–746.

93. PEARL ML, VALEA FA, FISCHER M, et al. A randomized controlled trial of early postoperative feeding in gynecologic oncology patients undergoing intra-abdominal surgery. Obstet Gynecol 1998;92:94–97.

94. CHUMILLAS S, PONCE JL, DELGADO F, et al. Prevention of postoperative pulmonary complications through respiratory rehabilitation: a controlled clinical study. Arch Phys Med Rehabil 1998;79:5–9.

95. HALL JC, TARALA RA, TAPPER J, et al. Prevention of respiratory complications after abdominal surgery: a randomised clinical trial. BMJ 1996;312:148–152.

96. SOPER DE, BUMP RC, HURT WG. Wound infection after abdominal hysterectomy: effect of the depth of subcutaneous tissue. Am J Obstet Gynecol 1995;173:465–469.

97. GALLUP DC, GALLUP DG, NOLAN TE, et al. Use of a subcutaneous closed drainage system and antibiotics in obese gynecologic patients. Am J Obstet Gynecol 1996;175:358–361.

98. ZULLO MA, MANCI N, ANGIOLI R, et al. Vesical dysfunctions after radical hysterectomy for cervical cancer: a critical review. Crit Rev Oncol Hematol 2003;48:287–293.

99. LIN HH, YU HJ, SHEU BC, et al. Importance of urodynamic study before radical hysterectomy for cervical cancer. Gynecol Oncol 2001;81:270–272.

100. LEE RB, PARK RC. Bladder dysfunction following radical hysterectomy. Gynecol Oncol 1981;11:304–308.

101. SHI HR, YANG XF, WEN JG. Urodynamic study of lower urinary tract function after radical hysterectomy in postoperative women of cervical cancer. Zhonghua Fu Chan Ke ZaZhi 2007;42:815–817.

102. MADEIRO AP, RUFINO AC, SARTORI MG, et al. The effects of bethanechol and cisapride on urodynamic parameters in patients undergoing radical hysterectomy for cervical cancer. A randomized, double-blind, placebo-controlled study. Int Urogynecol J Pelvic Floor Dysfunct 2006;17:248–252.

103. ZANOLLA R, MONZEGLIO C, CAMPO B, et al. Bladder and urethral dysfunction after radical abdominal hysterectomy: rehabilitative treatment. J Surg Oncol 1985;28:190–194.

104. BERGMARK K, AVALL-LUNDQVIST E, DICKMAN PW, et al. Vaginal changes and sexuality in women with a history of cervical cancer. N Engl J Med 1999;340:1383–1389.

105. GRUMANN M, ROBERTSON R, HACKER NF, et al. Sexual functioning in patients following radical hysterectomy for stage IB cancer of the cervix. Int J Gynecol Cancer 2001;11:372–380.

106. SAKAMOTO S, TAKAZAWA K. An improved radical hysterectomy with fewer urological complications and with no loss of therapeutic results for cervical cancer. Bailliers Clin Obstet Gynaecol 1999;2:953–962.

107. TRIMBOS JB, MAAS CP, DERUITER MC, et al. A nerve-sparing radical hysterectomy: guidelines and feasibility in Western patients. Int J Gynecol Cancer 2001;11:180–186.

108. PAPP Z, CSAPÓ Z, HUPUCZI P, et al. Nerve-sparing radical hysterectomy for stage IA2–IIB cervical cancer: 5-year survival of 501 consecutive cases. Eur J Gynaecol Oncol 2006;27:553–560.

109. LIKIC IS, KADIJA S, LADJEVIC NG, et al. Analysis of urologic complications after radical hysterectomy. Am J Obstet Gynecol 2008;199:644.e1–644.e3.

110. AYHAN A, TUNCER ZS, DOGAN L, et al. Results of treatment in 182 consecutive patients with genital fistulas. Int J Gynecol Obstet 1995;48:43–47.

111. GIBERTI C, GERMINALE F, LILLO M, et al. Obstetric and gynaecological ureteric injuries: treatment and results. Br J Urol 1996;77:21–26.

112. ROCK JA, JONES HW III. Operative injuries to the ureter. Vesicovaginal fistula and urethrovaginal fistula. In: ROCK JA, JONES HW III, editors. Te Linde's Operative Gynecology. Philadelphia, PA: Lippincott, Williams & Wilkins; 2008.

113. KOONINGS PP, HUFFMAN JL, SCHLAERTH JB. Uerteroscopy: a new asset in the management of postoperative ureterovaginal fistulas. Obstet Gynecol 1992;80(3):548–549.

114. DOWLING RA, CORRIERE JN Jr, SANDLER CM. Iatrogenic ureteral injury. J Urol 1986;135(5):912–915.

115. BERGMARK K, AVALL-LUNDQVIST E, DICKMAN PW, et al. Lymphedema and bladder-emptying difficulties after radical hysterectomy for early cervical cancer and among population controls. Int J Gynecol Cancer 2006;16:1130–1139.

116. RYAN M, STAINTON C, SLAYTOR EK, et al. Aetiology and prevalence of lower limb lymphoedema following treatment for gynaecological cancer. Aust N Z J Obstet Gynecol 2003;143:148–151.

117. TAM KF, LAM KW, CHAN KK, et al. Natural history of pelvic lymphocysts as observed by ultrasonography after bilateral pelvic lymphadenectomy. Ultrasound Obstet Gynecol 2008;32:87–90.

118. DARGENT D, MARTIN X, MATHEVET P. Laparoscopic assessment of sentinel lymph nodes in early cervical cancer. Gynecol Oncol 2000;79:411–415.

119. LEVENBACK C, COLEMAN RL, BURKE TW, et al. Lymphatic mapping and sentinel node identification in patients with cervix cancer undergoing radical hysterectomy and pelvic lymphadenectomy. J Clin Oncol 2002;20:688–693.

120. SILVA LB, SILVA-FILHO AL, TRAIMAN P, et al. Sentinel node detection in cervical cancer with (99m)Tc-phytate. Gynecol Oncol 2005;97:588–595.

121. FRUMOVITZ M, RAMIREZ PT, LEVENBACK CF. Lymphatic mapping and sentinel lymph node detection in women with cervical cancer. Gynecol Oncol 2008;110:S17–S20.

122. QUERLEU D, LEBLANC E, CASTELAIN B. Laparoscopic pelvic lymphadenectomy in the staging of early carcinoma of the cervix. Am J Obstet Gynecol 1991;164:579–585.

123. ROY M, PLANTE M, RENAUD MC. Laparoscopically assisted vaginal radical hysterectomy. Best Pract Res Clin Obstet Gynaecol 2005;19:377–386.

124. JACKSON KS, DAS N, NAIK R, et al. Laparoscopically assisted radical vaginal hysterectomy vs. Radical abdominal hysterectomy for cervical cancer: a match controlled study. Gynecol Oncol 2004;95:655–661.

125. MORGAN DJ, HUNTER DC, MCCRACKEN G, et al. Is laparoscopically assisted radical vaginal hysterectomy for cervical carcinoma safe? A case control study with follow up. BJOG 2007;114: 537–542.

126. RAMIREZ PT, SLOMOVITZ BM, SOLIMAN PT, et al. Total laparoscopic radical hysterectomy and lymphadenectomy: the M.D. Anderson Cancer Center experience. Gynecol Oncol 2006;102:252–255.

127. FRUMOVITZ M, DOS REIS R, SUN CC, et al. Comparison of total laparoscopic and abdominal radical hysterectomy for patients with early-stage cervical cancer. Obstet Gynecol 2007;110:96–102.

128. SERT BM, ABELER VM. Robotic-assisted laparoscopic radical hysterectomy (Piver type III) with pelvic node dissection—case report. Eur J Gynaecol Oncol 2006;27:531–533.

129. MAGRINA JF, KHO RM, WEAVER AL, et al. Robotic radical hysterectomy: comparison with laparoscopy and laparotomy. Gynecol Oncol 2008;109:86–91.

130. BOGGESS JF, GEHRIG PA, CANTRELL L, et al. A case-controlled study of robot-assisted type III radical hysterectomy with pelvic lymph node dissection compared with open radical hysterectomy. Am J Obstet Gynecol 2008;199:357.e1–357.e7.

131. MILLIKEN DA, SHEPHERD JH. Fertility preserving surgery for carcinoma of the cervix. Curr Opin Oncol 2008;20:575–580.

132. BEINER ME, HAUSPY J, ROSEN B, et al. Radical vaginal trachelectomy vs. radical hysterectomy for small early stage cervical cancer: a matched case-control study. Gynecol Oncol 2008;110:168–171.

133. DARGENT D. Radical trachelectomy: an operation that preserves the fertility of young women with invasive cervical cancer. Bull Acad Natl Med 2001;185:1295–1304.

134. HOSKINS WJ, PEREZ CA, YOUNG RC. Cancer in the pregnant patient. In: HOSKINS WJ, PEREZ CA, YOUNG RC, editors. Principles and Practice of Gynecologic Oncology. Philadelphia, PA: Lippincott, Williams & Wilkins; 2000.

135. DUGGAN B, MUDERSPACH LI, ROMAN LD, et al. Cervical cancer in pregnancy: reporting on planned delay in therapy. Obstet Gynecol 1993;82:598–602.

136. HOPKINS MP, MORLEY GW. The prognosis and management of cervical cancer associated with pregnancy. Obstet Gynecol 1992;80:9–13.

137. CREASMAN WT, RUTLEDGE FN, FLETCHER GH. Carcinoma of the cervix associated with pregnancy. Obstet Gynecol 1970;36:495–501.

138. SOOD AK, SOROSKY JI, KROGMAN S, et al. Surgical management of cervical cancer complicating pregnancy: a case-control study. Gynecol Oncol 1996;63:294–298.

139. SOROSKY JI, SQUATRITO R, NDUBISI BU, et al. Stage I squamous cell cervical carcinoma in pregnancy: planned delay in therapy awaiting feral maturity. Gynecol Oncol 1995;59:207–210.

140. FISHER HA, BENNET AH, RIVARD DJ, et al. Nonoperative supravesical urinary diversion in obstetrics and gynecology. Gynecol Oncol 1982;14:365–372.

141. CARTER J, RAMIREZ C, WAUGH R, et al. Percutaneous urinary diversion in gynecologic oncology. Gynecol Oncol 1991;40:248–252.

142. CODDINGTON CC, THOMAS JR, HOSKINS WJ. Percutaneous nephrostomy for ureteral obstruction in patients with gynecologic malignancy. Gynecol Oncol 1984;18:339–348.

143. DELGATO G. Urinary conduit diversion in advanced gynecologic malignancies. Gynecol Oncol 1978;6:217–222.

144. GRAHAM JB, ABAB RS. Ureteral obstruction due to radiation. Am J Obstet Gynecol 1967;99:409–412.

145. BRIN EN, SCHIFF M, WEISS RM. Palliative urinary diversion for pelvic malignancy. J Urol 1975;113:619–622.

146. TAYLOR PT, ANDERSEN WA. Untreated cervical cancer complicated by obstructive uropathy and oliguric renal failure. Gynecol Oncol 1981;11:162–174.

Chapter 10

Endometrial Cancer

R. Wendel Naumann, MD

INTRODUCTION

Uterine cancer is the most common malignancy arising in the female genital tract and is the second most common cause of death from gynecologic cancers. It is estimated that there were 40,100 new cases of uterine cancer in the United States resulting in 7470 deaths in 2008.[1]

It has long been recognized that excessive estrogens and obesity have been associated with endometrial cancer.[2,3] However, in 1983 Bokhman proposed a hypothesis that there were two distinct types of endometrial cancer.[4] The first and most common type was associated with obesity and is driven by an excess of estrogen as a result of aromatase activity in peripheral adipose tissue. These so called type I endometrial cancers are also associated with mutations in the PTEN tumor suppressor gene and abnormalities in the PI3K pathway. They are generally associated with a good overall prognosis.[5] Type II tumors are felt to develop through a separate pathway of tumorigenesis not associated with excess estrogen. These tumors are clinically much more aggressive and have often spread outside of the uterus at the time of diagnosis. Of these type II tumors, uterine papillary serous carcinoma (UPSC) is the most common subtype. While UPSC accounts for only about 10% of all uterine cancers, it is responsible for almost 40% of deaths from this disease.[6]

Over the past 15 years the incidence of endometrial cancer has climbed from an estimated 31,000 in 1993 to 40,100 in 2008.[1,7] This trend is expected to continue due to increasing obesity rates in the United States. Currently 49 states have obesity rates above 20% (as defined by a BMI of > 30) and three states have obesity rates over 30%.[8] Fortunately, despite the trend in obesity it is notable that the death rate from endometrial cancer has decreased from 4.18 per 100,000 to 4.12 per 100,000 an absolute decrease of 1.4% over a 15-year period.[1,7]

Gynecologic Oncology: Evidence-Based Perioperative and Supportive Care, Second Edition.
Edited by Scott E. Lentz, Allison E. Axtell and Steven A. Vasilev.
© 2011 John Wiley & Sons, Inc. Published 2011 by John Wiley & Sons, Inc.

FAMILIAL GENETIC SYNDROMES

Identifying families who are at increased risk for malignancy offers one of the greatest opportunities to institute increased screening, or in the case of endometrial cancer to undergo prophylactic surgery to prevent these cancers. Genetic predisposition to endometrial cancer has been noted in hereditary non-polyposis colon cancer (HNPCC) syndrome, also known as Lynch syndrome. This syndrome was originally described by Warthin in 1913 in a family that had a very strong history of endometrial and gastrointestinal cancers.[9] It is now known that the increased risk of cancer in the HNPCC syndrome is the result of a germ-line mutation in one of several genes that are responsible for DNA mismatch repair. The three most commonly mutated genes in this family are MLH-1, MSH-2, and MSH-6. The family originally described by Walthin has now been followed for many generations and has been documented with an MSH-2 mutation.[10]

HNPCC-related cancers often occur at a younger age than spontaneous cancers. Carrying an HNPCC mutation increases the lifetime risk of colon cancer to approximately 80%; the lifetime risk of endometrial cancer is reported to be as high as 60%. Other cancers that are increased in HNPCC include brain, stomach, hepatobiliary, small intestine, urinary tract, and ovary (Table 10.1).

Cancers that occur in individuals with an HNPCC mutation can be tested for microsatellite instability. These microsatellites are short tandem repeats of DNA. Because of the repeating nature of these loci, one of the repeat segments can loop and the next repeat can bind the DNA to create a DNA mismatch. Because tumors that as a result of an HNPCC mutation lack efficient DNA mismatch repair, these loops lead to variable length in these microsatellite loci, a phenomenon known as microsatellite instability.[13] An alternate approach to detect HNPCC is direct immunohistochemical staining for MLH-1, MSH-2, and MSH-6.[14] Both of these methods are over 90% sensitive for detecting HNPCC mutations.

Individuals who are less than 50 years of age who develop endometrial cancers should be considered for testing by either MSI or IHC, especially if they are not

Table 10.1 Risk of HNPCC Associated Cancers and Median Age of Onset

Cancer	Population Risk	HNPCC Mutation Risk	Mean Age
Colon	5.5%	80%	44 years
Endometrium	2.7%	20%–60%	46 years
Stomach	<1%	11–19%	56 years
Ovary	1.6%	9%–12%	43 years
Hepatobiliary	<1%	2%–7%	Not reported
Urinary tract	<1%	4%–5%	55 years
Small bowel	<1%	1%–4%	49 years
Brain/CNS	<1%	1%–3%	50 years

Adapted from Reference 11.

Table 10.2   When to Consider Testing Specimens for Microsatellite Instability (MSI) or Immunohistochemistry for MLH-1, MSH-2, or MSH-6 Deficiency

Colorectal cancer in an individual $<$ 50 years old
Presence of synchronous, metachronous colorectal, or other HNPCC associated tumors
Familial colorectal cancer (especially if $<$ 60 years)
HNPCC tumor with one or more first-degree relatives with an HNPCC tumor $<$ 50 years
HNPCC tumor with HNPCC tumors in two or more first- or second-degree relatives

Adapted from Reference 12.

obese or they have a family history of another HNPCC-related cancer (Tables 10.2 and 10.3). If these tests are unavailable, then genetic sequencing can be considered.

Cowden's syndrome is a rare disorder that is associated with a germline mutation in the putative tumor suppressor gene PTEN. This syndrome is associated with hamartomas as well as an increase in thyroid, breast, glioblastoma, and prostate cancers.[15] Because somatic mutations of PTEN are common in endometrial cancer, it was felt that germline PTEN mutations might also be associated with an elevated risk of endometrial cancer.[16] It does appear that there is some increased risk of endometrial cancer in women with Cowden's syndrome.[17] However, a retrospective review of over 200 endometrial cancers revealed no germ-line mutations in PTEN. This would at least suggest that germ-line mutations of PTEN are at most a rare cause of endometrial cancer.[16]

PRECURSOR LESIONS

It is currently believed that most cases of endometrial cancer begin with excessive hormonal stimulation leading to the development of endometrial hyperplasia preceding the diagnosis of malignancy. The current classification of endometrial hyperplasia is based on cytologic architecture (simple vs. complex) and the presence or absence of nuclear atypia.[18] In his series looking at the results of untreated patients, Kurman noted that nuclear atypia represented a greater risk of progressing to endometrial cancer than cytologic architecture. For women with both cytologic architecture

Table 10.3   Mutation Prevalence Based on Family History

	Family History (at least one first- or second-degree relative)	
	Negative	Positive
Colorectal cancer $\leq$ 50 years	7.2%	27.5%
Colorectal cancer $>$ 50 years	4.4%	14.1%
Endometrial cancer $\leq$ 50 years	7.0%	29.9%
Other HNPCC cancer	3.6%	14.3%
$\geq$ 2 HNPCC cancers	8.8%	45.8%

Adapted from Reference 11.

and nuclear atypia, the risk of developing endometrial cancer without treatment was 29%.[18]

The reproducibility distinguishing between hyperplasia and endometrial cancer has been reported to be relatively high among expert pathologists. However, there is substantial discordance in the diagnosis of the atypical hyperplasia suggesting this can be a difficult diagnosis.[19, 20] The discordance rate may be even higher outside of expert centers. This fact was highlighted in a recent report from the Gynecologic Oncology Group suggesting that the GOG pathologists agreed with the referring diagnosis of atypical endometrial hyperplasia only 38% of the time with a kappa value of only 0.28.[21] Agreement between the three expert pathologists was also poor with a kappa value of 0.40. The most common missed diagnosis in patients referred with atypical endometrial hyperplasia is endometrial cancer in 29% of cases. An additional 18% were noted to have simple hyperplasia and 7% had normal, cycling endometrium. There has been an increased interest in simplifying hyperplastic lesions into the benign hyperplasia associated with increased hormonal stimulation and endometrial intraepithelial carcinoma, which would represent a clonal proliferation that is felt to be premalignant but adoption of this system has not been widespread.[22]

In contrast to the type I endometrial cancers which are slow growing and related to excessive estrogen, UPSC appears to have a rapid progression from an intraepithelial process to a malignant state with extrauterine spread often occurring prior to the development of myometrial invasion or clinical symptoms. Precursor lesions of UPSC tumors have only recently been described. Although UPSC tumors can contain hormone receptors, more than 90% of these tumors arise in a background of atrophic endometrium.[23] The presence of a layer of malignant cells one to five cells thick has been noted adjacent to UPSC tumors in up to 80% of cases and can extend some distance from the primary tumors.[23, 24] These lesions have been termed endometrial intraepithelial carcinoma (EIC).[23] By itself, "intraepithelial carcinoma," is a misnomer. These lesions should be considered to have the potential for metastatic spread in the absence of invasion. Extrauterine disease is commonly reported in the absence of myometrial invasion with recurrence rates of up to 50% in this situation.[23, 25] For this reason, other terms for EIC have been proposed since this term could be taken as a premalignant lesion based on the nomenclature.

A lesion that is considered a precursor to EIC has also been discovered by examining endometrial biopsies of women taken several months to years before they developed UPSC.[26] While not visible grossly, microscopic lesions were noted with nuclear enlargement and mild nuclear atypia. This putative precursor lesion is described as endometrial glandular dysplasia. These foci of endometrial glandular dysplasia stain positive for both p53 and the nuclear proliferation marker MIB-1. They have been detected in 75% of women diagnosed with EIC and 47% of women with UPSC suggesting that there is a transition from endometrial glandular dysplasia to EIC prior to the development of invasive UPSC. Endometrial glandular dysplasia was seen in women who were on the average 3 years younger than those with UPSC and preceded the development of UPSC by an average of 33 months.[27]

As preinvasive lesions associated with USPC have only recently been described, there are no series that describe the outcome of nonoperative treatment. Because of the aggressive nature of the invasive component of these lesions, surgical intervention is prudent. Women with EIC should be considered to have an overt malignancy and undergo complete staging including a hysterectomy, bilateral salpingo-oophorectomy, full pelvic and para-aortic lymphadenectomy, peritoneal washings, as well as omentectomy.

PREOPERATIVE EVALUATION

Preoperative evaluation of women with endometrial cancer should focus on comorbid conditions. It has been recognized that 60% of preoperative tests are ordered without indication.[28] Routine testing should be discouraged unless there is a significant risk of abnormality and the utility of various preoperative tests have been evaluated.[29] Discontinuation of the longstanding practice of ordering routine preoperative tests is difficult. It has been demonstrated that hospital based protocols for preoperative testing can reduce routine preoperative test utilization up to 45% in low risk patients while not adversely effecting care.[30] This position has been supported by the Practice Advisory Task Force for Preanesthesia Evaluation.[31]

Hemoglobin

While no large series of patients with endometrial cancer has been reported, it has been noted that preoperative hemoglobin is abnormal in only 1.8% of cases with only 0.1% of these abnormalities influencing surgical management.[29] Justification for preoperative hemoglobin should include symptoms suggestive of anemia or history of significant or prolonged bleeding. Often hemoglobin is obtained as a baseline measurement prior to a surgical procedure. The value of the hemoglobin has been shown to predict the risk of postoperative transfusion.[32] In cases where significant blood loss can occur, this may help estimate the need for a blood type and cross match for transfusion. However, in the absence of significant history or symptoms, routine hemoglobin determinations have not been shown to influence outcomes and should not be obtained when minimal blood loss is expected.[29]

Electrolytes

Preoperative serum electrolytes have been noted to be abnormal in 12.7% of patients and abnormalities influenced perioperative management in 1.8% of cases.[29] The rationale for obtaining electrolytes is to identify cases of hypokalemia, which might lead to cardiac arrhythmias. However, in a series of more than 400 patients, it was noted that preoperative serum potassium was not predictive of intraoperative arrhythmias.[33] Similarly, there was no difference in serum electrolyte abnormalities in patients who developed supraventricular tachycardia after cardiac bypass surgery.[34] Therefore, in absence of renal failure or other medical conditions at risk for abnormalities of renal function, routine use of preoperative electrolytes should be discouraged unless patients are at significant risk of hypokalemia or arrhythmia because of medical conditions or drugs such as diuretics, digoxin, ACE inhibitors, chemotherapeutic agents or other medications which alter potassium. The Practice Advisory Task Force for Preanesthesia Evaluation has not set definitive age or requirements for these tests.[31]

Renal Function

In a review of preoperative patients, the prevalence of renal dysfunction was 8.2% with 2.6% of the findings influencing management.[29] Detection of renal dysfunction is significant given that it is now considered an intermediate cardiac risk factor by the American College of Cardiology similar to mild angina, or a history of a myocardial infarction.[35] Although the risk of renal dysfunction has been reported as high as 24% in patients prior to cardiac surgery, a risk of only 4% was noted prior to surgery for colon cancer.[36, 37] Because of the increased perioperative complications with renal failure it has been recommend to obtain a routine renal panel in patients over 50 years old, or when indicated by other risk factors such as long standing hypertension, diabetes, or coronary artery disease.[29] Also, testing should be performed in patients under 50 who have a history of potentially nephrotoxic drug use, such as NSAIDs.

Cardiac Evaluation

Cardiovascular events are the leading cause of mortality after major surgery. Because obesity, hypertension and diabetes are associated with endometrial cancer, an assessment of cardiovascular risk should be made and appropriate preoperative testing and referral should be made. Evaluation of signs and symptoms as well as the use of preoperative risk scoring systems should be utilized to determine when preoperative cardiac testing and consultation is required.[38] In general, women with a normal functional status (able to climb a flight of stairs or do light housework) should not need routine cardiac evaluation unless major cardiac risk factors are present such as a history of coronary artery disease, severe aortic stenosis, a history of congestive heart failure, or a significant arrhythmia. For women with a diminished functional status, cardiac testing should be considered for intermediate and high-risk procedures.[39]

A randomized trial using preoperative beta blockade with atenolol immediately prior to surgery and continued for up to 7 days while in the hospital showed a significant reduction in 2-year mortality from cardiovascular disease after major surgery.[40] Patients were included in this study if they had a previous MI, angina, or a positive stress test. Patients were also enrolled if they had two or more of the following risk factors; age $\geq$ 65 years old, hypertension, smoking, elevated cholesterol ($\geq$240 mg/dl), or diabetes. Unfortunately women are under represented in this trial and may require different risk stratification than men. It should be remembered that women with a positive stress test are only about half as likely to report symptoms of angina.[41] Given the association of hypertension, diabetes and age, it is likely many women with endometrial cancer would qualify as being at elevated risk of cardiac morbidity and should be considered for beta blockade. In absence of contraindications, it is reasonable to offer beta blockade to women who are at increased cardiac risk undergoing abdominal surgery for endometrial cancer. The need for this type of intervention after laparoscopic surgery for endometrial cancer is not known.

Chest X-Ray

With endometrial adenocarcinoma, the risk of abnormal findings on CXR in the absence of signs or symptoms of pulmonary involvement is low. Patients with uterine sarcomas and advanced endometrial cancer are more likely to have metastatic disease and may have unexpected findings on Chest X-ray. Patients with uterine papillary serous tumors are also more like to have plural effusions, but clinically significant effusions are likely to be detected on physical examination.

Based on the marked increase in abnormal findings on chest radiograph over the age of 50, routine testing has been suggested.[29,42] However, the Practice Advisory Task Force for Preanesthesia Evaluation stated that clinical characteristics such as smoking, COPD, recent infection, and cardiac disease should be taken into account in determining the need for chest radiograph but these conditions and arbitrary age should not be an absolute indication.[31] There is no clear evidence that obtaining a chest x-ray as a baseline test will alter patient outcome.

Diagnostic Imaging

Much of the literature involving preoperative imaging with computed tomography (CT) or magnetic resonance imaging (MRI) has focused on the ability to predict significant myometrial invasion. In a meta-analysis comparing CT, MRI, and ultrasound (U/S) there was no significant difference for predicting myometrial invasion between the modalities when the sensitivity and specificity were compared.[43] However, contrast-enhanced MRI did show an advantage over other modalities. ACOG now recommends routine staging in women with endometrial cancer with any significant myometrial invasion making such scanning unnecessary prior to most surgery for endometrial cancer.[44] CT scan is the modality of choice to investigate patients with abnormal findings on physical examination or signs and symptoms that could represent metastatic disease. Imaging also has a role in evaluating patients who are not surgical candidates or who present with advanced disease. As with all preoperative testing, a CT or MRI should only be obtained if it will alter treatment planning or surgical approach. Limitations with CT scans include a relative lack of sensitivity for detecting small pelvic lymph nodes.[45]

Tumor Markers

Elevated Ca-125 levels have been noted in women with endometrial cancer.[46] Several reports have now been published demonstrating that the sensitivity and specificity for an elevated Ca-125 to detect extrauterine disease is between 70% and 90%.[47–49]

Because extrauterine disease is relatively uncommon and it is recommended that all women with myometrial involvement undergo surgical staging, routine preoperative determination of Ca-125 is not warranted. However, it might be appropriate to measure Ca-125 in a patient who is medically inoperable to determine the risk of nodal metastasis. If patients are noted to have disease outside the uterus, the Ca-125 level can be helpful in monitor the response to treatment and checking for recurrent endometrial cancer.

Deep Venous Thrombosis Prophylaxis

Deep venous thrombosis is a risk after any surgery and may occur in up to 40% of women after major gynecologic surgery without any prophylaxis.[50] Patients with endometrial cancer may be at particularly high risk due to the average age, the presence of malignancy, and other co-factors such as morbid obesity and extensive pelvic surgery. ACOG has recently issued a practice bulletin outlining recommendations for prophylaxis after gynecologic surgery (Table 10.4). Patients at moderate or high risk for DVT should have some sort of prophylaxis based on currently available evidence. Randomized trials have supported the use of either sequential compression

Table 10.4   Recommendations for Thromboembolic Prophylaxis in Gynecologic Surgery

Risk	Surgery	Recommendation	Evidence Level
Low	Surgery < 30 minutes and age < 40 years	Early mobilization	Level C
Medium	Surgery < 30 minutes with other risk factors	Heparin 5000 units q 12°	Level A
		LMWH 40 mg q24°	Level A
	Surgery < 30 min and Age 40–60 years	SCD	Level A
	Major surgery < 40 years		
High	Surgery < 30 min and > 60 years	Heparin 5000 units q8°	Level A
	Major surgery and > 40 years	LMWH 40 mg q24°	Level A
	with other risk factors	SCD	Level A
	Major surgery > 60 years		
Very high	Major surgery > 60 years and	Heparin 5000 units q8°	Level A
	additional risk factors such as	LMWH 40 mg q24°	Level A
	cancer, history of DVT or PE,	SCD + heparin or LMWH	Level C
	or hypercoagulable state		
Laparoscopic surgery	Same as laparotomy	Same as laparotomy	Level C

Levels of evidence are after ACOG (Level A: consistent scientific evidence supports use, Level B: limited or inconsistent scientific evidence supports use, and Level C: limited scientific evidence based primarily on consensus and expert opinion); LMWH, low molecular weight heparin (enoxaparin or equivalent); SCD, sequential compression stockings; DVT, deep venous thrombosis; PE, pulmonary embolism. Adapted from Reference 56.

stockings or the use of either heparin or low molecular weight heparin in this population. For optimal prophylaxis, the graduated compression stockings should be applied prior to surgery and continued throughout the hospital stay. Ideally, heparin should be started 2 hours before the surgery. Preoperative heparin has been associated with an increase in minor bleeding such as wound hematomas.[51,52] Although studies have not demonstrated that preoperative heparin is associated with increase in intraoperative bleeding, there is some concern that this might be a problem in women with advanced gynecologic malignancies. There is little evidence from the gynecologic literature to suggest how the timing of heparin administration alters the effectiveness of this therapy. However, in orthopedic surgery, an increase in bleeding complications was noted when giving heparin prior to 6 hours after surgery and a decrease in efficacy if started more than 12 hours postprocedure.[53]

The use of sequential compression stockings may be appropriate in women having gynecologic surgery if heparin is contraindicated because of bleeding risk or regional anesthesia. It was noted that using sequential compression stockings alone the risk of DVT following abdominal hysterectomy for benign conditions was reduced to less than 1%, and for a hysterectomy and staging with pelvic and para-aortic lymphadenectomy the rate was about 4%.[54] The combination of graduated compression stockings and heparin has not been studied in a randomized fashion in gynecologic surgery. However, a Cochrane review has suggested that the combination may be more effective than heparin alone in colorectal surgery.[55]

Currently, there is insufficient data to compare the risk of DVT after laparoscopic surgery for endometrial cancer. In theory, laparoscopic surgery is associated with less pain and earlier mobilization although it may be associated with longer operative times. In a review of patients after laparoscopy or vaginal hysterectomy treated with sequential compression hose alone, it was noted that there were no episodes of venous thromboembolism in over 300 cases.[56] While the risk appears to be low in this group, the current ACOG recommendations are to use the same risk stratification after laparoscopic surgery as compared to laparotomy.[56]

STAGING

Endometrioid Adenocarcinoma

In 1988, FIGO adopted a surgical staging system in place of a clinical staging system after the results from GOG protocol #33 defined the risk of spread of endometrial cancer outside of the uterus.[57,58] This study examined the surgical pathologic spread patterns in women with previously untreated endometrial cancer that appeared to be confined to the uterus. This protocol included both endometrioid and non-endometrioid endometrial cancers. Overall, 22% of women with apparent stage I endometrial cancer were noted to have extrauterine spread. Predictors of lymphatic metastasis included histologic subtype (for para-aortic nodes), depth of myometrial invasion, tumor grade, peritoneal cytology, site of the tumor (fundus vs. isthmus cervix), adnexal involvement, and lymph-vascular space involvement. The strongest

Table 10.5 Risk of Pelvic Nodal Involvement Based on Depth of Invasion and Tumor Grade

	Grade 1	Grade 2	Grade 3
No invasion	0% (0/44)	3% (1/31)	0% (0/11)
Inner 1/3	3% (3/96)	5% (7/31)	9% (5/54)
Middle 1/3	0% (0/22)	9% (6/69)	4% (1/24)
Outer 1/3	11% (2/18)	19% (11/57)	34% (22/64)

Adapted from Reference 57.

predictors were the depth of myometrial invasion and the tumor grade. The risk of lymphatic spread to the pelvic and para-aortic lymph nodes based on the depth and grade of the tumor are given in Tables 10.5 and 10.6. Currently the FIGO staging system is based on the surgical evaluation of the uterus and the results of surgical staging (Fig. 10.1). The American Joint Commission on Cancer TMN staging system closely mirrors that of FIGO.[59] Current staging guidelines call for abdomino-pelvic washings and a complete pelvic and para-aortic lymphadenectomy, when there is significant risk of lymphatic spread.

In the two decades since the staging system was changed, there has been a great deal of controversy as to when the risk of lymphatic metastasis is high enough to justify lymphadenectomy and how thorough the lymphadenectomy should be.[60] In the low risk patients with stage IA or IB and grade 1 and 2 tumors, the overall risk of lymphatic involvement is less than 5%. Many have argued that these patients generally have a good prognosis and do not require staging.[61] However, proponents of more universal staging point out that this procedure has a limited morbidity, may have some therapeutic value,[62,63] and will detect the cohort of patients with low risk that would have been missed with staging based on risk stratification.[60] Several researchers have evaluated different strategies and have suggested that universal staging is a cost-effective strategy over risk stratification based on frozen section results.[64–66] An additional benefit to moving toward more frequent surgical staging is that it appears to decrease the recommendation for postoperative radiation.[67,68] Current trends in the United States suggest that gynecologic oncologists are now less

Table 10.6 Risk of Para-Aortic Nodal Involvement Based on Depth of Invasion and Tumor Grade

	Grade 1	Grade 2	Grade 3
No invasion	0% (0/44)	3% (1/31)	0% (0/11)
Inner 1/3	1% (1/96)	4% (5/31)	4% (2/54)
Middle 1/3	5% (1/22)	0% (0/69)	0% (0/24)
Outer 1/3	6% (1/18)	14% (8/57)	23% (15/64)

Adapted from Reference 57.

Stages

Stage I*	Tumor confined to the corpus uteri
1A*	No or less than half myometrial invasion
1B*	Invasion equal to or more than half of the myometrium
Stage II*	Tumor invades cervical stroma but does not extend beyond the uterus**
Stage III*	Local and/or regional spread of the tumor
IIIA*	Tumor invades the serosa of the corpus uteri and/or adnexae
IIIB*	Vaginal and/or parametrial involvement
IIIC*	Metastases to pelvic and/or para-aortic lymph nodes
IIIC1*	Positive pelvic nodes
IIIC2*	Positive para-aortic nodes with or without positive pelvic lymph nodes
Stage IV*	Tumor invades bladder and/or bowel mucosa, and/or distant metastases
IVA*	Tumor invasion of bladder and/or bowel mucosa
IVB*	Distant metastases, including intra-abdominal metastases and/or inguinal nodes

* Either G1, G2, or G3

** Endocervical glandular involvement only should be considered as Stage I and no longer as Stage II

* Positive cytology has to be reported separately without changing the stage

Rules Related to Staging

-Since corpus cancer is now surgically staged, procedures previously used for determination of stages are no longer applicable, such as the finding of fractional D&C to differentiate between stage I and stage II

-It is appreciated that there may be a small number of patients with corpus cancer who will be treated primarily with radiation therapy. If that is the case, the clinical staging adopted by FIGO in 1971 would still apply but designation of that staging system would be noted.

-Ideally, width of the myometrium should be measured along with the width of tumor invasion

Histopathology – Degree of Differentiation

G1 = 5% or less of a non-squamous on non-morular solid growth pattern

G2 = 6-50% of a non-squamous or non-morular solid growth pattern

G3 = more than 50% of a non-squamous or non-morular solid growth pattern

Notes on Pathologic Grading

-notable nuclear atypia, inappropriate for the architectural grade, raises the grade of a grade 1 or grade II tumor by 1

-In serous adenocarcinomas, clear cell adenocarcinomas, and squamous cell carcinomas, nuclear grading takes precedence

-Adenocarcinomas with squamous differentiation are graded according to the nuclear grade of the glandular component

Figure 10.1   FIGO staging of Endometrial Cancer [131].

likely to recommend pelvic radiation and more likely to perform a complete staging procedure including a complete lymphadenectomy.[69]

In high risk patients, recent data from the Mayo clinic has been used to justify a more aggressive approach in women at risk for para-aortic nodal metastasis. In their series, 22% of patients with endometrial cancer (endometrioid and non-endometrioid) had positive lymph nodes if high risk factors were present. In a breakdown of where the nodal metastasis occurred, 51% of the patients were found to have both pelvic and para-aortic involvement, 33% to have only pelvic involvement, and 16% to have isolated para-aortic nodes. Of interest was that 77% of patients with positive pelvic nodes had involvement above the IMA with 60% of these women having no positive nodes below the IMA. It was noted that 28% of patients with para-aortic nodal metastasis also had disease surrounding the gonadal vessels that were excised at the time of the staging procedure. While isolated para-aortic metastasis occurred in 16% of those who were node positive, it should be pointed out that this represented only 2% of the total population and 3.5% of the population that had a lymphadenectomy performed. It should also be noted that women with grade 1 or 2 endometrioid tumors with the disease limited to the inner 1/2 of the uterus if the primary tumor was less than 2 cm in diameter on frozen section were considered low risk for nodal spread and a formal staging procedure was not done on these women. This algorithm allowed omission of the lymphatic dissection in approximately one-fourth of the patients. A criticism of this approach has been that that even though the researchers achieved a high degree of accuracy in frozen section, this may not be reproducible in other institutions or hospitals.[70] In addition, the presence of lymph-vascular space involvement cannot easily be accessed on frozen section and is an important independent predictor of nodal metastasis.[71] Unfortunately, this trial does not give long-term follow-up on the patients without lymphatic assessment. Based on the data from GOG #33 one would expect a 3%–5% rate of pelvic lymphatic metastasis and a 1%–4% of para-aortic metastasis in this group of women (see Tables 10.5 and 10.6).

Other recent studies have questioned the benefit of routine staging in endometrial cancer. The ASTEC trial was presented in 2006 and recently published in 2009.[72] In this trial, 1408 women with endometrial cancer (endometrioid and non-endometrioid) apparently confined to the uterus were randomly assigned to either simple hysterectomy or hysterectomy with pelvic lymphadenectomy. The protocol called for a full dissection of the pelvic nodes, but the decision to perform a para-aortic node dissection was at the discretion of the investigator. The patients were then secondarily randomized to pelvic radiation or no therapy (without regard to the lymph node status). The use of vaginal radiation was also at the discretion of the investigators. No difference in overall survival was reported (HR = 1.05; 95% CI: 0.77–1.43; $P = 0.77$). While it is argued that this trial did not show a benefit for lymph node dissection, it is difficult to interpret the data since the choice of postoperative pelvic radiation was not decided on the basis of the intrauterine pathology or lymph node status and may have masked any potential benefit from lymphatic dissection. This makes this data difficult to apply to the United States where there is a trend toward using less radiation in women who undergo complete surgical staging. Also, the fact that the use of vaginal radiation was not controlled for further complicates interpretation of the results of this trial.

A recent Italian trial has also explored the utility of lymphadenectomy in early endometrial cancer.[73] This trial randomized over 500 women with endometrial cancer to lymphadenectomy versus no lymphadenectomy. In this trial, patients randomized to lymphadenectomy underwent a complete pelvic lymphadenectomy with a mean of 26 nodes recovered. Only 26% of the lymphadenectomy cohort had a para-aortic lymphadenectomy with a median of four lymph nodes removed. It should be noted that 22% of the patients in the no lymphadenectomy arm had some lymph node tissue evaluated. The protocol did not specify the requirements or type of postoperative adjuvant therapy. The results of the trial showed that rate of positive lymph node detection was higher in the lymphadenectomy group as expected (13.3% vs. 3.2%; 95% CI for difference 5.3% vs. 14.9%; $P < 0.001$). However, with a median follow-up of 48 months, the hazard ration for recurrence (HR $= 1.10$; 95% CI: 0.7–1.7; $P = 0.68$) and death (HR $= 1.20$; 95% CI: 0.7–2.7; $P = 0.5$) was not different between the two groups. The most common adjuvant therapy was pelvic radiation. This was given more often in the group without lymphadenectomy (29.6% vs. 22.4%; $P = 0.07$) and was more often pelvic radiation. Of note was that adjuvant chemotherapy was given at a slightly higher rate in the lymphadenectomy group and the simple hysterectomy group (14.4% vs. 10.0%, P value not reported). While some of the different in the adjuvant chemotherapy can be explained by the finding of positive nodes at the time of surgery, it would seem that the group with the simple hysterectomy may have been slightly more likely to receive chemotherapy in the absence of nodal metastasis.

It is unlikely that the issue of staging will ever be settled with a randomized trial since there is a wide variation in treatment patterns between the United States, where universal staging is more popular, and Europe, where simple hysterectomy followed by pelvic radiation is more popular. In addition, overall the rate of lymphatic metastasis is in the 5%–10% range. Therefore it may take an extremely large trial with very rigorous standardization of surgery and postoperative radiation to be adequately powered to answer such a question with direct evidence. Ultimately, one has to weigh the risk of lymphadenectomy, against the morbidity of the procedure and the consequences of not having the lymphatic staging information.

Uterine Papillary Serous Carcinoma

Patterns of spread for UPSC are different from those seen in endometrioid cancers. LVSI is common and lymph node metastasis are present in about 40% of patients overall and has been noted in 6% of cases without microscopic evidence of myometrial invasion.[74] In addition to being morphologically similar to papillary serous tumors of the ovary and fallopian tube, UPSC also tends to spread through the fallopian tube to the abdominal cavity with metastasis to the omentum. Gross abdominal spread was present in 26% of patients in one series and an additional 18% of patients had microscopic omental involvement.[75] While peritoneal cytology was predictive of disease in the omentum, there are cases of omental involvement when peritoneal cytology is negative. In a retrospective analysis, the risk of omental disease with positive cytology was 81%, but the omentum was positive 12% of the time when the cytology was negative.[76] Overall, an omentectomy was necessary to detect 25% of patients with stage IV UPSC that would have been missed by conventional staging without an omentectomy.

Because of the high rate of extrauterine metastasis with minimal myometrial invasion, the risk of recurrence in stage I is often over estimated in studies where formal staging was not performed. Recently, several series with more complete staging procedures have better defined the risk of recurrence in women without extrauterine spread. These studies have found that the risk of recurrence after an adequate staging procedure is similar to that of stage I grade 3 endometrioid cancers.[77] However, there is a significant difference in the risk of extrauterine disease at presentation and recurrence patterns with a predisposition for distant spread.

POSTOPERATIVE SURVEILLANCE

Follow-up of women after treatment of endometrial cancer is based more on tradition than on fact. Typical follow-up schema for women with gynecologic malignancies have included visits every 3 months followed by biannual visit until the patient is 5 years out from her diagnosis.[78] Aside from the psychological benefit of physician contact after the diagnosis and treatment of an endometrial cancer, the rationale of follow-up is to detect asymptomatic recurrences so that further treatment can be administered that that is curative or more effective when administered early when the recurrent cancer burden is small. Endometrial cancer is well suited for close follow-up as many recurrences are noted in the vagina and curative treatment with radiation can be offered to most patients with this condition. Isolated vaginal recurrence represents between 30% and 40% of all patients with recurrent endometrial cancer.[79, 80] In women with disease confined to the uterus and who had a complete surgical staging without postoperative therapy, the isolated vaginal failure rate was 7% and the majority of these women were cured with further therapy.[80, 81]

However, the utility of postoperative follow-up has been called into question because there is no significant difference in survival after the detection of symptomatic versus asymptomatic recurrent endometrial cancer.[82, 83] When one considers a relatively low risk population, it was noted that only 1 in 205 examinations detected a recurrence.[83] Routine vaginal cytology was responsible for detecting 6 cancers in 4830 vaginal cytology smears (1 in 805).[82] The cost per case of endometrial cancer detected was $19,200. However, it should be pointed out that women who do not receive pelvic radiation are more likely to present with an asymptomatic vaginal recurrence and are most likely to benefit from additional therapy. Therefore, local preferences for the use of adjuvant therapy could easily affect the outcome of this type of retrospective study. In GOG 99, the vaginal cuff recurrence rate was reduced from 7% to 2% in the women assigned to pelvic radiation and the only vaginal cuff recurrences noted in pelvic radiation therapy arm were in patients that did not receive the prescribed dose of radiation.[80]

When formulating a cost-effective strategy, it is important to know how recurrent endometrial cancer is detected. In a series of 39 patients who initially presented with stage I cancer and later were noted to have a recurrence, 41% had symptoms, 40% were diagnosed on physical examination, 3% on chest X-ray, 15% due to elevated Ca-125, and routine CT scan in 5%.[84]

Routine chest X-rays during follow-up are often ordered and can detect pulmonary metastases. Proponents of this practice argue that the lung is a common site of distant metastasis. Ca-125 levels have also been noted to be elevated in up to 60% of women at the time of diagnosis of recurrence.[85] However, both of these modalities are unlikely to detect recurrent cancer in a state where curative therapy can be offered. Therefore, routine tumor markers or imaging with routine X-ray, CT, MRI, or PET would not be a cost-effective follow-up strategy in endometrial cancer.

POSTOPERATIVE HORMONE REPLACEMENT

Estrogen replacement therapy is relatively contraindicated after surgery for endometrial cancer based on the theoretical risk of stimulating residual tumors since most endometrial cancers are associated with increased levels of estrogen[5] and unopposed estrogen use was linked to the development of endometrial cancer.[86] However, most women with endometrial cancer are cured of their disease and the estrogen-related type I tumors generally have the best prognosis.[4] Approximately 25% of women who develop endometrial cancer are premenopausal. For these reasons, it is reasonable to consider the issue of hormone replacement for symptomatic control of vasomotor induced hot flashes and genital atrophy. The GOG sponsored a randomized protocol (GOG #137) to evaluate the safety of estrogen replacement therapy after endometrial cancer.[87] This protocol was a randomized double blind trial and did not require women to undergo surgical staging. Patients were eligible after hysterectomy with any type of primary endometrial cancer that was confined to the uterus (FIGO stage I and II). The trial was originally designed for an 80% power to detect a 50% relative increase in recurrence risk on estrogen replacement therapy and the accrual goal was 2108 patients. During this trial it was announced that the combination hormone replacement arm Women's Health Initiative (WHI) Trial was being closed prematurely after an interim analysis showed in increased risk of breast cancer with no cardiovascular benefit.[88] Even thought the estrogen only arm of the WHI continued, the enrollment to the GOG trial was effected to the point where attainment of the accrual goal was unrealistic. For this reason, the study was discontinued after enrolling 1236 patients. Overall, the incidence of disease recurrence in this population was 1.3% in the placebo group and 1.5% in the estrogen replacement group (RR 1.27; 80% CI: 0.92–1.77; P = not significant). While this trial certainly suggests the replacement therapy is not associated with a dramatic increased risk of recurrence, it will likely be impossible to ever exclude a modest increased risk with estrogen therapy. For this reason, ACOG published a committee opinion stating that it is reasonable to offer hormone therapy to women after endometrial cancer after carefully considering the risks and benefits this medication.[89]

Although the cause is not known, African American women have a mortality rate from endometrial cancer approximately twice that of Caucasian women.[90] A post hoc analysis of the data from GOG #137 was performed to examine the risk of recurrent endometrial cancer in African American women. This review noted an 11-fold increase risk of mortality (95% CI: 2.9–43.6; P = 0.0005) in African American women when they were taking hormone replacement after adjusting for age, BMI, and tumor grade. Since these women were on a protocol, it would be assumed that the follow-up care would be relatively standardized and the reason for the excess mortality is unknown.

ADJUVANT THERAPY IN EARLY DISEASE

Hormonal Agents

Because normal endometrial cells are responsive to hormonal manipulation, it is likely that some endometrial cancers will respond to these agents. Because of the favorable side-effect profile of these agents, the use of hormonal agents in endometrial cancer has been investigated extensively. Four randomized studies have been conducted in women with early endometrial cancer in the adjuvant setting, and none of these trials showed an advantage to postoperative hormonal therapy with progestational agents.[91–94] In the largest trial it was noted that while the death rate from endometrial cancer was marginally improved in the group on progestin therapy, the death rate from nonmalignant disease was higher suggesting that the risk of the medication may have counteracted the effectiveness of this treatment.[94]

Radiation

Despite the high overall cure rate in FIGO stage I endometrial cancer, there remains much controversy concerning the use of adjuvant radiation therapy after surgery. Several studies have attempted to determine the optimal patients who should receive adjuvant radiation after surgery for endometrial cancer. Unfortunately, the different trial designs and treatment designs make these studies difficult to compare.

The first large randomized trial of postoperative external radiation in endometrial carcinoma was performed by Aalders.[95] This trial was open to all women who had adenocarcinoma of the endometrium that was apparently confined to the uterus. In this protocol, 540 women were randomized to either WPRT with 40 Gy or no further therapy after a hysterectomy and oophorectomy without lymphadenectomy. All patients in this trial were treated with 60 Gy of vaginal brachytherapy. Overall, there was a significant decrease in the risk of pelvic recurrence with the addition of WPRT (6.9% vs. 1.9%; $P < 0.01$) However, the total recurrence rate or mortality were reduced with the use of WPRT. The 5-year survival was 91% with brachytherapy alone and 89% with brachytherapy and WPRT, which was not statistically different. An improvement in survival was noted in the subgroup of women with deeply invasive high grade tumors. However, because the women in this trial were not completely staged, it is likely that this represents treatment of undetected occult lymphatic metastasis, which occur in over 20% of these women.[57]

The Postoperative Radiation Therapy in Endometrial Cancer (PORTEC) trial also randomized women with apparent stage I endometrial adenocarcinoma to no further treatment versus WPRT with 46 Gy.[96] The median follow-up for women in this trial is 52 months. This trial also did not require surgical staging and these women were not treated with vaginal brachytherapy on this trial. The PORTEC trial was limited to women with IB grade 2/3 and IC grade 1/2 tumors. Similar to the Aalders trial, there was a decrease in the vaginal/pelvic recurrence rate from 14% to 4%, but there was no difference in the overall survival (85 vs. 81%). This trial was powered to have an 86% chance of detecting a 10% difference in overall survival at 5 years. However, 50% of the deaths in this study were due to disease other than endometrial cancer. The improved pelvic control came at the expense of a 2% grade 3 or 4 gastrointestinal complication rate in the radiation group.

The GOG has published the results of a randomized study in patients with invasive stage I and occult stage II endometrial cancers. In this study, 334 women were randomized to whole pelvic adjuvant radiation after surgery or no further therapy.[80] Women who received pelvic radiation showed a significant reduction in the vaginal recurrence rate with no overall effect on survival. One of the strengths of this study was that all of the women had a complete surgical staging. However, because of a lower than expected recurrence rate and the fact that almost half of the deaths were not due to endometrial cancer, this study was powered to detect only a very large difference in overall survival (58% difference in hazard ratio; $\beta = 0.2$).

In an attempt to define a high intermediate risk subgroup that might have more benefit from the radiation, an analysis of data previously collected by the GOG showed that a subgroup with an expected 25% recurrence rate could be defined in patients with certain risk factors.[80,81] These risk factors include the presence of lymph-vascular space involvement, >50% myometrial invasion, or grade 2–3 tumors. Patients older than 50 years were noted to be at increased risk with two of these factors and patients older than 70 years were at increased risk with only one of these factors. These risk factors describe only 33% of the study population of GOG #99 but account for 67% of the deaths. When this high intermediate subgroup was analyzed in GOG #99, it was noted pelvic radiation was more effective in decreasing the local recurrence rate when compared to the overall group. The hazard ratio for death in the high intermediate risk group in the radiation arm was reduced to 0.73, but this did not reach statistical significance due to the small size of the subgroup.[80]

Pelvic radiation was highly effective in preventing vaginal cuff recurrences in GOG #99.[80] There were 31 recurrences noted in the 202 women on the no treatment arm. Of these 31 recurrences, 13 (6%) were isolated vaginal recurrences. Of the 190 women in the treatment arm, there were 13 recurrences and only 2 (1%) of these were isolated to the vagina. Interestingly, the two patients in the radiation group who had a vaginal cuff recurrence did not actually receive the prescribed pelvic radiation since this was an intent to treat analysis. Pelvic radiation decreased the local recurrence rate in the vagina in the low and low intermediate risk groups from 7% to 0%. In the high intermediate risk group, the rate was decreased from 13% to 5%. However, there was significant toxicity involved with the administration of 50.4 cGy of whole pelvic radiation, including two deaths thought to be secondary to treatment related bowel injury.

A fourth trial of Observation versus WPRT has recently been published. This trial was conducted jointly by the MRC (ASTEC Trial) and the NCIC (EN.5 Trial). The study design was complex and sought to answer two questions in women with endometrial cancer. The first part of the trial randomized women with endometrial cancer to staging versus no staging at the time of hysterectomy. Women without macroscopic disease were then secondarily randomized to WPRT versus no further treatment.

Several major problems are noted with this trial. First, the randomization to WPRT was done without respect to the status of the lymph nodes that were removed. This certainly could have the effect of counteracting the benefit of finding and treating early lymphatic spread. The use of vaginal brachytherapy was not part of the protocol and the decision to administer this treatment was left up to the treating institution and individual treatment centers. Just over half of the women received vaginal radiation as part of this trial. An additional problem with the study was that approximately 10% of women on this trial also had UPSC. This endometrial subtype has a marked increased risk for nodal metastasis and different spread patterns.[97]

Because of the lack of a proven survival advantage for WPRT in the low intermediate or high intermediate subgroups, vaginal cuff radiation after surgery for endometrial cancer was popularized after single institution trials of vaginal cuff irradiation showed very low rates of local recurrence.[98, 99] Recently, the second PORTEC trial was presented comparing vaginal brachytherapy with either 21 Gy in three HDR fractions or 30 Gy by LDR to 46 Gy of WPRT.[100] Women were eligible for this trial if they had IB grade 3, or IC grade 1 or 2 and were older than 60 years or had stage IIA disease at any age. In this trial, the rate of vaginal recurrence was less than 2% in both arms and overall 3-year survival was no different. However, this trial did not include patients with stage IC grade 3 tumors.

There is considerable variation in the approach to the vaginal cuff and this may influence the efficacy of this treatment modality. The majority of radiation oncologists now treat the upper half of the vagina, but some treat only the upper third. The most common prescription for high dose rate vaginal radiation is three fractions of 5.0–7.0 Gy each, calculated 0.5 cm below the vaginal surface using a high dose rate applicator.[101] A high rate of vaginal recurrence was described in a single study of vaginal cuff radiation, where only the upper 2 cm of the cuff was treated suggesting that the amount of vagina treated could potentially be important.[102]

An argument can be made to completely omit vaginal radiation after staging surgery for patients with stage I endometrial cancer. In all of the published trials, the risk of vaginal recurrence is less than 10% without radiation. Previous experience has shown that women who did not receive adjuvant radiation after surgery have demonstrated a long term disease-free survival of greater than 50% if recurrences are detected on follow-up examination and salvage radiation is given.[81]

In UPSC more than 50% of the recurrences have been noted to be extrapelvic. Even in patients who have had a complete surgical staging procedure with an omentectomy, the abdominal cavity is a common site of recurrence[103] This has led to either recommending whole abdominal radiation or a combination of vaginal radiation with or without pelvic radiation combined with chemotherapy as adjuvant therapy in early stage UPSC. One recent series that included both completely staged and unstaged patients demonstrated a marginally significant reduction in the pelvic failure rate from 29% to 14% with adjuvant teletherapy.[104] However, in a multivariate analysis, radiation was not shown to improve overall survival. In other studies, the size of the groups precludes any meaningful analysis of the effect of teletherapy on the recurrence rates in UPSC with either pelvic or abdominal fields.

There is some indication that brachytherapy might decrease local recurrence. In one series it was noted that none of the 38 patients who received radiation to the vaginal vault as part of the teletherapy or brachytherapy had a vaginal cuff recurrence as compared to 6 of the 31 (19%) who were not treated with radiation.[105] While local control can be achieved with minimal morbidity with vaginal cuff radiation therapy, it is doubtful that this will impact overall cure rates since it has been noted that all of the vaginal recurrences women in without adjuvant therapy were also associated with distal recurrence.[106]

Chemotherapy

Endometrioid Tumors

Radiation alone has been the traditional modality of choice for endometrial cancer. However, there has been an increased interest in chemotherapy as an adjuvant treatment in women with high risk disease limited to the uterus and for patients with advanced disease. Several trials have suggested that chemotherapy may be as effective as radiation in preventing pelvic recurrence and may be more effective in treating distant disease. A number of studies have also combined the two modalities in an attempt to improve outcome in women with high risk endometrial cancer.

The GOG performed the first randomized trial of adjuvant chemotherapy in women with endometrial cancer. GOG #34 was a randomized trial of adjuvant chemotherapy with doxorubicin in women who had risk factors for recurrence including deep myometrial invasion, nodal metastasis, cervical involvement, or adnexal metastasis.[107] During accrual to this protocol, it was amended so that surgical staging including sampling of the pelvic and para-aortic nodes was required. The protocol specified treatment with WPRT to 50 Gy with a para-aortic field if the para-aortic nodes were positive. After completion of radiation, patients were randomized to no further therapy or chemotherapy with doxorubicin at 45 mg/m with escalation to 60 mg/m^2 every 3 weeks to a cumulative dose of 500 mg/m^2. Accrual to this trial was very slow and after 8 years only 181 patients enrolled. The protocol was closed prematurely after it was determined that the enrollment goal would not be reached in a reasonable time frame. In addition, only 67 of the 92 women who were assigned to chemotherapy actually received any chemotherapy. Even if all of the patients on the chemotherapy arm had received their assigned treatment, it is estimated that the power the study to detect a difference in the two arms was reduced to less than 40%. It is not surprising that there was no difference in survival between the two arms. However, it was noted that there was an imbalance in randomization in the two arms with patients assigned to chemotherapy having more grade 3 tumors (39% vs. 27%) and a higher rate of nodal metastasis (35% vs. 28%). Even though there was no difference in the two arms with respect to survival, the imbalance in patient randomization may have handicapped the chemotherapy arm.

In 2006, an Italian trial was published comparing chemotherapy alone to radiation in women with high risk disease.[108] While the majority of women in this trial had stage IIIA and IIIC disease, approximately 33% had disease confined to the uterus.

Enrollment was limited to women with endometrioid adenocarcinoma and randomization was between WPRT (45 Gy) versus CAP [cyclophosphamide (600 mg/m^2), doxorubicin (45 mg/m^2), and cisplatin (50 mg/m^2)] every 4 weeks for fivecycles. This trial failed to demonstrate any difference in overall survival after a mean follow-up of almost 8 years.

The Japanese Gynecologic Oncology Group (JGOG) has published the results of a randomized trial of WPRT (45 Gy) versus cyclophosphamide (333 mg/m^2), doxorubicin (40 mg/m^2), and cisplatin (50 mg/m^2) for four cycles in patients with high intermediate risk and high risk endometrioid cancers.[109] Entrance criteria included women with stage I–III endometrioid tumors. Although staging was not required, 96% of patients enrolled had a pelvic lymphadenectomy and 29% had a para-aortic lymphadenectomy. The protocol required more than 50% myometrial invasion even in advanced tumors and 58% of women had stage IC cancers. The recurrence rate was about 15% in both groups after a median follow-up of approximately 60 months. When comparing the WPRT and chemotherapy arms, it was noted that the rates of pelvic recurrence (6.7% vs. 7.3%) and distant recurrence were similar (13.5% vs. 16.1%). The vaginal recurrence rate was higher in the chemotherapy arm (1.0% vs. 4.7%). There was no significant difference in the overall survival between the chemotherapy and radiation therapy arms. However, in the high risk groups (IC any grade over 70 years, IC grade 3 tumors, stage II and III), there was a statistically significant reduction in the hazard ratio for recurrence in the chemotherapy arm (HR = 0.44 (0.20 – 0.97; $P = 0.02$).

The preliminary results of the NSGO-EC-9501/EORTC-55991 trial have recently been presented. This study randomized 382 patients with high risk endometrial stage I–III endometrial cancers to radiation alone or radiation and chemotherapy. This trial enrolled women with both endometrioid and non-endometrioid cancers and who had high risk factors such as grade 3 tumors, $\geq 50\%$ myometrial invasion, positive pelvic lymph nodes, positive cytology, non-endometrioid tumors, or DNA nondiploidy. Staging with lymph node dissection was optional. The exact chemotherapy regimen was not specified but generally included a platinum-anthracycline combination. The order of chemotherapy and radiation was also not specified. Despite the fact that 27% of patients did not complete the prescribed chemotherapy regimen, there was an improvement in the hazard ration for PFS that was statistically significant (HR = 0.62; 95% CI: 0.40–0.97; $P = 0.03$). There was a trend in the hazard for overall survival (HR = 0.65; 95% CI: 0.40–1.06; $P = 0.08$).

RTOG 9708 was a pilot trial of concurrent chemotherapy and RT in women with high risk endometrial cancer.[110] Patients were eligible for this phase II trial if they had grade 2 or grade 3 endometrial adenocarcinoma with greater than 50% myometrial invasion, cervical involvement, or extrauterine disease confined to the pelvis. The treatment protocol specified 45 Gy of WPRT in 180 cGy fractions with concurrent cisplatin (50 mg/m^2) on days 1 and 28. Subsequently, patients were treated with cisplatin (50 mg/m^2) and paclitaxel (175 mg/m^2) every 4 weeks. Overall, 46 patients were included for this protocol. The toxicity was mainly hematologic although there was one grade 4 small bowel complication. At 2 years, the disease-free survival was 83% and the overall survival was 90%.

Similar to the NSGO/EROTC trial, the PORTEC group opened the third trial in 2006 and is now enrolling patients with high intermediate to high risk tumors to a protocol comparing concurrent chemoradiation and adjuvant chemotherapy to WPRT alone. Entrance criteria for patients with stage I endometrioid tumors include IB grade 3 tumors with LVSI or IC grade 3 tumors. Patients with stage IIA grade 3, IIIA and IIIC tumors are eligible. Women with UPSC or clear cell are eligible if they have more than 50% myometrial invasion. It is estimated that the protocol will take 5 years to accrue and results will probably not be reported before 2013.

The GOG is conducting a trial in the high intermediate risk group in stage I patients as defined in GOG 99. This randomized trial compares cuff radiation and 3 cycles of chemotherapy compared to WPRT in women who had approximately a 20% risk of recurrence GOG protocol 249. This trial opened for accrual in March 2009 with a target enrollment of 562 patients.

UPSC

Several large retrospective studies of UPSC have been reported that include only patients with surgical stage I disease.[103, 105, 106, 111] While all patients had pelvic and para-aortic lymphadenectomy, omentectomy or omental sampling was not done in all cases. Despite the bias introduced by retrospective analysis of adjuvant therapy, these are currently the best available studies to examine the impact of adjuvant therapy. Table 10.7 depicts the overall rate of recurrence comparing women who were treated with chemotherapy in these trials compared to all other women without chemotherapy. In this combined series, the recurrence rate was 9% compared to 37% in the patients who did not receive chemotherapy, regardless of whether or not they were treated with radiation. Given this apparent reduction in recurrence rate in early stage disease, it would be reasonable to recommend adjuvant chemotherapy to women with stage I UPSC. Some researchers have suggested when there is no residual tumor or when the cancer is present only in a polyp that chemotherapy may not be necessary.[112] However, given the small number of cases, it is difficult to make a definite recommendation in this group. One must weigh the relatively low risk of recurrence against the fact that recurrences have been noted after surgery alone for stage IA UPSC and that recurrence

Table 10.7   Risk of Recurrence in Women with Surgical Stage I[a] UPSC with and without Adjuvant Chemotherapy[105, 111]

Stage	N	Recurrence Risk	
		Chemotherapy	No Chemotherapy
IA	88	2/37 (5%)	10/47 (21%)
IB	94	5/63 (8%)	16/31 (52%)
IC	38	4/21 (19%)	9/16 (56%)
Total	220	11/121 (9%)	35/94 (37%)

All patients had pelvic and para-aortic lymphadenectomy with or without omentectomy.

in this situation is often fatal.[111] The optimal adjuvant chemotherapy regimen has also not been defined for this population, although a platinum and taxane combination for 3–6 cycles is commonly administered and well tolerated.

TREATMENT OF ADVANCED DISEASE

Role of Surgery

Surgery remains the cornerstone of therapy for all endometrial cancer, including UPSC. In ovarian cancer, the concept of maximal surgical effort has been associated with overall survival. Because relatively few patients present with advanced metastatic cancer, there is less data to support this concept in endometrial cancer. However, retrospective studies suggest that women with less than 1 cm of disease after surgery for advanced endometrial cancer have an improved outcome when compared to those who have suboptimal resection.[113,114]

A retrospective study combining patients from two institutions with advanced endometrial cancer with both endometrioid and non-endometrioid cancers showed that 83% patients could be optimally resected.[113] The patients who were suboptimally resected were at significantly higher risk for recurrence (HR = 3.66; 95% CI: 2.40–5.58; $P < 0.001$) and death (HR = 3.15; 95% CI: 1.98–5.01; $P < 0.001$). The amount of residual disease was a better predictor or outcome that all other variables including the type of postoperative therapy (radiation vs. chemotherapy), age, race stage, grade, and histologic subtype. In another retrospective analysis in women with UPSC showed that those women who had $\leq$ 1 cm residual disease had an improved overall survival.[114] In addition, those that had no residual disease had an even greater improvement in overall survival. With maximal surgical effort, optimal resection was completed in approximately half of the patients who presented with stage IV UPSC.

Hormonal

The GOG has conducted several trials of hormonal therapy in women with advanced or recurrent endometrial cancer. GOG #81 reviewed the dose response relationship with oral medroxyprogesterone acetate.[115] This trial randomized 299 patients to either 200 mg per day or 1000 mg per day. Of note was that the overall response rate was higher (25% vs. 15%), the duration of response was longer (3.2 months vs. 2.5 months), and the overall survival longer (11.1 months vs. 7.0 months) in the low dose group. These differences are of marginal statistical significance. Univariate predictors of response to progestational agents is shown in Table 10.8. The GOG also conducted a trial of high dose Megestrol at 800 mg/day (GOG #121). This agent was noted to have an overall response rate of 24%, consistent with other GOG trials of progestational agents.

GOG protocol 81-F was a phase II trial of tamoxifen 20 mg BID in women with advanced or recurrent endometrial cancer.[116] This protocol enrolled 68 patients.

Table 10.8 Factors Predicting Univariate Response
to Progestational Agents

Factor	Overall RR
Age	
< 60 years	27%
60–69 years	23%
≥ 70 years	13%
Grade	
1	37%
2	23%
3	9%
Progesterone Receptors	
< 50 fmol/mg	8%
≥ 50 fmol/mg	37%
Estrogen receptors	
< 50 fmol/mg	7%
≥ 50 fmol/mg	26%

Excerpted from Reference 115.

The overall response rate for this agent was 10% (90% CI: 5.7%–17.9%) with a duration of response of 1.9 months and an overall survival of 8.8 months. As with progestational agents, the response rate was higher in women with grade 1 tumors (23%) and very poor in high grade tumors (3%). Because of the modest response rates to this medication, it was felt that it might be more appropriate to use this medication sequentially with progestational agents. GOG 119 and GOG 153 investigated this concept. In these phase II trials, the overall response rate was slightly higher than seen in the single agent trials. In addition, phase II trials in recurrent endometrial cancer have also included danazol as well as a GnRH Analog (Goserelin) and an aromatase inhibitor (anastrozole). These agents all had minimal responses rates in advanced endometrial cancer. A summary of all of the GOG studies is shown in Table 10.9.

In light of limited response rates and duration of responses to hormonal therapies, these agents are probably best used in patients who have well-differentiated tumors that are known to be positive for hormone receptors. Although it is temping to use these agents for front line therapy for the well-differentiated tumor, it has been noted that response rates to chemotherapy are higher in well-differentiated tumors as well.[117] To date, the GOG has not had a randomized trial comparing a hormonal agent to a cytotoxic agent in endometrial cancer.

Radiation

The GOG conducted a trial (GOG #94) of whole abdominal radiation in women with stage III and IV endometrial cancers, which included women with both UPSC and endometrioid tumors.[124] The overall disease-free survival was similar between

Table 10.9   Summary of GOG Trials of Hormonal Agents in Advanced Endometrial Cancer

GOG Trial	Regimen	Overall RR	PFS	Survival
81 (Ref. 115)	MPA 200 mg/day	25%	3.2 months	11.1 months
	MPA 1000 mg/day	15%	2.5 months	7.0 months
81-F (Ref. 116)	TMX 20 mg bid	10%	1.9 months	8.8 months
119 (Ref. 118)	MPA 100 mg bid	33%	3.0 months	12.8 months
	TMX 20 mg bid			
	Alternating weekly			
121 (Ref. 117)	Megestrol 800 mg/day	24%	2.5 months	7.6 months
153 (Ref. 120)	Megestrol 80 mg bid	27%	2.7 months	14.0 months
	TMX 20 mg bid			
	Alternating q3weeks			
159 (Ref. 121)	Goserelin 3.6	12%	1.9 months	7.3 months
	mg/month			
168 (Ref. 122)	Anastrozole 1 mg/day	9%	Not stated	Not stated
180 (Ref. 123)	Danazol 100 mg qid	0%	1.9 months	14.4 months
		(27% stable		
		disease)		

the endometrioid and non-endometrioid tumors. However, the recurrence patterns were different with the non-endometrioid tumors having a much higher failure rate in the abdominal cavity and the lung. Another trial by the GOG (GOG #122) has compared radiation with chemotherapy in advanced endometrial cancer.[117] In this trial, whole abdominal radiation was compared to the combination of doxorubicin and cisplatin in women with stage III stage IV endometrial cancer who had no more than 2 cm of residual tumor after surgery. Approximately 20% of the women in this trial had UPSC. More women completed the radiation arm but the progression-free survival and overall survival were statistically superior in the chemotherapy arm of the trial. This has resulted in the use of chemotherapy as the standard of care for women with advanced endometrial cancer. Radiation has been used as adjuvant therapy after surgery in advanced UPSC. However, the results of these trials have been disappointing. A 3-year disease-free survival of only 32% was reported after the treatment of women with stage III/IV UPSC or clear cell carcinoma of the uterus treated with whole abdominal radiation.[125]

Although chemotherapy has been accepted as the optimal treatment modality for women with advanced endometrial cancer, there may be a role for local, regional, or tumor-directed radiation in women with advanced endometrial cancer, including UPSC. A recent GOG trial (GOG #184) compared cisplatin and doxorubicin to cisplatin, doxorubicin, and paclitaxel with all patients receiving tumor-directed radiation[126] It was noted that full dose chemotherapy with doxorubicin, cisplatin, and paclitaxel could be combined with radiation and was relatively well tolerated. However, when tumor-directed radiation was included in the treatment of women with advanced endometrial cancer, no benefit to the more aggressive and toxic three-drug regimen was noted. This is in contrast to an earlier GOG trial (GOG #177) where the same three-drug regimen was shown to have improved progression free and overall survival in a regiment that did not included planned radiation.[127] However, no trial has demonstrated that the addition of radiation to a chemotherapy regimen is superior to chemotherapy alone in advanced disease.

The optimal sequencing of chemotherapy and radiation has not been determined. There are several theoretical arguments for giving chemotherapy before radiation. This sequence will cause less neutropenia as radiation can decrease the pelvic bone marrow reserve. Also, chemotherapy can generally be started earlier after surgery may be more effective in treating subclinical metastasis. However, there are proponents of a "sandwich" technique where radiation is given between courses of chemotherapy and there are no prospective studies suggesting that radiation followed by chemotherapy is any less effective than giving the chemotherapy first.

Chemotherapy

While GOG #177 established the combination of cisplatin, doxorubicin, and paclitaxel as the gold standard for chemotherapy in advanced or recurrent endometrial cancer, the combination of paclitaxel and carboplatin is commonly used in the community.[69, 127] This regimen is better tolerated and many women with endometrial cancer have significant comorbidity including cardiac disease. Currently, the GOG is conducting a phase III noninferiority trial (GOG #209) comparing carboplatin and paclitaxel to the triple combination of paclitaxel, doxorubicin, and cisplatin. This trial included patients with endometrioid cancers as well as UPSC. Enrollment in this trial is completed but the data is not currently mature.

One retrospective trial combining chemotherapy and radiation has suggested there may a benefit to combination therapy, although in this study the benefit was limited to women with optimally resected disease.[113] Given the data, it is not clear from GOG 184 whether radiation and chemotherapy will improve survival or whether the combination will simply allow less toxic chemotherapy regimens to be given.

UPSC may not have the same response to chemotherapy as endometrioid adenocarcinomas. Studies using a combination of platinum, doxorubicin, and cyclophosphamide reported an overall response rate of between 18% and 27% in women with advanced or recurrent measurable disease.[128, 129] High response rates to paclitaxel as a single agent have suggested that this may be the most active agent against UPSC.[130] In the GOG trial (GOG #122) comparing whole abdominal radiation to cisplatin and doxorubicin, a subgroup analysis of the UPSC patients compared to the endometrioid patients suggests that the UPSC patients may not achieve as much benefit from chemotherapy as compared to endometrioid histology.[117] Although this study was not significantly powered to detect such a difference and these patients were not treated with paclitaxel, it does suggest that the UPSC may be less responsive to chemotherapy than other subtypes of endometrial cancer. However, a retrospective analysis of four GOG trials in endometrial cancer has suggested that while the PFS was decreased in these patients that the overall response rate to chemotherapy was the same between these histologic subtypes.[131]

Intraperitoneal cisplatin regimens have been reported in limited numbers of patients with advanced UPSC. Chambers reported that one patient with stage IVB disease was alive and NED after complete resection of disease and IP cisplatin with doxorubicin and cyclophosphamide. However, all other patients with disease outside of the uterus recurred with a median overall survival of 22 months.[132]

REFERENCES

1. JEMAL A, SIEGEL R, WARD E, et al. Cancer statistics, 2008. CA Cancer J Clin 2008;58:71–96.
2. GUSBERG SB. Precursors of corpus carcinoma: estrogens and adenomatous hyperplasia. Am J Obstet Gynecol 1947;54:905.
3. WAY S. The aetiology of carcinoma of the body of the uterus. J Obstet Gynaecol Brit Emp 1954;1:46–58.
4. BOKHMAN JV. Two pathogenetic types of endometrial carcinoma. Gynecol Oncol 1983;15:10–17.
5. MUTTER GL, BAAK JP, FITZGERALD JT, et al. Global expression changes of constitutive and hormonally regulated genes during endometrial neoplastic transformation. Gynecol Oncol 2001;83:177–185.
6. HAMILTON CA, CHEUNG MK, OSANN K, et al. Uterine papillary serous and clear cell carcinomas predict for poorer survival compared to grade 3 endometrioid corpus cancers. Br J Cancer 2006;94:642–646.
7. BORING CC, SQUIRES TS, TONG T. Cancer statistics, 1993. CA Cancer J Clin 1993;43:7–26.
8. Center for Disease Control. U.S. Obesity Trends 1985–2007. CDC; 2008.
9. WARTHIN SA. Heredity with reference to carcinoma as shown by the study of the cases examined in the pathological laboratory of the University of Michigan, 1895–1913. Archives of Internal Medicine 1913;12:546–555.
10. DOUGLAS JA, GRUBER SB, MEISTER KA, et al. History and molecular genetics of Lynch syndrome in family G: a century later. JAMA 2005;294:2195–2202.
11. JETER JM, KOHLMANN W, GRUBER SB. Genetics of colorectal cancer. Oncology (Williston Park) 2006;20:269–276.
12. UMAR A, BOLAND CR, TERDIMAN JP, et al. Revised Bethesda Guidelines for hereditary nonpolyposis colorectal cancer (Lynch syndrome) and microsatellite instability. J Natl Cancer Inst 2004;96:261–268.
13. PLOTZ G, ZEUZEM S, RAEDLE J. DNA mismatch repair and Lynch syndrome. J Mol Histol 2006;37:271–283.
14. STORMORKEN AT, BOWITZ-LOTHE IM, NOREN T, et al. Immunohistochemistry identifies carriers of mismatch repair gene defects causing hereditary nonpolyposis colorectal cancer. J Clin Oncol 2005;23:4705–4712.
15. LI J, YEN C, LIAW D, et al. PTEN, a putative protein tyrosine phosphatase gene mutated in human brain, breast, and prostate cancer. Science 1997;275:1943–1947.
16. BLACK D, BOGOMOLNIY F, ROBSON ME, et al. Evaluation of germline PTEN mutations in endometrial cancer patients. Gynecol Oncol 2005;96:21–24.
17. ENG C. Will the real Cowden syndrome please stand up: revised diagnostic criteria. J Med Genet 2000;37:828–830.
18. KURMAN RJ, KAMINSKI PF, NORRIS HJ. The behavior of endometrial hyperplasia. A long-term study of "untreated" hyperplasia in 170 patients. Cancer 1985;56:403–412.
19. BERGERON C, NOGALES FF, MASSEROLI M, et al. A multicentric European study testing the reproducibility of the WHO classification of endometrial hyperplasia with a proposal of a simplified working classification for biopsy and curettage specimens. Am J Surg Pathol 1999;23:1102–1108.
20. KENDALL BS, RONNETT BM, ISACSON C, et al. Reproducibility of the diagnosis of endometrial hyperplasia, atypical hyperplasia, and well-differentiated carcinoma. Am J Surg Pathol 1998;22:1012–1019.
21. ZAINO RJ, KAUDERER J, TRIMBLE CL, et al. Reproducibility of the diagnosis of atypical endometrial hyperplasia: a Gynecologic Oncology Group study. Cancer 2006;106:804–811.

22. MUTTER GL. Endometrial intraepithelial neoplasia (EIN): will it bring order to chaos? The Endometrial Collaborative Group. Gynecol Oncol 2000;76:287–290.

23. SHERMAN ME, BITTERMAN P, ROSENSHEIN NB, et al. Uterine serous carcinoma. A morphologically diverse neoplasm with unifying clinicopathologic features. Am J Surg Pathol 1992;16:600–610.

24. AMBROS RA, SHERMAN ME, ZAHN CM, et al. Endometrial intraepithelial carcinoma: a distinctive lesion specifically associated with tumors displaying serous differentiation. Hum Pathol 1995;26:1260–1267.

25. SLOMOVITZ BM, BURKE TW, EIFEL PJ, et al. Uterine papillary serous carcinoma (UPSC): a single institution review of 129 cases. Gynecol Oncol 2003;91:463–469.

26. ZHENG W, LIANG SX, YU H, et al. Endometrial glandular dysplasia: a newly defined precursor lesion of uterine papillary serous carcinoma. Part I: morphologic features. Int J Surg Pathol 2004;12:207–223.

27. ZHENG W, LIANG SX, YI X, et al. Occurrence of endometrial glandular dysplasia precedes uterine papillary serous carcinoma. Int J Gynecol Pathol 2007;26:38–52.

28. KAPLAN EB, SHEINER LB, BOECKMANN AJ, et al. The usefulness of preoperative laboratory screening. JAMA 1985;253:3576–3581.

29. SMETANA GW, MACPHERSON DS. The case against routine preoperative laboratory testing. Med Clin North Am 2003;87:7–40.

30. MANCUSO CA. Impact of new guidelines on physicians' ordering of preoperative tests. J Gen Intern Med 1999;14:166–172.

31. Practice advisory for preanesthesia evaluation: a report by the American Society of Anesthesiologists Task Force on Preanesthesia Evaluation. Anesthesiology 2002;96:485–496.

32. FARIS PM, SPENCE RK, LARHOLT KM, et al. The predictive power of baseline hemoglobin for transfusion risk in surgery patients. Orthopedics 1999;22:s135–s140.

33. HIRSCH IA, TOMLINSON DL, SLOGOFF S, et al. The overstated risk of preoperative hypokalemia. Anesth Analg 1988;67:131–136.

34. NALLY BR, DUNBAR SB, ZELLINGER M, et al. Supraventricular tachycardia after coronary artery bypass grafting surgery and fluid and electrolyte variables. Heart Lung 1996;25:31–36.

35. EAGLE KA, BERGER PB, CALKINS H, et al. ACC/AHA guideline update for perioperative cardiovascular evaluation for noncardiac surgery–executive summary: a report of the American College of Cardiology/American Heart Association Task Force on Practice Guidelines (Committee to Update the 1996 Guidelines on Perioperative Cardiovascular Evaluation for Noncardiac Surgery). J Am Coll Cardiol 2002;39:542–553.

36. ANDERSON RJ, O'BRIEN M, MAWHINNEY S, et al. Mild renal failure is associated with adverse outcome after cardiac valve surgery. Am J Kidney Dis 2000;35:1127–1134.

37. SKENDERIS BS 2ND, RODRIGUEZ-BIGAS M, WEBER TK, et al. Utility of routine postoperative laboratory studies in patients undergoing potentially curative resection for adenocarcinoma of the colon and rectum. Cancer Invest 1999;17:102–109.

38. GOLDMAN L, CALDERA DL, NUSSBAUM SR, et al. Multifactorial index of cardiac risk in noncardiac surgical procedures. N Engl J Med 1977;297:845–850.

39. JOHNSON BE, PORTER J. Preoperative evaluation of the gynecologic patient: considerations for improved outcomes. Obstet Gynecol 2008;111:1183–1194.

40. MANGANO DT, LAYUG EL, WALLACE A, et al. Effect of atenolol on mortality and cardiovascular morbidity after noncardiac surgery. Multicenter Study of Perioperative Ischemia Research Group. N Engl J Med 1996;335:1713–1720.

41. ALEXANDER KP, SHAW LJ, SHAW LK, et al. Value of exercise treadmill testing in women. J Am Coll Cardiol 1998;32:1657–1664.

42. GAGNER M, CHIASSON A. Preoperative chest x-ray films in elective surgery: a valid screening tool. Can J Surg 1990;33:271–274.

43. KINKEL K, KAJI Y, YU KK, et al. Radiologic staging in patients with endometrial cancer: a meta-analysis. Radiology 1999;212:711–718.

44. ACOG practice bulletin, clinical management guidelines for obstetrician-gynecologists, number 65, August 2005: management of endometrial cancer. Obstet Gynecol 2005;106:413–425.

45. AKIN O, MIRONOV S, PANDIT-TASKAR N, et al. Imaging of uterine cancer. Radiol Clin North Am 2007;45:167–182.

46. NILOFF JM, KLUG TL, SCHAETZL E, et al. Elevation of serum CA125 in carcinomas of the fallopian tube, endometrium, and endocervix. Am J Obstet Gynecol 1984;148:1057–1058.

47. HSIEH CH, CHANGCHIEN CC, LIN H, et al. Can a preoperative CA 125 level be a criterion for full pelvic lymphadenectomy in surgical staging of endometrial cancer? Gynecol Oncol 2002;86: 28–33.

48. PATSNER B, MANN WJ, COHEN H, et al. Predictive value of preoperative serum CA 125 levels in clinically localized and advanced endometrial carcinoma. Am J Obstet Gynecol 1988;158: 399–402.

49. SOOD AK, BULLER RE, BURGER RA, et al. Value of preoperative CA 125 level in the management of uterine cancer and prediction of clinical outcome. Obstet Gynecol 1997;90:441–447.

50. GEERTS WH, PINEO GF, HEIT JA, et al. Prevention of venous thromboembolism: the Seventh ACCP Conference on Antithrombotic and Thrombolytic Therapy. Chest 2004;126:338S–400S.

51. CLAGETT GP, REISCH JS. Prevention of venous thromboembolism in general surgical patients. Results of meta-analysis. Ann Surg 1988;208:227–240.

52. CLARKE-PEARSON DL, DELONG ER, SYNAN IS, et al. Complications of low-dose heparin prophylaxis in gynecologic oncology surgery. Obstet Gynecol 1984;64:689–694.

53. RASKOB GE, HIRSH J. Controversies in timing of the first dose of anticoagulant prophylaxis against venous thromboembolism after major orthopedic surgery. Chest 2003;124:379S–385S.

54. CLARKE-PEARSON DL, DODGE RK, SYNAN I, et al. Venous thromboembolism prophylaxis: patients at high risk to fail intermittent pneumatic compression. Obstet Gynecol 2003;101:157–163.

55. WILLE-JORGENSEN P, RASMUSSEN MS, ANDERSEN BR, et al. Heparins and mechanical methods for thromboprophylaxis in colorectal surgery. Cochrane Database Syst Rev 2003;CD001217.

56. ACOG Practice Bulletin No. 84: Prevention of deep vein thrombosis and pulmonary embolism. Obstet Gynecol 2007;110:429–440.

57. CREASMAN WT, MORROW CP, BUNDY BN, et al. Surgical pathologic spread patterns of endometrial cancer. A Gynecologic Oncology Group Study. Cancer 1987;60:2035–2041.

58. FIGO. FIGO stages—1988 Revision. Gynecol Oncol 1988;35:125.

59. GREENE FL, PAGE DL, FLEMING ID, et al. AJCC Cancer Staging Manual. 6th ed. New York: Springer-Verlag; 2002.

60. ORR JW JR, NAUMANN WR, ESCOBAR P. "Attitude is a little thing that makes a big difference" Winston Churchill. Gynecol Oncol 2008;109:147–151; author reply 151–153.

61. AALDERS JG, THOMAS G. Endometrial cancer—revisiting the importance of pelvic and para aortic lymph nodes. Gynecol Oncol 2007;104:222–231.

62. CHAN JK, CHEUNG MK, HUH WK, et al. Therapeutic role of lymph node resection in endometrioid corpus cancer: a study of 12,333 patients. Cancer 2006;107:1823–1830.

63. KILGORE LC, PARTRIDGE EE, ALVAREZ RD, et al. Adenocarcinoma of the endometrium: survival comparisons of patients with and without pelvic node sampling. Gynecol Oncol 1995;56:29–33.

64. ASHIH H, GUSTILO-ASHBY T, MYERS ER, et al. Cost-effectiveness of treatment of early stage endometrial cancer. [see comments]. Gynecologic Oncology 1999;74:208–216.

65. BARNES MN, ROLAND PY, ALVAREZ RD, et al. A comparison of treatment stratagies for endometrial adenocarcinoma: a decision analysis [Abstract]. Gynecol Oncol 1998;68:125.

66. FANNING J, FIRESTEIN SL. Cost-effective analysis of complete lymphadenectomy and brachytherapy in early endometrial cancer [Abstract]. Gynecol Oncol 1998;68:128.

67. NAUMANN RW, HIGGINS RV, HALL JB. The use of adjuvant radiation therapy by members of the Society of Gynecologic Oncologists. Gynecol Oncol 1999;75:4–9.

68. ROLAND PY, KELLY FJ, KULWICKI CY, et al. The benefits of a gynecologic oncologist: a pattern of care study for endometrial cancer treatment. Gynecol Oncol 2004;93:125–130.

69. NAUMANN RW, COLEMAN RL. The use of adjuvant radiation therapy in early endometrial cancer by members of the Society of Gynecologic Oncologists in 2005. Gynecol Oncol 2007;105:7–12.

70. ORR JW JR, TAYLOR PT JR. Surgical management of endometrial cancer: how much is enough? Gynecol Oncol 2008;109:1–3.

71. MARIANI A, WEBB MJ, KEENEY GL, et al. Low-risk corpus cancer: is lymphadenectomy or radiotherapy necessary? Am J Obstet Gynecol 2000;182:1506–1519.

72. KITCHENER H, SWART AM, QIAN Q, et al. Efficacy of systematic pelvic lymphadenectomy in endometrial cancer (MRC ASTEC trial): a randomised study. Lancet 2009;373:125–136.

73. PANICI P, BASILE S, MANESCHI F, et al. Systematic pelvic lymphadenectomy versus no lymphadenectomy in early-stage endometrial carcinoma: randomized clinicial trial. J Natl Cancer Inst 2008;100:1707.

74. GOFF BA, KATO D, SCHMIDT RA, et al. Uterine papillary serous carcinoma: patterns of metastatic spread. Gynecol Oncol 1994;54:264–268.

75. GEISLER JP, GEISLER HE, MELTON ME, et al. What staging surgery should be performed on patients with uterine papillary serous carcinoma? Gynecol Oncol 1999;74:465–467.

76. CHAN JK, LOIZZI V, YOUSSEF M, et al. Significance of comprehensive surgical staging in noninvasive papillary serous carcinoma of the endometrium. Gynecol Oncol 2003;90:181–185.

77. CREASMAN WT, KOHLER MF, ODICINO F, et al. Prognosis of papillary serous, clear cell, and grade 3 stage I carcinoma of the endometrium. Gynecol Oncol 2004;95:593–596.

78. BARNHILL D, O'CONNOR D, FARLEY J, et al. Clinical surveillance of gynecologic cancer patients. Gynecol Oncol 1992;46:275–280.

79. BERCHUCK A, ANSPACH C, EVANS AC, et al. Postsurgical surveillance of patients with FIGO stage I/II endometrial adenocarcinoma. Gynecol Oncol 1995;59:20–24.

80. KEYS HM, ROBERTS JA, BRUNETTO VL, et al. A phase III trial of surgery with or without adjunctive external pelvic radiation therapy in intermediate risk endometrial adenocarcinoma: a Gynecologic Oncology Group study. Gynecol Oncol 2004;92:744–751.

81. MORROW CP, BUNDY BN, KURMAN RJ, et al. Relationship between surgical-pathological risk factors and outcome in clinical stage I and II carcinoma of the endometrium: a Gynecologic Oncology Group study. Gynecol Oncol 1991;40:55–65.

82. AGBOOLA OO, GRUNFELD E, COYLE D, et al. Costs and benefits of routine follow-up after curative treatment for endometrial cancer. CMAJ 1997;157:879–886.

83. SHUMSKY AG, STUART GC, BRASHER PM, et al. An evaluation of routine follow-up of patients treated for endometrial carcinoma. Gynecol Oncol 1994;55:229–233.

84. REDDOCH JM, BURKE TW, MORRIS M, et al. Surveillance for recurrent endometrial carcinoma: development of a follow-up scheme. Gynecol Oncol 1995;59:221–225.

85. ROSE PG, SOMMERS RM, REALE FR, et al. Serial serum CA 125 measurements for evaluation of recurrence in patients with endometrial carcinoma. Obstet Gynecol 1994;84:12–16.

86. SMITH DC, PRENTICE R, THOMPSON DJ, et al. Association of exogenous estrogen and endometrial carcinoma. N Engl J Med 1975;293:1164–1167.

87. BARAKAT RR, BUNDY BN, SPIRTOS NM, et al. Randomized double-blind trial of estrogen replacement therapy versus placebo in stage I or II endometrial cancer: a gynecologic oncology group study. J Clin Oncol 2006;24:587–592.

88. ROSSOUW JE, ANDERSON GL, PRENTICE RL, et al. Risks and benefits of estrogen plus progestin in healthy postmenopausal women: principal results from the women's health initiative randomized controlled trial. JAMA 2002;288:321–333.

89. ACOG committee opinion. Hormone replacement therapy in women treated for endometrial cancer. Number 234, May 2000 (replaces number 126, August 1993). Int J Gynaecol Obstet 2001;73:283–284.

90. GHAFOOR A, JEMAL A, COKKINIDES V, et al. Cancer statistics for African Americans. CA Cancer J Clin 2002;52:326–341.

91. LEWIS GC JR, SLACK NH, MORTEL R, et al. Adjuvant progestogen therapy in the primary definitive treatment of endometrial cancer. Gynecol Oncol 1974;2:368–376.

92. MACDONALD RR, THOROGOOD J, MASON MK. A randomized trial of progestogens in the primary treatment of endometrial carcinoma. Br J Obstet Gynaecol 1988;95:166–174.

93. MALKASIAN GD JR, BURES J. Adjuvant progesterone therapy for stage I endometrial carcinoma. Int J Gynaecol Obstet 1978;16:48–49.

94. VERGOTE I, KJORSTAD K, ABELER V, et al. A randomized trial of adjuvant progestagen in early endometrial cancer. Cancer 1989;64:1011–1016.

95. AALDERS J, ABELER V, KOLSTAD P, et al. Postoperative external irradiation and prognostic parameters in stage I endometrial carcinoma: clinical and histopathologic study of 540 patients. Obstet Gynecol 1980;56:419–427.

96. CREUTZBERG CL, VAN PUTTEN WL, KOPER PC, et al. Surgery and postoperative radiotherapy versus surgery alone for patients with stage-1 endometrial carcinoma: multicentre randomised trial. PORTEC Study Group. Post operative radiation therapy in endometrial carcinoma. Lancet 2000;355:1404–1411.

97. NAUMANN RW. Uterine papillary serous carcinoma: state of the state. Curr Oncol Rep 2008;10:505–511.

98. CHADHA M, NANAVATI PJ, LIU P, et al. Patterns of failure in endometrial carcinoma stage IB grade 3 and IC patients treated with postoperative vaginal vault brachytherapy. Gynecol Oncol 1999;75:103–107.

99. PIVER MS, HEMPLING RE. A prospective trial of postoperative vaginal radium/cesium for grade 1–2 less than 50% myometrial invasion and pelvic radiation therapy for grade 3 or deep myometrial invasion in surgical stage I endometrial adenocarcinoma. Cancer 1990;66:1133–1138.

100. NOUT R, PUTTER H, JURGENLIEMK-SCHLZ I, et al. Vaginal brachytherapy versus external beam pelvic radiotherapy for high-intermediate risk endometrial cancer: results of the randomized PORTEC-2 trial. J Clin Oncol 2008;26:LBA5503.

101. SMALL W JR, ERICKSON B, KWAKWA F. American Brachytherapy Society survey regarding practice patterns of postoperative irradiation for endometrial cancer: current status of vaginal brachytherapy. Int J Radiat Oncol Biol Phys 2005;63:1502–1507.

102. NG TY, PERRIN LC, NICKLIN JL, et al. Local recurrence in high-risk node-negative stage I endometrial carcinoma treated with postoperative vaginal vault brachytherapy. Gynecol Oncol 2000;79:490–494.

103. HAVRILESKY LJ, SECORD AA, BAE-JUMP V, et al. Outcomes in surgical stage I uterine papillary serous carcinoma. Gynecol Oncol 2007;105:677–682.

104. GOLDBERG H, MILLER RC, ABDAH-BORTNYAK R, et al. Outcome after combined modality treatment for uterine papillary serous carcinoma: a study by the rare cancer network (RCN). Gynecol Oncol 2008;108:298–305.

105. KELLY MG, O'MALLEY DM, HUI P, et al. Improved survival in surgical stage I patients with uterine papillary serous carcinoma (UPSC) treated with adjuvant platinum-based chemotherapy. Gynecol Oncol 2005;98:353–359.

106. HUH WK, POWELL M, LEATH CA 3RD, et al. Uterine papillary serous carcinoma: comparisons of outcomes in surgical Stage I patients with and without adjuvant therapy. Gynecol Oncol 2003;91:470–475.

107. MORROW CP, BUNDY BN, HOMESLEY HD, et al. Doxorubicin as an adjuvant following surgery and radiation therapy in patients with high-risk endometrial carcinoma, stage I and occult stage II: a Gynecologic Oncology Group Study. Gynecol Oncol 1990;36:166–171.

108. MAGGI R, LISSONI A, SPINA F, et al. Adjuvant chemotherapy vs radiotherapy in high-risk endometrial carcinoma: results of a randomised trial. Br J Cancer 2006;95:266–271.

109. SUSUMU N, SAGAE S, UDAGAWA Y, et al. Randomized phase III trial of pelvic radiotherapy versus cisplatin-based combined chemotherapy in patients with intermediate- and high-risk endometrial cancer: a Japanese Gynecologic Oncology Group study. Gynecol Oncol 2008;108:226–233.

110. GREVEN K, WINTER K, UNDERHILL K, et al. Preliminary analysis of RTOG 9708: Adjuvant postoperative radiotherapy combined with cisplatin/paclitaxel chemotherapy after surgery for patients with high-risk endometrial cancer. Int J Radiat Oncol Biol Phys 2004;59:168–173.

111. FADER AN, DRAKE RD, O'MALLEY DM, et al. Platinum/taxane-based chemotherapy with or without radiation therapy favorably impacts survival outcomes in stage I uterine papillary serous carcinoma. Cancer 2009;115:2119–2127.

112. KELLY MG, O'MALLEY DM, HUI P, et al. Patients with uterine papillary serous cancers may benefit from adjuvant platinum-based chemoradiation. Gynecol Oncol 2004;95:469–473.

113. ALVAREZ SECORD A, HAVRILESKY LJ, BAE-JUMP V, et al. The role of multi-modality adjuvant chemotherapy and radiation in women with advanced stage endometrial cancer. Gynecol Oncol 2007;107:285–291.

114. Bristow RE, Duska LR, Muntz FJ. The role of cytoreductive surgery in the management of stage IV uterine papillary serous carcinoma. Gynecol Oncol 2001;81:92–99.

115. Thigpen JT, Brady MF, Alvarez RD, et al. Oral medroxyprogesterone acetate in the treatment of advanced or recurrent endometrial carcinoma: a dose-response study by the Gynecologic Oncology Group. J Clin Oncol 1999;17:1736–1744.

116. Thigpen T, Brady MF, Homesley HD, et al. Tamoxifen in the treatment of advanced or recurrent endometrial carcinoma: a Gynecologic Oncology Group study. J Clin Oncol 2001;19: 364–367.

117. Randall ME, Filiaci VL, Muss H, et al. Randomized phase III trial of whole-abdominal irradiation versus doxorubicin and cisplatin chemotherapy in advanced endometrial carcinoma: a Gynecologic Oncology Group Study. J Clin Oncol 2006;24:36–44.

118. Whitney CW, Brunetto VL, Zaino RJ, et al. Phase II study of medroxyprogesterone acetate plus tamoxifen in advanced endometrial carcinoma: a Gynecologic Oncology Group study. Gynecol Oncol 2004;92:4–9.

119. Lentz SS, Brady MF, Major FJ, et al. High-dose megestrol acetate in advanced or recurrent endometrial carcinoma: a Gynecologic Oncology Group Study. J Clin Oncol 1996;14:357–361.

120. Fiorica JV, Brunetto VL, Hanjani P, et al. Phase II trial of alternating courses of megestrol acetate and tamoxifen in advanced endometrial carcinoma: a Gynecologic Oncology Group study. Gynecol Oncol 2004;92:10–14.

121. Asbury RF, Brunetto VL, Lee RB, et al. Goserelin acetate as treatment for recurrent endometrial carcinoma: a Gynecologic Oncology Group study. Am J Clin Oncol 2002;25:557–560.

122. Rose PG, Brunetto VL, VanLe L, et al. A phase II trial of anastrozole in advanced recurrent or persistent endometrial carcinoma: a Gynecologic Oncology Group study. Gynecol Oncol 2000;78:212–216.

123. Covens A, Brunetto VL, Markman M, et al. Phase II trial of danazol in advanced, recurrent, or persistent endometrial cancer: a Gynecologic Oncology Group study. Gynecol Oncol 2003;89:470–474.

124. Sutton G, Axelrod JH, Bundy BN, et al. Whole abdominal radiotherapy in the adjuvant treatment of patients with stage III and IV endometrial cancer: a gynecologic oncology group study. Gynecol Oncol 2005;97:755–763.

125. Smith RS, Kapp DS, Chen Q, et al. Treatment of high-risk uterine cancer with whole abdominopelvic radiation therapy. Int J Radiat Oncol Biol Phys 2000;48:767–778.

126. Homesley HD, Filiaci VL, Gibbons SK, et al. Randomized phase III trial in advanced endometrial carcinoma of surgery and volume-directed radiation followed by cisplatin and doxorubicin with or without paclitaxel: A Gynecologic Oncology Group study. Gynecol Oncol 2008;108:S1.

127. Fleming GF, Brunetto VL, Cella D, et al. Phase III trial of doxorubicin plus cisplatin with or without paclitaxel plus filgrastim in advanced endometrial carcinoma: a Gynecologic Oncology Group Study. J Clin Oncol 2004;22:2159–2166.

128. Levenback C, Burke TW, Silva E, et al. Uterine papillary serous carcinoma (UPSC) treated with cisplatin, doxorubicin, and cyclophosphamide (PAC). Gynecol Oncol 1992;46:317–321.

129. Price FV, Chambers SK, Carcangiu ML, et al. Intravenous cisplatin, doxorubicin, and cyclophosphamide in the treatment of uterine papillary serous carcinoma (UPSC). Gynecol Oncol 1993;51:383–389.

130. Ramondetta L, Burke TW, Levenback C, et al. Treatment of uterine papillary serous carcinoma with paclitaxel. Gynecol Oncol 2001;82:156–161.

131. McMeekin DS, Filiaci VL, Thigpen JT, et al. The relationship between histology and outcome in advanced and recurrent endometrial cancer patients participating in first-line chemotherapy trials: a Gynecologic Oncology Group study. Gynecol Oncol 2007;106:16–22.

132. Chambers JT, Chambers SK, Kohorn EI, et al. Uterine papillary serous carcinoma treated with intraperitoneal cisplatin and intravenous doxorubicin and cyclophosphamide. Gynecol Oncol 1996;60:438–442.

Chapter 11

Pelvic Masses and Ovarian Carcinoma

Margarett C. Ellison, MD

INTRODUCTION

Although only 6%–11% of pelvic masses in premenopausal and 29%–35% postmenopausal are malignant, because ovarian cancer is the most significant disease in the differential of a pelvic mass the evaluation of pelvic masses should be taken quite seriously.[1] Ovarian cancer remains the third most frequent gynecologic malignancy and is the gynecologic malignancy with the highest mortality rate in developed countries.[2] Pelvic masses occur in women of all ages. In asymptomatic women aged 25–40 years the prevalence on ultrasound is about 7.8%.[1] The most important aspect of evaluating a woman with a pelvic mass is the necessity of making decisions without a firm diagnosis. This is because until a microscopic examination of the tissue from the mass is made, many possibilities exist, including physiologic changes, congenital masses, nonneoplastic lesions, benign and cancerous neoplasms of the ovary, benign and cancerous neoplasms of other pelvic organs, and cancers metastatic to pelvic organs. In this chapter, perioperative decision making regarding the woman with a pelvic mass is viewed from two aspects: the first in which a cancer diagnosis is uncertain, and the second in which ovarian cancer is known to be present.

OVARIAN CANCER DIAGNOSIS UNCERTAIN

This clinical grouping is much larger than that in which a certain diagnosis exists, and can be further subdivided into (1) patients with pelvic masses at low risk for representing ovarian cancer and (2) pelvic masses at high risk for representing ovarian cancer.

There have been several attempts at creating algorithms for managing women with pelvic masses. Most have developed a clinical profile from the history and

Gynecologic Oncology: Evidence-Based Perioperative and Supportive Care, Second Edition.
Edited by Scott E. Lentz, Allison E. Axtell and Steven A. Vasilev.
© 2011 John Wiley & Sons, Inc. Published 2011 by John Wiley & Sons, Inc.

Table 11.1 Risk of Malignancy Index

					Malignancy Likelihood Ratio	
RMI[a] Score	Sensitivity	95% CI	Specificity	95% CI	Positive	Negative
150	85%	71%–95%	94%	87%–98%	14	16
200	85%	71%–95%	97%	91%–99%	42	15
250	78%	62%–89%	99%	95%–100%	77	22

[a]RMI = U × M × Serum CA125, where U = 0 for ultrasound score of 0 and M = 1 if premenopausal; U = 1 for ultrasound score of 1 and M = 3 if postmenopausal; U = 3 for ultrasound score of 2–5.

physical examination, the determination of a serum CA-125 level, or other tumor markers, and details of an ultrasound examination of the pelvis, and sometimes other factors to triage patients.[3–5] Factors in the history which would suggest a noncancerous etiology for a pelvic mass are young age, postmenarchal but premenopausal status, the use and length of use of oral contraceptives in the past, tubal ligation, and parity. On physical examination, small size, mobility, and nonsolid smooth uniform character on palpation of the mass generally suggest a benign process. Serum CA-125 levels less than 35 U/mL in a premenopausal woman and less than 20 U/mL in a postmenopausal woman are reassuring. In young girls and women under the age of 30 there is risk that an ovarian germ cell cancer may be present. That diagnosis could be anticipated by other tumor markers, namely lactate dehydrogenase, alpha-feto protein, and human chorionic gonadotropin.[6] A number of ultrasound characteristics have been shown to indicate high risk for the presence of an ovarian cancer. They include solid areas in the tumor, thickened septa in multilocular cysts, ascites, bilateral ovarian involvement, and large size. Using the color flow Doppler technique, a decreased vascular resistance has been suggested as a high risk finding for cancer.[7] Perhaps the best multiple factor scoring system, summarized in Table 11.1, is that proposed by Jacobs.[3] This risk of malignancy index (RMI) profile integrates the menopausal status, the serum CA-125 level in units per cubic centimeter, and an ultrasound grading system. Ultrasound grading assigned one point each for (1) multilocular cyst, (2) solid areas, (3) evidence of metastases, (4) ascites, and (5) bilateral lesions. Use of this clinical profile produces a sensitivity of 85% and a specificity of 97% if the RMI is set at 200, and a very high likelihood of representing cancer (LR = 77) if the result exceeds 250. A recent study from Australia confirmed an RMI of >200 had a sensitivity of 84%, specificity of 77%, positive predictive value of 76%, and negative predictive value of 85% in detecting both borderline and invasive ovarian tumors. The false negative rate for invasive tumors was 9%. Forty-one percent of benign tumors were appropriately triaged to general obstetrician-gynecologists.[8] The most frequent errors in applying this scoring system occur in young women whose endometriotic pelvic mass or masses produce high levels (potentially over 1000 U/cc) of CA-125. This would naturally cause the scoring system to reflect a high risk for ovarian cancer, which, in fact, would not be found. The other potential error group is the pre- and postmenopausal women whose ovarian cancers are among the 20% or so which do not produce CA-125.

Pelvic Masses at Low Risk for Representing Ovarian Cancer

Ultrasound examinations have provided a new group of female patients for consideration of pelvic mass lesions, and those are newborn girls. Sometimes fetal ultrasound examination detects the presence of a cystic pelvic abdominal mass.[9] Most masses identified antenatally in this manner demonstrate involution over the next month or so following delivery.

In premenarchal girls, subclinical cystic masses are identified on occasion by ultrasound done for other reasons. Despite the difficulties in explaining a physiological origin for cystic masses less than 8 cm in size, a short period of observation is probably warranted in this group.

During the reproductive years, unilateral cystic masses over 5 cm in size which persist through a menstrual cycle or into the second trimester of pregnancy are unlikely to be physiologic and are best considered for removal.[10] Smaller masses incidentally discovered on ultrasound examinations, which persist through a period of 3 or more months, may warrant enough clinical suspicion to recommend removal.

Menopausal women with cystic pelvic masses are at significant risk for harboring a benign or malignant ovarian neoplasm. The standard treatment has been to approach such lesions surgically. Recently there has been a growing interest in defining a group of menopausal women whose pelvic masses can be safely observed without surgical intervention. Generally speaking, these are women who have unilocular pelvic cystic masses less than 5 cm in diameter (although less than 3 cm may represent a safer upper limit) with normal serum CA-125 determinations. There seems to be little risk that such lesions represent or will evolve into ovarian cancers. Similarly, there seems to be little risk if such a mass stays stable over a period of time that increased growth or adnexal accidents such as rupture, hemorrhage, or torsion will occur. This necessitates, however, indefinite long-term follow-up with physical examinations, ultrasound determinations, and CA-125 determinations. Although this concept seems to have merit, no one has shown comparative data illustrating whether removal or follow-up is superior.[11]

For patients with a pathologic mass of low malignancy risk, a straightforward elective surgical operation to serve as a diagnosis and therapy for the mass is indicated. In this group of patients the very low risk of cancer being present allows for some latitude in surgical planning. An emphasis on minimally invasive surgical maneuvers, including laparoscopically directed surgery, could be employed. Elective decompression of the cystic mass to facilitate removal, preservation of fertility by unilateral oophorectomy, or of ovarian tissue itself by cystectomy is a reasonable undertaking in premenopausal women in this setting.[12, 13] In postmenopausal women it is still wise to consider a bilateral salpingo-oophorectomy combined with a hysterectomy as definitive treatment in this low risk situation. This recommendation has received recent support by an elegant analysis performed by the group at the University of California at San Francisco.[14]

Pelvic Masses at High Risk for Representing Ovarian Cancer

The definition of a pelvic mass at high risk for representing a cancer is arbitrary and debated. The previously cited definition of Jacobs is one attempt to divide high from low risk masses. The three important decisions to make in this setting are, first, what further diagnostic work-up should be considered, second, what intraoperative contingencies need to be planned for, and finally, what preparations for therapy need to be undertaken.[15]

DIAGNOSTIC CONSIDERATIONS

The diagnostic modalities, which should be applied to reach this point, are the history and physical examination, a serum CA-125 determination, and an ultrasound examination of the pelvis. In anticipation of major clinical intervention, preoperative testing should be initiated as discussed in Chapters 8 and 9. If the woman is in her childbearing years, pregnancy testing should be undertaken, a recent Pap smear result should be available, and a test for occult blood in the stool should be considered. Aside from testing for occult blood in the stool, further routine evaluation of the intestinal tract in the presence of a high risk pelvic mass is not justified. However, if significant gastrointestinal symptoms and signs are elicited, they should become a matter of focus and could lead to upper or lower gastrointestinal endoscopy and/or upper gastrointestinal series or barium enema evaluation.[16] Particular clinical scenarios where this could be important would be with a tender, relatively fixed pelvic mass in a woman over the age of 35 in which case diverticulitis could be a consideration, or the finding of bilateral ovarian masses largely solid in character, which may represent a gastrointestinal (gastric) cancer becoming clinically evident by metastasis to the ovaries (Krukenberg's tumors).

Another clinical question, which faces every pelvic surgeon regarding a pelvic mass, is whether the mass compromises the lower urinary tract or not. If the pelvic mass is large, immobile, or there is demonstrated distortion of pelvic organs on examination, then outlining the bladder as it interfaces with the mass and the position and number of ureters in relation to the mass are important determinations. Intravenous urography is a straightforward method of discerning these issues. However, a more elaborate way of defining these is with computerized tomography (CT) or magnetic resonance imaging.[17] Although it is more expensive, it may also provide more information for intraoperative decision making. Particularly important in the setting of the high risk pelvic mass is the possible demonstration of retroperitoneal lymph node involvement, intraperitoneal metastasis to the omentum, the peritoneum, the subdiaphragmatic spaces, as well as intrahepatic and intrasplenic lesions.

Preanesthetic tests (a chest X-ray and electrocardiogram) as well as provision for blood transfusions are usual hospital requirements prior to major surgery.[18] Assuming a woman is in stable health with adequate cardiopulmonary reserve, following the diagnostic work-up, an exploratory laparatomy should be scheduled for the diagnosis and treatment of the pelvic mass. The ideal situation is that the surgery be undertaken by a team of gynecologic oncologists who are fully capable of addressing complete removal of the pelvic tumor mass and of addressing the anatomic sites that contain or are at risk for containing metastasis so that a firm diagnostic basis can be provided for further treatment and that further treatment can be given in the best situation possible (i.e., little or no residual cancer).[19–24] Except for the rare deep hepatic parenchyma metastasis, or pleural-based metastasis, such a surgical team could handle whatever organ involvement or metastatic sites might be detected. However, if the surgery must take place without access to a surgical team capable of optimal cytoreduction, information from a CT scan and other extended diagnostic tests could be considered as "screening tests" for possible referral for such surgery. It is important to note, however, that CT is not very good at detecting intra-abdominal metastasis or retroperitoneal lymph node metastasis, especially if they are small in size. As noted, it is uncommon that involvement of solid structures such as the liver or spleen would be encountered in this setting. Outcomes in terms of disease-free interval and overall survival have been found to be superior when initial debulking surgery is performed by a gynecologic oncologist when compared with a general surgeon and/ or general obstetrician-gynecologist.[25]

Preparation for surgery. Reasonable provisions for this group would include assessing the risk for blood transfusion and anticipating an inpatient hospital stay. A pathologist should be available for specimen examination to include rapid frozen section analysis. A clear plan should be delineated covering the circumstances under which ovarian function or fertility would be terminated, considering age and patient preference. Prophylactic measures should be initiated as discussed in Chapters 9 and 11.

The Gynecologic Oncology Group (GOG) in their surgical procedures manual best defines the surgical procedures judged essential to address an ovarian cancer discovered intraoperatively (Tables 11.2 and 11.3). This manual was developed as a consensus for standardizing research based on intraoperative data regarding ovarian cancer.

Under certain circumstances, health status will be severely affected by the pelvic mass. The most common direct indicator of a mass markedly affecting health is the presence of clinical ascites. Undertaking surgery in such women can lead to a need for multifocal excavations of large metastatic sites and potential for incomplete removal of metastasis. It is not at all uncommon for such women to reaccumulate ascites rapidly and for over a period of a few days following the surgery. In this setting a confusing clinical picture of oliguria, inconsistent central venous pressures, inconsistent arterial blood pressures, and abdominal distention can cause a confusing clinical picture where heart failure, respiratory failure, internal hemorrhage, and renal failure are not easily sorted out. Preoperative consideration for an intensive care unit (ICU) with possible central venous or Swan Ganz catheter monitoring is

Table 11.2   Ovarian Cancer Surgical Staging Procedure[a]

---

1. The abdominal incision must be adequate to explore the entire abdominal cavity and allow safe cytoreductive surgery. A vertical incision is recommended but not required.

2. The volume of any free peritoneal fluid should be estimated. Free peritoneal fluid is to be aspirated for cytology. If no free peritoneal fluid is present, separate peritoneal washings will be obtained from the pelvis, paracolic gutters, and infradiaphragmatic area. These may be submitted separately or as a single specimen. Patients with stage III or IV disease do not require cytologic assessment.

3. All peritoneal surfaces including the undersurface of both diaphragms and the serosa and mesentery of the entire gastrointestinal tract will be visualized for evidence of metastatic disease.

4. Careful inspection of the omentum and removal if possible of at least the infracolic omentum will be accomplished. At minimum, a biopsy of the omentum is required.

5. If possible, an extrafascial total abdominal hysterectomy and a bilateral salpingo-oophorectomy will be performed. If these are not possible, a biopsy of the ovary and sampling of the endometrium must be performed. In selected situations of apparent low stage disease in a woman desiring reproductive potential, a unilateral salpingo-oophorectomy may be appropriate.

6. If possible, all remaining gross disease within the abdominal cavity is resected.

7. If there is no evidence of disease beyond the ovary or pelvis, the following must be done:
   (a) Peritoneal biopsies from
   - Cul-de-sac
   - Vesical peritoneum
   - Right and left pelvic sidewalls
   - Right and left paracolic gutters
   (b) Biopsy and scraping of the right diaphragm
   (c) Selective bilateral pelvic and para-aortic node dissection

8. Selective pelvic and para-aortic node dissection must be done in the following situations:
   (a) Patients with tumor nodules outside the pelvis which are less than or equal to 2 cm
   (b) Patients with stage IV disease and those with tumor nodules outside the pelvis which are greater than 2 cm do not require node dissection, unless the only nodule greater than 2 cm is a lymph node, in which case it must be biopsied.

---

[a]Excerpted and modified from the GOG Surgical Manual.

probably a wise plan for such patients. However, in the only review published addressing this issue specifically, the intraoperative course was more predictive than preoperative condition with respect to extended use of ICU resources beyond 24 hours.[26] Cardiac, pulmonary, renal, or systemic diseases such as diabetes known to be present preoperatively heighten the concern for intra- and postoperative problems. A long anesthetic accompanied by extensive fluid shifts with compromised organ systems can well require extended postoperative endotracheal intubation and respiratory ventilator support.[26, 27] Such intervention and risk-taking is reasonable in many

Table 11.3 Reassessment Laparotomy (Second Look) for Ovarian Cancer[a]

Indications	1. To assess completeness of response to chemotherapy
	2. To resect residual disease
Timing	After therapy, patients exhibiting a complete response or a partial response will undergo a restaging laparotomy.
Incision	The abdominal incision must be adequate to explore the entire abdominal cavity and allow safe cytoreductive surgery. A vertical incision is recommended but not required.
Ascites	If present, ascites must be examined cytologically.
Washings	If ascites is not present, washings must be obtained immediately upon entry into the peritoneal cavity from the pelvis, right and left paracolic gutters, and the subdiaphragmatic space. These may be submitted separately or as a single specimen. Patients who have histologically confirmed persistent disease do not require cytologic assessment.
Exploration	All peritoneal surfaces must be visually examined including direct inspection of the diaphragm. The location and exact size of tumor nodules must be described. Biopsy proof of residual disease is necessary.
	If no tumor is visualized, routine biopsies must be performed from:
	• Right and left pelvic sidewalls
	• Cul-de-sac and vesical peritoneum
	• Right and left abdominal gutter peritoneums
	• Undersurface of the right hemi-diaphragm (or scraping of the diaphragm may be submitted as an alternative)
	• Residual omentum
	• Adhesive bands, abnormally scarred areas
	• Retro-peritoneum: If lymph node dissection was performed at the initial staging procedure and was negative, resampling is not required. If the lymph nodes were positive, or were not done at the time of initial surgery, pelvic and para-aortic node dissection should be performed.
Laparoscopy	Laparoscopic evaluation of the peritoneal cavity is acceptable as a second look surgery if histologically confirmed persistent disease can be seen and biopsied. If no disease is seen, then exploratory laparotomy is mandatory for purposes of GOG protocol activity.

[a]Excerpted and modified from the GOG Surgical Manual.

women with metastatic ovarian cancer because it is widely held that return to health and length of life with subsequent postoperative treatment are directly related to the amount of residual cancer remaining at the end of the surgical operation.

The most common nonvital disability that surrounds ovarian cancer surgery is the issue of an enterostomy or colostomy. The use of gastrointestinal stapling devices have allowed for safe performance of coloproctostomies, which are frequently an issue with large pelvic cancers. In fact, it should be an unusual circumstance in which a permanent intestinal stoma is necessary in the setting of a planned first operation for a metastatic ovarian cancer.

When a woman with a high risk pelvic mass is medically compromised, a surgical operation of any sort may be too hazardous. Here an extended diagnostic work-up would seem to be indicated because one may be forced to act on a presumptive diagnosis, since biopsy information from the tumor mass would require the surgery that is contraindicated. Imaging-guided needle biopsy has been problematic in the evaluation of pelvic masses. Intervening vital structures, masses comprised mostly of cyst fluid, and the risk of intraperitoneal spill of malignant cells are all cited as difficulties, the latter being controversial in terms of clinical implications. In this setting one may choose to follow a patient hoping that her physical situation can be improved so that the surgery could be undertaken in a period of weeks or a few months. This would be most applicable in cases where there is no evidence of metastasis. In the presence of ascites or of metastatic masses, it may be best to proceed with chemotherapy for a presumed ovarian cancer. Recently, an interest has developed regarding neoadjuvant chemotherapy that involves several chemotherapy courses following a surgical operation of modest extent during which the histologic diagnosis of metastatic ovarian cancer has been established. Complete cytoreductive surgery is then performed following response to chemotherapy.[28, 29] Whether this will prove to be a better approach to ovarian cancer than the traditional one of a primary definitive surgical attempt followed by chemotherapy is not clear at present. There is, however, enough merit from this experience to warrant beginning the chemotherapy in medically compromised patients with presumed metastatic ovarian cancers. Sometimes patients burdened with acute heart failure, the ravages of cerebral vascular accidents, the disabilities of pleural effusions with respiratory compromise, and immobility from ascites may have their general health status improved such that they become, after a short interval of chemotherapy, an acceptable surgical candidate. Should that not be the case, then those who respond to the initial courses of chemotherapy could continue and represent the sole method of management. As a final point, those women who present with a setting likely indicative of ovarian cancer but do not respond to the chemotherapy are unlikely to benefit from any surgical interventions.

OVARIAN CANCER DIAGNOSIS CERTAIN

Following (Initial) Incomplete Surgery

Presumed Nonmetastatic

When the primary surgical procedure provides the diagnosis of low malignant potential or invasive carcinoma of the ovary but incomplete staging information, the oncologist must decide whether another surgical operation is warranted to provide necessary information upon which to base further treatment. This is especially difficult because there is usually some degree of information available regarding staging. In patients with presumed stage I neoplasms, information regarding exploration of the abdomen, the status of the omentum, and the clinical status of lymph nodes is usually present to some extent. There are no published or universally agreed upon guidelines regarding which combinations of data suffice in this setting (i.e., exploration, with or without omental biopsy/omentectomy, with or without target biopsies, with or without lymph node removal, with or without peritoneal cytology). Recent reports describe management of such cases with a second laparoscopic staging operation, involving inspection of all accessible peritoneal surfaces omentectomy, pelvic and para-aortic lymphadenectomies, and peritoneal cytologic washings. This has the advantage of gathering all of the information in a surgical operation, which is of much less physical impact, and total cost than an exploratory laparotomy, and it can probably be applied to most incompletely staged patients.

Some presumably stage I patients will have enough worrisome factors already known (that is, the presence of malignant cells in ascitic fluid or high grade cancers penetrating the tumor capsule) that chemotherapy is warranted.[30] In such patients, one can make a case for deferring the staging surgery until after the completion of chemotherapy, with a reassessment or second look surgery.

Known Metastatic

In this case, metastatic ovarian cancer is encountered which was not anticipated. The diagnosis has been established and usually some therapeutic intervention has taken place. Often an adnexectomy or hysterectomy/adnexectomy or even surgical correction of a bowel obstruction with or without an intestinal stoma has been performed. In many cases the intraperitoneal metastases are left largely unaddressed.

To the extent that the initial surgery was minor in scope (e.g., mini-laparotomy or laparoscopy), recovery is prompt and uncomplicated, and a major cytoreduction seems possible, it is best to proceed in a medically fit patient, with a definitive surgery prior to chemotherapy.

If the initial surgery is followed by slow recovery, complications, or the identification of unresectable metastases, delaying the cytoreductive surgery and beginning chemotherapy seems prudent. This clinical setting is another scenario for neoadjuvant chemotherapy consideration.[28, 29]

Adjuvant Therapy

Intravenous Chemotherapy

Since 1996 intravenous with paclitaxel and platinum chemotherapy for advanced stage of ovarian cancer has been the mainstay of treatment. Prior to this era, cyclophosphamide and cisplatin were the standard of care. In 1996, the GOG completed its trial of IV cisplatin and cyclophospamide vs. IV cisplatin and paclitaxel.[31] In this trial, 386 eligible women with suboptimally debulked stage III or stage IV patients were randomized to receive either IV cisplatin and cyclophosphamide or IV cisplatin and paclitaxel, which resulted in an improved response rate of 73% vs. 60%, improved progression-free interval of 18 vs. 13 months, and overall survival improvement of 38 vs. 24 months in the paclitaxel group over the cyclophosphamide group.[31] Although there were more allergic reactions, alopecia, neutropenia, and fever in the paclitaxel group, the improvement in survival, progression-free interval, and response rate was felt to be worth this relative increase in toxicity and therefore this regimen became the standard of care until 2003.[31]

In 2003, GOG 158 results were published, which compared IV carboplatin and paclitaxel to IV cisplatin and paclitaxel.[32] GOG 158 found not only less toxicity and easier administration, but also a survival advantage of relative risk of death of 0.84 in the carboplatin arm.[32] In light of these trial results, paclitaxel and carboplatin intravenous therapy for six cycles after debulking has become the gold standard to which all other therapies are compared currently.

Intraperitoneal Therapy

After initial cytoreductive surgery, if residual disease is less than 1 cm or preferably microscopic only, then intraperitoneal chemotherapy has emerged as the first-line standard of care for these patients. Three randomized controlled trials have led to this conclusion. The most recent trial completed, GOG 172, which compared IV taxol and IV cisplatin to IV taxol followed by IP cisplatin on day 2 and IP taxol on Day 8.[33] In this study of 415 eligible patients, there was a statistically significant increase in leukopenia, gastrointestinal toxicity, neutropenia, infection, fatigue, metabolic abnormalities, and pain in the IP arm; however, there was a significant improvement in progression-free interval and overall survival compared to the control arm of 5 months and 16 months, respectively.[33] These benefits were found even though only 42% of patients were able to receive the proscribed six cycles of intraperitoneal therapy.[33] Criticisms of the trial are that the control arm containing cisplatin instead of carboplatin may have contributed to some of the improvement in survival, since GOG 158 showed a survival advantage in those patients who received carboplatin vs. cisplatin. In addition, many have argued that the added toxicity of IP therapy is not worth the benefit, although quality of life surveys were equivalent at 1-year posttreatment.[33] Clearly further trials are needed to improve tolerability of future IP regiments and to determine whether the trend toward improved progression-free interval and overall survival is real.

Prior IP trials yielded difficult-to-interpret data. GOG 104 which evaluated patients with 0–2 cm residual disease compared IV cyclophosphamide and IV cisplatin vs. IP cisplatin and IV cyclophosphamide.[34] Although there was an overall survival benefit of 41 vs. 49 months, this benefit was not seen in the group in which one would expect to see it the most, the subset of patients with less than 0.5 cm residual disease.[34] The subsequent trial, GOG 114, which compared IV cisplatin and paclitaxel as the control arm and an experimental arm of two cycles of carboplatin at an AUC of 9 IV followed by IP cisplatin and IV paclitaxel for six cycles in patients with less than 1 cm residual disease showed an overall progression-free survival benefit but no statistically significant survival benefit.[35]

Maintenance Therapy

Although ovarian cancer generally has an excellent initial response rate to chemotherapy, these responses are not durable and in the overwhelming majority of patients who present with advanced disease it will recur at some point in the future. This has led researchers to propose the concept of maintenance or consolidation therapy for patients who have a clinical complete response after initial therapy. An attempt to evaluate the premise that prolonged consolidation chemotherapy is better was made in the SWOG/GOG trial (GOG 178) which compared 3 vs. 12 monthly courses of paclitaxel after a complete clinical response to platinum and taxane therapy.[36] Because at the interim analysis there was an improvement in progression-free interval of 28 vs. 21 months in the 12-month arm, the study was closed and further survival data could not be determined.[36] Controversy exists over whether an additional 9 months on treatment yields an improvement in quality of life given the improvement in progression-free interval of only 7 months. This is as of yet a question that remains unanswered.

During Postoperative Chemotherapy

Refractory   Up to 20% of patients with metastases will exhibit progression of their disease during chemotherapy. Surgical intervention in an attempt to salvage the situation risks significant morbidity. There is little evidence that survival can be affected in this group by further surgery.[37]

Following Postoperative Chemotherapy

Persistence   Patients whose measurable disease has remained stable at the conclusion of primary chemotherapy should also be considered refractory to such chemotherapy, although the clinical situation may have less immediate peril. Since these patients represent a minority of the refractory patient population, little is known regarding the impact of surgical intervention. Relatively healthy individuals, who have a few large isolated metastases noted on imaging studies or on examination may represent an exception. Surgical intervention may be considered if these are judged amenable to complete resection.

Persistence of disease following postoperative chemotherapy can represent a spectrum from a partial response, to stable disease at the end of planned chemotherapy. In the absence of clinically measurable disease, persistence can also be inferred by a serum CA-125 level that has failed to normalize during treatment.[38] In these situations a second look laparotomy for diagnostic purposes is superfluous. Resistance to first-line chemotherapeutic agents is clear and an elective cytoreductive surgery for widespread disease will prove futile, with the possible exception of isolated disease resection as noted above. This group of patients is most similar to those with refractory disease, although the threat to health and life is less immediate. Elective therapeutic interventions should generally be medical, not surgical. This area requires further study, and will likely evolve as a result of development of more effective primary and secondary salvage chemotherapy regimens.

Persistence can also be determined by finding residual cancer at the time of second look laparotomy. Of all the postchemotherapy scenarios, this is the one in which an aggressive therapeutic approach can best be justified. This is so because at the time of discovery a significant proportion of the surgical risks have already been taken. Also, the disease burden for cytoreduction is usually modest, in that it is subclinical. This usually means a partial response has been achieved and salvage therapy can be applied in an optimal residual disease setting.

Whether the knowledge gained regarding disease status and/or the tumor removal translates to a survival advantage is debated. Retrospective analyses have spoken strongly both for[39] and against[40] an advantage, but are severely limited in drawing meaningful conclusions due to study design. Other prospective studies including randomized trials have failed to show an advantage,[41–43] but are also burdened by problems with study design and questionable chemotherapeutic choices, for both initial and salvage regimens. Thus the bulk of available data rests with conflicting Level II and minimal Level I evidence.

There does seem to be general agreement that (1) some positive second look patients will experience prolonged (i.e., greater than 5 years) survival and (2) large volume disease at second look is an ominous finding. What is not clear is the relative impacts of therapies at and subsequent to the second look and what subgroups of patients and tumor types stand to benefit most from the second look.[44]

No Evidence of Disease   Many patients with metastatic ovarian carcinoma will complete first-line chemotherapy and present no evidence of their cancer (i.e. physical examination is normal, serum tumor markers have normalized, and imaging studies reveal no abnormalities). Performing a laparotomy on patients with previously documented metastatic disease but with a normal physical examination and serum CA-125 will demonstrate persistent cancer in approximately 50%[45,46] (see Table 11.3).

Barter's[45] collective review suggests that CT scans add little precision to decision making because of a false negative rate of 28% and a false positive rate of 6%. There is little evidence that magnetic resonance imaging or sonography is superior to CT imaging for evaluation of persistence.[47] The role of spiral CT scanning is yet to be investigated.

Newer approaches employing radioisotope-labeled monoclonal antibodies such as indium-labeled TAG-72 may offer promise for the future. Current experience suggests the sensitivity of this method to be about 60%, not equal to the sensitivity of second look laparotomy. Currently, this modality seems most useful where there is already strong evidence that occult cancer is present.

Thus, it seems that second look laparotomy at this point offers the best information regarding disease status. Two groups of patients are derived from this endeavor: those with no evidence of disease and those with persistent cancer. In the group of women with no evidence of persisting disease (approximately 50%), approaches such as no further therapy, consolidation therapy by continuing the same chemotherapy, or consolidation therapy by changing treatment have been tried. Interest in continuing treatment in some form is supported by long-term follow-up of patients with negative second look, which suggests recurrence rates may eventually approach 50%.[49,50]

It is important to note also that in this group where at least 50% will experience extended disease-free survival, serious postoperative complications are uncommon.

Surgical mortality is estimated to be 0.1%.[45] Significant morbidities include ileus and infections, each occurring with an incidence as high as 15%.[51]

Second look laparoscopy has been suggested as a means to reduce morbidity and total costs with no loss in reliability as opposed to laparotomy.[52] There is no long-term information on the outcome of negative second look laparoscopy. There have also been concerns voiced concerning possible increased morbidity from laparoscopy because of extensive adhesions, which limit exposure and conceal visceral injury.[39, 53]

In the other 50% of women who harbor persistent disease, management decisions can be made on a sound basis and without delay. There is also the opportunity for secondary cytoreduction during reassessment surgery, as mentioned previously.[54]

Asymptomatic Recurrence   Women being followed after chemotherapy may have a sequence of follow-up tumor markers, may have interval scans, and will have interval physical examinations, all of which can elicit findings suggestive of recurrence. Patients with evidence of asymptomatic recurrence of ovarian cancer should be considered for surgical intervention. This becomes more of a consideration if the appearance of the putative recurrence is late (i.e., longer than 6 months from chemotherapy), if it is unifocal or is confined to a region, and if there are no significant adverse sequelae from the initial surgery and chemotherapy. The same principles for cytoreductive surgery apply in this setting as they would in the initial surgical setting for properly selected patients. The goals may include increased disease-free interval and QALY (quality adjusted life year) gain after completion of therapeutic intervention.

A recently completed randomized trial in asymptomatic recurrence has fueled the debate over when to institute second-line therapy. The MRCOV05/EORTC 5955 trial involved 529 women who were predominantly (81%) with stage 3/4 ovarian cancer, all with complete clinical responses after primary therapy. These women were divided into two groups, and were followed with CA-125 measurements every 3 months. Patients were not informed of their laboratory results, but were randomized to immediate notification once CA-125 reached 2× the upper limit of normal, or to treatment only when clinical manifestations of recurrence appeared. The primary outcome measure was overall survival. Results showed that treatment was instituted 5 months earlier in the immediate treatment arm, but the overall survival was no different between the two arms (median overall survival 41 months). The authors concluded that "earlier institution of chemotherapy did not induce a longer remission . . . or improve survival" in these ovarian cancer patients. They even suggested that CA-125 may have no role for follow-up in patients who achieve a complete clinical response.[55]

Symptomatic Recurrence   Most symptomatic recurrences of ovarian cancer are related to obstruction of the intestinal tract. Exploratory laparotomy will usually be performed in the hope that a decisive surgical maneuver can be performed to overcome the obstruction, either by by-pass, resection and anastamosis, or creation of an intestinal stoma.[54] This occurs often enough that it is worthwhile to consider, as long as the limitations of such an approach are clearly understood. The likelihood of creating multiple enterotomies during dissection, of not relieving the obstruction, of creating a stoma with a significantly shortened intestinal tract, or of settling for placement of a gastrostomy or jejunostomy tube for drainage only is very high. Worst of all, coalescent metastases affecting most or all of the intestinal tract are often encountered such that one may be left with only damaged bowel segments and an unrelieved obstruction. These are all sobering realities to such surgery. Marginal analysis (i.e., high morbidity and cost for one additional unit of benefit) of this situation suggests that few patients will benefit overall. Therefore, one is left with highly individualized patient selection, which may result in an acceptable outcome. It is critical to appreciate that these decisions are made in the face of no real alternative other than terminal care. Medical management of bowel obstruction in this setting, with or without chemotherapy and intravenous hyperalimentation, is even less effective.[56]

Randomized controlled trials are lacking in areas related to primary, much less secondary, cytoreductive surgery and the associated scenarios described above. However, given the spectrum of clinical management problems, it is unlikely that all questions will be answered at Level I certainty. Thus, patient management should be based on individual assessment of risk and cost to benefit, with an emphasis on clinical trial participation.

REFERENCES

1. BORGFELDT C, ANDOLF E. Transvaginal ultrasound ovarian findings in a random sample of women 25–40 years old. Ultrasound Obstet Gynecol 1999;13:345–350.
2. ORIEL K, HARTENBACK E, et al. Trends in United States ovarian cancer mortality. Obstet Gynecol 1999;93:30–33.
3. JACOBS I, ORAM D, FAIRBANKS J, et al. A risk of malignancy index incorporating CA-125, ultrasound, and menopausal status for the accurate preoperative diagnosis of ovarian cancer. Br J Obstet Gynaecol 1990;97:922–929.
4. LERNER JP, TIMOR-TRITSCH IE, FEDERMAN A, et al. Transvaginal ultrasonographic characterization of ovarian masses with an improved weighted scoring system. Am J Obstet Gynecol 1994;170:81–85.
5. FINKLER NJ, BENACERRAF B, LAVIN Pt, et al. Comparison of serum CA-125 clinical impression and ultrasound in the preoperative evaluation of ovarian masses. Obstet Gynecol 1988;72:659–671.
6. SCHWARTZ PG. The role of tumor markers in the preoperative diagnosis of ovarian cysts. Clin Obstet Gynecol 1993;36 (2).
7. YORUK P, DUNDAR O, et al. Comparison of the risk of malignancy index and self-constructed logistic regression models in preoperative evaluation of adnexal masses. J Ultrasound Med 2008; 27(10):1469–1477.
8. CHIA YN, MARSDEN DE, et al. Triage of ovarian masses. Aust N Z J Obstet Gynaecol 2008; 48(3):322–328.
9. MILLER DM, BLAKE JM, STRINGER DA, et al. Prepubertal ovarian cyst formation: five years experience. Obstet Gynecol 1993;81:434–438.
10. NIH Consensus Conference. Ovarian cancer screening treatment and follow-up. JAMA 1995;276:491–498.
11. GOLDSTEIN SR. Conservative management of small postmenopausal cystic masses. Clin Obstet Gynecol 1993;36.
12. HASSON HM. Laparoscopic management of ovarian cysts. J Reprod Med. 1990;35:863–867.

13. GRANBERG S. Relationship of macroscopic appearance to the histologic diagnosis of ovarian tumors. Clin Obstet Gynecol 1993;36(2):363–374.

14. GROVER CM, KUPPERMAN M, KAHN JG, et al. Concurrent hysterectomy at bilateral salpingo-oophorectomy: benefits, risks, and costs. Obstet Gynecol 1996;88:907–913.

15. Society of Gynecologic Oncologists Clinical Practice Guidelines. Practice guidelines: ovarian cancer. Oncology 1998; 129–133.

16. SALTZMAN AK, CARTER JR, FOWLER NM, et al. The utility of preoperative screening colonoscopy in gynecologic oncology. Gynecol Oncol 1995;56:181–186.

17. BUIST MR, GOLDING RP, BURGER CW, et al. Comparative evaluation of diagnostic methods in ovarian carcinoma with emphasis on CT and MRI. Gynecol Oncol 1994;52:191–198.

18. BROOKS S. Preoperative evaluation of patients with suspected ovarian cancer. Gynecol Oncol 1994;55:580–590.

19. NGUYEN HN, AVERETTE HE, HOSKINS W, et al. National Survey of Ovarian Carcinoma Part V. The impact of physician's specialty on patients' survival. Cancer 1993;72(2):3663–3670.

20. EISENKOP SM, SPIRTOS NM, MONTAG TW, et al. The impact of subspecialty training on the management of advanced ovarian cancer. Gynecol Oncol 1992;47:203–209.

21. LIU PC, BENJAMIN I, MORGAN MA, et al. Effect of surgical debulking on survival in stage IV ovarian cancer. Gynecol Oncol 1997;64:4–8.

22. LE T, KREPART GV, LOTOCKI RJ, et al. Does debulking surgery improve survival in biologically aggressive ovarian carcinoma? Gynecol Oncol 1997;67:208–214.

23. MUNKARAH AR, HALLUM AV, MORRIS M, et al. Prognostic significance of residual disease in patients with stage IV epithelial ovarian cancer. Gynecol Oncol 1997;64:13–17.

24. CURTIN JP, MALIK R, VENKATRAMAN E, et al. Stage IV ovarian cancer: impact of surgical debulking. Gynecol Oncol 1997;64:9–12.

25. CHAN JK, KAPP DS, et al. Influence of the gynecologic oncologist on the survival of ovarian cancer patients. Obstet Gynecol 2007;109(6):1342–1350.

26. AMIR M, SHABOT M, KARLAN BY. Surgical intensive care unit care after ovarian cancer surgery: an analysis of indications. Am J Obstet Gynecol 1997;176:1389–1393.

27. VAN LE L, FAKHRY S, WALTON LA, et al. Use of APAC HE II scoring system to determine mortality of gynecologic oncologic patients in the intensive care unit. Oncol Gynecol 1995;85:53–59.

28. SHAPIRO F, SCHNEIDER J, MARKMAN M, et al. High intensity intravenous cyclophosphamide and cisplatin, interim surgical debulking and intraperitoneal cisplatin in advanced ovarian carcinoma: a pilot trial with ten year followup. Gynecol Oncol 1997;67:39–45.

29. VANDERBURG MEL, VANLENT M, BUYSE M, et al. The effect of debulking surgery after induction chemotherapy on the prognosis in advanced epethelial ovarian cancer. N Engl J Med 1995;10:629–634.

30. SCHILDER RJ, BOENTE MP, CORN BW, et al. The management of early ovarian cancer. Oncology 1995;9:171–182.

31. McGUIRE W, HOSKINS W, et al. Cyclophosphamide and cisplatin compared with paclitaxel and cisplatin in patients with stage III and stage IV ovarian cancer. N Engl J Med 1996;334(1):1–6.

32. OZOLS R, BUNDY B, et al. Phase III trial of carboplatin and paclitaxel compared with cisplatin and paclitaxel in patients with optimally resected stage III ovarian cancer: a Gynecologic Oncology Group study. J Clin Oncol 2003;21(17):3194–3200.

33. ARMSTRONG D, BUNDY B, et al. Intraperitoneal cisplatin and paclitaxel in ovarian cancer. New Engl J Med 2006;354(1):34–43.

34. ALBERTS D, LIU P, et al. Intraperitoneal cisplatin plus intravenous cyclophospamide versus intravenous cisplatin and intravenous cyclophosphamide for stage III ovarian cancer. N Engl J Med 1996;335:1950–1955.

35. MARKMAN M, BUNDY B, et al. Phase III trial of standard dose intravenous cisplatin plus paclitaxel versus moderately high dose carboplatin followed by intravenous pacilitaxel and intraperitoneal cisplatin in small volume stage III ovarian carcinoma: an intergroup study of the GOG, SWOG, and ECOG. J Clin Oncol 2001;19:1001–1007.

36. MARKMAN M, LIU P, et al. Phase III randomized trial of 12 versus 3 months of maintenance paclitaxel in patients with advanced ovarian cancer after complete response to platinum and paclitaxel-based

chemotherapy: a Southwest Oncology Group and Gynecologic Oncology Group trial. J Clin Oncol 2003;21:2460–2465.

37. MORRIS M, GERSHENSON DM, WHARTON JT. Secondary cytoreductive surgery in epithelial ovarian cancer: nonresponders to first line therapy. Gynecol Oncol 1989;33:1–5.

38. MARKMAN M. CA-125: an evolving role in the management of ovarian cancer (Editorial). J Clin Oncol 1996;14:1411–1412.

39. FRIEDMAN RL, EISENKOP SM, WANG HJ. Second look laparotomy for ovarian cancer provides reliable prognostic information and improves survival. Gynecol Oncol 1997;67:88–94.

40. CHAMBERS SK, CHAMBERS KTR, KOBORIS EL, et al. Evaluation of the role of second look surgery in ovarian cancer. Obstet Gynecol 1988;71(3):404–408.

41. LEUSLEY D, LAWTON F, BLACKLEDGE G, et al. Failure of second look laparotomy to influence survival in epithelial ovarian cancer. Lancet 1988;2:599–602.

42. RAJJI KS, McKINNA JA, BECKER GH, et al. Second look operations in the planned management of advanced ovarian carcinoma. Am J Obstet Gynecol 1982;144:650–654.

43. FIORENTINO MV, NICOLETTA MO, TUMOLO S, et al. Uselessness of surgical second look in epithelial ovarian cancer: a randomized study. Proc ASCO 1994;13:259.

44. BOOKMAN MA, OZOLS RF. Factoring outcomes in ovarian cancer. J Clin Oncol 1996;14:325–327.

45. BARTER JF, BARNES WA. Second look laparotomy In: RUBIN SC, SUTTON GP, editors. Ovarian Cancer. New York, McGraw-Hill; 1993. p 269–300.

46. RUBIN SC. Second look laparotomy. In: MARKMAN M, HODKINS WJ, editors. Cancer of the Ovary. New York, Raven Press; 1993. p 179–186.

47. COPELAND LJ, VACCARELLO L, LEWANDOWSKI GS. Second look laparotomy in epithelial ovarian cancer. Obstet Gynecol Clin North Am 1994;21(1):155–166.

48. SURWIT EA, CHILDERS JM, KRAG DN, et al. Clinical assessment of immunoscrintigraphy in ovarian cancer. Gynecol Oncol 1993;48:285–292.

49. COPELAND LJ, GERSHENSON DJ. Ovarian cancer recurrences in patients with no macroscopic tumor at second look laparatomy. Obstet and Gynecol 1986;68:873–877.

50. RUBIN SC, HOGKINS WN, SAIGO PE, et al. Prognostic factors for recurrence following negative second look laparotomy in ovarian cancer patients treated with platinum-based chemotherapy. Gynecol Oncol 1991;42:137–141.

51. GALLUP DG, TALLEDO OE, DUDZINSKI MR, et al. Another look at the second assessment procedure for ovarian epithelial carcinoma. Am J Obstet Gynecol 1987;157:590–594.

52. CHILDERS JM, LAUG J, SURWIT EA, et al. Laparoscopic surgical staging of ovarian cancer. Gynecol Oncol 1995;59:23–33.

53. ROME R, FORTUNE DW, AUST NZ. The role of second look laparotomy in the management of patients with ovarian carcinoma. J Obstet Gynecol 1988;28:318–322.

54. RUBIN SE, LEWIS JJ. Second look surgery in ovarian carcinoma. Crit Rev Oncol Hematol 1988;8:75–91.

55. RUSTIN GJ, VAN DER BURG ME, et al. A randomized trial in ovarian cancer (OC) of early treatment of relapse based on conventional clinical indicators (MRC OV05/EORTC 55955). J Clin Oncol 2009;(suppl: Abstr 1).

56. ABU-RUSTUM NR, BARAKAT RR, VENKATRAMAN E, et al. Chemotherapy and total parenteral nutrition for advanced ovarian cancer with bowel obstruction. Gynecol Oncol 1997;64:493–495.

Chapter 12

Molar Gestation

Allison E. Axtell, MD and Steven A. Vasilev, MD, MBA

INTRODUCTION

Mortality and severe complications due to molar pregnancy are rare in the United States today, largely because of earlier recognition and timely treatment.[1] Moreover, this early recognition and improved postevacuation follow-up has resulted in earlier diagnosis of the malignant sequelae of molar gestation, choriocarcinoma, and invasive mole.

This chapter addresses molar gestation related perioperative problems and their evidence-based management. With few exceptions, the conditions discussed arise in patients with complete rather than partial molar gestation. Often, coexisting problems arise and may be due to multiple etiologies. For example, cardiorespiratory insufficiency has been blamed on trophoblastic embolization, cardiogenic and noncardiogenic pulmonary edema, thyrotoxicosis, and iatrogenic fluid overload.[2] Hematologic, endocrinologic, neurologic, and infectious complications occur in up to 70% of patients.[3] Central to all these problems is the presence and relative volume of molar tissue in utero. The goal is early diagnosis and expeditious evacuation of the molar gestation, along with supportive and preventative measures.

TROPHOBLASTIC EMBOLIZATION AND CARDIORESPIRATORY INSUFFICIENCY

Sudden hypoxemia or tachypnea with associated tachycardia occurs in 2%–11% of molar gestations. This incidence increases to 27% in patients who present with a molar pregnancy exceeding 16 weeks gestation.[2,4,5] Although this condition most often spontaneously resolves, maternal deaths have been reported.[2] Most often the acute cardiorespiratory insufficiency is clinically ascribed to trophoblastic embolization. While the etiology is more likely multifactorial, there are many reports of presumed or documented pulmonary trophoblastic deportation. Some result in cardiac failure

Gynecologic Oncology: Evidence-Based Perioperative and Supportive Care, Second Edition.
Edited by Scott E. Lentz, Allison E. Axtell and Steven A. Vasilev.
© 2011 John Wiley & Sons, Inc. Published 2011 by John Wiley & Sons, Inc.

and death.[6–11] However, the occurrence of clinical embolism, well documented or not, approximates only 3%.[6–11] Thus, it is doubtful that this is the main cause of cardiorespiratory insufficiency in these patients.

According to data from autopsy and central catheterization series, the magnitude of trophoblastic deportation varies markedly. The term *embolism* should be reserved for clinically significant deportation.[6–13] Trophoblastic embolization appears to occur most often in patients with a large for dates uterus, particularly if the uterine size exceeds 16–20 weeks.[2, 3]

Trophoblastic deportation has been associated temporally with uterine manipulation.[10] However, because all methods of evacuation increase uterine activity, this factor is not highly controllable. Suction dilatation and curettage, which increases uterine activity indirectly, has become a standard for molar evacuation[14] (**Level II-1**). Most molar pregnancies can be safely evacuated by suction curettage.[15, 16] However, if a fetus and mole gestation are slated for termination, a dilatation and evacuation (D&E) may be required as a supplement under some circumstances. Although D&E is widely considered to be statistically the safest method of termination for a fetus greater than 16 weeks gestation, there is no evidence which directly supports this approach in the case of combined fetus-mole pregnancies.[17] A recommendation to perform a D&E in this situation is purely by extrapolation, and several caveats are in order. First of all, the safety of this approach depends on the orientation of the molar pregnancy in utero and the degree of fetal gestational development. Pre- and intraoperative ultrasonography may be instrumental in preventing or decreasing complications. Second, if the fetus is trisomic, its growth is usually quite retarded such that suction evacuation is adequate. Third, the evacuation of a large fetus-mole gestation is often incited or accompanied by pregnancy-induced hypertension (PIH) and its comorbidities and sequelae. In the presence of such a clinical presentation, hysterotomy may be advised as an alternative.

Oxytocin or prostaglandin induction as the primary evacuation method is far less desirable because of a potential for increased deportation and sudden uncontrolled hemorrhage.[3] Furthermore, tissue is often retained so that curettage is still required in addition to the induced evacuation. However, the perioperative addition of oxytocin at the initiation of suction curettage may cause contraction of the myometrium around venous sinusoids as the uterus is emptied. This may decrease the degree of deportation[3, 9] as well as decrease blood loss.

Hysterectomy, usually with the molar pregnancy *in situ*, may be considered in those patients without significant medical complications from the molar gestation who are hemodynamically stable and who do not desire further fertility[18] (**Level II-2**). This approach reduces the risk of malignant sequelae from 20% to approximately 3.5%.[18–21] Whether or not trophoblastic embolization risk is decreased remains controversial.

Invasive monitoring data in patients undergoing molar evacuation refute trophoblastic embolization as a common cause of acute cardiorespiratory insufficiency. When embolization occurs, symptoms are likely dose-related as opposed to being anaphylactoid in nature.[12, 13] Despite the findings of transient cardiorespiratory dysfunction and pulmonary edema, several small series failed to identify unequivocally the presence of circulating trophoblastic cells in patients with pulmonary complications.[12, 13] Therefore, pulmonary insufficiency associated with hydatidiform mole is more likely due to factors other than trophoblastic deportation as discussed below (**Level II-3**).

PULMONARY EDEMA

Etiologic factors contributing to pulmonary edema may include (1) cardiac depression by anesthetic agents, (2) preexisting dilutional anemia, (3) iatrogenic fluid overload, (4) thyrotoxicosis, (5) PIH, and (6) heart failure due to either trophoblastic embolization or preexisting cardiopulmonary disease.

General anesthesia with nitrous oxide, fentanyl, or other narcotics can transiently depress ventricular performance.[22] Limited data in patients with molar gestations greater than 16-week size, monitored perioperatively with pulmonary artery catheters, confirm this effect.[12, 13] A low colloid osmotic pressure to pulmonary capillary wedge pressure gradient combined with aggressive volume resuscitation, in the presence of depressed myocardial function, may exacerbate the development of pulmonary edema.[23]

Relative or dilutional anemia due to plasma volume expansion may exist in molar gestation, just as in normal pregnancy, becoming more pronounced in the second trimester[24–26] (**Level II-1**). This is a physiologic response which acts to provide a reserve for hemorrhage, among other protective effects.[27] Due to the hypervolemia, a large patient can lose up to 2 L of blood at delivery without serious sequelae.[28] One notable exception is seen in patients with coexisting PIH in which a hypovolemic state may be present[29, 30] (**Level II-1**). This may be reflected by hemoconcentration and a falsely "normal" hematocrit determination.

Estimated "blood loss" at evacuation of a molar pregnancy includes sanguinous molar tissue which should not be included in the estimate of circulating blood volume loss. While preexisting severe anemia may be corrected with packed red blood cells (PRBCs), any attempt to replace potentially overestimated losses with whole blood or other large volume infusion in an already hypervolemic state will increase the likelihood of developing pulmonary edema. Patients with PIH or hypertension, in whom there may be an increase in systemic vascular resistance (SVR) and a contracted blood volume, tolerate acute volume loads even less well.[12]

An inverse relationship between the intrinsic work capability of the left heart, measured by left ventricular stroke work index and SVR, has been documented in eclamptic patients.[31] Therefore, if uncertainty exists as to the patient's volume status, especially in those already symptomatic or with coexisting severe PIH, use of a pulmonary artery catheter should be considered[32] (**Level II-2**).

Thyrotoxicosis can contribute to pulmonary edema as a known cause of high output cardiac failure.[33] The adverse effect of thyrotoxicosis would be especially important in patients with already limited cardiac reserve from the aforementioned factors. Those reported cases in which cardiac failure or acute dyspnea complicated hyperthyroidism have resolved spontaneously after evacuation. Several of these patients were being treated medically for hyperthyroidism for a prolonged time period with a known molar gestation *in situ*. Their adverse outcome emphasizes the need to evacuate a molar gestation as soon as possible rather than to attempt protracted medical treatment.

Several small series have reported molar pregnancy complicated by acute respiratory distress syndrome (ARDS). ARDS may coexist with or be complicated by sepsis, disseminated intravascular coagulation (DIC), PIH, and pneumothorax.[4,34]

Risk factors for the development of pulmonary edema in molar pregnancy have been summarized by Morrow.[5] These include advancing patient age, advanced molar gestation, thecalutein cysts, large uterine size, hypertension, extensive uterine hemorrhage, and anemia. Evaluation of pulmonary edema in these patients should begin with the recognition of these risk factors and the maintenance of a high index of suspicion. Conversely, a high index of suspicion for molar gestation should be maintained when a woman of childbearing age presents with pulmonary edema. In one case report, a patient with infiltrates due to pulmonary edema was mistakenly treated for presumed pneumonia for a week prior to the discovery of a molar gestation.[2]

In light of the above factors and syndromes, laboratory determinations and preoperative preparation should be expeditious. The evaluation should include a complete blood count (CBC), serum electrolytes, and a urinalysis, including a test for protein as part of screening for PIH. Thyroid function tests may be sent, but evacuation should not be delayed pending results. A chest X-ray should be obtained for all patients. Findings may include pulmonary infiltrates or effusions with variable appearance[34] (**Level II-1**). Those in the high risk group for pulmonary complications or with symptoms of respiratory insufficiency should have pulse oximetry measurements taken. In a hemodynamically unstable patient with poor peripheral perfusion, arterial blood gas measurements may be indicated if the Hb is <3 g/dL or hypotension exists at <30 mm Hg[35,36] (**Level II-1**). Finally, a central venous pressure (CVP) or pulmonary artery catheter should be considered in especially high risk or symptomatic patients. CVP monitoring may be sufficient in some patients. However, the extensive added information made possible by flow-directed catheters far outweigh the slight additional risk from placement, making its use preferable in most high risk or unstable instances[37,38] (**Level II-2**).

ANEMIA

The consequences of dilutional or relative anemia have already been discussed. Its development is due to an increase in plasma volume out of proportion to RBC production, resulting in a hypervolemic state.[24,25] Increasing levels of circulating beta human chorionic gonadotropin (beta-hCG) do not suppress bone marrow production of RBCs as initially suspected.[25] In most patients, a bone marrow evaluation reveals normoblastic cells.[25] However, dietary deficiencies in iron or folate may result in mixed anemia indices. Development of morning sickness or hyperemesis gravidarum may further affect adequate nutrition. Acute and chronic blood loss can also contribute or be a major factor if excessive. Except in rare instances of DIC, hemolysis is not a significant factor.[25]

If correction of severe anemia is required, replacement should generally be with PRBCs slowly infused, to avoid fluid overload. The decision to transfuse should be based on symptoms and findings and not on any absolute hemoglobin or hematocrit values that may be misleading in view of pregnancy-related dilutional anemia. Furthermore, hemoglobin/hematocrit values provide no information regarding tissue oxygenation or oxygen-carrying capacity. In light of this, several physiologic tissue oxygenation indicators proposed as transfusion triggers for normovolemic anemia are an oxygen extraction ratio (O_2ER) $> 50\%$ and blood lactate > 4 mmol/L.[39] In hypovolemic anemia, volume resuscitation is indicated, but transfusion to a normotensive end point may actually promote continued blood loss.[40] The key is early and adequate resuscitation with appropriate volume in order to stave off persistent microvascular hypoperfusion as manifested by the no reflow phenomenon.[41]

COAGULOPATHY

Deaths have been reported due to DIC complicating molar pregnancy.[42] Although not yet isolated, factors released by hydatidiform moles are known to have thromboplastic and fibrinolytic activity.[43] *In vitro* studies have shown procoagulant activity in molar vesicle fluid at the level of factor X.[44] This activity is similar to that described for amniotic fluid. Spillage of these factors into uterine maternal blood spaces may account for focal necrosis and uterine bleeding.[44,45]

Prostanoids produced by various tumors may cause platelet aggregation and activation of coagulation cascades.[46] However, even though vesicular fluid contains thromboxane and prostacyclin in high concentrations, plasma levels of these substances remain low.[46] Therefore, a systemic effect is unlikely. The coexistence of ARDS and DIC has been documented, and deposition of platelets on damaged pulmonary epithelium has been reported, but a cause-and-effect relationship has not been established.[47]

In view of the above, the evaluation of high risk molar gestation patients should include a coagulation screen (**Level II-3**). Results may include a decreased platelet count, prolonged clotting time, prolonged partial thromboplastin time (PTT), or prolonged prothrombin time (PT). Confirmatory studies with fibrin degradation products and fibrin split products should not delay evacuation, which remains the cornerstone of therapy. Sepsis as an etiology for DIC should also be considered, appropriate cultures taken, and antibiotics started as indicated. Finally, use of oxytocin immediately before suction evacuation may decrease the release of thromboplastins and reduce the risk of coagulopathy[9] (**Level II-3**).

PREGNANCY-INDUCED HYPERTENSION/ECLAMPSIA

Pregnancy-induced hypertension (PIH) occurs in 12%–50% of molar pregnancies. However, only 57 cases of eclampsia have been reported, with 7 fatalities. In a review of these cases, Newman[48] noted that completeness of records and diagnostic accuracy was variable. However, several salient features can be gleaned from these reports, which emphasize the need for early evacuation. In most cases, multiple seizures were noted, 70% of which occurred before evacuation. Prolonged delay in evacuation of the molar gestation was common. All three components of the classic PIH triad (elevated blood pressure, proteinuria, and edema) were present in most patients. These patients usually met "severe PIH" criteria by blood pressure or proteinuria, although decreased platelets were documented in only one patient. However, there are also many reports that detail atypical presentation, with hypertension as the only finding. Acosta-Sison[49] noted that 100% of the hypertensive patients in their series had an enlarged uterus, at or above the umbilicus. They emphasized the importance of tumor volume and uterine size rather than weeks of amenorrhea as a risk factor. Parodoxically, PIH incidence in patients with molar pregnancy is higher in multiparous women.

Any pregnant patient presenting in the second trimester with evidence of PIH should be promptly evaluated with ultrasound for the presence of a molar gestation.[19]

If PIH is diagnosed, appropriate prophylactic measures with magnesium sulfate should be initiated. Any delay in evacuation will contribute to increased morbidity and mortality.

HYPERTHYROIDISM

Since first noted by Tisne in 1955, there have been numerous reports of hyperthyroidism in patients with molar gestation.[50–56] Chemically, hyperthyroidism is evidenced by an elevated free thyroxine index and an increased plasma free T_4 level. Clinical evidence may include agitation and sinus tachycardia or atrial fibrillation. This may progress to thyroid crisis evidenced by fever, severe agitation, and high output heart failure. Left untreated, this can in turn progress to coma and fatal hypotension.

Fortunately, clinical hyperthyroidism is rare in molar pregnancy, and the etiology of thyroid hyperfunction remains unclear. The level of thyroid-stimulating hormone (TSH) is low or normal in these patients, and a secondary thyroid-stimulating factor has not been isolated. Initially beta-hCG was reported as being the causative factor.[51] This has not been substantiated in larger clinical studies.[52] Some *in vitro* evidence supports the fact that beta-hCG binds to TSH receptors in the human thyroid gland.[53,54] However, the methodology has been questioned, and others have reported contradicting data.[55] Because the thyroid-stimulating activity of beta-hCG has been estimated at 1/4000 that of TSH, it may have an effect in very high concentration. Higher beta-hCG levels, seen with large molar gestations, are more often associated with pronounced hyperthyroidism. Upon evacuation, clinical and laboratory evidence of hyperthyroidism quickly resolves.

If clinically suspected, evacuation should not be delayed in awaiting confirmatory thyroid function tests or in an attempt to medically control thyroid hyperfunction. Beta blockade with intravenous propranolol, initially 1 mg every 5 minutes until tachyarrhythmia is controlled, can be adjusted to 20–120 mg four times per day. Additionally, sodium or potassium iodide may be administered intravenously (500–1000 mg every 12 hours) to block release of thyroxine and thus reduce the circulating levels of triodothyronine. In the event of iodine allergy, lithium (300 mg PO every 8 hours) may be used as a substitute. Prior to evacuation, administration of propylthiouracil and awaiting its effects on thyroid hormone synthesis is unwarranted (**Level II-3**).

HYPEREMESIS GRAVIDARUM

The presence of hyperemesis in the pregnant patient after the first trimester should arouse suspicion for the presence of hydatidiform mole. This late occurrence of severe nausea and emesis may be related to elevated beta-hCG levels and hyperthyroidism, although the relationship has not been completely elucidated.[56–58] Excessive emesis and poor dietary intake secondary to nausea lead to electrolyte imbalance and dehydration, which should be treated as indicated.

ENDOMYOMETRITIS

Infection of molar tissue and endomyometritis complicate up to 20% of molar gestations evacuated electively and up to 56% of those requiring suction evacuation.[3] The mechanism is probably an ascending bacterial invasion through an open cervical os in the presence of chronic bleeding. Instrumentation for evacuation increases the risk. Extrapolation from elective and spontaneous abortion data suggests that broad-spectrum antibiotics sufficient to cover both gram-negative and anaerobic bacteria should be administered if infection is suspected.[59] Based on similar elective abortion data, prophylactic intravenous antibiotics should be administered in high risk cases and could be considered for all cases[60] (**Level I**). Evacuation should be performed as soon as therapeutic levels of antibiotics are established.

POSTEVACUATION DELAYED BLEEDING

Follow-up after evacuation of a molar gestation includes beta-hCG titers and routine examinations as discussed elsewhere[19, 20] (**Level I**). During such follow-up, recurrence of vaginal bleeding more often represents development of malignant sequelae rather than retained molar trophoblastic tissue. This is usually reflected by an abnormal hCG regression curve. Of course, if the bleeding occurs soon after the initial evacuation, incomplete suction curettage could be suspected and re-curettage may be indicated. This scenario can often be avoided by a very minimal and careful sharp curettage with a large curette following the initial suction evacuation.

As the beta-hCG level normalizes, delayed bleeding may simply represent resurgence of normal menses. Thus, in the face of a normal regression curve with delayed bleeding, an extensive work-up leading to possible re-curettage is unwarranted[19, 20, 61] (**Level I**).

When delayed bleeding occurs in conjunction with an abnormal hCG regression curve, a metastatic work-up should be performed to detect persistent or malignant gestational trophoblastic disease (GTD). An abnormal hCG regression curve as defined by the International Federation of Gynecologists and Obstetricians (FIGO) is (1) a serum hCG concentration that plateaus (decline of less than 10% for at least four values over 3 weeks), (2) a serum hCG concentration that rises (increase in more than 10% of three values over 2 weeks), (3) persistence of detectable hCG for more than 6 months after molar evacuation.[62] This work-up would include a pelvic exam, peripheral blood counts, assessment of renal and liver function, as well as a radiologic evaluation. Given the fact that the most common site of metastatic disease is the chest, a chest X-ray or a chest CT scan is required in addition to a pelvic ultrasound. The chest CT scan is the more sensitive of the two tests as 40% of patients with a negative chest X-ray will have detectable metastasis on a chest CT scan.[63] The second most common site of metastatic disease is the vagina. Patients with metastasis to the vagina or lungs or choriocarcinoma should undergo further imaging of the liver and brain. Asymptomatic women with negative pelvic exams and normal chest imaging need no further metastatic evaluation.[64] If persistent tissue is identified on pelvic ultrasound, consideration should be given to repeat curettage. Repeat curettage can alleviate abnormal bleeding as well as identify those patients with malignant transformation to choriocarcinoma. In addition, up to 40% of patients with persistent GTD limited to the uterus who undergo repeat evacuation can avoid adjuvant chemotherapy completely[65] (**Level II-3**).

MANAGEMENT GUIDELINES FOR MOLAR PREGNANCY EVACUATION

Therapeutic Goals

1. Complete and expeditious uterine evacuation
2. Prevent volume overload and cardiorespiratory compromise
3. Avoid or be prepared to treat massive hemorrhage
4. Recognize and provide supportive care for PIH and hyperthyroidism

Evidence-Based Management Guidelines

1. Establish IV access (16- to 18-gauge angiocath) running isotonic crystalloid (**Level II-2**)
2. Laboratory: CBC, quantitative beta-hCG routine (**Level I**); coagulation screen (fibrinogen, PT, PTT, platelet count, fibrin split products) in high risk patients (**Level II-2**)
3. Blood bank: Two units of PRBC "type and cross" or "type and screen" for greater than or less than 14- to 16-week gestation, respectively (also depending on preevacuation blood indices) (**Level I-2**)
4. Correct severe preevacuation anemia, avoiding hypervolemia
5. Chest X-ray if uterus is greater than 14–16 weeks gestation (**Level II-1**)

6. Pulse oximetry, arterial blood gas if severe anemia or hypotension (**Level II-1**)

7. Central line cordis if uterus is greater than 14–16 weeks gestation for rapid fluid infusion capability; pulmonary artery catheter if high risk/clinically unstable (**Level II-2**)

8. $MgSO_4$ if superimposed PIH (**Level I**)

9. Beta blockade for evidence of thyroid storm (**Level I**)

10. Carefully use suction/curettage, without preevacuation uterine sounding, followed by large curette sharp gentle curettage (**Level II-1**)

11. Begin oxytocin infusion at curettage and continue for 24 hours or until vaginal bleeding subsides (administer methergine if no contraindication as alternative) (**Level III**)

12. Match intake and output, discounting sanguinous molar tissue

13. Laparotomy tray in the OR

14. Hysterectomy if completed childbearing (**Level II-2**)

15. If clinical hyperthyroidism suspected, treat with beta-blockade and iodides as indicated and evacuate (**Level II-3**)

16. Observe carefully for evidence of respiratory distress

REFERENCES

1. Soto-Wright V, Bernstein M, Goldstein DP, et al. The changing clinical presentation of complete molar pregnancy. Obstet Gynecol 1995;86(5):775.
2. Twiggs LB, Morrow CP, Schlaerth JB. Acute pulmonary complications of molar pregnancy. Am J Obstet Gynecol 1979;135:189.
3. Schlaerth JB, Morrow CP, Montz FJ, et al. Initial management of hydatidiform mole. Am J Obstet Gynecol 1988;158(6):1299.
4. Orr JW, Austin JM, Hatch KD, et al. Acute pulmonary edema associated with molar pregnancies: a high risk factor for development of persistent trophoblastic disease. Am J Obstet Gynecol 1980;136:412.
5. Morrow CP, Kletzky DA, DiSaia JJ, et al. Clinical and laboratory correlates of molar pregnancy and trophoblastic disease. Am J Obstet Gynecol 1977;128:424.
6. Trotter RF, Tieche HL. Maternal death due to pulmonary embolism of trophoblastic cells. Am J Obstet Gynecol 1956;71:1114.
7. Lipp RG, Kindschi JD, Schmitz R. Death from pulmonary embolism associated with hydatidiform mole. Am J Obstet Gynecol 1962;83:1644.
8. Kohorn EI, McGinn RC, Gee BL, et al. Pulmonary embolization of trophoblastic tissue in molar pregnancy. Obstet Gynecol 1978;51(Suppl):165.
9. Kohorn EI, Richard CM, Bernard LG, et al. Pulmonary embolisation of trophoblastic tissue in molar pregnancy. Scand J Clin Lab Invest 1978;23:191.
10. Wagner D. Trophoblastic cells in the blood stream with normal and abnormal pregnancy. Acta Cytol 1968;12:137.
11. Kohorn EI. Clinical management and the neoplastic sequelae of trophoblastic embolization associated with hydatidiform mole. Obstet Gynecol Surv 1987;42:484.

12. HANKINS GD, WENDELL GD, SNYDER RR, et al. Trophoblastic embolization during molar evacuation: central hemodynamic observations. Obstet Gynecol 1987;69:368.

13. COTTON DB, BERNSTEIN SG, READ JA, et al. Hemodynamic observations in evacuation of molar pregnancy. Am J Obstet Gynecol 1980;138:6.

14. BRANDES JM, GRUNSTEIN S, PERETZ A. Suction evacuation of the uterine cavity in hydatidiform mole. Obstet Gynecol 1966;28:689.

15. GOLDSTEIN DP, BERKOWITZ RS. Current management of complete and partial molar pregnancy. J Reprod Med 1994;39:139–143.

16. BERKOWITZ RS, GOLDSTEIN DP, DUBESHTER B, et al. Management of complete molar pregnancy. J Reprod Med 1987;32:634–638.

17. GRIMES DA, CATES W JR. The composite efficacy and safety of intraamniotic prostaglandin F2 and hypertonic saline for second trimester abortion. J Reprod Med 1979;22:248–252.

18. BAHAR AM, EL-ASHNEI MS, SENTHILSEL VAN A. Hydatidiform mole in the elderly: hysterectomy or evacuation. Int J Obstet Gynecol 1989;23:233–237.

19. MORROW CP, CURTIN JP, TOWNSEND DE, editors. Synopsis of gynecologic oncology. 4th ed. New York, Churchill Livingstone Inc; 1993. p 317.

20. SOPER JT, LEWIS JL, HAMMOND CB. Gestational trophoblastic disease. In: HOSKINS WJ, PEREZ CA, YOUNG RC, editors. Principles and Practice of Gynecologic Oncology. Philadelphia, PA: Lippincott-Raven Publishers; 1997. p 1050.

21. CURRY SL, HANMARD CB, TYREY L, et al. Hydatidiform mole: diagnosis, management, and long-term followup of 347 patients. Obstet Gynecol 1975;45:1.

22. STOELTING RK, GIBBS PS, CREASSER CW, et al. Hemodynamic and ventilatory responses to fentanyl, frentanyl-droperidol, and nitrous vs oxide in patients with acquired valvular disease. Anesthesiology 1975;42:319.

23. RACKOW EC, FEIN IA, LEPPO J. Colloid osmotic pressure as a prognostic indicator of pulmonary edema and mortality in the critically ill. Chest 1977;72:709.

24. CHESLEY LC. Plasma and red cell volumes during pregnancy. Am J Obstet Gynecol 1972;112:440.

25. PRITCHARD JW. Blood volume changes in pregnancy and puerperium IV. Anemia associated with hydatidiform mole. Am J Obstet Gynecol 1965;91:621.

26. LILEY AW. Clinical and laboratory evidence of variations in maternal plasma volume in pregnancy. Int J Gynaecol Obstet 1970;8:358.

27. GOODLIN RC. Why treat "physiologic" anemia of pregnancy? J Reprod Med 1982;27:639.

28. PRITCHARD JA. Changes in the blood volume during pregnancy and delivery. Anesthesiology 1965;26:393.

29. BENEDETTI TJ, TWIGGS LB, MORROW CP. Pre- and postevacuation metabolic studies of hydatidiform mole and serve pregnancy induced hypertension. J Reprod Med 1980;25:133.

30. SOFFRONOFF EC, KAUFMANN BM, CONNAUGHTON JF. Intavascular volume determinations of pregnancy. Am J Obstet Gynecol 1977;127:4.

31. HANKIN GDV, WENDEL GD JR, CUNNINGHAM FG, et al. Longitudinal evaluation of hemodynamic changes in eclampsia. Am J Obstet Gynecol 1984;150:506.

32. COTTON DB, GONIK B, DORMAN K, et al. Cardiovascular alterations in severe pregnancy induced hypertension: relationship of central venous pressure to pulmonary capillary wedge pressure. Am J Obstet Gynecol 1985;151:762.

33. HIGGINS HP, HERSCHMANN JM, KENIMER JG, et al. The thyrotoxicosis of hydatidiform mole. Ann Intern Med 1975;83:307.

34. HUBERMAN RP, FON GT, BEIN ME. Benign molar pregnancies: pulmonary complications. AJR Am J Roentgenol 1982;138:71.

35. SEVERINGHAUS JW, SPELLMAN MJ. Pulse oximeter failure thresholds in hypotension and vasoconstriction. Anesthesiology 1990;73:532.

36. JAY GD, HUGHES L, RENZI FP. Pulse oximetry is accurate in acute anemia from hemorrhage. Ann Emerg Med 1994;24:32.

37. SCOTT WL. Complications associated with central venous catheters. Chest 1988;91:1221.

38. PATEL C, LABBY V, VENUS B, et al. Acute complications of pulmonary artery catheter insertion in critically ill patients. Crit Care Med 1986;14:195.
39. LEVY P, CHAVEZ RP, CRYSTAL GJ, et al. Oxygen extraction ratio: a valid indicator of transfusion need in limited coronary vascular reserve? J Trauma 1992;32:769–774.
40. American College of Physicians. Practice strategies for elective red blood cell transfusions. Ann Intern Med 1992;116:403–406.
41. Consensus Conference. Perioperative red blood cell transfusion. JAMA 1988;260:2700–2703.
42. TSAKOK FHM, KOH S, ILANCHERAN A, et al. Maternal death associated with hydatidiform molar pregnancy. Int J Gynaecol Obstet 1983;21:485.
43. TSAKOK FHM, RATNAM SS, CHEW SC, et al. Thromboplastic and fibrinolytic activity of hydatidiform molar tissue and vesicular fluid. J Obstet Gynecol 1977;86:233.
44. KAPLAN SS, SZULMAN AE, SURTI U. Effect of hydatidiform molar vesicular fluid on blood coagulation. Am J Obstet Gynecol 1985;153:703.
45. ROY AC, KARIM MM, KOTTEGODA SR, et al. Thromboxane A$_2$ and prostacyclin levels in molar pregnancy. Br J Obstet Gynaecol 1984;91:908.
46. HONN KV, BOCKMAN RS, MARNETT LJ. Protaglandins and cancer: a review of tumor initiation through tumor metastasis. Prostaglandins 1981;21:833.
47. BONE RC, FRANCIS PB, PIERCE AK. Intravascular coagulation associated with adult respiratory distress syndrome. Am J Med 1976;61:585.
48. NEWMAN RB, EDDY GL. Association of eclampsia and hydatidiform mole: case report and review of the literature. Obstet Gynecol Surv 1988;43:185.
49. ACOSTA-SISON H. The relationship of hydatidiform mole to pre-eclampsia and eclampsia. A study of 85 cases. Am J Obstet Gynecol 1956;71:1279.
50. TISNE L, BARZALATTO J, STEVERSON C. Estudio d funcion tirodea durante el estado gravido-puerperal con el yodo radioactive. Bol Soc Chil Obstet Ginecol 1955;20:246.
51. KENIMER JG, HERSHMAN JM, HIGGINS HP. The thyrotropin in hydatidiform moles is human chorionic gonadotropin. J Clin Endocrin Metab 1975;40:480–489.
52. AMIR SM, OSATHANONAH R, BERKOWITZ RS, et al. Human chorionic gonadotropin and thyroid function in patients with hydatidiform mole. Am J Obstet Gynecol 1984;150:723.
53. SILVERBERG J, O'DONNELL J, SUGERONYA A, et al. Effect of human thyroid tissue in vitro. J Clin Endocrinol Metab 1978;46:420.
54. CARAYON P, LEFORT G, NISULA B. Interaction of human chorionic gonadotropin and human luteinizing hormone with human thyroid membranes. Endocrinology 1980;106:1907.
55. AMIR SM, KANE P, OSATHANODH R. Divergent responses by human and mouse thyroid to human chorionic gonadotropin in vitro. Program of the Sixty-fourth Annual Meeting of the Endocrine Society, 1982. Abstract 1222.
56. NGOWNGARMRATANA S, SUNTHORNTHEPVARAKUL T, KANCHANAWAT S. Thyroid function and human chorionic gonadotropin in patients with hydatidiform mole. J Med Assoc Thai 1997;80(11):693.
57. SOULES MR, HUGHES CL JR, GARCIA JA, et al. Nausea vomiting of pregnancy: role of human chorionic gonadotropin and 17-hydroxyprogesterone. Obstet Gynecol 1980;55:696.
58. TAREEN AK, BASEER A, JAFFRY HF, et al. Thyroid hormone in hyperemesis gravidarum. J Obstet Gynaecol 1995;21(5):497–501.
59. BURKMAN RT, ATIENZA MF, KING TM. Culture and treatment in endometritis following elective abortion. Am J Obstet Gynecol 1977;128:556.
60. HENRIQUES CU, WILKEN-JENSEN C, THORSEN P, et al. A randomised controlled trial of prophylaxis of post-abortal infection: ceftriaxone versus placebo. Br J Obstet Gynaecol. 1994;101(7):610.
61. LAO TTH, LEE FHC, YEUNG SSL. Repeat curettage after evacuation of a hydatidiform mole. Acta Obstet Gynecol Scand 1987;66:305.
62. KOHORN EI. The new FIGO 200 staging and risk factor scoring system for gestational trophoblastic disease: description and critical assessment. Int J Gynecol Oncol 2001;11:73.
63. GAMER EI, GARRET A, GOLDSTEIN DP, et al. Significance of chest computed tomography findings in evaluation and treatment of persistent gestational trophoblastic neoplasia. J Reprod Med 2004;49:411.

64. ACOG Practice Bulletin #53. Diagnosis and treatment of gestational trophoblastic disease. Obstet Gynecol 2004;103:1365.

65. PEZECHKI M, HANDCOCK BW, SILCOCKS P, et al. The role of repeat uterine evacuation in the management of persistent gestational trophoblastic disease. Gynecol Oncol 2004;95:423–429.

ADDITIONAL POSSIBLE TOPICS FOR FUTURE EDITIONS

66. Frequency of problems decreased due to early Dx and US.
67. US use and CXR use and other tests.
68. GTN issues : higher Betas and TL cysts.
69. Critical care issues: great imitator, no need for craniotomy, chemo issues and IS vs IT and XRT/brain indications.
70. Fetus and mole:% viable and if have% to term and how.
71. Periop of D&E, US position of fetus and mole.

- **Neurologic Sequelae**
- Hemothorax
- Fetus and Mole

Chapter 13

Perioperative Issues in the Management of Vulvar Cancer

Kathryn F. McGonigle, MD and Maliaka W. Amneus, MD

INTRODUCTION AND BACKGROUND

Perioperative issues surrounding the care of patients with vulvar malignancy have evolved rapidly over the last few decades. Improvements in surgical technique, less radical surgery, improved perioperative management, and better antibiotic therapies have dramatically decreased complications associated with the treatment of vulvar cancer. These changes have been associated with a reduction of both immediate and delayed morbidity, shorter hospital stay and recovery time, and less interference with body image and sexual function.

Treatment of vulvar cancer depends on the stage at presentation, histologic type, size of lesion, and location of the primary lesion on the vulva relative to the midline and relative to anatomic structures including the urethra, bladder, anus, and rectum. In addition, treatment is influenced by the status of regional lymph nodes. The focus of this chapter is not on specific management of patients on the basis of these factors, but on perioperative issues in patients with vulvar cancer. Surgery is the primary treatment for vulvar cancer, particularly early stage disease. Radiation therapy and or chemotherapy are sometimes used prior to or after surgical treatment depending on the extent of disease and may be pivotal in optimizing chance for cure. However, their use is commonly associated with an increased risk of perioperative complications.

LESS RADICAL SURGERY

Over the last several decades numerous modifications in surgical technique have been incorporated into the management of vulvar cancer. The classic approach to vulvar cancer, regardless of size or location of the primary lesion, was radical vulvectomy with bilateral inguinal-femoral lymphadenectomy using an en bloc technique. This

Gynecologic Oncology: Evidence-Based Perioperative and Supportive Care, Second Edition. Edited by Scott E. Lentz, Allison E. Axtell and Steven A. Vasilev. © 2011 John Wiley & Sons, Inc. Published 2011 by John Wiley & Sons, Inc.

approach for the treatment of vulvar cancer and its regional lymphatics was initially proposed by Basset in 1912 and successfully implemented by Taussig and Way several decades later.[1,2] Subsequently, the modified Basset procedure (butterfly incision) was introduced. This incision involved the removal of 2–3 cm of skin over the groin from the anterior-superior iliac spine to the pubic tubercle and crossing anteriorly and inferiorly to the inguinal ligament incorporating the underlying lymphatic tissue along with the radical vulvectomy specimen. These extensive en bloc procedures were associated with appreciable morbidity and prolonged hospitalizations with wound complication rates that approached 60%.[3] In one series, the modified Basset procedure was associated with impairment of primary wound healing in 85%, varying degrees of lymphedema in 69%, and thrombophlebitis in 9% of patients.[4] Operative mortality was also high, in the range of 2.6%–5.7%.[5,6] Because of the substantial morbidity and prolonged hospitalization associated with the en bloc procedures, gynecologic cancer surgeons have been inspired to examine modifications to this classic surgical approach to vulvar cancer. The acceptance of these modifications and incorporation into the care of vulvar cancer patients has been based on multiple observational and nonrandomized studies demonstrating a reduction in morbidity without demonstrating a reduction in patient cure.

As early as 1940, Taussig suggested that radical vulvectomy and inguinal lymphadenectomy be performed through three separate incisions.[1] This technique was not accepted into the general management of vulvar cancer until many decades later when gynecologic cancer surgeons described performing a three-incision technique. Compared with the en bloc incision in historical controls, a significant reduction in morbidity was observed.[7–9] In one series, there was a reduction in groin breakdown from 70% using the en bloc technique to 20% using the three-incision technique.[10] In another study, wound breakdown decreased from 64% to 38%, wound infection from 21% to 14%, and lymphocyst formation from 28% to 14%.[11] The reduction in perioperative morbidity was not associated with an obvious increase in skin bridge or local recurrences.[9,11] Numerous studies suggest that more conservative surgery has been associated with a marked reduction in hospital stay, blood loss, operating time, blood transfusion, and other perioperative morbidities.[4,10–12] Modifications of surgery for vulvar cancer were initially performed in a very select group of patients with early vulvar cancer, but over time, these techniques have been more widely applied in patients with larger and more extensive and invasive primary vulvar cancers (**Level III**). As the surgical management of vulvar cancer evolved, further modifications were introduced. A prospective, nonrandomized, noncontrolled Gynecologic Oncology Group (GOG) study treated stage I vulvar cancer patients with modified radical hemivulvectomy and ipsilateral superficial inguinal lymphadenectomy.[13] Compared with historical controls, the authors noted an increased failure in the vulva, but 8 of 10 patients were salvaged by a second operation. They also noted recurrences in both the contralateral groin and the ipsilateral groin among 9 of 121 patients. Acute and long-term complications were lower than historical controls. Wound separation, hematoma, or infection occurred in 28.9% of 121 patients and only 19% developed lymphedema, the majority of cases of being mild. Compared with historical controls, there was a significantly increased risk of recurrence, but not death. The authors suggested this modified surgical approach is an appropriate alternative to the traditional radical operation for selective vulvar cancer patients.[13] More recently, further modifications have occurred including radical local excision of the primary vulvar lesion with a 1- to 2-cm margin and unilateral inguinal-femoral lymphadenectomy for the more invasive lateralized lesion.[14] Since there are no randomized, prospective studies, it is possible that the more conservative approach is associated with a slightly higher risk of local recurrence (**Level III**). Way's classic technique of inguinal-femoral lymphadenectomy included removal of superficial groin nodes with sartorius muscle fascia, cribiform fascia over the femoral vessels, adductor longus fascia and pectineus muscle fascia. Over the last several decades, investigators have found that preservation of the fascia lata is a satisfactory method for groin lymphadenectomy, without obvious evidence of compromising the patient's survival. Another proposed modification of the groin dissection is omission of the deep femoral node dissection in the absence of groin metastases in superficial inguinal nodes. Some have suggested that the risk of lymphedema and infection may be reduced with this approach, but this is unproven.[15] The safety of this modification has been seriously questioned. In a prospective, noncontrolled GOG study, four women among 121 vulvar cancer patients died after recurrence in the groin subjected to superficial lymphadenectomy with negative superficial nodes. These and similar reported cases suggest possible involvement of femoral nodes in the absence of superficial groin involvement.[13] Because patients with groin recurrences have a dismal prognosis with greater than 80% mortality and because of the absence of any compelling evidence that eliminating the deep groin dissection results in a decrease in morbidity, this approach has not gained widespread approval[16,17] (**Level III**). A further surgical modification is the elimination of pelvic lymphadenectomy in the majority of patients with vulvar cancer. Because pelvic node involvement is exceedingly rare in the absence of positive groin nodes, it has been suggested that pelvic lymphadenectomy be reserved for patients with involvement of groin nodes only.[4,18] Subsequently, data from a randomized prospective GOG study suggested there may be little to no role of pelvic lymphadenectomy in vulvar cancer patients. In this study, patients undergoing groin and pelvic lymphadenectomy fared worse than those treated with radiation therapy. As a result, the authors suggested that even in the setting of involved groin nodes, pelvic lymphadenectomy should not be performed, but rather the patient should be treated with postoperative pelvic and groin irradiation[5] (**Level II-2**).

Although some have reported no increased morbidity from the addition of pelvic lymphadenectomy to radical vulvectomy and bilateral groin dissection, others have not verified this.[6,19–21] One study suggested that operative mortality could be reduced by 2% if pelvic lymphadenectomy were omitted and another study found that major complications were twice as common in patients undergoing pelvic lymphadenectomy.[6,20,21] There is a growing body of evidence suggesting that involvement of the pelvic lymph nodes is associated with a dismal chance of survival not improved by pelvic lymphadenectomy. The role of pelvic lymphadenectomy in the management of vulvar cancer appears to be limited. Indications may include patients with prior radiation therapy to the pelvic or other contraindication to pelvic radiation therapy. These observations have been made based on Level I[5] and III evidence.

For patients with advanced or recurrent vulvar cancer, the ultraradical surgical approach (exenterative surgery) to the treatment of advanced vulvar cancer has historically been associated with a 7% postoperative mortality in combined series. Furthermore, the loss of organ function or impairment of sexual function is significant.[10] Based on favorable results in uncontrolled series and in other solid tumors (head and neck cancer and anal carcinoma), the GOG has studied the use of chemotherapy in conjunction with radiation therapy to reduce the radicality of surgery required for patients with advanced (T3 and T4) vulvar cancers.[22] This approach to patients with advanced disease has decreased the extensiveness of surgery required. In many cases organ preservation has been possible when treatment otherwise would have necessitated pelvic exenteration. The use of radiation therapy in the management of advanced vulvar cancer is outside the scope of this chapter, and the reader is referred to text specifically devoted to this management strategy.

Sentinel Lymph Node Biopsy

A further modification of surgery being examined for vulvar cancer patients is the use of intraoperative lymphatic mapping techniques to identify the initial lymph node (the sentinel node) in the regional lymphatic basin. Numerous published studies of patients with solid malignancies support the efficacy of these techniques in identifying the sentinel node.[23–26] Given the high potential morbidity of inguinal-femoral lymphadenectomy, a less invasive technique that would allow surgeons to identify patients in whom complete lymphadenectomy can be safely omitted would be a welcome addition to the diagnostic and therapeutic armamentarium.[27] Of note, this method is not intended for use in patients with clinically suspicious or histologically confirmed positive lymph nodes, and current data is largely confined to squamous cell histology.[28] The most common techniques for sentinel lymph node detection involve the use of blue dye and/or ^{99m}Technicium (^{99m}Tc)-labeled sulfur colloid (lymphoscintigraphy). Using blue dye, 2–4 mL of blue dye (e.g., isosulfan blue, methylene blue, Patent blue) is injected into the tissue around the perimeter of the primary vulvar cancer. After a short period of time (5–10 minutes), the groin(s) is (are) explored. Blue-stained lymphatics are identified and dissected to the sentinel node, which is then removed. Using lymphoscintigraphy, ^{99m}Tc-labeled sulfur colloid is similarly injected around the perimeter of the tumor the day prior to the operative procedure. Following injection, imaging of the injection site and draining node basin is performed and the location of the node(s) is marked on the skin. Intraoperatively, the "hot node" is identified using a handheld gamma probe.

In recent years, data on the use of sentinal lymph node biopsy in vulvar cancer has greatly expanded. In 2005, Selman et al.[29] published a systematic review in which they assessed the accuracy of sentinel node biopsy in vulvar cancer. The analysis included 16 prospective studies that utilized dye and/or ^{99m}Tc. Pooled analysis revealed that the use of blue dye alone was able to identify the sentinel node in 52%–95% of groins, while the use of ^{99m}Tc was able to identify the sentinel node in 73%–100% of groins. The accuracy of was high, with a pooled sensitivity of 97% (95% CI 91–100) and a negative likelihood ratio of 0.12 (95% CI 0.053–0.28) for ^{99m}Tc and a pooled sensitivity of 95% (95% CI 82–99%) with a negative likelihood ratio of 0.16 (95% CI 0.07–0.32) for blue dye alone. A total of two false negative results were noted in each group. In Hampl et al.,[30] the most recent and largest multicenter trial investigating the accuracy of sentinel lymph node biopsy in vulvar cancer which included 127 patients (227 groins), identification of the sentinel node(s) was successful in 125 patients (98.4%). Sensitivity was 92.3%, with a false negative rate of 7.7%. A significant limitation of the study is the lack of consistency in the method of sentinel node detection, with blue dye alone, ^{99m}Tc alone, or ^{99m}Tc with blue dye being utilized. In the largest study of sentinel node accuracy in vulvar cancer in which combined blue dye injection and ^{99m}Tc lymphoscintigraphy was used in all patients, identification of the sentinel node(s) was successful in 100% of patients and there were no false negative results.[31]

Given the high mortality rate associated with groin recurrence, false negative results in the sentinel lymph node procedure are very concerning. The three false negative results in the Hampl study are the only reported false negative results from large (greater than 20 patients) prospective studies in which ^{99m}Tc was used. Interestingly, all three of these lesions were located in the midline, highlighting a potential pitfall in sentinel node detection in vulvar cancer. This was explored in a study by Louis-Sylvestre et al.[32] who performed sentinel node identification on 17 patients with midline vulvar cancers using ^{99m}Tc. All patients underwent a complete bilateral lymphadenectomy. They found that in 13 of 17 patients, lymphoscintigraphy and intraoperative identification localized sentinel nodes to only one side. In 3 out of these 13 patients, metastatic nodes were found on the side where no sentinel nodes were identified. It has been suggested that in midline tumors, if sentinel nodes are not identified in both groins, consideration should be given to abandoning the sentinel node procedure.[30, 33]

The results of the GROINSS-V trial, the largest prospective study on the use of sentinel node biopsy in vulvar cancer, were recently published in 2008 by van der Zee et al. This report included 403 patients who underwent sentinel lymph node procedures using both ^{99m}Tc and blue dye in 623 groins. Complete inguinal-femoral lymphadenectomy was omitted in patients who were found to have negative sentinel nodes. The goals of the study were to assess the safety of omitting inguinal-femoral lymphadenectomy in patients with a negative sentinel node, as well as to compare morbidity of sentinel node dissection versus complete lymphadenectomy. The groin recurrence rate was 3% overall and only 2.3% in the subset of patients with unifocal disease. This compares favorably with the published recurrence rate after complete lymphadenectomy of 0%–8.7%. Improved short- and long-term morbidity were also demonstrated for patients undergoing sentinel lymph node biopsy only compared to those undergoing sentinel lymph node dissection and complete lymphadenectomy. Given that a randomized trial comparing complete lymphadenectomy to sentinel lymph node dissection followed by complete lymphadenectomy only in patients with positive sentinel nodes is unlikely to ever be performed, the GROINSS-V study is likely to be the best data available to address the safety of the sentinel lymph node procedure in vulvar cancer when performed by surgeons who have proven to be proficient at the procedure. Results of GOG 173, a trial designed to assess the accuracy of sentinel lymph node biopsy in a community-based setting that does not require demonstrated proficiency at the procedure, are eagerly awaited and will also contribute significantly to the body of evidence regarding the use of sentinel lymph node biopsy in vulvar cancer.[34] Given the data from the GROINSS-V study, when performed by a "quality controlled multidisciplinary team" sentinel lymph node biopsy appears to be a safe and less morbid alternative to complete lymphadenectomy in patients with early stage vulvar cancer. The safety of this technique in the community setting remains to be proven. These observations are made based on Level II-1 evidence.

COMPLICATIONS OF THERAPY

Early Complications

Wound Breakdown or Cellulitis

By far the most common and serious complications associated with the surgical treatment of vulvar cancer, particularly the en bloc classical surgical procedures, have been infectious. The large size of the wounds, reduction in residual vascular supply, coupled with the shearing forces during flexion and extension of the lower extremities compromise wound healing and result in suboptimal adherence of tissue to the underlying structures. The result is accumulation of lymphatic fluid, skin and soft tissue infection, and possible necrosis of the compromised cutaneous flaps.[4] Efforts to reduce complications have primarily focused on less radical surgery. Other perioperative treatment modalities, including the use of groin suction catheters for evacuation of subcutaneous fluid and debris, selective use of sartorius muscle flaps, and improved antibiotics, have also led to a decrease in infectious complications.

Perioperative morbidity from wound breakdown may be significant, and in rare cases death may occur as a result of sepsis.[22] The risk of wound breakdown after surgery for vulvar cancer is directly related to the extent of the surgery and underlying disease processes that may impair wound healing. With the classic en bloc radical vulvectomy and bilateral inguinal-femoral lymphadenectomy, wound breakdown was as high as 60%–70%.[35] With the three-incision technique of radical vulvectomy and groin dissection the risk of wound breakdown was reduced to approximately 20%.[10] The risk has been even further reduced with more conservative surgical modifications limiting the amount of resection, such as radical hemivulvectomy or radical local excision. The risk of breakdown is also related to surgical technique and is clearly increased with tension on the wound. Factors that may impair wound healing and increase infectious complications include diabetes mellitus, peripheral vascular disease, history of parenteral drug use, chronic malnutrition, steroid use, or alcoholism. Optimizing glucose control in the diabetic patient is important to minimize risk of infectious complications. Prior radiation therapy to the groins and/or vulva also significantly increases risk for wound breakdown. These issues will be further discussed in the section on "Wound Healing."

Some have suggested using hyperbaric oxygen therapy following radical vulvectomy to improve wound healing.[36] In a nonrandomized, prospective study, the authors noted a reduction in wound breakdown for patients undergoing radical vulvectomy with lymph node dissection and hyperbaric oxygen therapy compared with historical controls. There is no randomized prospective data on the use of hyperbaric oxygen in this setting. Because of limited Level III data, its use to reduce wound complications in vulvar cancer patients should be considered experimental.

In one large retrospective series, the risk of complications in the groin did not correlate with the extent of the vulvar surgery and similarly the addition of groin lymphadenectomy did not increase the risk of vulvar complications.[37] Sparing of the saphenous vein did not appear to affect postoperative groin wound breakdown or cellulitis occurring in 24% of patients in whom the vessel was sacrificed compared with 18% whose vein was spared.[38] Sartorius muscle transposition may decrease the risk of groin wound complications in vulvar cancer patients. A retrospective analysis of the effect of sartorius transposition on wound morbidity following inguinal-femoral lymphadenectomy through separate incisions suggested there may be some benefit on risk of wound infection. In this study, the incidence of groin cellulitis or wound breakdown was less in patients undergoing sartorius transposition than those who did not have the procedure performed, 41% vs. 66%, respectively ($p = 0.03$).[38] Also reported is anecdotal success using the sartorius transposition in the treatment of infected groin wounds with vascular grafts after reconstructive vascular surgery.[39,40] However, its use in vulvar cancer patients after groin wound infection has not been described. Selective use of sartorius muscle transposition after groin dissection may be appropriate based on limited Level III data.

For the vulvar wound, drains are not routinely used and perioperative care consists of keeping the wound clean and dry. Cleansing with warm saline or water should be started approximately 24 hours postoperatively. After cleaning the wound, excess moisture is removed with a towel. Since the vulva tends to be a very moist area, the moisture is minimized by using a heating lamp or blow dryer. This should be performed two to three times daily and after bowel movements depending on the size and location of the wound. The groins are routinely drained and the drains are not removed until there is less than 30–40 cc/day of drainage. Particularly in the immediate postoperative period, it is essential that the groin flaps remain adherent to the underlying tissues. This is accomplished using compression dressing and drains and may prevent a fluid collection that could lead to an abscess or lymphocyst formation, or increase the risk of flap necrosis. Either wall suction or bulb suction is appropriate, but if bulb suction is used, vigilance to maintain continued suction is essential. Some have suggested that wall suction might be preferable, particularly in the first two to three postoperative days. When evidence of either groin or vulvar infection occurs such as drainage, induration, or erythema, the wound must be inspected to exclude an abscess collection and broad-spectrum antibiotics should be instituted. If an abscess is present, it should be drained and the wound opened.

Wound Healing

In general, wound healing mechanisms may be divided into four phases—early, intermediate, later, and a final phase. The early phase includes those changes occurring over the initial 3 days after a surgical incision. During this phase of wound healing, the change in the tensional or compressional state of the tissue is immediately communicated to local connective tissue cells. There are also mechanisms of hemostasis including vasoconstriction and retraction mediated through the sympathetic nervous system and possibly prostaglandins. In addition, immediately following the production of a wound, the coagulation cascade is initiated and clot formation occurs. In addition to its role in the clotting cascade, fibrin serves as a lattice to facilitate adhesion, migration, and phagocytic processes of leukocytes during inflammation. It also provides a scaffold for subsequent angiogenesis. Platelet aggregation is initiated primarily by exposure of subendothelial collagen. Finally, inflammation occurs during the early phase of wound healing and is the key modulator of the healing process. Inflammation is associated with initial vasoconstriction, followed by a more prolonged vasodilation of postcapillary venules. During this phase there is a cellular response with an inflammatory cell influx of neutrophils, monocytes, macrophages, and lymphocytes for scavenging the wound. Mediators of inflammation are also released from the plasma and tissues, including kinins, complements, histamine, serotonins, prostaglandins, fibronectins, lysosomal proteases, and lymphokines.[41–43]

During the intermediate phase of wound healing, fibroblast migration and proliferation occur. In addition, angiogenesis is stimulated by the release of growth factors, low oxygen tension, high lactate, and a low pH. Epithelialization occurs by mobilization, migration, mitosis, and differentiation. Epithelial cells immediately adjacent to the wound mobilize. Cellular migration is visible at 24 hours following injury. During cellular migration, fixed basal cells adjacent to the wound begin mitosis, resulting in resurfacing of the wound. As the new epithelial layer becomes complete and begins to thicken, normal cellular differentiation from basal to surface layers resumes. The stratification of epithelial layers occurs within 48–72 hours.[41–43]

During the later phase of wound healing, collagen synthesis occurs. This process does not begin for 3–5 days after the surgical incision. Collagen is a fibrous protein and is the major component of scar tissue. The formation of glycosaminoglycan occurs and functions to act as a "glue" to the subepithelial tissues. Wound contraction as part of the later phase of healing plays a minimal role in the healing of a surgically created linear incision.[41–43]

During the final phase of wound healing, scar remodeling occurs. Collagen synthesis and collagen degradation are in a finely controlled state of equilibrium during normal tissue repair. The tensile strength of a wound can be correlated with collagen synthesis only up to 45 days after injury. Despite no increase in net collagen synthesis, cutaneous scars continue to increase in breaking strength and tensile strength for months. Tensile strength results from collagen cross-linking. Even in optimal circumstances, wound strength never reaches that of normal skin.[41–43]

There are numerous factors that may adversely affect wound healing. In vulvar cancer patients, bacterial infection is the most common and is defined as the presence of greater than 10^5 organisms per gram of tissue in a wound where clinical signs of infection are present. At this level, wound healing may be inhibited or complicated because of competition for nutrition or destruction of cells by bacterial toxins, increased collagen lysis, decreased tissue oxygen tension, and a continued presence of an inflammatory reaction.[44] Other factors in patients with vulvar cancer that may impair wound healing include alcoholism, diabetes, glucocorticoids, hematoma formation, severe malnutrition, older age, prior radiation therapy, cigarette smoking, and suboptimal surgical technique. Chronic alcohol use is associated with slower wound healing and slower collagen accumulation. The use of glucocorticoids is associated with a decrease in the inflammatory response, less collagen formation, and delay in angiogenesis. These effects are seen whether steroids are used topically or given systemically, and are markedly potentiated by even mild malnutrition.[45] Although there have been no carefully controlled human trials that clearly demonstrate the deleterious effect of therapeutic steroid doses on wound healing, retrospective data suggests that many episodes of nonhealing have been associated with steroid use. Based on Level III data, we recommend that steroid administration be limited to those clinical situations in which it is absolutely necessary.

The diabetic has many problems that predispose to wound healing complications, including neuropathy (more mechanical trauma), microangiopathy, and an increased risk of infection.[46–48] One factor implicated in poor wound healing is the impaired circulation secondary to large and small vessel occlusive disease in which the blood supply to the healing wound is impaired.[46] Diabetics have been found to have five times the risk of infection in clean incision than nondiabetics. Well-controlled diabetics are more resistant to wound infection than poorly controlled diabetics. In the poorly controlled diabetic, a major component of this phenomenon is the impaired inflammatory response caused by hyperglycemia. In addition, all aspects of leukocyte function are impaired, especially phagocytosis.[47] Hyperglycemia is also associated with a general suppression of both humoral and cellular immunity. In animal models, these immunologic defects can largely be reversed by good control of blood glucose, but relevant human data are not available.[47] In addition, collagen accumulates at a slower rate, and breaking strength is diminished. Insulin may improve the decrease in collagen synthesis.[48]

Massive loss of body weight and malnutrition impair wound healing. Protein depletion and vitamin deficiencies may impair collagen synthesis.[49,50] Malnutrition has long been implicated in poor wound healing. In animal models, loss of 15%–20% of lean body mass can result in a decrease in wound breaking strength and colonic bursting pressure. A prospective, randomized trial of preoperative total parenteral nutrition in patients with gastrointestinal malignancies reported a significant reduction in postoperative morbidity and mortality.[49] Another study that evaluated the pooled results of prospective, randomized trials of perioperative total parenteral nutrition in cancer patients concluded that the use of parenteral nutrition can reduce the incidence of major surgical morbidity and mortality, at the expense of an increased risk of infection.[50] At present, it is generally agreed that nutritional support may have a beneficial effect on wound healing in nutritionally depleted patients, but has no such effect in well-nourished patients and may even increase risk of complications. Parenteral nutrition should be used selectively in patients with documented malnutrition. This recommendation is made based on Level I through Level III evidence.

Older age is associated with slower wound healing.[51] Cigarette smoking impairs wound healing, probably by several mechanisms. Smoking is associated with decreased tissue oxygenation due to elevated carboxyhemoglobin levels. Endothelial changes and increased platelet adhesiveness occur and can lead to additional limitation of local blood flow. It is not entirely clear how nicotine impairs wound healing.[52]

The effect of prior radiation therapy in the wound healing process can be seen in all aspects of the repair process. The problems with wound healing and ulceration after radiation have been historically related to relative ischemia of the irradiated tissue due to an obliterative endarteritis of the microvasculature with resulting reduction in blood supply.[53] More recent experiments suggest that the change is due to a diminished transcutaneous oxygen pressure, although this is controversial.[54] Radiation also affects cells of the hematopoietic system and this might account for the delayed inflammatory process. It also affects cells that participate in wound remodeling and repair. Radiation has a direct effect on structural collagen with a marked reduction in tensile strength. As a result, radiated wounds have a higher risk of wound dehiscence, wound infection, and overall delay in wound healing. Data from animal studies suggest that many of the adverse effects of radiation on wound healing may be reversed through the administration of high doses of vitamin A. However, only anecdotal evidence is available in humans.[55]

Finally, meticulous surgical technique is required to minimize the risk of wound complications. Delicate tissue handling, particularly the delicate skin flaps in the groin dissection, is essential. Meticulous hemostasis, asepsis, minimizing the amount of foreign bodies (sutures), and avoiding dead space are also important. Hematoma increases the likelihood of bacterial infection since neutrophils do not migrate effectively into an avascular hematoma and a small inoculum of bacteria in a hematoma could multiply without limitation by host defense mechanisms. These clinical observations on wound healing have been made based on Level III evidence.

Necrotizing Soft Tissue Infections and Necrotizing Fasciitis

Necrotizing soft tissue infections may occur in the vulva or groin after surgical treatment of vulvar cancer or in a patient who has not recently had surgery. Management is similar regardless of events preceding the patient's presentation. Necrotizing soft tissue infections after radical vulvar surgery may present initially with only localized minimal pain and a deceptively benign appearance, but usually an infectious process is obvious in the wound.[58–61] Local signs of infection such as edema, erythema, crepitis, or bullae may or may not be present. Signs of deep tissue infection may be evident such as cyanosis or bronzing of the skin. Induration is common and crepitance may be present when a gas-producing organism is present. As the inflammatory process progresses, thrombosis of the perforating vessels to the skin may occur, resulting in breakdown of the overlying skin and sometimes associated paresthesias. The fascia and muscle may become involved. Systemic manifestations of sepsis may develop concurrently, but bacteremia is rarely identified. Wound culture usually reveals a polymicrobial infection, particularly in infections occurring postoperatively. Organisms that are commonly isolated include Bacteroides, coliforms, Klebsiella, Proteus, Group A *B*-hemolytic Streptococcus, staphylococcus, peptostreptococcus, and clostridia.[62,63]

Because the patient may present either with an obvious vulvar wound infection or with minimal cutaneous manifestations of a necrotizing soft tissue infection, a high index of suspicion is needed in order to make an early diagnosis. Certainly, if the patient with an apparent cellulitis fails to respond to standard therapy with appropriate antibiotics and wound care, a suspicion of a more extensive infection should be considered. Radiologic studies are seldom helpful in making the diagnosis of a necrotizing soft tissue infection.[64]

Whenever the diagnosis is considered, management initially consists of aggressive resuscitative measures and broad-spectrum antibiotic therapy, prior to proceeding to the operating room for surgical exploration. Some have suggested the use of frozen tissue sections to help make the diagnosis.[65] Surgical exploration and debridement should not be delayed even if the patient remains in septic shock since the sepsis will not resolve until excision of the infected tissue is performed.[64]

Surgical exploration of the vulvar wound should be thorough and include direct visual examination of the underlying muscle and fascia. The presence and extent of undermining, a manifestation of subcutaneous and fascial necrosis, should be assessed. All necrotic tissue, including muscle or fascia, is excised until healthy viable tissue is seen.[66] The wound is packed open and kept moist with saline and is reexplored in the operating room daily until progression of necrosis has ceased. Depending on the primary focus and extent of the necrotizing infection, there may be involvement of the anal sphincter and/or urethra, but if possible these are preserved. Patients with disruption of the anal sphincter or colonic perforation require diversion of stool.[64]

Necrotizing soft tissue infections untreated will progress to extensive tissue necrosis, florid sepsis, and death. The overall mortality rate for patients with all types of necrotizing soft tissue infections is approximately 38%.[58] In general, the literature supports the association of factors that contribute to death including diabetes mellitus, increased age, delay in diagnosis, and failure to control infection at first operation (i.e., inadequate debridement). Delay of surgical intervention is consistently a factor associated with increased mortality.[64] One study of 33 male and female patients with necrotizing fasciitis found that the time from diagnosis of an infectious process to operative intervention was higher for those who died, 11.7 days compared with 6.0 days for those who survived.[67] Similarly, McHenry et al. found that in 65 patients with necrotizing soft tissue infections, the average time from admission to operation was 90 hours in nonsurvivors and 25 hours in survivors ($p = 0.0002$).[68]

Observational clinical and animal studies have suggested that hyperbaric oxygen therapy may be beneficial in the treatment of necrotizing soft tissue infections.[69–71] Several mechanisms are postulated by which hyperbaric oxygen may improve wound healing and a detailed discussion of these is beyond the scope of this chapter.[62,72–74]

Animal models of necrotizing soft tissue infections using intramuscular injection of clostridia have shown an advantage of hyperbaric oxygen when used early after inoculation, with less tissue loss and decreased mortality rates.[75,76] Limited data on the use of hyperbaric oxygen in humans with necrotizing soft tissue infections is available and there has never been a controlled, randomized, prospective study in humans. Riseman et al. examined the use of hyperbaric oxygen therapy for necrotizing fasciitis in a retrospective fashion in 29 patients treated either with or without hyperbaric oxygen. The first group of patients received surgical therapy and antibiotics and the second group also received hyperbaric oxygen therapy. Patients treated with hyperbaric oxygen were more seriously ill but had a significantly lower mortality, 23% compared with 66% in the group not receiving hyperbaric oxygen therapy.[70] Preservation of tissue may be a significant benefit of hyperbaric oxygen therapy in the treatment of necrotizing fasciitis. Riseman et al. found that in addition to a reduction in mortality, the addition of hyperbaric oxygen significantly reduced the number of debridements required to achieve wound control.[70] Others have demonstrated a reduction in amputation rate from 75% to 20% among patients with necrotizing soft tissue infections of the extremity.[77]

There are serious potential complications of hyperbaric oxygen therapy and its administration is complex. Baratrauma may aggravate sinusitis, cause tympanic membrane rupture, pneumothorax, or air embolism. Oxygen may be toxic to the lungs or central nervous system and reversible visual changes may occur. In the hemodynamically unstable patient, the hyperbaric oxygen chamber makes resuscitation difficult. Patient claustrophobia may limit its practical use.[64] Patients with diabetes require particularly close monitoring with hyperbaric oxygen since dextrose metabolism is enhanced. As a result, patients may be more susceptible to hypoglycemic seizures.[78] These observations on the use of hyperbaric oxygen in patients with necrotizing soft tissue infections are made based on Level III evidence, and its use in clinical practice should be considered experimental.

Osteomyelitis Pubis

After surgery for vulvar cancer, partial necrosis or osteomyelitis of the pubic bone is a rare but serious infection that usually results from a contiguous focus of infection weeks or months after a surgical procedure. Associated morbidity is significant and rarely may lead to fulminant sepsis and death.[37] In one large series of patients undergoing radical vulvectomy, the rate of osteomyelitis was 2%.[12] In a series of four patients who developed osteomyelitis of the pubic bone after radical vulvectomy, the mean hospital stay was increased by 5.6 weeks.[79] Two to four months after surgery, the patients presented with pain and tenderness over the pubic symphysis, difficulty ambulating, and evidence of infection in the pubic or vulvar area. Plain X-ray films showed abnormalities of the pubic bone in all cases. In a review of the literature, the infecting organism was *Staphylococcus aureus* in 60% of cases and in the other 40%, gram-negative organisms were etiologic.[79] Management includes wound and bone cultures, drainage and debridement, and intravenous antibiotics. The more serious cases involving bone necrosis require surgical resection of the necrotic bone.

Femoral Vessel Rupture or Hemorrhage

Femoral vessel rupture with hemorrhage is a rare, but serious, complication of groin dissection. Groin wound breakdown is more common in patients undergoing more radical surgery and when the groin breaks down, femoral vessels may be exposed, increasing the risk of vessel rupture, a potentially catastrophic event.[80] Rarely, femoral vessel rupture may result in perioperative death in patients with vulvar cancer.[22] One retrospective study suggested that sartorius muscle transposition may be associated with a decreased risk of this occurrence.[35] In patients with groin wound breakdown, rupture of a femoral vessel occurred on four occasions among 50 patients (9%) who did not have sartorius muscle transposition after inguinal-femoral lymphadenectomy. In three cases, there was rupture of the artery and in one case, rupture of the vein. No femoral vessel rupture occurred in over 200 patients who underwent sartorius muscle transposition.[35] Some of the disadvantages of sartorius muscle transposition include an increase in operative time, risk of femoral nerve injury, and lower extremity pain with associated limitation of mobility. In an effort to evaluate the effectiveness of alternative surgical techniques to protect the femoral vessels after inguinal-femoral lymphadenectomy, authors have examined the use of dura mater grafts and artificial dura film to cover the femoral vessels.[81, 82] The use of dura mater to cover the femoral vessels was examined in 20 patients who underwent inguinal-femoral lymphadenectomy. Among 38 groins, the 3 groin wounds that broke down healed satisfactorily without exposing the femoral vessels. The authors suggest that coverage of the femoral vessels with dura mater is a safe and effective alternative to sartorius muscle transposition.[81] In contrast, the use of artificial dura film to cover femoral vessels in 11 patients was associated with an unacceptable complication rate, with 9 of 11 patients experiencing infectious complications. In the 3 patients who suffered groin breakdown, removal of the dura film was necessary.[82] Sartorius muscle transposition or placement of dura mater to cover the femoral vessels may decrease the risk of femoral vessel rupture, but data is very limited and only Level III evidence is available. We recommend the use of sartorius muscle transposition in selective cases of patients at high risk for infectious morbidity after inguinal-femoral lymphadenectomy.

Thromboembolic/Arterial Occlusion

Deep venous thrombosis and pulmonary embolism are major complications following gynecologic cancer surgery. Using ^{125}I fibrinogen leg counting to detect deep vein thrombi, studies have shown that 17%–45% of patients develop thrombosis after surgery for gynecologic cancer.[83, 84] In a retrospective review of 281 patients with early uterine or cervical cancer, Clarke-Pearson et al. found that clinically significant thromboemboli were encountered in 7.8% of patients postoperatively.[85] Approximately 1%–2.5% of patients with a gynecologic malignancy will die from a postoperative pulmonary embolism.[85, 86] Radical surgery for vulvar cancer appears to be a significant risk factor for the development of postoperative venous thrombosis. In a prospective analysis, authors examined variables associated with postoperative deep venous thrombosis in 411 patients undergoing gynecologic surgery using ^{125}I fibrinogen leg counting.[83] Seventy-two (17.5%) of the 411 patients developed ^{125}I fibrinogen evidence of postoperative deep venous thrombosis. Frequency of deep venous thrombosis was highest in patients undergoing radical vulvectomy with inguinal lymphadenectomy and pelvic exenteration, occurring in 32% and 88% of patients, respectively. Patients undergoing radiation therapy prior to surgery also appear to be at an increased risk of postoperative thromboembolic disease.[85]

Risk of postoperative thrombosis in gynecologic oncology patients is reduced by the use of intermittent pneumatic calf compression devices instituted in the operating room and continued for the first five postoperative days.[87] Low dose perioperative heparin has also been shown to reduce the risk of thrombosis, but its use may increase the risk of bleeding and lymphocyst formation.[88,89] The patient must be followed closely for evidence of venous thrombosis throughout the postoperative recovery period. The routine use of intermittent pneumatic compression devices in patients undergoing surgery for vulvar cancer is recommended based on Level I evidence. The use of prophylactic heparin therapy should be considered on a case by case basis, acknowledging there may be some increased risk of perioperative complications.

Lower extremity arterial occlusion after radical vulvar surgery is a rare but serious event.[90] Predisposing factors may be a prior history of thromboembolic disease and groin infection after surgery. Limited Level III evidence supports these observations. Following inguinal-femoral lymphadenectomy for vulvar cancer, the patient should be examined for presence of pulses or signs of arterial ischemia that may represent femoral artery thrombosis, particularly in the first 24 hours postoperatively.[91] Treatment consists of anticoagulation and sometimes vascular thrombectomy.

Lymphocyst

Formation of a lymphocyst in the groin is a potential complication of inguinal-femoral lymphadenectomy. A lymphocyst is a lymph-filled space without a distinct epithelial lining. Lymphocysts occur after inguinal-femoral lymphadenectomy in 2%–28% of cases.[11,12,15,20,92] Piver et al. suggested that prophylactic mini-dose heparin may be associated with an increase in occurrence of inguinal lymphocysts after radical vulvectomy and inguinal lymphadenectomy occurring in 43% of those receiving versus 0% not receiving heparin.[89] Other factors that have been found to be associated with the development of pelvic lymphocysts, but whose association with inguinal lymphocysts has not been examined, include previous radiation therapy, lymph node metastases, and pregnancy.[93–97] The risk of lymphocyst formation does not appear to be related to the extent of the vulvar surgery.[37] Furthermore, sparing of the saphenous vein did not appear to affect the occurrence of lymphocyst formation.[38]

The formation of lymphocysts cannot always be avoided, even with meticulous surgical technique and optimal perioperative care. Modification of groin dissection with a three-incision technique compared with an en bloc procedure was not found to reduce this complication.[98] Inguinal drains placed at the time of surgery and compression dressings in the first 24 hours after surgery are thought to decrease the risk of lymphocyst formation. It has been suggested that added protection against lymphocyst formation is given by leaving the drain in place after discontinuing the suction, allowing it to be advanced slowly over several days.[91]

Inguinal lymphocysts can cause a significant amount of discomfort. The median time for their development has been reported to be 7.5 days after lymphadenectomy.[89] Although small lymphocysts usually resolve spontaneously, persistent large lymphocysts may contribute to thigh and leg edema, are prone to become infected, or cause necrosis of the overlying skin.[91] Thus, large and/or symptomatic lymphocysts should be treated. Information about the management of inguinal lymphocysts is scant compared with pelvic lymphocysts. The management of pelvic lymphocysts has involved percutaneous drainage, sclerotherapy, and, if unsuccessful, laparotomy and marsupialization.[99–102] Most inguinal lymphocysts should be managed, at least initially by drainage.[103] In most cases, daily aspiration of lymphocyst fluid may result in resolution, but there is a significant risk of infection. Anecdotal experience with insertion of a rubber drain for approximately 7 days and use of antibiotic therapy have successfully resulted in resolution of inguinal lymphocysts. If these methods are ineffective, sclerotherapy should be considered. Bleomycin sclerotherapy has been used to successfully manage inguinal lymphocysts.[104] The sclerosing action of antibiotics is thought to be secondary to induction of an inflammatory reaction. Although not reported for inguinal lymphocysts, Gilliland et al. have successfully used 10% povidone–iodine solution for sclerosis of pelvic lymphocysts.[105] It has also been suggested that absolute ethanol may be used as a sclerosing solution. Rarely, open drainage is necessary and will result in slow healing of groin lymphocysts.[91] The muscle paddle of a myocutaneous flap may be used to fill dead space after open drainage of a lymphocyst and will readily accept a skin graft.[106] These observations and recommendations are made based on Level III evidence.

Delayed Complications

Lymphedema

Lymphedema is a common and particularly problematic long-term complication of groin dissection. Its frequency after inguinal-femoral lymphadenectomy generally varies from 7% to 19%.[10–13, 15] Lymphedema occurs to some degree in almost every patient, commonly temporarily. Patients receiving radiation therapy to the groins in addition to surgical dissection are at an increased risk of lymphedema. In addition, concurrent pelvic node dissection, obesity, postoperative deep venous thrombosis, and varicosities increase the risk of lymphedema after groin dissection.[91] Some have suggested fitting the patient for knee-length antiedema stockings either before surgery or in the early postoperative period to decrease the occurrence of lymphedema, but there are no studies to document the efficacy of this practice.[91]

It has been suggested that preservation of the long saphenous vein decreases the risk of postoperative lymphedema, but there is no data to support the efficacy of this therapy. In a retrospective study of wound morbidity after inguinal-femoral lymphadenectomy through separate incisions, lymphedema occurred in 36% of patients who had preservation of the saphenous vein compared with 21% in whom the vessel was sacrificed.[38] Similarly, Lin et al. in a retrospective study of patients undergoing groin dissection found that lymphedema occurred in 17% of patients who had preservation of the long saphenous vein versus 13% in whom the vein was sacrified.[98] In the same study, the authors noted that omission of the deep femoral node dissection was not of significant benefit in reducing lower extremity edema. Furthermore, they found that performance of an en bloc or three-incision technique did not affect the occurrence of lymphedema in patients undergoing groin dissection, occurring in 13% and 15%, respectively.[98] The extent of vulvar surgery was not found to influence the risk of lymphedema.[37] Furthermore, the incidence of lymphedema was not greater in patients developing groin necrosis, lymphocysts, or vulvar complications compared with those without complications.[37]

Available medical and surgical treatments of lymphedema are unsatisfactory. Management consists of elevation of legs, the use of thigh high stockings, and in more severe cases the use of mechanical stockings to compress the edema out of the lower extremities. The patient should be instructed to avoid standing still for any period of time and avoid exposure to hot weather.[91] Prompt antibiotic treatment of cellulitis is important. Within approximately 2 years, collateral lymphatic pathways usually become established and there may be an improvement of lymphedema. Formation of collateral lymphatic may take a significantly longer period of time in radiated tissues. Surgical intervention may be necessary for complications of severe chronic lymphedema. These observations and recommendations are made based on Level III evidence.

Hernia and Prolapse

Hernia formation after radical vulvar surgery with inguinal-femoral lymphadenectomy may occur, usually perineal, vaginal, inguinal, or femoral. After completion of the inguinal node dissection, the external inguinal ring and the femoral canal should be examined for evidence of looseness and presence of a hernia sac. If the inguinal ring is not snug, it is tightened with permanent suture or for the femoral canal, sutures are placed between the inguinal ligament and the lacunar ligament to tighten the femoral canal. Care must be taken to avoid compromising the diameter of the femoral vein.[91] A rare but serious complication of a strangulated femoral hernia has been reported in a patient undergoing laparoscopic pelvic lymphadenectomy after groin node dissection.[80] It is possible that the increased abdominal pressure associated with insufflation of gas into the peritoneal cavity was a predisposing factor in this case.

Rectocele, cystocele, and uterine prolapse have been reported to complicate vulvectomy in 5%–25% of patients.[107–109] Calame et al. found that 17% of 58 patients undergoing surgery for vulvar cancer developed some form of pelvic floor defect, with surgical repair required in most.[109] Magrina et al. examined complications in 225 patients with vulvar cancer undergoing radical versus modified radical surgery.[37] Cystocele and rectocele formation occurred in 16% and 12% of patients undergoing radical vulvar surgery compared with 2% and 1% of patients in the modified surgical group. Stress urinary incontinence occurred in 16% of patients in the radical surgery group compared with 8% of patients undergoing modified radical vulvar surgery. The authors suggest that radical extirpation of the labia and perineum, the advancement of the vaginal walls to effect closure, and the resulting tension of the vulvar wound may contribute to these occurrences.[37] These complications are typically late, but can appear within a few weeks of surgery or even in the immediate postoperative period. It has been suggested they occur predominantly in patients with preexisting pelvic floor defects and may be aggravated by tension on the vagina from the operative closure. One expert recommended that a perineorrhaphy be routinely performed after radical vulvectomy to reduce the risk of this occurrence, but the efficacy of this approach is unproven.[91] These observations are made based on Level III evidence.

Urinary or Stool Incontinence

Excision of the distal portion of the urethra as part of radical excision of a vulvar cancer may result in stress or total incontinence.[107] As a general rule, up to 2 cm of the distal urethra can be resected without producing incontinence, and anecdotal experience suggests that more of the posterior wall of the urethra can be removed than the anterior wall. When the functional length of the urethra is inadequate or marginal, incontinence may be avoided by combining the meatal resection with plication of the urethra and bladder neck or by performing a retropubic bladder neck suspension.[91] Care must be taken with closure of skin surrounding the urethra since the position of the urethra and urinary stream may be distorted. Leaving a small area of tissue open anterior to the urethra may minimize this occurrence.[91] When distortion of the urinary stream occurs, the patient may respond to urethral dilation postoperatively or surgical correction may be necessary. These observations are made based on Level III evidence.

After partial or total excision of the anal sphincter, stool incontinence may occur and diverting colostomy may be necessary. For posterior vulvar lesions, in order to get a minimum 1-cm margin, shaving off the anterior portion of the anal sphincter may be necessary. This can usually be performed without producing anal incontinence. However, about 10% of women have a very thin perineal body, severely limiting the depth of resection that can be performed without damaging the integrity of the sphincter.[91] When necessary, the entire anterior quadrant of the external anal sphincter and perineal body can be removed as a wedge without necessarily producing fecal incontinence, particularly when there is good levator tone. In such cases, the patient should be instructed to institute constipating measures postoperatively. Plication of the levator muscles may improve continence of stool, but incontinence of flatus will almost invariably occur. In some cases, surgical repair of the external sphincter can be performed with some symptomatic relief.[91] These observations are made based on Level III evidence.

Radiation Necrosis and Fistula

Radionecrosis of the vulva is an uncommon event in the modern management of vulvar cancer because the disease is primarily treated surgically and because of improved radiation techniques. The vulvar skin is, however, notoriously less tolerant of radiation therapy than skin covering other areas of the body and as a result is subject to an increase in complications. Reasons may include moisture, friction, nonflat surface, and a larger proportion of end arteries than in other areas of skin. Patients exposed to low energy radiation therapy, an older technique that delivered most of the energy to the skin or slightly below the skin, were found to have a significant increased risk of radiation skin complications. In contrast, modern megavoltage radiotherapy is less commonly associated with radionecrosis of skin and the injury tends to be much deeper than that seen with low energy radiation therapy. These issues will be further discussed in the section on "Radiation Therapy."

Minor chronic radiation-induced injury to the skin is manifested by hyperpigmentation, dryness, telangiectasias, induration, decreased resilience, thinning of epidermis, and loss of normal adnexal structures.[110–112] The most serious chronic effects on skin and soft tissues are related to slowly progressive fibrosis and an obliterative vasculitis.[113] As a result, subcutaneous tissues become progressively ischemic and viability of overlying epithelium cannot be maintained.[110] Bacterial overgrowth in ischemic soft tissues may result in frank tissue necrosis.[110] The result is a radionecrotic wound and usually presents 6–18 months after completion of radiation, although a latent period of up to 20 years may occur.[113,114] Radionecrotic wounds demonstrate little ability to contract or epithelialize and may slowly increase in size as ischemia progresses and bacterial contamination continues.[114]

When radionecrosis involves the lower genital tract, the patient is commonly in severe pain and suffers from a foul discharge. Traditional initial conservative therapy consists of narcotic analgesics, antibiotics, local debridement, and intensive local care.[115] However, conservative therapy rarely leads to resolution of the radionecrosis. Such treatment was not associated with even partial healing in any of 12 patients with vaginal or vulvar radionecrosis.[116] Systemic antibiotics may be of limited value in the initial treatment of radionecrotic wounds because of poor tissue perfusion, but may be of greater value during definitive wound closure.

Treatment of chronic radionecrotic wound begins with control of pain and correction of underlying systemic factors that may be contributing to poor wound healing such as poor nutrition, control of diabetes, and smoking. Radical surgical excision of the radionecrotic wound is usually necessary. When surgical debridement is undertaken, all necrotic tissue should be removed down to a bleeding base.[110,111] If bone is infected and exposed within the wound, removal of either the outer cortex or the entire bone may be necessary.[106,117] In the chronic wound that is poorly drained or grossly infected or very large, staged surgical excision may be necessary.[118] In such cases, superficial debridement of necrotic material to promote wound drainage should be performed initially. Recurrent cancer should be excluded by performing biopsies of nonnecrotic tissue at the edge of the ulcer. Depending on the site of the radionecrotic lesion, urinary or fecal diversion may be required. In some cases necrosis may progress to form a fistula.

Definitive closure of the radionecrotic wound should usually be performed immediately after excision. Delaying closure until there is adequate growth of granulation tissue over the wound base usually fails since capillary or fibroblastic proliferation does not occur in the radiation-damaged tissue normally. The result is continued ischemia and bacterial regrowth that leads to further wound breakdown.[110] Radiated tissues are not pliable and will not tolerate even very minimal tension on the wound or disruption will occur.[114] In rare cases, primary closure may be appropriate, but usually well-vascularized tissue must be used and brought in to close the ischemic defects.[119] Simple skin graft is commonly inadequate for coverage of the wound since soft tissues may have a poor blood supply. Split-thickness skin grafting for radiation ulcer treatment had a 100% complication rate in nine cases, defined as the need for further surgery. The complication rate for local full-thickness flaps was similarly very high.[119] As a result, myocutaneous flaps are usually necessary. Techniques of wound coverage of the vulva are similar to those discussed in the section on "Vulvar Reconstruction." In general, they include random pattern skin flaps, myocutaneous flaps, or free flaps. The importance of complete excision of radiation-damaged tissue so that a myocutaneous flap can be sewn into normal tissue both on the underside and at the periphery must be emphasized.[119] Complications of healing even with a myocutaneous flap may occur because after excision of the ulcer, there is a radiated bed that accepts the myocutaneous flap poorly. These observations and recommendations concerning the radionecrotic wound have been made based on Level III evidence.

Pentoxifylline is a drug that has been used anecdotally to improve healing of radionecrotic wounds. Pentoxifylline is a methylxanthine derivative that produces dose-related hemorrheologic effects, lowers blood viscosity, improves erythrocyte flexibility, and increases tissue oxygenation. Twenty-six patients with late radiation complications of the head and neck were treated with oral pentoxifylline. Nine of 12 patients with soft tissue necrosis completely healed. Five patients with mucosal pain had resolution of their symptoms. Radiation fibrosis improved in 67% of patients.[120] In another series, 12 patients with 15 sites of late radiation necrosis of soft tissues were treated with pentoxifylline. Thirteen of 15 (87%) of the necroses had healed completely, and one was partially healed. Furthermore, the time course of healing was significantly less than the duration of nonhealing prior to pentoxifylline, 9 weeks vs. 30 weeks on average.[120] These anecdotal data suggest that pentoxifylline may accelerate healing of radiation-associated soft tissue necrosis and reverse some late radiation injuries. Since the risks associated with administration of the drug are minimal, its use in patients with radionecrotic wounds should be considered despite the lack of randomized prospective evidence supporting its efficacy.

The use of hyperbaric oxygen has been studied with some anecdotal success in treatment of radionecrosis of some head and neck radionecrotic wounds.[122, 123] The experience of using hyperbaric oxygen for radionecrotic wounds at other locations has been more limited.[116, 124] As a result, its use in radionecrotic wounds of the vulva cannot be recommended outside of a research study.

VULVAR RECONSTRUCTION

Despite the more conservative surgical approach to vulvar cancer that is common practice today, there are still cases where primary closure of the skin may not be possible. This is more commonly problematic with a large lesion or one in an unfavorable location for closure. In some cases, although closure may be technically feasible, risk of breakdown may be unacceptably high because of tension on the suture line or scarring and disfigurement of the vulva may be excessive. In such cases, reconstruction of the vulva should be performed using local tissues such as skin flaps or with myocutaneous flaps, usually at the time of the original surgery.

The random pattern skin flap is relatively simple and useful for closure of a wound that is not too large. These flaps are at risk for ischemia since they lack an anatomically identifiable vascular pedicle and rely on a dermal-subdermal vascular plexus between skin and fascia. Their marginal vascular supply requires that these flaps be short with a maximum length-to-width ratio of 2:1 or flap necrosis will occur.[106, 118] In addition, they should be avoided in the irradiated patient, since the proximity of the flap donor site to the wound makes radiation damage likely within the flap itself.[106, 114]

Local advancement flaps such as the rhomboid flap may be used to cover a vulvar wound that otherwise would be closed under significant tension. The flap derives its blood supply from the underlying subcutaneous vascular network. The flap must maintain a 1.0- to 1.5-cm layer of attached subcutaneous tissue. Unilateral or bilateral flaps may be used. Burke et al. described the use of rhomboid flaps in 13 patients who underwent extensive vulvar resections.[125] Two of 13 patients had minor wound disruptions and there were no other early or delayed complications. With this technique, approximately 15%–20% of patients may have minor separation of wounds with rare cases of major wound disruption (<5%).[126, 127] Others have used the Z-plasty full-thickness pedicle flap for similar indications. Close attention to the design of the flap is necessary since the base of the flap should be twice as long as the length of the flap to ensure adequate blood supply to the distal flap.[91]

The axial pattern skin flap is formed by a longitudinally orientated vascular pedicle traveling superficially to the deep fascia.[106, 128] Adding a random flap to the end of an axial flap results in an improved blood supply that allows for a significant increase in the length–width ratio of the flap of up to 4:1.[118] One example of an axial flap is the groin flap, based on the superficial circumflex iliac artery.[128] Unfortunately, its vascular pedicle is frequently ligated during the course of genitourinary surgery, limiting its usefulness in vulvar reconstruction.[106]

Mayer and Rodriguez described the use of bilateral axial pedicle skin flaps based on the superficial external pudendal artery to successfully close a vulvar defect.[129] Skin-fascial flaps such as the gluteal thigh flap provide another option for wound coverage and are formed by large paddles of skin and deep fascia supplied by vascular pedicles that branch from major extremity or truncal vessels.[106, 130] This flap is useful for closure of perineal and sacral defects.

Myocutaneous flaps are based on the vascular pedicle of a major muscle that is elevated and transposed together with its overlying skin paddle to an adjacent site.[131–135] Depending on the size of the defect, its location, and prior radiation history, this may be the technique of choice to close vulvar or groin wounds. Because of its excellent blood supply from an anatomically distinct vascular pedicle, this type of flap tends to be more resistant to infection and be quite durable. Myocutaneous flaps may be either transposition flaps or free flaps. Muscle perforating vessels allow survival of the skin that is transferred with the muscle.[136] Variations of the myocutancous flap include creation of a muscle flap by deletion of the skin island.

Selection of the myocutaneous flap is based on its reliability, location to the defect, potential disability from donor muscle loss, and other anatomic factors.[136] The gracilis muscle flap is commonly used for repair of wounds of the perineum and groin.[137] It is supplied by the medial circumflex branch of the profunda femoris artery and the flap may be rotated medially and superiorly. The skin island is raised from the proximal or middle thigh. Since the adductor longus and magnus muscles remain intact, there is no functional impairment in the leg.[106] The rectus abdominus muscle is a very versatile flap with a dual blood supply from both the superior and inferior epigastric arteries and as a result may be transposed in either direction. Its skin island may be harvested in a transverse or longitudinal orientation and when used to cover vulvar or groin defects is based on the deep inferior epigastric artery.[91, 135, 138–141] Many surgeons' experience with the rectus abdominus flap has been more favorable than with the gracilis myocutaneous flap. The flap is more reliable and provides quality surface restoration and revascularization of wound.

The rectus femoris muscle, supplied primarily by the descending branch of the lateral circumflex femoral artery, can be used for groin wounds with little or no loss of function in the ipsilateral leg.[106] Other myocutaneous flaps include the gluteus maximus flap, best suited for covering defects in the posterior vulva and perineum, and the tensor fascia lata muscle flap, used primarily for covering a predominantly anterior defect.[91]

A free pedicle flap allows for closure of a wound distant from the flap donor site through microvascular reanastomosis of its vascular pedicle to vessels in proximity to the recipient wound.[142] This is rarely performed for closure of vulvar wounds since local myocutaneous flaps tend to be readily available.

RADIATION THERAPY

Traditionally, radiation therapy has been considered to have a limited role in the primary management of vulvar cancer. Radiation techniques used in the past were associated with poor survival and severe acute skin reactions were common. Vulva and perineal tissues were thought to be intolerant of radiation therapy. With the introduction of megavoltage external-beam equipment and the judicious use of electrons or interstitial brachytherapy, there has been an overall improvement in vulvar tissue tolerance to radiation therapy. As a result, radiation therapy is used more commonly to treat vulvar cancer.[143–145]

Even with modern radiation techniques, interruption of radiation therapy to the vulva is often necessary in the third or fourth week to relieve symptoms of severe moist desquamation of the perineal region. In addition, delay of therapy is common due to symptoms of cystitis or proctitis.[146] Overall, radiation therapy should be used selectively for vulvar cancer because of complications of radiation fibrosis, lymphedema, skin ulceration, and other severe morbidity.

Radiation therapy plays many roles in the treatment of patients with vulvar cancer: (1) to decrease locoregional failures after surgery in patients undergoing radical local excision and bilateral inguinal-femoral lymphadenectomy with close surgical margins or involved inguinal lymph nodes, (2) to serve as an alternative to inguinal or pelvic lymph node dissection in patients with clinically negative nodes, (3) to reduce the extent of surgery required in patients with stage III and IV disease (e.g., lesion that extends to vital structures such as the anus, rectum or proximal urethra, bladder), (4) to treat patients before surgery for locally extensive tumors that may be considered inoperable initially (e.g., fixed groin nodes), and (5) to treat recurrent disease.[146, 147] In patients receiving preoperative radiation therapy, less radical surgery may be performed to resect the disease or unresectable nodes may be rendered resectable. In patients with recurrent vulvar cancer, radiation therapy has been used with limited success.[148-150] Treatment-related morbidity may be significant including rectovaginal fistula, proctitis, rectal stricture, bone vaginal or skin necrosis, and groin abscess.[146]

The use of chemotherapy synchronous with radiation therapy to treat locally advanced vulvar cancer has stemmed from its success in patients with locally advanced anal and head and neck cancers. Concurrent radiation therapy and chemotherapy for carcinoma of the anus yields an 80% complete response rate and 75% cure rate for lesions of less than 8 cm diameter, results similar to those obtained with surgery, but with preservation of a functional anus.[151] These excellent preliminary results have led investigators to utilize this technique for locally advanced vulvar cancer to improve treatment outcome and reduce need for ultraradical surgery.[152-154] Leiserowitz et al. studied the use of chemoradiation therapy in 23 patients with locally advanced squamous cell carcinoma of the vulva with clinically uninvolved groin nodes. Subsequent groin surgery was not performed. No patient failed in the groin and their were no cases of lymphedema, vascular insufficiency, neurological injury, or aseptic necrosis of the femur.[155] Moore et al. reported preliminary results of a phase II prospective GOG study of preoperative chemoradiation for advanced vulvar cancer.[22] Seventy-three patients with T3 or T4 primary tumors were treated with concurrent cisplatin/5-fluorouracil and radiation therapy followed by surgical excision of the residual primary tumor plus inguinal-femoral lymph node dissection. At the time of surgery, 33 of 71 (46.5%) of the patients had no visible vulvar cancer. For patients with residual cancer, complete resection was almost always possible, except in 2.8% of patients. Toxicity was acceptable.[22] This and other studies suggest that preoperative chemoradiotherapy in advanced squamous cell carcinoma of the vulva is feasible and may reduce the need for more radical surgery, including pelvic exenteration. The use of this technique is recommended based on Level II and III evidence.

REFERENCES

1. TAUSSIG FJ. Cancer of the vulva: an analysis of 155 cases (1911–1940). Am J Obstet Gynecol 1940;40:764.
2. WAY S. The anatomy of the lymphatic drainage of the vulva and its influence on the radical operation for carcinoma. Ann R Coll Surg Engl 1948;3:187.

3. MORLEY GW. Infiltrative carcinoma of the vulva: results of surgical treatment. Am J Obstet Gynecol 1976;124:874.
4. PODRATZ KC, SYMMONDS RE, TAYLOR WF, et al. Carcinoma of the vulva: analysis of treatment and survival. Obstet Gynecol 1983;61:63–74.
5. HOMESLEY HD, BUNDY BN, SEDLIS A, et al. Assessment of current International Federation of Gynecology and Obstetrics staging of vulvar carcinoma relative to prognostic factors for survival (a Gynecologic Oncology Group study). Am J Obstet Gynecol 1991;164:998–1004.
6. IVERSEN T, ABELER V, CHRISTENSEN A, et al. Squamous cell carcinoma of the vulva: a review of 424 patients, 1956–1974. Gynecol Oncol 1980;9:271–279.
7. BALLON SC, LAMB EJ. Separate incisions in the treatment of carcinoma of the vulva. Surg Gynecol Obstet 1975;140:81–84.
8. FLANNELLY GM, FOLEY ME, LENEHAN PM, et al. Obstet Gynecol 1992;79:307–309.
9. HACKER NF, LEUCHTER RS, BEREK JS, et al. Radical vulvectomy and bilateral inguinal lymphadenectomy through separate groin incisions. Obstet Gynecol 1981;58:574–579.
10. CAVANAGH D, FIORICA JV, HOFFMAN MS, et al. Invasive carcinoma of the vulva. Changing trends in surgical management. Am J Obstet Gynecol 1990;163:1007–1015.
11. HOPKINS MP, REID GC, MORLEY GW. Radical vulvectomy—the decision for the incision. Cancer 1993;72:799–803.
12. SUTTON GP, MISER MR, STEHMAN FB, et al. Trends in the operative management of invasive squamous carcinoma of the vulva at Indiana University, 1974–1988. Am J Obstet Gynecol 1991;164: 1472–1482.
13. STEHMAN FB, BUNDY BN, DVORETSKY PM, et al. Early stage I carcinoma of the vulva treated with ipsilateral inguinal lymphadenectomy and modified radical hemivulvectomy: a prospective study of the Gynecology Oncology Group. Obstet Gynecol 1992;79:490–497.
14. HEAPS JM, FU YS, MONTZ FJ, et al. Surgical-pathologic variables predictive of local recurrence in squamous cell carcinoma of the vulva. Gynecol Oncol 1990;38:309–314.
15. BURKE TW, STRINGER CA, GERSHENSON DM, et al. Radical wide excision and selective inguinal node dissection for squamous cell carcinoma of the vulva. Gynecol Oncol 1990;38:328–332.
16. HACKER NF, NIEBERG RK, BEREK JS, et al. Superficially invasive vulvar cancer with nodal metastases. Gynecol Oncol 1983;15:65–77.
17. HACKER NF, BEREK JS, LAGASSE LD, et al. Individualization of treatment for stage I squamous cell vulvar carcinoma. Obstet Gynecol 1984;63:155–162.
18. HACKER NF, BEREK JS, LAGASSE LD, et al. Management of regional lymph nodes and their prognostic influence in vulvar cancer. Obstet Gynecol 1983;61:408–412.
19. KRUPP PJ, BOHM JW. Lymph gland metastases in invasive squamous cell cancer of the vulva. Am J Obstet Gynecol 1978;130:943.
20. FIGGE DC, GAUDENZ R. Invasive carcinoma of the vulva. Am J Obstet Gynecol 1974;106:1117.
21. MORRIS JM. A formula for selective lymphadenectomy. Obstet Gynecol 1977;50:152.
22. MOORE DH, THOMAS GM, MONTANA GS, et al. Preoperative chemoradiation for advanced vulvar cancer: a phase II study of the Gynecologic Oncology Group. Int J Rad Oncol Biol Phys 1988;42: 79–85.
23. KELEMEN PR, VANHERLE AJ, GIULIANO AE. Sentinel lymphadenectomy in thyroid malignant neoplasms. Arch Surg 1998;133:288–292.
24. STADELMANN WK, JAVAHERI S, CRUSE CW, et al. The use of selective lymphadenectomy in squamous cell carcinoma of the wrist: a case report. J Hand Surg 1997;22:726–731.
25. COX CE, HADDAD F, BASS S, et al. Lymphatic mapping in the treatment of breast cancer. Oncol 1998;12:1283–1298.
26. LEONG SP, STEINMETZ I, HABIB FA, et al. Optimal selection sentinel lymph node dissection in primary malignant melanoma. Arch Surg 1997;132:666–672.
27. AYHAN A, CELIK H, DURSUN P. Lymphatic mapping and sentinel node biopsy in gynecological cancers: a critical review of the literature. World J Surg Oncol 2008;6(53).
28. KNOPP S, NESLAND JM, TROPE C. SLNB and the importance of micrometastases in vulvar squamous cell carcinoma. Surg Oncol 2008;17:219–225.
29. SELMAN TJ, LUESLAY DM, ACHESON N, et al. A systematic review of the accuracy of diagnostic tests for inguinal lymph node status in vulvar cancer. Gynecol Oncol 2005;99:206–214.

30. HAMPL M, HANTSCHMANN P, MICHELS W, et al. Validation of the accuracy of the sentinel lymph node procedure in patients with vulvar cancer: results of a multicenter study in Germany. Gynecol Oncol 2008;111:282–288.

31. de HULLU JA, HOLLEMA H, PIERS DA, et al. Sentinel lymph node procedure is highly accurate in squamous cell carcinoma of the vulva. J Clin Oncol 2000;18(15):2811–2816.

32. LOUIS-SYLVESTRE C, EVANGELISTA E, LEONARD F, et al. Sentinel node localization should be interpreted with caution in midline vulvar cancer. Gynecol Oncol 2005;97:151–154.

33. LEVENBACK CF, VAN DER ZEE AGJ, ROB L, et al. Sentinel lymph node biopsy in patient with gynecologic cancers. Expert panel statement from the International Sentinel Node Society Meeting, February 21, 2008. Gynecol Oncol 2009;114:151–156.

34. LEVENBACK C. Update of sentinel lymph node biopsy in gynecologic cancers. Gynecol Oncol 2008;111:S42–S43.

35. CAVANAGH D, ROBERTS WS, BRYSON SC, et al. Changing trends in the surgical treatment of invasive carcinoma of the vulva. Surg Gynecol Obstet 1986;162:164–168.

36. REEDY MB, CAPEN CV, BAKER DP, et al. Hyperbaric oxygen therapy following radical vulvectomy: an adjunctive therapy to improve wound healing. Gynecol Oncol 1994;53:13–16.

37. MAGRINA JF, GONZALEZ-BOSQUET J, WEAVER AL, et al. Primary squamous cell cancer of the vulva: radical versus modified radical vulvar surgery. Gynecol Oncol 1998;71:116–121.

38. PALEY PJ, JOHNSON PR, ADCOCK LL, et al. The effect of sartorius transposition on wound morbidity following inguinal-femoral lymphadenectomy. Gynecol Oncol 1997;64:237–241.

39. GOMES MN, SPEAR SL. Pedicled muscle flaps in the management of infected aortofemoral grafts. Cardiovasc Surg 1994;2:70–77.

40. PEREZ-BURKHARDT JL, GONZALEZ-FAJARDO JA, CARPINTERO LA, et al. Sartorius myoplasty for the treatment of infected groins with vascular grafts. J Cardiovasc Surg 1995;36:581–585.

41. COHEN IK, DIEGELMAN RF, LINDBLAD WJ. Wound Healing—Biochemical and Clinical Aspects. Philadelphia, PA: WB Saunders Company; 1992.

42. FORREST L. Current concepts in soft tissue connective tissue wound healing. Br J Surg 1983;70:133–140.

43. NEMETH AJ. Dermatologic Clinics—Wound Healing. Philadelphia, PA: WB Saunders Company; 1993.

44. THOMSON PD, SMITH DJ. What is infection? Am J Surg 1994;167:7S–11S.

45. PEACOCK EE. Wound Repair. 3rd ed. Philadelphia, PA: WB Saunders Company; 1984. p 128.

46. DUNCAN HJ, FARIS IB. Skin vascular resistance and skin perfusion pressure as predictors of healing of ischemic lesions of the lower limb: influences of diabetes mellitus, hypertension, and age. Surgery 1986;99:432.

47. ROBERTSON HD, POLK HC. The mechanism of infection in patients with diabetes mellitus: a review of leukocyte malfunction. Surgery 1974;75:123.

48. YUE DK, McLENNAN S, MARSH M, et al. Effects of experimental diabetes, uremia, and malnutrition on wound healing. Diabetes 1987;36:295.

49. MULLER JM, BRENNER U, DIENST C, et al. Preoperative parenteral feeding in patients with gastrointestinal carcinoma. Lancet 1982;1:68.

50. KLEIN S, SIMES J, BALCKBURN GL, et al. Total parenteral nutrition and cancer clinical trials. Cancer 1986;58:1378.

51. EAGLSTEIN WH. Wound healing and aging. Clin Geriatr Med 1989;5:183.

52. SHERWIN MA, GASTWIRTH CM. Detrimental effects of cigarette smoking on lower extremity wound healing. J Foot Surg 1990;29:84–87.

53. WOLBACH SB. Summary of the effects of repeated roentgen ray exposure upon human skin, antecedent to the formation of carcinoma. Am J Roentgenol 1925;13:139–143.

54. MUSTOE TA, PORRAS-REYES BH. Modulation of wound healing response in chronic irradiated tissues. Clin Plast Surg 1993;20:466–472.

55. LEVENSON SM, GRUBER CA, RETTURA G, et al. Supplemental vitamin A prevents the acute radiation-induced defect in wound healing. Ann Surg 1984;200:494.

56. BAILEY AJ, TROMANS WJ. Effects of ionizing radiation on the ultrastructure of collagen fibrils. Radiat Res 1964;23:145.

57. GRANT RA, COX RW, KENT CM. The effects of gamma radiation on the structure of native and cross-linked collagen fibers. J Anat 1973;115:29.

58. AHRENHOLZ DH. Surgical spectrum. Clinical skin and soft tissue infection. Physicians World Communications [Monograph], West Point, PA: Merck Sharpe and Dohme; 1988. p 16–24.

59. BAXTER CR. Surgical management of soft tissue infections. Surg Clin North Am 1972;52:1483.

60. DELLINGER EP. Severe necrotizing soft-tissue infections. JAMA 1981;246:15–17.

61. KAISER RE, CERRA FB. Progressive necrotizing surgical infections—a unified approach. J Trauma 1981;21:349.

62. BAKKER DJ. Clostridial myonecrosis. In: DAVIS JC, HUNT TK, editors. Problem Wounds. The Role of Oxygen. New York: Elsevier; 1988. p 153.

63. BASKIN LS, CARROLL PR, COTTOLICA EV, et al. Necrotizing soft tissue infections of the perineum and genitalia: bacteriology, treatment, and risk assessment. Br J Urol 1990;54:524.

64. SUTHERLAND ME, MEYER AA. Necrotizing soft-tissue infections. Surg Clin North Am 1994;74: 591–606.

65. STAMENKOVIC I, LEW PD. Early recognition of potentially fatal necrotizing fasciitis. The use of frozen-section biopsy. NEJM 1984;310:1689–1693.

66. WILSON B. Necrotizing fasciitis. Am Surg 1970;217:109.

67. PESSA ME, HOWARD RJ. Necrotizing fasciitis. Surg Gynecol Obstet 1985;161:357–361.

68. MCHENRY CR, PIOTROWSKI JJ, PETRINIC D, et al. Determinants of mortality for necrotizing soft-tissue infections. Ann Surg 1995;221:558–563.

69. GRIM PS, GOTTLIEB LJ, BODDIE A, et al. Hyperbaric oxygen therapy. JAMA 1990;263:2216.

70. RISEMAN JA, ZAMBONI WA, CURTIS A, et al. Hyperbaric oxygen therapy for necrotizing fasciitis reduces mortality and the need for debridements. Surgery 1990;108:847–850.

71. RUDGE FW. The role of hyperbaric oxygenation in the treatment of clostridial myonecrosis. Mil Med 1993;158:80–83.

72. FORMAN HJ, THOMAS MJ. Oxidant production and bactericidal activity of phagocytes. Annu Rev Physiol 1986;48:669.

73. NYLANDER G, LEWIS D, NORDSTROM H, et al. Reduction of postischemic edema with hyperbaric oxygen. Plast Reconstr Surg 1985;76:596.

74. KNIGHTON DR, SILVER JA, HUNT TK. Regulation of wound healing angiogenesis; effect of oxygen gradients and improved oxygen concentration. Surgery 1981;89:262.

75. HILL GB, OSTERHOUT S. Experimental effects of hyperbaric oxygen on selected clostridial species: II. In vivo studies in mice. J Infect Dis 1972;125:26.

76. HOLLAND JA, HILL GB, WOLFE WG, et al. Experimental and clinical experience with hyperbaric oxygen in the treatment of clostridial myonecrosis. Surgery 1975;77:75.

77. JACKSON RW, WADDELL JP. Hyperbaric oxygen in the management of clostridial myonecrosis (gas gangrene). Clinic Orthop 1973;96:271–276.

78. LOVE TL, SCHNURE JJ, LANKIN EC, et al. Glucose intolerance in man during prolonged exposure to a hyperbaric-hyperoxic environment. Diabetes 1975;20:282–285.

79. HOYME UB, TAMIMI HK, ESCHENBACH DA, et al. Osteomyelitis pubis after radical gynecologic operations. Obstet Gynecol 1984;63:47S.

80. MAGRINA JF, TAHERY MM, HEPPELL J, et al. Femoral hernia: a complication of laparoscopic pelvic lymphadenectomy after groin node dissection. J Laparoendosc Adv Surg Tech 1997;7: 191–193.

81. FIORICA JV, ROBERTS WS, LAPOLLA JP, et al. Femoral vessel coverage with dura mater after inguino-femoral lymphadenectomy. Gynecol Oncol 1991;42:217–221.

82. FINAN MA, FIORICA JV, ROBERTS WS, et al. Artificial dura film for femoral vessel coverage after inguinal-femoral lymphadenectomy. Gynecol Oncol 1994;55:333–335.

83. CLARKE-PEARSON DL, DELONG ER, SYNAN IS, et al. Variables associated with postoperative deep venous thrombosis: a prospective study of 411 gynecology patients and creation of a prognostic model. Obstet Gynecol 1987;69:146–150.

84. CRANDON AJ, KOUTTS J. Incidence of postoperative deep vein thrombosis in gynecologic oncology. Aust N Z J Obstet Gynaecol 1983;23:216–219.

85. CLARKE-PEARSON DL, JELOVSEK FR, CREASMAN WT. Thromboembolism complicating surgery for cervical and uterine malignancy: incidence, risk factors, and prophylaxis. Obstet Gynecol 1983;61:87–94.

86. JONES HW III. Treatment of adenocarcinoma of the endometrium. Obstet Gynecol Surv 1975;30: 147–169.

87. CLARKE-PEARSON DL, SYNAN IS, HINSHAW WM, et al. Prevention of postoperative venous thromboembolism by external pneumatic calf compression in patients with gynecologic malignancy. Obstet Gynecol 1984;63:92–98.

88. CLARKE-PEARSON DL, SYNAN IS, DODGE R, et al. A randomized trial of low-dose heparin and intermittent pneumatic calf compression for the prevention of deep venous thrombosis after gynecologic oncology surgery. Am J Obstet Gynecol 1993;168:1146–1154.

89. PIVER MS, MALFETANO JH, LELE SB, et al. Prophylactic anticoagulation as a possible cause of inguinal lymphocyst after radical vulvectomy and inguinal lymphadenectomy. Obstet Gynecol 1983;62:17–21.

90. LEVENBACK C, BURKE TW, RUBIN SC, et al. Arterial occlusion complicating treatment of gynecologic cancer: a case series. Gynecol Oncol 1996;63:40–46.

91. MORROW CP, CURTIN JP, editors. Gynecologic Cancer Surgery. New York: Churchill Livingstone; 1996. p 329–377, 381–450.

92. RUTLEDGE F, SMITH JP, FRANKLIN EW. Carcinoma of the vulva. Am J Obstet Gynecol 1973;106: 1117–1130.

93. DODD GD, RUTLEDGE F, WALLACE S. Postoperative pelvic lymphocyst. Am J Roentgenol 1970;108: 312–323.

94. MORI N. Clinical and experimental studies on so-called lymphocyst which develops after radical hysterectomy in cancer of uterine cervix. J Jpn Obstet Gynecol Soc 1955;2:178.

95. GRAY MJ, PLENTL AA, TAYLOR HC. The lymphocyst: a complication of pelvic lymph node dissection. Am J Obstet Gynecol 1958: 75:1059–1062.

96. RUTLEDGE F, DODD GD, KASILAG FB. Lymphocysts: a complication of radical pelvic surgery. Am J Obstet Gynecol 1959;77:1165–1175.

97. FERGUSON JH, MACLURE JG. Lymphocele following lymphadenectomy. Am J Obstet Gynecol 1961;82:783–791.

98. LIN JY, DUBESHTER B, ANGEL C, et al. Morbidity and recurrence with modifications of radical vulvectomy and groin dissection. Gynecol Oncol 1992;47:80–86.

99. MANN W, VOGEL F, PATSUER B, et al. Management of lymphocysts after radical gynecologic surgery. Gynecol Oncol 1987;33:248–250.

100. CHOO YC, WONG LC, WONG KP, et al. The management of intractable lymphocyst following radical hysterectomy. Gynecol Oncol 1986;24:309–317.

101. CONTE M, PANIC PB, GUARIGLIA L, et al. Pelvic lymphocele following radical paraortic and pelvic lymphadenectomy for cervical carcinoma: incidence, rate and percutaneous management. Obstet Gynecol 1990;76:268–271.

102. OSTROWSKI MJ. Intracavitary therapy with bleomycin for the treatment of malignant pleural effusion. J Surg Oncol Suppl 1989;1:7–13.

103. DALY JW, POMERANCE AJ. Groin dissection with prevention of tissue loss and postoperative infection. Obstet Gynecol 1979;53:395–398.

104. KHORRAN O, STERN JL. Bleomycin sclerotherapy of an intractable inguinal lymphocyst. Gynecol Oncol 1993;50:244–246.

105. GILLILAND JD, SPIES JB, BROWN SB, et al. Lymphoceles: percutaneous treatment with povidone-iodine sclerosis. Radiology 1989;171:227.

106. MATHES SJ, HURWITZ DJ. Repair of chronic radiation wounds of the pelvis. World J Surg 1986;10:269–280.

107. REID GC, DELANCEY JO, HOPKINS MP, et al. Urinary incontinence following radical vulvectomy. Obstet Gynecol 1990;75:852–858.

108. Ansink AC, vanTinteren M, Artsen EJ, et al. Outcome, complications and follow-up in surgically treated squamous cell carcinoma of the vulva 1956–1982. Eur J Obstet Gynecol Reprod Biol 1991;42:137.

109. Calame RJ. Pelvic relaxation as a complication of the radical vulvectomy. Obstet Gynecol 1980;55:716.

110. Luce EA. The irradiated wound. Surg Clin North Am 1984;64:821–829.

111. Robinson DW. Surgical problems in the excision and repair of radiated tissue. Plast Reconstr Surg 1975;55:41–49.

112. Cox JD, Byhardt RW, Wilson JF, et al. Complications of radiation therapy and factors in their prevention. World J Surg 1986;10:171–188.

113. Kinsella TJ, Bloomer WD. New therapeutic strategies in radiation therapy. JAMA 1981;245: 1669–1674.

114. Reinish JF, Pucket CL. Management of radiation wounds. Surg Clin North Am 1984;64:795–802.

115. Williams JA Jr, Clarke D, Dennis WA, et al. The treatment of pelvic soft tissue radiation necrosis with hyperbaric oxygen. Am J Obstet Gynecol 1992;167:412–416.

116. Roberts WS, Hoffman MS, LaPolla JP, et al. Management of radionecrosis of the vulva and distal vagina. Am J Obstet Gynecol 1991;164:1235–1238.

117. Arnold PG, Pairolero PC. Surgical management of the radiated chest wall. Plast Reconstr Surg 1986;77:605–612.

118. Lynch DJ, Whitte RR IV. Management of the chronic radiation wound. Surg Clin North Am 1982;64:795–802.

119. Rudolph R. Complications of surgery for radiotherapy skin damage. Plast Reconstr Surg 1982;70:179–183.

120. Futran ND, Trotti A, Gwede C. Pentoxifylline in the treatment of radiation-related soft tissue injury: preliminary observations. Laryngoscope 1997;107:391–395.

121. Dion MW, Hussey DH, Doornbos JF, et al. Preliminary results of a pilot study of pentoxifylline in the treatment of late radiation soft tissue necrosis. Int J Radiat Oncol Biol Phys 1990;19:401–407.

122. Mainous EG, Hart GB. Osteoradionecrosis of the mandible: treatment with hyperbaric oxygen. Arch Otolaryngol 1975;101:173–177.

123. Farmer JC, Shelton DL, Angelillo JD, et al. Treatment of radiation-induced tissue injury by hyperbaric oxygen. Ann Otol Rhinol Laryngol 1978;87:707–715.

124. Shupak A, Shoshani O, Goldenberg I, et al. Necrotizing fasciitis: an indication for hyperbaric oxygenation therapy? Surgery 1995;118:873–878.

125. Burke TW, Morris M, Levenback C, et al. Closure of complex vulvar defects using local rhomboid flaps. Obstet Gynecol 1994;84:1043–1047.

126. Barnhill DR, Hoskins WJ, Metz P. Use of the rhomboid flap after partial vulvectomy. Obstet Gynecol 1983;62:444–447.

127. Helm CW, Hatch KD, Partridge EE, et al. The rhomboid flap for repair of the perineal defect after radical vulvar surgery. Gynecol Oncol 1993;50:164–167.

128. McGregor IA, Jackson IT. The groin flap. Br J Plast Surg 1972;25:3–16.

129. Mayer AR, Rodriguez RL. Vulvar reconstruction using a pedicle flap based on the superficial external pudendal artery. Obstet Gynecol 1991;78:964–968.

130. Ponten B. The fasciocutaneous flap: its use in soft tissue defects of the lower leg. Br J Plast Surg 1981;34:215–220.

131. Brown RG, Jurkiewicz MJ. Reconstructive surgery in the cancer patient. Curr Probl Cancer 1977;2:3–73.

132. McCraw JB, Dibbell DG, Carraway JH. Clinical definition of independent myocutaneous vascular territories. Plast Reconstr Surg 1977;60:341–352.

133. Vasconez LO, McCraw JB, editors. Myocutaneous flaps. Clin Plast Surg 1980;7:1–134.

134. Mathes SJ, Nahai F. Clinical applications for muscle and myocutaneous flaps. St. Louis: CV Mosby Company; 1982.

135. Tobin GR, Day TG. Vaginal and pelvic reconstruction with distally based rectus abdominis myocutaneous flaps. Vaginal Pelvic Reconstr 1988;81:62–70.

136. TOBIN GR. Myocutaneous and muscle flap reconstruction of problem wounds. Surg Clin North Am 1984;64:667–681.

137. BALLON SC, DONALDSON RC, ROBERTS JA, et al. Reconstruction of the vulva using a myocutaneous graft. Gynecol Oncol 1979;7:123–127.

138. PURSELL SH, DAY TG, TOBIN GR. Distally based rectus abdominis flap for reconstruction in radical gynecologic procedures. Gynecol Oncol 1990;37:234–238.

139. DEHAAS WG, MILLER MJ, TEMPLE WJ, et al. Perianal wound closure with the rectus abdominis musculocutaneous flap after tumor ablation. Ann Surg Oncol 1995;2:400–406.

140. MCALLISTER E, WELLS K, CHAET M, et al. Perineal reconstruction after surgical extirpation of pelvic malignancies using the transpelvic transverse rectus abdominal myocutaneous flap. Ann Surg Oncol 1994;1:164–168.

141. BARE RL, ASSIMOS DG, MCCULLOUGH DL, et al. Inguinal lymphadenectomy and primary groin reconstruction using rectus abdominus muscle flaps in patients with penile cancer. Urology 1994;44:557–561.

142. DANIEL RK, TAYLOR GI. Distant transfer of an island flap by microvascular anastomoses: a clinical technique. Plast Reconstr Surg 1973;52:111–117.

143. BACKSTROM A, EDSMYR F, WICKLUND H. Radiotherapy of carcinoma of vulva. Acta Obstet Gynecol Scan 1972;51:109–115.

144. DALY JW, MILLION RR. Radical vulvectomy combined with elective node irradiation for TXN0 squamous carcinoma of the vulva. Cancer 1974;34:161–165.

145. FRANKENDAL B, LARSSON LG, WESTLING P. Carcinoma of the vulva. Acta Radio 1973;12:165–174.

146. PEREZ CA, GRISBY PW, GALAKATOS A, et al. Radiation therapy in management of carcinoma of the vulva with emphasis on conservation therapy. Cancer 1993;71:3707–3716.

147. BORONOW RC, HICKMAN BT, REAGAN MT, et al. Combined therapy as an alternative to exenteration for locally advanced vulvovaginal cancer. Am J Clin Oncol 1987;10:171–181.

148. TILMANS AS, SUTTON GP, LOOK KY, et al. Recurrent squamous carcinoma of the vulva. Am J Obstet Gynecol 1992;167:1383–1388.

149. PIURA B, MASOTINA A, MURDOCH J, et al. Recurrent squamous cell carcinoma of the vulva: a study of 73 cases. Gynecol Oncol 1993;48:189–195.

150. HOPKINS MP, REID GC, MORLEY GW. The surgical management of recurrent squamous cell carcinoma of the vulva. Obstet Gynecol 1990;75:1001–1005.

151. HUSSAIN M, AL-SARRAF M. Anal carcinomas: new combined modality treatment approaches. Oncology 1988;2:42.

152. KOH W-J, WALLACE HJ, GREER BE, et al. Combined radiotherapy and chemotherapy in the management of local-regionally advanced vulvar cancer. Int J Radiat Oncol Biol Phys 1993;26:809.

153. RUSSEL AH, MESIC JB, SCUDDER SA, et al. Synchronous radiation and cytotoxic chemotherapy for locally advanced or recurrent squamous cancer of the vulvar. Gynecol Oncol 1992;47:14–20.

154. THOMAS G, DEMBO A, DEPETRILLO A, et al. Concurrent radiation and chemotherapy in vulvar carcinoma. Gynecol Oncol 1989;34:263.

155. LEISEROWITZ GS, RUSSELL AH, KINNEY WK, et al. Prophylactic chemoradiation of inguinofemoral lymph nodes in patients with locally extensive vulvar cancer. Gynecol Oncol 1997;66:509–514.

Part Four

Complimentary Medicine/Supportive Care

Chapter 14

Perioperative Psychosocial Considerations

Judith McKay, PhD and Steven A. Vasilev, MD, MBA

INTRODUCTION

Traditionally, healing has been associated with bringing a patient back into a sense of wholeness. Hippocrates' concept of health centered on an innate harmony within the individual. Restoring the harmony of the individual parts was the goal of medicine. The World Health Organization defines health as a "state of complete mental and social well-being."[1]

Surgery involves the cutting away of some part of the patient and, while it may be an unwanted or diseased part, it often represents a loss that must be adapted to. In no other type of surgery do these losses have as great an impact on the psychological, functional, and social existence of the patient as in gynecologic surgery.

Added to the generic fear that all surgery patients face regarding the physical trauma, general anesthetic, and the worry of what will be discovered, the residual effects of gynecologic surgery have been found to have ramifications far beyond the physical significance and effect of the operation.[2] High proportions of patients receiving radical gynecologic surgery report depression and anxiety postoperatively,[3–5] temporary or permanent loss of sexual function,[6–9] problems with body image,[10] in addition to gender identity problems associated with reproductive/menopausal issues, lowered libido, and decreased sexual confidence.[10–13] However, radical pelvic surgery leads to better preservation of sexual function than radiation therapy.[14] In addition, not all studies report bleak outcomes. For example, long-term survivors of cervical cancer can and do achieve sexually fulfilling lives.[15] It is also important to note that these psychological effects are not related only to radical gynecologic surgery. A simple hysterectomy can require a huge emotional adjustment on the part of the patient with regard to her femininity, her body image, even perhaps causing her to question her purpose in life. It is absolutely crucial that the surgeon recognize

Gynecologic Oncology: Evidence-Based Perioperative and Supportive Care, Second Edition. Edited by Scott E. Lentz, Allison E. Axtell and Steven A. Vasilev.
© 2011 John Wiley & Sons, Inc. Published 2011 by John Wiley & Sons, Inc.

and administer to these other aspects of loss and healing that are concomitant to this type of surgery (**Level II-2**).

The good news is that although patients are usually hesitant to initiate conversations around these concerns, they readily respond to and are able to discuss their problems when they are brought up by their physician, nurse-practitioner, or other member of the health-care team.[16] The other hopeful aspect is that a trained sex-therapist is not necessary to implement very supportive and beneficial strategies for this group of patients.

St. Bartholomew's Hospital in London provides a senior nurse with basic counseling training on an outpatient basis to see patients at their first routine postoperative checkup to screen for depression, anxiety, and sexual concerns. With regard to sexual dysfunction, the responsibility lies both with the physician, to initiate discussion about the possibility of these concerns and to provide relevant information, and with the couple, to address and be willing to work together to achieve a maximally satisfying sexual interaction.[17]

As early as 1980, Derogatis noted that with the expanded awareness and experience of sexuality at all ages, patients will demand not only that their disease process be treated, but that "they will require and expect therapeutic interventions which will assist them in becoming psychosexually, as well as physically, rehabilitated."[18]

In designing the ideal treatment, therefore, the surgeon must be aware that "his object is not only to save life, but also to help make the life he saves worth living."[11] This is especially true when considering treatment options for patients with cervical cancer. Although curing the disease is the primary objective, the surgeon needs to be mindful of the effect of surgery on other organs. The vagina is not essential to life, but the mutilation, shortening, or complete occlusion of the vagina may have such significance to the patient as to compromise postsurgical emotional and psychosocial adjustment.[11] In any gynecologic surgery the surgeon needs to consider the broader impact of the treatment and what it will mean to the specific patient in question.

SEXUAL/EMOTIONAL PROBLEMS

Frequency of Sexual/Emotional Reactions

Cain[12] found that the diagnosis and treatment of cervical, endometrial, ovarian, vaginal, or vulvar cancer significantly affected the mood level of patients. He and his colleagues interviewed 60 women within a month of being diagnosed with carcinoma. As a group they reported significantly more depressed feelings than a large sample randomly selected from the community.

Since it was felt that psychosocial disabilities might correlate with the site, stage and grade of cancer, as well as treatment, data were grouped by these variables. Women with ovarian cancer, women receiving triple agent chemotherapy, and women with grade 3 tumors of the uterus and ovary approached the level of depression typically obtained by patients entering outpatient psychiatric clinics as measured by the Hamilton Depression Scale, the Hamilton Anxiety Scale, and the Psychosocial Adjustment to Illness Scale. The women with gynecological cancer and treatment scored significantly higher on these measures than a large sample of women from the community without cancer. Many of these impairments such as ability to work, to perform domestic chores, or to function sexually resulted not from physical limitations, but from the patients' psychosocial reaction to the cancer and its treatment.

Twenty-nine of the 60 women interviewed described a regular and satisfying sexual relationship before the diagnosis. After diagnosis, all 29 women ceased to have sexual intercourse. "Either they were told to abstain following surgery or they believed sexual intercourse would exacerbate vaginal bleeding or vaginal discharge."[12]

Abitol[19] and Jensen[20] suggest that sexual function is often not taken into consideration especially with older women, since it is usually assumed that "intercourse is an unsuitable indulgence for any woman of or beyond middle age."[21] However, many early studies[22–24] have observed that women between 60 and 93 are sexually active, and if they are not, it is most usually not due to lack of interest, but rather the absence of a partner or the partner's inability to have sex. Starr and Weiner[25] surveyed 800 subjects from 60 to 91 years (65% were women) and found that the majority remained sexually active. The older women in the study were interested in sex and wanted to feel and be perceived as sexual.

In comparing the posttreatment sexual functioning of 97 patients with invasive carcinoma of the cervix (stages I and II of the International Classification), Abitol[19] found that in 22 out of the 28 patients treated with radiotherapy there was significant disturbance of sexual function. Only 2 of the 32 surgical patients experienced sexual interference. Of the 15 patients treated with both surgery and radiotherapy, 5 mentioned problems with sexual function. Abitol concludes, "Whenever the five-year cure rate is similar with different modes of therapy and the possibility of complication is limited, preference should be given to radical surgery over radiotherapy."

Although Abitol's point, that sexual functioning is an important aspect when choosing treatment options, is well taken, it should be noted that in Abitol's study, treatment groups were unmatched in terms of cancer staging. Also, the low evidence (6%) of sexual dysfunction among surgical subjects is markedly lower than that found in uncomplicated hysterectomy studies, which is surprising since with the compounding factors of malignancy and the more extensive procedure of a Wertheim hysterectomy, one would predict greater sexual dysfunction in this group.[17]

Although in 90% of the patients in Abitol's study[19] there was some relationship between pelvic findings and sexual activity, this relationship was inverse in about 10%: three women claimed a normal sexual life with a practically obliterated vagina, and five women complained of marked difficulty in spite of a normal vagina. Twombly[26] points out that sexual function may depend primarily on the motivation of the patient to succeed as well as her conception of gratifying sexual activity.

In another study of 96 women (between 41 and 50 years of age) treated surgically for cervical cancer, 34% abstained completely from sexual activity because of "dyspareunia or psychic factors." This was at a 1- to 2-year follow-up.[27]

Weijmar Schultz[17] reviewed 44 posttreatment studies summarizing the posttreatment psychosocial functioning of gynecological cancer patients. In all of the studies in which the patient compared her preoperative and postoperative states retrospectively, sexual functioning was considered to have deteriorated after treatment.

In spite of major physical limitations and significant emotional strain, the patients attempted to maintain a sexual life.[27] Schultz discovered several prognostic variables with regard to postoperative sexual dysfunction: the magnitude of surgical intervention, the pretreatment libidinal level, age, presence of a stable relationship, and partnership-related factors such as availability, attitude, and health.

In Schultz's review it was found that with the cervical cancer patients there was a difference between treatment groups in the degree of posttreatment sexual disruption, with the major negative factor being inclusion of radiation therapy in the treatment. However, a recent pilot study by the same group showed objective evidence that sexual function can be preserved after radiation using vaginal plethysmography.[28]

After radical vulvectomy,[5, 13, 29, 30] as many as 50%–80% of the women in these studies had stopped all sexual activity. However, in a cohort of 10 women treated for vulvar cancer by radical vulvectomy, 8 of the 10 couples accomplished complete or partial sexual rehabilitation.[31] One of the women in this group became pregnant and had an uncomplicated vaginal delivery after the radical vulvectomy. It was felt that this high level of sexual rehabilitation was due to the fact that adequate information was offered to the patients and a safe venue for discussion was provided, although even these factors were not enough to guarantee a successful resumption of sexual activities with the entire group (**Level II-2; 1**).

Andersen[29] did a study in 1988 comparing 42 women treated for vulvar cancer (6 treated with laser or chemotherapy, 26 treated with wide local excision, 9 with total vulvectomy, and 1 with radical vulvectomy) and 42 healthy women. The treatment group did have disruption in the excitement and resolution phases of sexual function, but did not lose their desire for sexual activity. There was two to three times more sexual dysfunction in this group compared to the healthy group. Thirty percent of the treatment group was sexually inactive at follow-up ranging from 1 to 10 years after surgery. The severity of the surgical intervention correlated with the sexual outcome: the more extensive the treatment, the greater the disruption of the desire and resolution phases of the sexual response cycle.

In an interesting study of 308 women treated for breast cancer or genital cancer, Wenderlein found that patients with gynecological cancer have a 50% higher incidence of sexual problems and anxiety about sexual activity than do mastectomy patients.[32]

Feelings of guilt are common with cervical cancer patients as most have heard from the media that this is a viral sexually transmitted disease.[30, 33] Guilt can also be experienced when vulval irritation, vaginal discharge, and bleeding are exacerbated by sexual contact. This could obviously be easily mitigated to some extent by the simple provision of information and the open discussion of some of the very painful conclusions patients have adopted. Again, this discussion will have to be initiated by the physician or some member of the health-care team as the patient is usually too embarrassed to mention her concerns.[6, 34]

In a comparative study of 16 women treated for breast cancer (stage II, treated by surgery and chemotherapy), 16 women treated for gynecological cancer (treated by surgery or surgery and radiotherapy), and 16 healthy women, 82% of the gynecological cancer sample reported poorer body image in contrast to 31% of the breast cancer patients. Although frequency of sexual behavior and level of sexual arousal were lower for both patient groups compared to healthy outpatients, there were no differences on indicants of sexual desire or orgasm.[3]

In Great Britain 105 women were retrospectively questioned about their psychosexual functioning after treatment for cancer of the cervix and vulva by radical vulvectomy, Wertheim's hysterectomy, and pelvic exenteration.[6] Ninety percent of the women in relationships had been sexually active prior to surgery. Sixty-six percent of those sexually active women had sexual function problems more than 6 months after surgery and 15% never resumed intercourse (two women had colpectomies and were not included). Eighty-two percent of those aged less than 50 years who had radiotherapy suffered sexual dysfunction.

Lack of desire was the most prevalent problem. Fifty percent of the women felt that their sexual relationship had deteriorated, yet only 16% felt that their marriage had worsened. Forty-six percent felt moderately to severely distressed. The authors comment, "As well as organic causes there is a strong psychogenic element brought about by loss of fertility, disfigurement, depression and anxiety about one's desirability as a sexual partner."[6] Again, a stable relationship helped mitigate the severity of the problems, and young, single women were at highest risk.

Sewell,[33] using a semistructured interview and psychometric measures with 15 patients treated for vulvar cancer, found that sexual functioning and body image are significant problems postoperatively even though intercourse is possible. Women reported levels of sexual arousal in the eighth percentile and body image at the fourth percentile. Although they reported levels of sexual activity comparable to healthy women preoperatively, postoperatively their sexual activity was half that of the normative sample. This sample did, however, report higher frequency of sexual activity as compared to a sample of patients who had a pelvic exenteration.[13] The vulvectomy patients' psychological distress as measured by the Symptom Checklist[35] were 1–1.5 standard deviations above the mean expected for normal, healthy individuals. Scores on the Beck Depression Inventory[36] indicated mild to moderate levels of depression in these patients.

A survey questionnaire of 18 patients treated with wide local excision rather than vulvectomy for microinvasive disease was reported by DiSaia and colleagues.[37] All women maintained their sexual responsiveness, in contrast to two radical vulvectomy patients who reported loss of orgasmic ability and dyspareunia.

Lack of Postsurgical Education

As cited above, many patients experience a myriad of psychosocial problems after gynecologic surgery including sexual dysfunction, depression, anxiety, poor body image, and lack of confidence in their femininity. These factors have been shown to be significantly improved with education and open discussion (**Level I; 2 and Level III**). However, the paucity of information given to patients and the lack of any provision for discussion of sexual function and how it might be effected subsequent to surgical procedures is alarming.

Andersen[29] found that in a cohort of 42 women treated surgically for vulvar cancer, 60%–84% received no information regarding sexual outcome. Jenkins[10] interviewed 27 sexually active women following surgical and radiotherapy treatment for endometrial and cervical cancer who experienced significant negative changes on four indicators of sexual function: frequency of intercourse, orgasm, and feelings of desire and enjoyment. Fifty-nine percent of this group received no information at all about sexual or psychological sequelae to surgery. Eight-eight percent of these women wanted sexual discussion initiated by their physician or nurse.

When interviewing 50 patients treated for cervical cancer, Vincent[38] reported that 70% of the women had received no information on the sexual implications of their disease either before or after treatment. Fifty-six percent wanted more information on sexual functioning than they received, and 79% of them said they would not ask their physician about these concerns.

In another study by Krueger et al.,[39] almost half of the 108 patients wanted nurses to initiate discussion about the effect of hysterectomy on sexuality.

Many studies have reported that women are inadequately prepared for the sexual outcome of their treatment, and that they find it difficult or impossible to ask health-care workers about this aspect of treatment. Patients report that they feel they should be grateful just to be alive, and that they are being presumptuous to ask for more in terms of quality of life.

In addition, if a woman is uninformed about her body and does not have the appropriate vocabulary with which to describe her experience, she will be more reticent to discuss these matters. In the past, if a patient has not voiced concerns, health-care givers have assumed that there were none.[5,30] It is imperative that the physician and his staff understand the danger of this assumption.

Cultural factors can also have a significant impact on the patient's feelings that she is entitled to have pleasurable sex and that it is her responsibility and right to address the problem if she is not.

Corney et al.[6] found in their interview of 105 women treated for gynecological cancer that over a quarter of the patients felt they would have benefited from more information, and 50% felt that more information should have been given to their husbands. Corney notes, "Other difficulties such as loss of libido, anorgasmia and anxiety about one's sexual desirability are unlikely to be discussed spontaneously by the woman. Nevertheless, we were impressed that women will talk about very intimate aspects of sexuality if they feel that there is a willingness to discuss the subject." Women in this study were accepting of the necessity of making the adjustments necessary to adapt to disfigurement and sexual limitations (only five of the women reported postsurgically that they wished they had not had surgery), but they expressed a real need for, and lack of, adequate explanation and discussion of alternative means of sexual expression, if appropriate.

In a study of 27 women treated for endometrial and cervical cancer with surgery and radiation therapy, Jenkins[10] found that 95% had not received any information on sexual functioning in spite of the fact that as a group they showed significant decrease in the actual frequency of intercourse, orgasm, and in their feelings of desire and enjoyment subsequent to treatment. Seventy-six percent reported dyspareunia, 60% vaginal dryness, and 53% narrowed or shortened vagina. Eighty-eight percent of the sample indicated that they would have liked a health-care professional to initiate discussion regarding sexual functioning and the possible effects of surgery. Education about potential negative sexual outcomes after surgery may enhance satisfaction with hysterectomy, independent of whether negative sexual outcomes were experienced.[40]

Treatment

Capone[41] compared two groups of patients diagnosed with cancer of the genital organs. Both groups were interviewed using a semistructured interview followed by the administration of three psychometric measures assessing psychological distress, affective state, and self-concept.

Return to employment and frequency of intercourse were two additional behavioral measures. One group ($N = 56$) received counseling a minimum of four times during their hospital stay aimed at developing realistic expectations and adaptive behavioral coping techniques. Patients were given an arena and permission to express feelings of anger, concern, and fears related to treatment or death. They were given information regarding their disease and possible treatment sequelae. Self-esteem, femininity, and interpersonal relationships were also covered during the counseling sessions.

For sexually active patients, a sexual rehabilitation component was added. Discussions of sexuality and sexual concerns were initiated early and continued throughout treatment. Counseling dealt with sexual misconceptions and fears and methods of working with anxieties associated with resumption of sexual activity. For those women whose medical treatment precluded a return to prior sexual activities, options and alternatives were discussed and realistic expectations set.

A control group ($N = 41$) was interviewed and assessed using the same procedures as were used for the experimental group. Patients in the control group were not counseled.

It was found that the intervention had a significant effect in reducing sexual dysfunction and in enhancing the rate of return to pretreatment frequency of intercourse. Counseled patients who had been employed before treatment returned to work at a 2:1 ratio over the noncounseled group. There were no significant differences between the groups on the emotional measures. The subjects in the control group repeatedly emphasized the lack of opportunity for discussion of sexual adjustment, which replicates the findings of Sadoughi's group[42] that the sexual concerns of chronically ill patients are not addressed.

When looking at the need for more counseling, especially regarding sexual functioning, Corney[43] suggests that a senior nurse with basic counseling training be available for postoperative outpatient visits. In addition, it was advised that medical staff also be aware of this need and be able to focus and initiate discussion about sexual matters with the patients as well. Thus, offering emotional support might not mean additional staff, but instead a heightened awareness on the part of all staff members that these issues are of extreme importance to the patient even though she might not initiate discussion of them. It simply requires a broadening of focus to consider the patient's emotional needs as well as her physical status.

Lamont's group in the Department of Obstetrics and Gynecology at McMaster University[44] has established a team approach with exenterative surgery patients utilizing a surgical assessment, a psychosexual assessment, and ongoing education for the patient and her partner (if she has one). The team includes two oncologists, an anesthetist, an enterostomal therapist, and a psychosexual counselor. Prior to surgery, the surgeon discusses the acceptability of an ileo-conduit and/or colostomy. The loss of sexually responsive tissues is discussed and the patient is offered the option of the creation of a neovagina. Dempsey[4] reported that all but one of his patients refused constructive vaginal surgery on the grounds that sexual function without reproductive capacity does not justify additional surgery. Lamont, however, found that only one couple did not want a neovagina constructed at the time of surgery. The higher level of willingness of Lamont's patients to have constructive surgery may be due to the availability of extensive counseling, which emphasized the importance of and gave permission to the patient for an ongoing, healthy sex life postsurgically. Lamont did find that sexual functioning is not a priority at the time the decision is made for exenteration. However, 6–9 months after surgery, when the patient begins to accept that she will survive, she will then focus on rehabilitation of a wider range of functions in her life. The best opportunity for preserving coital functioning occurs at the time of the original surgery.[44] It is therefore imperative for the health-care team to predict these changes to allow the patient to make the most informed choice with regard to her surgical options.

In Lamont's model the surgeon assumes the responsibility for conveying the impact of the surgical procedures on the patient's life. The surgeon ascertains the effectiveness of the communication by getting feedback from the patient as to her understanding. If the patient agrees to surgery, a psychosexual assessment is done.

The psychosexual assessment is carried out again with both the patient and her partner present. It includes gathering information about the present sexual relationship and the patient's comfort with her sexuality. It is also an educational interchange. Information is given to the couple on the sexual rehabilitation of the exenterative patient in general. This establishes a relationship between the therapist and the couple and also sets the expectation that the patient will be sexually rehabilitated. The patient is also given the opportunity to discuss the surgery and recovery process with previous exenteration patients preoperatively.

This discussion is extremely helpful to the patient and the team in clarifying the importance of the patient's decision and in establishing realistic expectations concerning the recovery process. It also gives the message to the patient and her partner that the quality of her life, especially her sexual life, is important to the team and gives her permission and familiarity with discussing these often sensitive arenas of her functioning with various health-care givers.

The enterostomal therapist also meets the patient preoperatively to discuss the care and placement of the ostomy. Postoperative meetings in hospital are also available as is counseling on an outpatient basis. Postoperative counseling is provided, encouraging the patient to be active and involved in the specific strategies of her recovery process, including dilation of the neovagina and the need for sexual activity to hasten recovery.

Counseling afforded the patient to discuss any further problems relative to her surgery, ostomy care, or sexual rehabilitation. Visits vary from every 2–4 weeks in the first 6 months to every 3–6 months after that. If the patient and her partner are identifying problems, the surgeon and the sex therapist are available to supervise self-examination in the office with either the patient alone or with her partner if needed.

Although radical pelvic surgery means loss of sexually responsive tissue, women who lose their vagina and clitoris can often learn to have complete sexual response with stimulation of other erogenous areas, i.e., anus, urethra, ostomy of the ileoconduit or colostomy, or even stimulation of the scar tissue in the area of the vulva. With counseling, the patient can learn that there are a wide range of sexually stimulating behaviors that she and her partner need to explore in order to maintain satisfying sexual function. Lack of sexual response and happiness in the woman who has been presurgically well adjusted sexually may well have to do more with her feelings of being unattractive or the absence of information or support to deal with postoperative psychological reactions than actual physical limitations.[9]

The Lamont report involved a group of 12 patients, and because the number was so small, few conclusions could be drawn. In this group, three neovaginas were constructed from peritoneum, five from sigmoid colon, and two from ileum. One patient did not need a neovagina because half of her vagina was preserved at the time of surgery. Eight of the women in this study were judged to have good adjustment preoperatively, and of these, seven resumed sexual activity and enjoyed good postoperative adjustment. Six of the seven patients were orgasmic within 6 months of their surgery. One patient was too newly discharged to be able to make an adequate assessment of her sexual functioning. One patient's postoperative adjustment was limited because of her emphasis on coital interaction, little opportunity to communicate with her partner about other sexual behaviors, and difficulty in accepting the care of her neovagina. The other three were not sexually active preoperatively. Two of these three remained inactive, and one was not assessed prior to Lamont's report.[44] In another series of patients who underwent pelvic exenteration with myocutaneous flap vaginal reconstruction, five surviving patients were very satisfied with their sexual function and were sexually active at the time of their interview.[45]

Patients need to be encouraged to not only engage in continued coital activity, but as well to explore various aspects of foreplay (with an emphasis on "play") allowing the couple to develop a range of stimulating experiences that will promote the same feelings and responses they enjoyed prior to surgery. Lamont and his group feel that the most important factor in sexual rehabilitation is an educated partner who is accepting of the patient's surgery and who is willing to support her feelings of loss and who will reinforce her feelings of her own femininity and self-esteem. Too often, if there is any sexual assessment, counseling, or education, the partner is left out.

ISSUES OF DEATH AND DYING

Patient's Mortality

Often a physician is hesitant to bring up issues of mortality, fearing that the suggestion might frighten a patient or cause the patient to lose confidence in the surgeon or the proposed intervention. If there is the chance of cancer involvement or cancer is diagnosed preoperatively, the patient's fears may realistically be heightened. Interestingly, in the 1950s patients were usually not told of their diagnosis of cancer, which put the surgeon in a difficult position when obtaining the informed consent for surgery. The diagnosis was kept from the patient as it was deemed too painful for the patient to handle.[47]

Since then, psychological responses of patients to life-threatening diagnoses and procedures have been examined more closely. Strain and Grossman[48] identified concerns of patients preoperatively as occurring within the broad categories of fears around turning one's life over to strangers, separation from the familiar environment of home and family, loss of control or death under anesthesia, being partially awake during surgery, and damage to body parts. In addition to these specific fears, a patient may have more generalized reactions of feeling hopeless, helpless, and angry.

More extreme emotional reactions are exhibited with patients who have a history of anxiety, a high need for control, or specific negative associations around surgery. The relationship established with the surgeon preoperatively in laying the foundation for the patient to expect direct, understandable information on her condition and the sense that her emotional reactions and concerns are important is crucial. Dr. S. J. Stehlin notes, "If the doctor–patient relationship is one in which each feels free to communicate with the other, . . . once the essentials of truth are explained in the proper manner, the way becomes clear for the next phase . . . hope. A patient can tolerate knowing he is incurable; he cannot tolerate hopelessness"[49] (**Level III**).

Discussing candidly with a patient that there is always a possibility of death or complications that would render her incompetent to make decisions for herself at some later date allows the patient to establish what her choices are from a position of power. It is important to discuss the advantages of the patient's recording her wishes in writing via Advance Directives, a Durable Power of Attorney and the provisions of a Will, when she is healthy and competent, as opposed to having her family or hospital administration guess at what she would want in a time of crisis.

If dealt with compassionately and gently, this can be an empowering process for the patient at a time when she may feel that most of the control in her life is being eroded away. It can also be an important precedent for establishing trust between patient and surgeon by way of direct, honest communication while discussing matters of the greatest import. The patient learns through this interaction that her wishes are being asked for and listened to.[49]

The preoperative consultation visit with the surgeon is the appropriate venue to assess the patient's emotional stability, her concerns, and to establish what the patient's wishes are in case of complications. As a part of securing the informed consent, it is important for the surgeon to explain clearly, and in layman's terms, all aspects of the proposed treatment and to allow the patient adequate time for questions and the expression of her fears about death and doubts and concerns about treatment. If the surgeon feels that the patient is significantly apprehensive or unable to face or discuss her mortality or the possibility of complications, a referral to a social worker or psychologist may be appropriate to provide support and increase the patient's feelings of safety. Personal confrontation of one's mortality is never easy, but the earlier and the more fully these issues are discussed, the easier the entire process will be for the surgeon, the patient, and her family.

In instances when the patient has not had a chance to complete Advance Directives, or "Do Not Resuscitate" (DNR) orders, and family members are left to make decisions about treatment without the guidance of having written instructions on the patient's wishes, many states have adopted Health Care Surrogate Acts which delineate, in a specified order, those individuals who may make decisions on behalf of a patient. In the states without such statutes, frequently a member of the family or a close friend may serve as a surrogate decision maker. Obviously, the patient's current condition and the expected outcome of resuscitation will be the primary variables to consider in making DNR decisions. However, when recovery is doubtful, it should be the responsibility of the attending physician to convey that information and to guide the patient's surrogate in attempting to ensure that the course of treatment is consistent with the known views of the patient, as reflected in oral statements, lifestyle commitments, and values. If the family member or friend is having difficulty with the decision, a referral to either a psychologist or social worker may be indicated to allow the surrogate decision maker to come to as clear a choice as possible with a minimum amount of guilt. Ferreting out the probable choices of the patient, were she competent, may take more time than the surgeon has available, but a timely referral can honor the needs of the family member in making these potentially guilt-producing decisions.

When in the course of surgery physical evidence of advanced disease and poor prognosis is discovered, the earlier foundation of honest communication about issues of death and dying will be of utmost benefit. In this case the postoperative period not only involves recovery from the procedures but also confrontation with and adaptation to loss and possible death.

This process resembles anticipatory grieving and often involves the five stages of grief identified in the 1960s by Elizabeth Kubler-Ross of denial, anger, bargaining, depression, and acceptance.[50] Sometimes suicidal thinking will emerge in the patient's attempt to take control of a process she may believe is hopeless.

In order to interact honestly and humanely, it is important for the physician to examine his or her own attitudes toward death. Implicit throughout the medical student's training is the theme that "every death corresponds to a failure, either of the individual physician or, more commonly, of medicine as a whole."[51]

In a pilot study, Feifel[52] found that compared to a control group of patients and other nonprofessionals, physicians thought less about death, but were more afraid of death. Seeing death as the "enemy," which would be natural in this philosophical formulation, will jeopardize the surgeon's ability to discuss in an empathic, supportive way the possibility of a patient's death. It is imperative, therefore, for each physician to examine his or her own relationship and feelings about death so as to better model an acceptance of death as an integral part of life as opposed to seeing death as a failure or an indignity that can be avoided if one is an "exceptional patient."

Fetal Death

Sometimes in the process of gynecologic treatment elective fetal termination will be required. Death of a child is one of the greatest human tragedies. Often physicians do not regard the interruption of fetal development as a significant loss compared to the death of an infant or child. Mothers are often plagued with guilt and suffer as much, if not more, adjustment to the loss of a fetus if that loss is a result of her own health requirements. Usually only the physician can provide the kind of information necessary to allay her guilt.[53]

In a retrospective study of 26 families who had experienced perinatal death (7 stillborn infants: >20 weeks gestation and 19 live-born infants, none of whom went home from the hospital), Rowe[54] found that only seven of the mothers interviewed were satisfied with the information they had received from their physician. Six mothers had a prolonged grief reaction of 12–20 months. There was a direct correlation between the degree of dissatisfaction and the mother's lack of understanding and/or her morbid grief response. A mother's level of dissatisfaction was not significantly related to her age, her economic class or marital status, the duration of survival of the infant, the cause of death, or the presence of a healthy child in the family. Mothers were more likely to feel dissatisfied if they had received no follow-up contact by a physician, either in person or by phone.

Rowe suggests it is not enough for a physician to simply inform the parents of the death of their child, whether a fetus or live-born. The physician has the "equal responsibility to present the information in a meaningful and empathetic context, in a personal interview if at all possible."[54] Rowe also recommends having a social worker assume responsibility for maintaining continuing communication with a family after they have had a perinatal loss.

Cullberg[55] found that one third of mothers experiencing a perinatal death suffer a morbid grief reaction. In his survey, 19 out of 56 mothers who were studied 1–2 years after the deaths of their neonates had developed severe psychiatric disorders. The period of mental symptomatology was longer in those women whose feelings of grief were initially suppressed or denied. Koop[56] has suggested some guidelines (see Table 14.1) for the physician when discussing with parents the loss of a fetus or infant. When parents were asked what their most desperate need was after a miscarriage, stillbirth, or death of a neonate, the most common response was the need to talk about it.[53] At the same time, grieving parents perceive many behaviors to be thoughtless or insensitive. Physicians and nurses may benefit from increased training in bereavement support.[57]

In our culture, death is not talked about. Giles[58] observed that physicians dealt with perinatal death by treating the mother's physical symptoms and prescribing sedatives liberally. They avoided, in about half of the cases, discussing the baby's

Table 14.1   Optimum Communication of Miscarriage, Stillbirth, or Death of Neonate

- The news should be given to both parents and they should be the first to know.
- The information should be conveyed in a private place where the parents will feel comfortable expressing any emotions they feel.
- The news should be factual, understandable, and delivered by the surgeon directly.
- Clichés of avoidance and denial such as "Forget about this" or "You can always have another child" are to be avoided.

Adapted from Reference 56.

death. When grieving parents feel they cannot share their feelings with friends and family, the physician may be the one avenue for the expression of their grief. Therapeutic listening, giving the patient permission to express her feelings, and providing ongoing resources for support are an important part of the physician's role as counselor/consoler. Giving the patient permission to seek grief counseling through individual or group work may be appropriate. There are many bereavement groups available, some of which have been formed for the specific purpose of dealing with infant death. Providing the patient with a referral to a social worker or psychologist who can help the patient find a support group during this difficult adjustment period is often beneficial.

Herzog[59] has suggested that there are three stages of grief work (see Table 14.2). Although the surgeon's role cannot obviously encompass all of these stages, the initial interaction and support that are conveyed by the physician may permit the patient and her family to express their grieving in healthy ways and seek additional avenues of expression as needed for completing the grieving process.

PSYCHOLOGICAL COMPLICATIONS IN INTENSIVE CARE UNIT

Postoperative stress in the intensive care unit (ICU) can have a significant impact on the mental and emotional status of the gynecologic surgery patient, which in turn can affect her physical state. In fact, Hackett[60] mentions that psychological reactions to surgery postoperatively "frequently trouble the surgeon, harass the nursing staff, impede the course of recovery, and may be fully as dangerous as the infections or embolic complications of surgery." The source of these complications can be classified as extrinsic or intrinsic.

Table 14.2   Three Stages of Grief Work

Resuscitation	Working through the initial shock during the first 24 hours
Rehabilitation	Consultation and discussion with family members for the first 6 months
Renewal	Healthy tapering of the mourning process from 6 months on

Adapted from Reference 59.

Extrinsic Factors

Extrinsic factors have to do with the environment, the external milieu in which the surgical patient finds herself. The ICU may evoke fear and anxiety in the patient if the technology and equipment are perceived as intimidating or even harmful and overtax the already diminished resources of the patient. Extensive intravenous lines, arterial lines, monitoring wires, oxygen masks, and ventilator assistance equipment can create a feeling in the patient of being "tied down" or "trapped" and can increase feelings of helplessness.[61] Fully half of all ICU patients recall significant discomfort.[62]

Twenty-four-hour management plans, employment of multiple invasive procedures, the use of omnipresent monitors, chronic high noise level, lack of privacy, continual activity, and light combine to create the paradoxical combination of sensory monotony and sensory overload, as well as sleep deprivation, in the patient. The combination of these myriad stressors on the critically ill patient can contribute to the development of postoperative depression, anxiety, or delirium which is sometimes referred to as "ICU delirium," "ICU syndrome," or "ICU psychosis."[63]

Intrinsic Factors

Factors intrinsic to the patient which increase the likelihood of psychological complications postsurgically are those which inhibit the patient's ability to adapt to stress.

Increased age correlates with higher risk. Patients over 50 years of age have a higher probability of developing delirium postoperatively.[64] Senile patients may show a deterioration of postoperative psychological functioning without a lucid interval.[65]

Prior psychiatric history is also associated with higher probabilities of psychological complications. Patients with depression, psychosomatic disease, sleep disturbance, anxiety disorder, phobias, or panic attacks have more limited resources to deal with the many stressors associated with gynecologic surgery and the subsequent physical, emotional, and sexual adaptations required.

Many of the drugs used after surgery may be potentiating factors for the development of depression, anxiety, delirium, or psychosis in a predisposed patient. Anticholinergic drugs, antitussives, tricyclic antidepressants, antihistamines, and anti-Parkinson agents are capable of promoting major psychological disturbance.[66]

Patients who have been addicted to drugs or alcohol or who have had cerebral damage, previous episodes of delirium or chronic cardiovascular, metabolic, respiratory, or renal illness are at higher risk for developing delirium. Metabolic and hemodynamic instabilities as a result of gastrointestinal hemorrhage, anoxia, liver failure, septic shock, respiratory failure, myocardial infarction, severe burns, drug overdoses, acid–base imbalances, electrolyte imbalances, infections, and pulmonary embolus have been correlated with instances of delirium. Sex does not appear to be a predisposing factor in the development of ICU delirium; the incidence is similar among men and women.[67]

It is thus important for the physician to assess all of the predisposing factors that might be contributing to the patient's psychological imbalance, including

Table 14.3   Psychological Risk Factors in ICU

Extrinsic

- Extensive and invasive equipment
- Noise pollution
- Lack of privacy
- Continual activity
- Anonymity
- Twenty-four hour lighting
- Sleep deprivation

Intrinsic

- Increased age
- Depression
- Anxiety—panic attacks
- Prior patterns of sleep disturbance
- Significant psychopathology
- Phobias
- Multiple psychotropic drugs
- Addictive patterns—drugs/alcohol

environmental, pharmacological, and medically related factors, as well as inherent psychological variabilities and coping abilities, before designing a treatment plan (see Table 14.3) (**Levels II-3, III**).

Delirium

The reversible, confusional state known as "ICU psychosis" or "ICU syndrome" is characterized by disorientation with regard to time, place, and person, difficulty in logical thinking, anxiety, apathy, sleep disturbance, incoherence, fear, excitement, illusions, hallucinations, and delusions. In more extreme cases, agitation, paranoia, and belligerence may cause the patient to be at risk to herself or others. Delirium differs from psychosis in that there is no consistent structure to the ideas as is found in psychotic states and there is no steady regressiveness. Instead, there is a fluctuation of consciousness with some intervals of lucidity.

Timely psychopharmacological intervention may be of great benefit. However, the differential diagnosis is very extensive. Thus, the specific etiology must be identified prior to administering such agents. It is beyond the intent of this chapter to specifically address drugs and dosages in detail. An aging but excellent review of assessment and management is provided in a *Society of Critical Care Medicine New Horizons* monograph.[65] A more recent review includes newer available options.[68]

Postoperative delirium usually manifests as early as the second or third postoperative day and generally resolves within 48 hours after discharge from the unit.[63,69] A lucid period of 2–3 days usually precedes the onset. The incidence in conscious patients admitted to critical care settings is estimated by Belitz[70] at 12.5%–38%. However, in a random sampling of 200 general surgical patients, Titchener[71] found that delirium was found in 78% of the patients. A more recent review of the literature suggests that risk factors for the development of intensive care delirium are understudied and underreported in the literature.[72]

It has also been noted that some procedures "characteristically eventuate an affectual disturbance; hysterectomy particularly is indicted."[73] Thus, because of the very emotionally laden nature of gynecologic surgery, one might predict a higher incidence of delirium postoperatively.

Treatment and Prevention of ICU Delirium

Preoperative assessment of a patient's predisposition to develop delirium can be ascertained by the physician or nurse. If any of the predisposing, psychological, or behavioral issues are evident, extra effort can be made to reassure and educate the patient as to the feelings and impaired perception that might develop and to emphasize the importance for the patient to inform nursing staff if she notices any of the associated experiences.

Early intervention (either pharmacological or behavioral) has been shown to be effective and can obviate the development of more extreme symptoms.[65,74] If drug use is an issue preoperatively, detoxification may have to be completed before surgery can be undertaken.[67]

Personalizing nursing care has been found to greatly reduce the risk of the development of delirium. Arranging for continuity of care so that some type of rapport can be established between the patient and her nursing staff is crucial to reassure the patient. Depersonalization is often cited as a contributor to the development of delirium. "The more technological the environment—and the more technological the intervention—the greater is the need for human contact, for human responses to fundamentally human needs."[75] The use of names to continually reorient the patient as to who they are and who is taking care of them can be a simple reassurance available to the nursing staff. Giving permission to the family to touch their loved one and making the patient more accessible to gentle contact are often necessary in the intimidating environment of the ICU. Numerous researchers have cited the benefit of personal interactions between the patient and health-care workers in helping to prevent delirium.[67,73,76]

Parker[63] found that patients experiencing delirium who were moved to a side room or transferred to a general medical floor and were allowed to interact with family members for extended periods of time did better than those who were simply treated with pharmacological sedation and soft cloth restraints.

Delirium is twice as frequent in windowless ICUs.[77,78] If possible, natural lighting should be relied upon as much as possible. Continuous lighting disturbs the structure by which the patient organizes the passage of time, inhibits the natural sleep cycle, and contributes to a sense of monotony which can be extremely disorienting. Large calendars and clocks with digital read-outs in clear view will help the patient orient herself in time.[65]

It has been pointed out that if health-care workers react to the patient's delirium with calm acceptance promoted by discussion of the factors contributing to the delirium, the use of restraints can usually be avoided. Often the use of restraints compounds the patient's feelings of depersonalization and helplessness, thus exacerbating the symptoms.

Phenothiazines are an effective remedy for postoperative delirium.[79,80] Hale suggests low dosages of perphenazine and haloperidol.[81] These medications lessen agitation, induce sleep, and help in managing the more belligerent patients. Minor tranquilizers such as the benzodiazapenes are only found to be transiently effective, and often require dosages that cause sedation.

Anxiety

Heightened vigilance, insomnia, agitation, and tremulousness are frequently manifested symptoms of anxiety. Hackett[82] feels that anxiety is consistently underdiagnosed in the ICU. He attributes this to the hesitancy on the part of the patient to report feelings of anxiety because of associations with being "weak," especially in lower socioeconomic groups. Another factor in undermedicating anxiety is the failure of the physician to observe anxiety in patients who are reluctant to reveal it. The doctor usually relies on the patient's complaints of anxiety, objective and obvious signs of anxiety such as sweating or agitation, or the report of a nurse or family member.

Data suggest[83] that it is most unusual to have an ICU patient complain of anxiety or request additional sedation. Many physicians hesitate to ascertain the level of their patient's anxiety by direct questioning, as the questioning might be felt to be suggestive that the physician feels the patient should be frightened or anxious. This being the case, Hackett suggests that it is safest to assume that *all* patients are anxious to some degree, and treat them accordingly.

Treatment and Prevention of Anxiety

If there are any opportunities to increase the patient's sense of personal control, Easton[67] suggests that this eases the patient's feelings of being immersed in a situation which is dangerous, depersonalized, and unpredictable. Simple choices, such as the scheduling of a shower or the time of day they engage in physical therapy, can be surprisingly empowering to a patient.

Hale[81] found that therapy involving a discussion of the frightening aspects of the patient's treatment and concerns about the future can also serve to enhance the patient's flagging ability to cope and to ease anxiety. Reassuring a patient that anxiety, and sometimes delusional thinking, is a transient occurrence suffered by many patients postoperatively can allay fears that the patient might jump to regarding the loss of their sanity or the permanent impairment of memory or cognition.

The training of patients in meditation or self-hypnosis was found to reduce intraoperative and postoperative anxiety in ambulatory surgery patients.[84] When patients were trained using progressive relaxation techniques, length of stay was reduced and fewer analgesics were utilized by abdominal surgery patients.[85]

Consultations involving the judicious use of major tranquilizers and psychotherapy can also alleviate the patient's symptoms. Early referral for psychological or psychiatric intervention is recommended.

Depression

Depression, characterized by marked withdrawal, insomnia, lassitude, a sense of hopelessness, and sometimes suicidal ideation, can also surface as a reaction to the stresses of surgery. Depression subsequent to surgery for a benign condition with no complications usually diminishes by the third postoperative day.[86] The magnitude of the depressive reaction is often correlated with the significance of the disease process uncovered during surgery, and also the amount of postoperative pain experienced by the patient.[87]

The prospects of a lengthy, debilitating illness can often prompt a patient to worry about being a "burden" on the family and promote a sense of hopelessness in the patient.[88] Suicidal ideation is common with this type of reaction when the patient is feeling that there is no point in continuing, or that a painful death is all that they have to look forward to. Again, early detection of these feelings is crucial in order to more adequately provide treatment.

Treatment of Postsurgical Depression

Often, supportive therapy, encouraging the patient to focus on the joyful aspects of her life that she has to be grateful for in spite of her losses, can be sufficient to allow her to rally her usual ego defenses and cope with the situation at hand. A therapeutic consultation in which a patient is given permission to cry and openly express her despair can be extremely beneficial. Normalizing her reactions and giving her a safe, neutral venue to express her feelings of fear and concerns for the future can allow the patient a cathartic experience as well as give the health-care giver valuable information as to the level of her depression.

It is sometimes necessary to provide ongoing psychological support for a patient after she is discharged if her depressive symptoms continue until the time of discharge. Families need help in planning care at home, especially if the patient is expressing suicidal thoughts or a sense of despair and hopelessness.

In addition to supportive therapeutic interventions in hospital, the use of antidepressants is often very helpful. If a patient has a preoperative history of taking an antidepressant, some psychiatrists and anesthesiologists suggest the conservative approach of suspending the use of all psychotropic drugs 2 weeks before surgery.[89]

Jacobsen and Holland[90] suggest, instead of utilizing such a general approach, that the anesthesiologist and the psychiatrist confer prior to surgery to generate a plan based on the particular patient's needs and the drug involved.

The earlier the psychopharmaceutical or therapeutic intervention is initiated, the more effective is its impact. In two meta-analyses[91,92] of psychological interventions facilitating adjustment to surgical procedures, the authors concluded that brief psychological interventions were superior to standard hospital care in reducing postoperative pain and in increasing satisfaction with care and psychological well-being. Patients who received psychological preparation were discharged an average of 2 days sooner than patients who received standard care. The surgeon should continuously be mindful of the emotional well-being of the patient in order to make the appropriate referrals in a timely fashion and, if possible, provide psychological preparation for the stressful event preoperatively to avoid more significant emotional reactions including depression.

SUMMARY

In summary, it is apparent that many women who have been treated with a wide range of gynecologic surgeries suffer sexual dysfunction, lowered libido, depression, anxiety, disruption in work activity, lowered self-esteem, poor body image, loss of femininity, and insecurity about sexual desirability.[6] In spite of the suffering, few women are willing to initiate discussion over these concerns especially if they are sexual concerns. In addition, although their partners are also troubled by the problems of sexual dysfunction, and many feel anxious or selfish about reengaging in sexual activity and worry that they will be unable to answer the patient's changed sexual needs postsurgery, even less attention is directed to educating the patient's partner.

While many of the aspects of sexual dysfunction, negative mood, and lack of confidence are directly correlated with amount of physical disfigurement and loss of physical function, there are many studies that show that this is not a direct correlation. Some studies quoted in this chapter show that even with complete pelvic exenteration, patients report being satisfied with the level of physical intimacy enjoyed postsurgery (**Levels II-3, III**).

While the lack of attention to these psychological factors is alarming, it is encouraging to note that simple counseling programs, the provision of adequate information, and a venue for discussion of sexual and psychological issues can greatly improve the patient's experience. As Jenkins[10] points out, "Data indicate that counselling and information should be part of the natural preparation for treatment.... A patient cannot be expected to initiate a discussion she does not know is needed." Therefore, all patients, irrespective of age or relationship status, should be provided with information regarding anatomical and hormonal changes postsurgery, and how these changes will effect emotions and sexual functioning. This information should be delivered to the patient and her partner, if she has one, before surgery. As problems develop postsurgically, staff should be available on an individual basis to counsel the

Table 14.4 Counseling for Gynecologic Surgery Patients

Goals

- To initiate discussion, predict possible treatment sequelae and provide support, information, and normalization of the myriad physical and emotional changes concomitant to gynecologic surgery. When patients are forewarned that they may have feelings of depression and loss, they feel more in control.
- To inform patient that her psychosocial functioning is an important aspect of healing.

Intervention
Immediate

1. Evaluation
   - Assess degree of psychological distress
   - Ascertain prior psychiatric history
2. Provide appropriate consultations
   - Psychology—Train in coping techniques for anxiety, provide supportive therapy for depression, grief work
   - Psychiatry—Psychotropic medications for significant anxiety, depression
   - Nursing staff—Discuss in detail predicted body and hormonal changes and adjustments required
   - Enterostomal therapist—Discuss care and placement of ostomy
   - Sex therapy consultation—Discuss in detail with patient and her partner about effects of surgery on sex life

One-month postsurgery

- Sexual counseling with patient and partner
- Supportive follow-up regarding emotional reactions of patient

Six-month postsurgery

- Ascertain overall psychosocial adjustment to surgery
- Provide consults as necessary

---

patient and give specific therapeutic recommendations. (See Table 14.4 for suggested elements and timing of psychosocial counseling for gynecologic surgery patients.)

Establishing, from the first preoperative visit, a pattern of direct and honest communication regarding the patient's mortality and the specific steps she needs to take to ensure that her wishes will be met no matter what the complications provides a foundation of trust and a sense of caring which will go a long way to softening the experience of surgery and the possible psychological sequelae.

It is important for physicians to examine their own comfort levels when discussing issues of death and complications as well as sexual and emotional issues with their patients. If this is difficult (and this may have more to do with time management than comfort level), it is imperative that resources be made available to the patient on a routine basis to explore these issues. The patient's partner should be involved in at least one of these sessions. Printed information, videotapes, and blocks of time specifically allotted to psychosocial counseling relative to surgical sequelae will allow the patient to see that her emotional, sexual, and social functioning is important to the health-care team.

Effective physicians will be aware that a successful surgical procedure depends on more than the skillful manipulation of body parts. A surgeon may be a brilliant technician, but a great physician needs to address the broader spectrum of healing. Recognizing the patient in her wholeness will allow the physician to administer to all of a patient's needs.

REFERENCES

1. World Health Organization. WHO Chron 1943;1:29.
2. CLARK J. Psychosocial responses of the patient. In: GROENWALD S, FROGGE MH, GOODMAN M, editors. Cancer Nursing Principles and Practice. 3rd ed. Boston: Jones & Bartlett; 1993.
3. ANDERSEN BL, JOCHIMSEN PR. Sexual functioning among breast cancer, gynecologic cancer and healthy women. J Consult Clin Psychol 1985;53:25–32.
4. DEMPSEY GM, BUCHSBAUM HJ, MORRISON J. Psychosocial adjustment to pelvic exenteration. Gynecol Oncol 1975;3:325–334.
5. MOTH I, ANDREASSON B, JENSEN SB, et al. Sexual function and somatopsychic reactions after vulvectomy. Dan Med Bull 1983;30:27–30.
6. CORNEY RH, CROWTHER ME, EVERETT H, et al. Psychosexual dysfunction in women with gynecological cancer following radical pelvic surgery. Br J Obstet Gynaecol 1993;100:73–78.
7. ANDERSEN BL, ANDERSON B, DEPROSSE C. Controlled prospective longitudinal study of women with cancer: II. Psychological outcomes. J Consult Clin Psychol 1989;57:692–697.
8. WEIJMAR SCHULTZ WCM, VAN DE WIEL HBM, BOUMA J, et al. Psychosexual functioning after the treatment of cancer of the vulva: a longitudinal study. Cancer 1990;66:402–407.
9. VAN DE WEIL HBM, WEIJMAR SCHULTZ WCM, HALLENSLEBEN A, et al. Sexual functioning of women treated for cancer of the vulva. Sex Marital Ther 1990;5; 73–82.
10. JENKINS B. Patient's reported sexual changes after treatment for gynecological cancer. Oncol Nurs Forum 1988;15:349–354.
11. VASICKA A, POPOVICH NR, BRAUSCH CC. Obstet Gynecol 1958;11:403.
12. CAIN EN, KOHORN EI, QUINLAN DM, et al. Psychosocial reactions to the diagnosis of gynecologic cancer. Obstet Gynaecol 1983;62:635–641.
13. ANDERSEN BL, HACKER NF. Psychosexual adjustment after vulvar surgery. Obstet Gynaecol 1983;62:462–475.
14. FRUMOVITZ M, SUNN CC, SCHOVER LR, et al. Quality of life and sexual functioning in cervical cancer survivors. J Clin Oncol 2005;23(30):7428–7436.
15. GREENWALD HP, MCCORKLE R. Sexuality and sexual function in long-term survivors of cervical cancer. J Womens Health (Larchmt) 2008;17(6):955–963.
16. WILSON-BARNETT J. Providing relevant information for patients and families. In: CORNEY R, editor. Developing Communication and Counselling Skills in Medicine. London: Routledge; 1991.
17. WEIJMAR SCHULTZ WCM, BRANSFIELD DD, VAN DE WIEL HBM, et al. Sexual outcome following female genital cancer treatment: a critical review of methods of investigation and results. Sex Marital Ther 1992;7:29–64.
18. DEROGATIS LR. Breast and gynecologic cancers: their unique impact on body image and sexual identity in women. In: VAETH JM, editor. Frontiers of Radiation Therapy and Oncology. Vol. 14. Basel:S. Karger; 1980. p 1–11.
19. ABITOL MM, DAVENPORT JH. Sexual dysfunction after therapy for cervical carcinoma. Am J Obstet Gynecol 1974;119:181–189.

20. Jensen PT, Groenvold M, Klee MC, et al. Early stage cervical carcinoma, radical hysterectomy and sexual function. A longitudinal study. Cancer 2004;100(1):97–106.
21. Masters WH, Johnson VE. Human Sexual Response. Boston:Little, Brown and Company; 1966.
22. Kinsey AC, Pomeroy WB, Martin CE, et al. Sexual Behavior in the Human Female. Philadelphia, PA:W.B. Saunders Company; 1953.
23. Pfeiffer E, Verwoerdt A, Wang HS. Arch Gen Psychiatry 1968;19:753.
24. Newman G, Nichols CR. JAMA 1960;173:33.
25. Starr BD, Weiner MB. The Starr–Weiner Report on Sex and Sexuality in the Mature Years. New York:McGraw-Hill; 1981.
26. Twombly GH. J Sex Res 1968;4:275.
27. Kos L.(1978) As reported in Weijmar Schultz WCM, Bransfield DD, Van de Wiel HBM, Bouma J. Sexual outcome following female genital cancer treatment: a critical review of methods of investigation and results. Sex Marital Ther 1992;7:29–64.
28. Pras E, Wouda J, Willemse PH, et al. Pilot study of vaginal plethysmography in women treated with radiotherapy for gynecological cancer. Gynecol Oncol 2003;91(3):540–546.
29. Andersen BL, Turnquist D, Lapolla J, et al. Sexual functioning after treatment of in situ vulvar cancer, preliminary report. Obstet Gynaecol 1988;71:15–19.
30. Stellman RE, Goodwin JM, Robinson J, et al. Psychological effects of vulvectomy. Psychosomatics 1984;25:779–783.
31. Weijmar Schultz WCM, Wifma K, Vande Wiel HBM, et al. Sexual rehabilitation of radical vulvectomy patients, a pilot study. J Psychosom Obstet Gynaecol 1986;5:119–126.
32. Wenderlein JM.(1979) As reported in Weijmar Schultz WCM, Bransfield DD, Van de Wiel HBM, Bouma J. Sexual outcome following female genital cancer treatment: a critical review of methods of investigation and results. Sex Marital Ther 1992;7:29–64.
33. Sewell HH, Edwards DW. Pelvic genital cancer: body image and sexuality. Front Radiat Ther Oncol 1980;14:35–41.
34. Sanders S, Pedro LW, Bantum EO, et al. Couples surviving prostate cancer: long-term intimacy needs and concerns following treatment. Clin J Oncol Nurs 2006;10(4):503–508.
35. Derogatis LR. The SCL-90R Administration, Scoring and Procedures Manual—II. Maryland:Clinical Psychometric Research, 1983.
36. Beck AT, Ward CH, Mendelson M, et al. An inventory for measuring depression. Arch Gen Psychiatry 1961;4:561–571.
37. DiSaia PJ, Creasman WT, Rich WM. An alternate approach to early cancer of the vulva. Am J Obstet Gynecol 1979;133: 825.
38. Vincent CE, Vincent B, Greiss FC, et al. Some marital-sexual concomitants of carcinoma of the cervix. South Med J 1975;68:552–558.
39. Krueger JC, Hassell J, Goggins DB. Relationship between nurse counselling and sexual adjustment after hysterectomy. Nurs Res 1979;28(3):145–150.
40. Bradford A, Meston C. Sexual outcomes and satisfaction with hysterectomy: influence of patient education. J Sex Med 2007;4(1):106–114.
41. Capone MA, Good RW, Westie KS, et al. Psychosocial rehabilitation of gynecologic oncology patients. Arch Phys Med Rehabil 1980;61:128–132.
42. Sadoughi W, Leshner M, Fine HL. Sexual adjustment in chronically ill and physically disabled population. Arch Phys Med Rehabil 1971;52:311–317.
43. Corney R, Everett H, Howells A, et al. The care of patients undergoing surgery for gynecological cancer: the need for information, emotional support and counselling. J Adv Nurs 1992;17:667–671.
44. Lamont JA, De Petrillo AD, Sargeant EJ. Psychosexual rehabilitation and exenterative surgery. Gynecol Oncol 1978;6:236–242.
45. Mirhashemi R, Averette HE, Penalver MA, et al. Vaginal reconstruction at the time of pelvic exenteration: a surgical and psychosexual analysis of techniques. Gynecol Oncol 2002;87(1):39–45.
46. Grinder RR. Sex and cancer. Med Aspects Human Sex 1976; 10:130.
47. Jacobsen P, Holland JC. Psychological reactions to cancer surgery. In Holland JC, Rowland JH, editors. Handbook of Psychooncology. New York:Oxford University Press; 1989.

48. STRAIN JJ, GROSSMAN S. Psychological Care of the Medically Ill. New York:Appleton-Century Crofts; 1975.
49. STEHLIN SJ, PEACH KH. Psychological aspects of cancer therapy. JAMA 1966;197:140–144.
50. KUBLER-ROSS E. On Death and Dying. New York:Macmillan Publishing; 1969.
51. BOHROD MG. Uses of the autopsy. JAMA 1974;193:810–812.
52. FEIFEL H. The functions of attitudes toward death. In: Death and Dying: Attitudes of Patient and Doctor. New York: Group for the Advancement of Psychiatry; 1965.
53. KNAPP RJ, PEPPERS LG. Doctor–patient relationships in fetal/infant death encounters. J Med Educ 1979;54:775–780.
54. ROWE J, CLYMAN R, GREEN C, et al. Pediatrics 1978;62(2):166–170.
55. CULLBERG J. Mental reactions of women to perinatal death. In: MORRIS N, editor. Proceedings of the Third International Congress of Psychosomatic Medicine in Obstetrics and Gynecology. New York: S. Karger; 1972.
56. KOOP CE. The seriously ill or dying child: supporting the patient and family. In: SCHNAPER N, et al., editors. Management of the Dying Patient and His Family. New York:MSS Information Corp.; 1974.
57. GOLD KJ. Navigating care after a baby dies: a systematic review of parent experiences with health providers. J Perinatol 2007;27(4):230–237.
58. GILES PFH. Reactions of women to perinatal death. Aust N Z J Obstet Gynaecol 1970; 10:207.
59. HERZOG AA. A clinical study of parental response to adolescent death by suicide with recommendations for approaching the survivors. In: FARBEROW NL, editor. Proceedings of the Fourth International Conference for Suicide Prevention. Los Angeles: Delmar Publications; 1968.
60. HACKETT TP, WEISMAN AD. Psychiatric management of operative syndromes: II. Psychodynamic factors in formulation and management. Psychosom Med 1960;22:256–372.
61. HALM MA, ALPEN MA. The impact of technology on patients and families. Adv Clin Nurs Res 1993;28:443–457.
62. VAN DE LEUR JP, VAN DER SCHANS CP, LOEF BG, et al. Discomfort and factual recollection in intensive care unit patients. Crit Care 2004;8(6):R467–R473.
63. PARKER DL, HODGE JR. Delirium in a coronary care unit. JAMA 1967;201(9):132–133.
64. HELLER SS, FRANK KA, MAIM JR. Psychiatric complications of open heart surgery. N Engl J Med 1970;283:1015–1019.
65. FRICCHIONE G, KOHANE DS, DALY R, et al. Psychopharmacology in the intensive care unit. New Horiz 1998;6:353–362.
66. ALTSCHULE MD. Postoperative psychosis: a biochemical disorder. Med Counterpoint 1969; 23–27.
67. EASTON C, MACKENZIE F. Sensory-perceptual alternations: delirium in the intensive care unit. Heart Lung 1988;17:229–237.
68. MORANDI A, JACKSON JC, ELY EW. Delirium in the intensive care unit. Int Rev Psychiatry 2009;21(1):43–58.
69. BALLARD KS. Identification of environmental stressors for patients in a surgical intensive care unit. Issues Ment Health Nurs 1981;3:89–108.
70. BELITZ J. Minimizing the psychological complications of patients who require mechanical ventilation. Crit Care Nurs 1983;3(3):42–46.
71. TITCHENER JL, ZWERLING I, GOTTSCHALK L, et al. Psychosis in surgical patients. Surg Gynecol Obstet 1956;102:59–65.
72. VAN ROMPAEY B, SCHUURMANS MJ, SHORTRIDGE-BAGGETT LM, et al. Risk factors for intensive care delirium: a systematic review. Intensive Crit Care Nurs 2008;24(2):98–107.
73. LAZARUS HR, HAGENS JH. Prevention of psychosis following open heart surgery. Am J Psychiatry 1968;124:76–81.
74. LAYNE OL Jr, YUDOFSKY SC. Postoperative psychosis in cardiotomy patients: the role of organic psychiatric factors. N Engl J Med 1971;284:518–520.
75. CURTIN L. Nursing: high-touch in a high-tech world. Nurs Manage 1984;15:7–8.
76. KORNFIELD DS, HELLER SS, FRANK KA, et al. Personality and psychological factors in postcardiotomy delirium. Arch Gen Psychiatry 1974;31:249–253.
77. KEEP P, JAMES J, INMAN M. Windows in the intensive therapy unit. Anesthesia 1980;35:257–261.

78. Wilson LM. Intensive care delirium. Arch Intern Med 1971;130:225–226.

79. McKegney FP. The intensive care syndrome: the definition, treatment and prevention of a new "disease of medical progress." Conn Med 1966;30:633–636.

80. Blachly PH, Starr A. Postcardiotomy delirium. Am J Psychiatry 1965;121:371–375.

81. Hale M, Koss N, Kerstein M, et al. Psychiatric complications in a surgical ICU. Crit Care Med 1977;5(4):199–203.

82. Hackett TP, Cassem NH, Wishnie H. Detection and treatment of anxiety in the coronary care unit. Am Heart J 1969;78(6):727–730.

83. Sgroi S, Holland J, Marwit SJ. Psychological reactions to catastrophic illness: comparison of patients treated in intensive care unit and medical ward. Presented at Twenty-fifth Annual Meeting. Am Psychosomatic Soc., March 29, 1968.

84. Domar AD, Noe JM, Benson H. The pre-operative use of the relaxation response with ambulatory surgery patients. J Human Stress 1987;13:101–107.

85. Wilson JF. Behavioral preparation for surgery: benefit or harm. J Behav Med 1981;4:79–102.

86. Chapman CR, Cox GB. Anxiety, pain and depression surrounding elective surgery: a multivariate comparison of abdominal surgery patients with kidney donors and recipients. J Psychosom Res 1977;21:1–15.

87. Massie MJ, Holland JC. The cancer patient with pain: psychiatric complications and their management. Med Clin North Am 1987;71:243–258.

88. Schmale AH. Giving up as a final common pathway to changes in health. Adv Psychosom Med 1972;8: 20.

89. DiGiacomo JN. Preoperative considerations concerning psychotropic drugs. Med Psychiatry 1985;2:4–6.

90. Jacobsen P, Holland JC. Psychological reactions to cancer surgery. In: Holland JC, Rowland, JH, editors. Handbook of Psychooncology. New York:Oxford University Press; 1980.

91. Mumford E, Schlesinger HJ, Glass GV. The effects of psychological intervention on recovery from surgery and heart attacks: an analysis of the literature. Am J Public Health 1982;72:141–151.

92. Devine EC, Cook TD. Clinical and cost-saving effects of psychoeducational interventions with surgical patients: a meta-analysis. Res Nurs Health 1986;9:89–105.

Chapter 15

Pain Management in Gynecologic Oncology

Laszlo Z. Galffy, MD and Clayton A. Varga, MD, MHSM

INTRODUCTION

Pain is one of the most feared consequences perceived by patients suffering from cancer.[25,42,58] It is estimated that 50%–60% of patients with incurable disease and as many as 90% of patients with advanced disease experience moderate to severe pain.[44,49,63,64,74] Patients with gynecological tumors most frequently complain of pelvic or abdominal pain but may also experience pain at a variety of locations. There is strong evidence that the undertreatment of pain in patients with gynecological tumors is still quite high.[46,59,62] In the perioperative period, cancer pain, surgically related pain, or both may need to be addressed.

Unrelieved pain causes avoidable suffering, diminishes activity, appetite, and impairs sleep. It will further compromise an already debilitated patient. It may also lead to depression, loss of hope, and may signify inexorable progress of a fearsome and fatal disease. Suffering and a feeling of hopelessness can lead patients to reject potentially beneficial active treatment programs and increases the risk for suicide.[25,26,42] Even in the stable patient with ostensibly cured disease, untreated pain impairs productivity, performance of family and social roles, and decreases the quality of life.[21,24,33,35]

Current treatment paradigms allow for the vast majority of cancer patients to achieve comfort with relatively simple pharmacological measures, the cornerstone of which is the use of opiate analgesics. Almost all patients can be rendered comfortable using a comprehensive approach to pain management. This would include the use of opiate analgesics, co-analgesics, and surgical and rehabilitative interventions.[23,41,56,60,66,68,73]

The cancer patient may experience acute as well as chronic pain. Pain may be directly tumor related (about 65%), secondary to treatment (about 25%) such as

Gynecologic Oncology: Evidence-Based Perioperative and Supportive Care, Second Edition. Edited by Scott E. Lentz, Allison E. Axtell and Steven A. Vasilev.
© 2011 John Wiley & Sons, Inc. Published 2011 by John Wiley & Sons, Inc.

surgery or chemotherapy, or completely unrelated to the cancer (about 10%) as in the case of acute or chronic back pain.[37,48,65] Overlap may be very significant when cancer patients receive surgical care.

Optimal treatment of pain necessitates that a detailed assessment of the patients and their pain complaints be carried out in order to fully understand the etiology of the pain. Pain should be categorized by its physiologic mechanism as nociceptive (somatic or visceral), neuropathic, or mixed. This differentiation then allows the tailoring of treatment in a more specific fashion.[3,51] Consideration should be given not just to alleviating the patient's pain, but to doing so in a manner that produces the fewest side effects and leaves the patient with the highest functional status and best possible quality of life.

CLINICAL ASSESSMENT

Presentation of Pain in the Patient with Gynecologic Cancer

Identification of the types of presentation of pain in the patient with gynecologic cancer will direct the overall management strategy. Proper diagnosis of the type(s) of pain a given patient has will determine the use of optimal pharmacological and non-pharmacological pain control measures. Frequent reassessment of both the patient's pain and the overall condition is necessary, given the dynamic nature of the course of the disease and its associated pain syndromes.[9,10,51]

At the time of initial diagnosis of gynecological cancers, metastases are present in 70% of cases.[67,70] There is a paucity of well-conducted studies on the incidence of pain as the initial or presenting symptom. Pain can be caused by the primary mass or by metastases. The three most common gynecologic cancers—epithelial ovarian, cervical, and endometrial—may be associated with organ parenchymal metastases (liver, lungs, pleura, and less frequently the brain), skeletal, and lymph node metastases.[70]

Epithelial ovarian carcinoma is diagnosed in 75%–85% of patients at the time of peritoneal spread (stage III), with the most common presenting symptom being vague abdominal pain or discomfort.

Cervical cancer usually presents with vaginal bleeding or discharge. However, pain in the lumbosacral and gluteal area due to parametrial spread or lymph node involvement can be the initial presenting symptom in some advanced stage patients.

Endometrial cancer usually presents early with abnormal bleeding but may be associated with pelvic pain when extrauterine spread is evident. At this point, pelvic and para-aortic node involvement may be associated with lumbosacral and gluteal pain.

Breast cancer may be associated with treatment or metastasis-related pain, including that due to pelvic masses.

Table 15.1   Types of Patients with Cancer Pain

1. Patients with tumor-related pain
2. Patients with therapy-related pain
3. Nonmalignant pain in the patient with cancer
4. Pregnant patients with cancer pain
5. Substance abusers with cancer pain
6. Psychiatric conditions associated with cancer pain
7. The dying patient with cancer pain

The principal types of pain presentation are listed in the following seven categories[48,64] (Table 15.1):

1. *Tumor-related pain*—Pain in this case is caused by infiltration of soft tissue, bony, or neurological structures. Pain may be the main symptom. It has a special significance as marker of the disease. Recurring pain often signifies recurring disease and effective treatment of cancer "cures" the pain. It can be acute, chronic, or chronically maintained acute or incident pain. It may be maintained or amplified by the associated immunologic and neuroendocrine changes characteristic of some types of tumors (Table 15.2).

2. *Therapy-related pain*—Pain may be caused by surgery, radiation, chemotherapy, or various adjuvant therapies such as antibiotic therapy, hormonal therapy, or steroid withdrawal. This pain is present in approximately 25% of patients suffering from cancer. Chronic tumor and cancer therapy–related pain becomes an aspect of global suffering, along with immobility, sleep disturbance, and depression (Table 15.3).

3. *Nonmalignancy-related pain in the patient with cancer*—With or without cancer pain, there may be concomitant nonmalignancy-related pain occurring in 10% of patients.[37] For successful treatment, it is important to establish the correct etiology and to avoid confusion with cancer-related pain. Preexisting chronic pain in a patient who subsequently develops cancer poses difficult diagnostic and therapeutic problems. This group of patients is at high risk for developing escalating pain syndromes, therapy- and procedure-related complications, and further functional incapacity. A subgroup in this category is that of AIDS-related pain syndromes (Table 15.4).

4. *Cancer pain in the pregnant patient*—Pain may be related to gynecological malignancies or tumors of other organs and systems. Personal decisions regarding abortion and efforts to minimize effects on the fetus will direct the use of available therapeutic options.

5. *Drug abuse/addiction preceding cancer pain*—In this group, pain is frequently undertreated and the diagnosis of cancer delayed. Appropriate opioid therapy should not be withheld. Cure of the cancer and control of cancer-related symptoms should be temporally coordinated with treatment of the addiction and psychological and social rehabilitation.[58]

Table 15.2   Tumor-Related Pain Syndromes

A. Nociceptive pain syndromes
   1. Visceral nociceptive
      1.1. Abdominal pain (poorly localized) due to
- infiltration of the peritoneum
- bowel obstruction
- biliary/pancreatic duct obstruction
- ureteral obstruction
- stretch, compression of, or torsion of organ capsules or suspensive structures (e.g., right upper quadrant pain from distention of hepatic capsules)

   2. Somatic nociceptive
      2.1. Involving soft tissues
- invasion of muscle and connective tissue structures
- invasion of mucous membrane
- invasion of the skin and subcutaneous tissue

      2.2. Involving bone and joints
         2.2.1. Pathological fractures of
- long bones
- vertebra
- atlantoaxial syndrome
  - C7-T1 syndrome
  - T12-L1 syndrome
  - sacral syndrome

         2.2.2. Incident pain related to mobilization of involved bone
- from bone itself
- due to reflex muscle spasm
- from connective tissue

         2.2.3. Invasion of the skull
- orbital syndrome
- parasellar syndrome
- sphenoid sinus syndrome
- middle cranial fossa syndrome
- clivus syndrome
- jugular foramen syndrome
- occipital condyle syndrome

         2.2.4. Generalized bone pain
- multiple metastases
- bone marrow replacement by tumor

6. *Cancer pain in patients with psychiatric conditions*—This group also presents diagnostic and therapeutic challenges since these patients may have increased difficulty in accurately reporting or describing their pain. Their complaints can change in a manner or degree disproportionate to changes in the course of the disease. They may either under- or overreport the intensity of their pain.

Table 15.3 Therapy-Related Pain Syndromes

1. Postoperative pain syndromes
    1.1. Acute postoperative pain
    1.2. Postmastectomy syndrome
    1.3. Postthoracotomy syndrome
    1.4. Postradical neck dissection syndrome
    1.5. Postnephrectomy syndrome
    1.6. Phantom limb and stump pain syndrome
2. Postchemotherapy pain syndromes
    2.1. Mucositis
    2.2. Polymyalgias and polyarthralgias
    2.3. Pain secondary to tumor embolization
    2.4. Peripheral neuropathy
    2.5. Steroid pseudorheumatism
    2.6. Aseptic bone necrosis
3. Postradiation pain syndromes
    3.1 Enteritis or proctitis
    3.2 Radiation fibrosis of the lumbosacral plexus
    3.3 Radiation fibrosis of the branchial plexus
    3.4 Radiation myelopathy
    3.5 Radiation-induced peripheral nerve tumors

Mental status changes, more frequent in the elderly population, may impair diagnostic accuracy, and limit therapeutic choices.[24,45]

7. *Dying patient with cancer pain*—The main therapeutic goal is maintaining the patient's comfort and addressing all the available modalities of easing the patient's and the family's suffering. Adequate pain control is of foremost importance and all available techniques in an optimal time frame should be attempted.[36,72,74]

PAIN ASSESSMENT

The International Association for the Study of Pain has defined pain as "an unpleasant sensory and emotional experience associated with actual or potential tissue damage

Table 15.4 Pain Indirectly Related or Unrelated to Cancer

1. Pain associated with degenerative joint disease of the cervical and lumbar spine
2. Myofascial pain
3. Postherpetic neuralgia
4. Chronic headache syndromes
5. Diabetic neuropathy
6. Pain associated with other therapies (i.e., Synercid)

or described in terms of such damage." The activity produced in the afferent nervous system by a stimulus originating in damaged tissues or damaged nerves is described as nociception.[1]

Intense and sustained nociceptive input will result in reflex responses at several levels. Segmental and suprasegmental reflex responses produce increased general sympathetic tone. This will result in vasoconstriction in the cutaneous and splanchnic vessels, increased stroke volume and heart rate, increased blood pressure, and increased metabolic rate and oxygen consumption. Decrease in gastrointestinal and urinary tract tone may progress to delayed gastric emptying and ileus and urinary retention. It also causes increased skeletal muscle tone, which may progress to muscle spasms. Catabolic endocrine responses to nociceptive input are represented by increases in stress hormone levels and decreases in insulin and testosterone levels. Metabolic responses include changes in protein, carbohydrate, and fat metabolism, water retention, decreased functional extracellular fluid, and fluid shifts to the vascular and cellular compartments. Stimulation of the respiratory center results in hyperventilation, a response which may be overcome by splinting.

The patient's perception of pain and interpretation of its meaning is a complex phenomenon. It involves, along with physiologic processes (such as pain perception, pain transmission, and modulation), psychological, emotional, and behavioral changes. Pain intensity is influenced by multiple factors and may not be directly proportional to the extent of the injury. Pain perception consists of a complicated interplay between sensory impulses in the central nervous system ascending pathways and activation of descending inhibitory systems. The diencephalic and cortical responses lead to anxiety, causing further increase in general sympathetic tone, increased blood viscosity, clotting time, fibrinolysis, and platelet aggregation, increasing the risk of thromboembolism and other coagulation disorders.

Given this complicated framework, it should be emphasized that there is no single effective approach to pain management. Diagnosis and management of pain should be strictly individualized, taking into account the stage of the disease, the presence of concomitant pathophysiologic states, the type of pain, and the psychological and sociocultural characteristics of the patient. Cancer pain assessment should be ongoing and active, necessitating frequent reassessment of pain quality, pain intensity, and treatment effectiveness.

CHARACTERISTICS OF PAIN

Pain assessment should include information about the temporal, physiologic, topographic, and etiologic characteristics of pain. On the basis of temporal characteristics, pain can be discriminated into acute pain and chronic pain:

1. *Acute pain*—This pain has a well-defined onset in time, usually an obvious cause, limited duration, and is responsive to the available analgesic treatments. It has a protective function and it is regarded as being a symptom. It is usually focal, experienced at the site of the injury, self-limited, and with mild or no associated psychological disturbance. It is associated with obvious

pain-related behavior, such as immobility, grimacing, and moaning. Severe acute pain is associated with all the physiological changes described above. Its prognosis is generally excellent.

2. *Chronic pain*—This pain is defined as pain lasting for more than 3 months, usually without a well-defined onset and a fluctuating course. Chronic pain may no longer serve any useful purpose as a warning sign of continued tissue damage and in this regard may be considered a disease process unto itself. Pain behavior may or may not be obvious and sympathetic hyperactivity may not be present. Patients may present with anger or depression, along with sleep disturbance, and may complain of symptoms involving uninjured tissue sites. Chronic pain may lead to physical disability from disuse such as muscular atrophy, contractures, and trophic changes. Treatment often requires multidisciplinary management efforts including intense physical therapy, vocational rehabilitation, and early psychological assessment and intervention.[53]

On a *physiologic* basis, pain can be discriminated into nociceptive pain and neuropathic pain:

1. *Nociceptive pain*—This pain is of two types, somatic nociceptive pain and visceral nociceptive pain. Nociceptive pain responds well to opiate analgesics and to interventions directed to the resolution of the initiating lesion. Nerve blocks or other procedures that interrupt nociception may also be effective.
   - *Somatic nociceptive pain*—This is the result of nociceptor activation in the skin and subcutaneous tissues. The pain is associated with a lesion that can be identified and is commensurate with its extent. It is often described as an aching or pressure-like sensation; however, it can be throbbing or stabbing too. It is described as well localized and sharp with stimulation of the affected tissue. Examples are postsurgical pain and pain caused by skeletal metastasis.
   - *Visceral nociceptive pain*—This has a cramping, poorly localized character resulting from distension, stretching, compression, or infiltration of the abdominal and thoracic organs. It is often referred to areas that are localized far from the site of the lesion, such as a shoulder pain caused by irritation of the diaphragm. Pain due to obstruction of a hollow viscus is described as crampy or gnawing. Involvement of organ capsules or peritoneal appendages may cause aching, throbbing or sharp pain.
2. *Neuropathic pain*—This pain is the result of abnormal somatosensory processing in the periphery or the central nervous system. It results from direct injury to the nerves as a consequence of tumor invasion or from therapy-induced neural injury. It is often associated with loss of motor and sensory function along with sympathetic dysfunction. The pain occurs in the absence of detectable tissue damaging processes. It may present as an abnormal, unpleasant sensation (i.e., dysesthesia), frequently with a burning quality, and a brief shooting-stabbing component. Its onset is delayed relative to the precipitating injury. Mild stimulation of the skin can be painful (i.e., allodynia).

Repeated stimulation with an identical stimulus causes progressive build-up of pain intensity (i.e., hyperpathia), and the pain persists after the eliciting stimulus is withdrawn (i.e., after-reaction.) Its hallmark is a dysesthetic and unfamiliar sensation perceived in an area of motor or sensory deficit.

There is disagreement in the literature about the response of neuropathic pain to opiate analgesics. It was initially felt that neuropathic pain was relatively nonresponsive to treatment with opiates. More recent studies, however, have called this finding into question.[53] Neuropathic pain is sometimes responsive to treatment with adjuvants, such as anticonvulsants, antidepressants, or antiarrhythmics. Preemptive analgesia may be useful in preventing the development of neuropathic pain syndromes.[53]

Topographically pain can be *localized, multifocal,* or *generalized.* This distinction is important in determining the usefulness of specific therapies, such as nerve block or neurosurgical interventions. *Localized pain* should be differentiated from *referred pain*, which could be

- pain referred along the course of an injured peripheral nerve,
- pain referred along the course of the fibers of a damaged nerve root ("radicular pain"),
- pain referred to nondermatomal parts of the body from lesions involving the spinal cord or central pathways ("funicular pain"), and
- pain referred in a nondermatomal fashion from a visceral source (e.g., jaw from myocardium or shoulder from diaphragmatic irritation).

Etiologic characterization refers to the cause–effect relationships, which are usually obvious in acute pain. In chronic pain, however, it may be difficult to link the pain to a specific injury. It is important that the etiology of the pain is considered in evaluation of cancer patients because this approach can lead to identification of an underlying recurrence and also guides therapy. Previously unsuspected new lesions can be identified by analysis of changing pain patterns in more than 60% of cancer patients.[51]

COMMON CANCER PAIN SYNDROMES

Tumor-Related Pain Syndromes

Common cancer pain syndromes are listed in Table 15.2. Visceral pain syndromes that the gynecological cancer patient may experience are familiar to most clinicians. The distinction between visceral and some somatic or neuropathic pain syndromes is not always clear. Involvement of the celiac plexus causes a boring, dull epigastric pain. This pain radiates to the back in the upper lumbar or lower thoracic area and is by convention considered visceral rather than neuropathic.[63] Tumor infiltration of the bladder and deep pelvic masses may cause suprapubic and perineal pain. Pain in the deep pelvis may also result from sacral plexus involvement. Tumor invasion of the pelvis may cause pain referred to the inguinal region and anterior thigh. Metastases in the epidural space can cause focal back pain, which may present as the initial symptom. This pain is often confused in older patients with nonmalignancy associated back pain. Tumor invasion of paravertebral or retroperitoneal chest wall regions can cause mononeuropathies. Infiltration of the brachial plexus may manifest as rapidly increasing pain in the shoulder and upper extremity, associated with motor and sensory dysfunction.

Primary or metastatic invasion of bone causes several specific pain syndromes. Pain due to metastasis to the skull base can manifest as the first complaint, preceding neurological signs and symptoms. Jugular foramen syndrome consists of occipital headaches, exacerbated by head movement, referred to the vertex and the shoulder and arm on the same side.[50] Pain associated with hoarseness, dysarthria, and cranial nerve–related symptoms from the 6th to the 12th nerves is typical for clivus metastases. Breast cancer can cause a constant, dull pain radiating to both shoulders, originating at the spinous processes of C7-T1. Involvement of the first lumbar vertebrae may cause referred pain to the sacroiliac region or superior iliac crest, along with mid backache exacerbated by sitting or laying and relieved by standing up.

Pain Associated with Cancer Therapy

Treatment-induced pain can be acute or chronic (Table 15.3). Acute therapy–related pain includes postsurgical pain, along with the mucositis of chemotherapy and the pain of radiation esophagitis.

Chronic cancer therapy–related pain poses a diagnostic challenge. The distinction between recurring disease–related symptoms and complications from therapy is often impossible to make. For example, postmastectomy pain manifests as a burning sensation in the axilla, upper arm, or anterior chest wall, exacerbated by movement. It is a result of surgical or postsurgical damage to the intercostobrachial nerve. In some cases, the severity of pain with movement may lead to such limited use of the arm that the patient may develop a frozen shoulder.

Chemotherapy can cause a polyneuropathy, manifested by pain in the hands and feet, which is burning in character. Lymphedema, numbness, and pain are characteristic for radiation fibrosis of the brachial plexus. Radiation fibrosis of the lumbosacral plexus may cause pain in the anterior thigh and perineum. One of the radiation-related injuries most difficult to treat is radiation myelopathy, characterized by a localized or referred area of dysesthesia, below the level of cord damage.

Pain Unrelated to Cancer or Cancer Therapy

Pain unrelated to cancer or cancer therapy (Table 15.4) most often manifests as back pain or neck pain related to degenerative joint disease of the cervical or lumbar spine. Postherpetic neuralgia may cause severe neuropathic pain, which often precedes the presence of skin lesions. Early diagnosis and aggressive treatment with Acyclovir, along with treatment of the pain, are recommended and may prevent the development of postherpetic neuralgia. Severe generalized pain syndromes can be present in patients treated for surgical or other therapy-related complications. As an example, therapy of VRE (vancomycin–resistant enterococcus faecium) infections with Synercid may cause elevation of the liver enzymes, along with severe arthralgias and myalgias. This pain does respond well to treatment with opiates.

MEASUREMENT OF PAIN

Pain measurement is inherently subjective and based on patient's self-report. The simplest techniques of pain measurement rely on a single dimension, such as pain intensity. Pain intensity is measured by using numerical or linear analog scales (Fig. 15.1). These are usually clinically satisfactory. Verbal descriptors of pain intensity such as mild, moderate, severe, and excruciating, or representations of facial expressions are less sensitive. The restricted number of possible responses causes

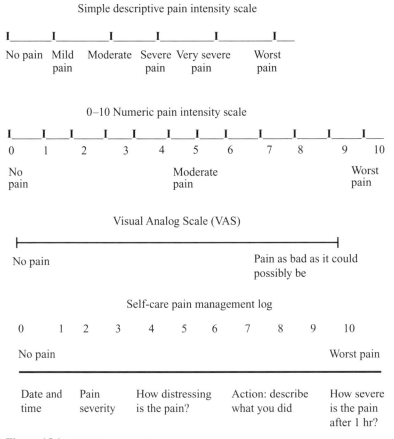

Figure 15.1   Pain intensity scales.

clustering to the middle of the scale.[3, 14] Follow-up and a self-care pain management log can be used (Fig. 15.1)

More complex assessments of pain involve multiple dimension reporting via pain questionnaires (such as the McGill pain questionnaire) coupled with a pain intensity score and a patient pain map (Fig. 15.1) In patients with chronic pain, psychometric testing is indicated as part of the initial workup. Commonly used techniques are the Minnesota Multiphasic Personality Inventory, Beck Depression Inventory, and Wisconsin Brief Pain Inventory. A measure of functional status such as the SPF 36 may also be indicated. Table 15.5 lists the components of a comprehensive initial pain assessment protocol.

MANAGEMENT OF PAIN

Common barriers to adequate cancer pain management are listed in Table 15.6. In the management of gynecologic cancer pain, a variety of options are available, including surgery, radiotherapy, chemotherapy, peripheral and neuraxial blockade, and pharmacological interventions. The suggested management interventions for cancer pain are presented in Figures 15.2 to 15.4.

Pharmacological Management

Drug therapy is the cornerstone of cancer pain management because of its effectiveness, comparatively lower risk, and economic advantages. The three major classes of drugs used alone or in combination are the NSAIDs and acetaminophen, the opiate analgesics, and the adjuvant analgesics.

Several principles outline the best approach to using medication in cancer pain management. The medication regimen must be individualized to the needs of the patient. The simplest dosage schedules and the least invasive route of administration should be used first. According to the World Health Organization *three-step analgesic ladder* developed in the early 1980s, acetaminophen or an NSAID should be the first step in managing mild to moderate pain. United States formularies are largely limited to oral administration of the NSAIDs, with the only parenteral nonsteroidal analgesic available being Ketorolac. The second step on the ladder is adding an opiate and adjusting the dose according to the severity of pain. The third step is the use of strong opiate agonists, with or without the use of nonopioid or adjuvant therapy. The co-analgesics, which may be used in any step, include anticonvulsants, antidepressants, anxiolytics, steroids, dextroamphetamine, phenothiazines, antiarrhythmics, alpha-1 antagonists, and alpha-2 agonists.[16, 29, 38]

The preferred route of analgesic administration is oral. Rectal and transdermal routes should be considered when the patient cannot take medications orally, before considering systemic parenteral administration. There is strong evidence against the appropriateness of intramuscular administration of analgesics, given the unpredictable absorption rate, duration of action, and the unpleasant and potentially harmful

Table 15.5 Initial Pain Assessment

A. Assessment of pain intensity and character

1. Onset and temporal pattern—When did your pain start? How often does it occur? Has its intensity changed?

2. Location—Where is your pain? Is there more than one site?

3. Description—What does your pain feel like? What words would you use to describe your pain?

4. Intensity—On a scale of 0–10, with 0 being no pain and 10 being the worst pain you can imagine, how much does it hurt right now? How much does it hurt at its worst? How much does it hurt as its best?

5. Aggravating and relieving factors—What makes your pain better? What makes your pain worse?

6. Previous treatment—What types of treatments have you tried to relieve your pain? Were they and are they effective?

7. Effect—How does the pain affect physical and social function?

B. Psychosocial assessment

1. Effect and understanding of the cancer diagnosis and cancer treatment on the patient and the caregiver

2. The meaning of the pain to the patient and the family

3. Significant past instances of pain and their effect on the patient

4. The patient's typical coping responses to stress or pain

5. The patient's knowledge of, curiosity about, preferences for, and expectations about pain management methods

6. The patient's concerns about using controlled substances such as opioids, anxiolytics, or stimulants

7. The economic effect of the pain and its treatment

8. Changes in mood that have occurred as a result of the pain (e.g., depression, anxiety)

C. Physical and neurological examination

1. Examine site of pain and evaluate common referral patterns

2. Perform pertinent neurologic evaluation
   - Head and neck pain—cranial nerve and funduscopic evaluation
   - Back and neck pain—motor and sensory function in limbs; rectal and urinary sphincter function

D. Diagnostic evaluation

1. Evaluate recurrence or progression of disease or tissue injury related to cancer treatment
   - Tumor markers and other blood tests
   - Radiologic studies
   - Neurophysiologic (e.g., electromyography) testing

2. Perform appropriate radiologic studies and correlate normal and abnormal findings with physical and neurologic examination

3. Recognize limitations of diagnostic studies
   - Bone scan—false negatives in myeloma, lymphoma, previous radiotherapy sites
   - CT scan—good definition of bone and soft tissue but difficult to image entire spine
   - MRI scan—bone definition not as good as CT; better images of spine and brain

Reference 1.

Table 15.6   Barriers to Cancer Pain Management

Problems related to health-care professionals
Inadequate knowledge of pain management
Poor assessment of pain
Concern about regulation of controlled substances
Fear of patient addiction
Concern about side effects of analgesics
Concern about patients becoming tolerant to analgesics

Problems related to patients
Reluctant to report pain
Concern about distracting physicians from treatment of underlying disease
Concern about not being a "good" patient
Reluctance to take pain medications
Fear of addiction or of being thought of as an addict
Worries about unmanageable side effects
Concern about becoming tolerant to pain medications

Problems related to the health-care system
Low priority given to cancer pain treatment; inadequate reimbursement
The most appropriate treatment may not be reimbursed or may be too
    costly for patients and their families
Restrictive regulation of controlled substances; problems of availability of
    treatment or access to it

Reference 1.

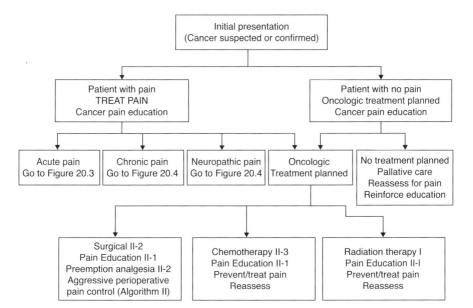

Figure 15.2   Management of pain in the patient with gynecologic cancer pain.

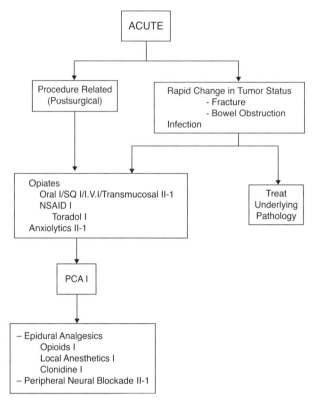

Figure 15.3   Management of acute procedure-related and tumor complication-induced pain.

side effects caused by the injection.[46] Consideration of epidural or intrathecal analgesic systems should follow failure of maximal systemic doses of opiates to relieve pain, despite proper management of opiate-induced side effects.

Nonopiate Analgesics

Nonopiate analgesics constitute a group of compounds that differ in chemical structure and pharmacological properties. Dosing data for these agents is listed in Table 15.7. Initially the group consisted of acetaminophen and the NSAIDs. Recently other types of nonopiate analgesics are being added, such as Tramadol, which has a combination of weak mu-1 agonist and serotonergic activity. Newer drugs, not yet released, target tumor necrosis factor-alpha and interleukin-mediated mechanisms of nociception.

Acetaminophen is an oral analgesic with the potency of aspirin. It has antipyretic activity, but its anti-inflammatory potency as well as its anti-platelet activity are minimal. It causes minimal gastric irritation, but it may cause severe hepato-toxicity. Acetaminophen is used in combination with opiates in several commercially available

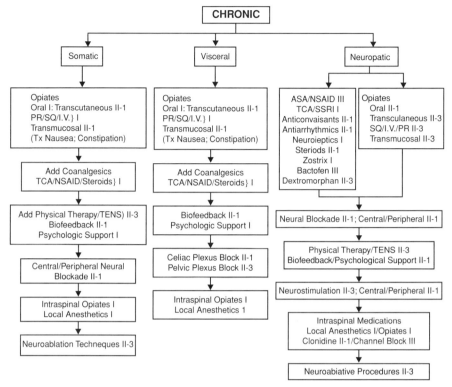

Figure 15.4   Management of chronic pain due to somatic, visceral, or neuropathic stimuli.

combination analgesics. It is the first line of treatment for mild to moderate pain. It can be administered orally or rectally and the total daily dose for adults should be limited to 4000 mg.

NSAIDs are a group of structurally diverse compounds that have a common mechanism of action, consisting of central and peripheral cyclo-oxygenase activity inhibition, which blocks prostanoid synthesis.[47] Cyclo-oxygenase has two main isoenzymes, which are inhibited to varying degrees by the available nonsteroidal anti-inflammatory drugs. Inhibition of COX-1 is linked to gastrointestinal ulcerations, while inhibition of COX-2 is not. Recent development of selective COX-2 inhibitors may lead to important progress in analgesic therapy. The available NSAIDs vary from being COX-1 selective (flurbiprofen, ketoprofen), to nonselective (ibuprofen, naproxen) or COX-2 selective (mefenamic acid, diclofenac). Mefenamic acid is unique in its ability to inhibit production of both prostaglandins and leukotrienes. Enhanced production of leukotrienes is responsible for anaphylactoid reactions to NSAIDs.[43,56]

The main side effects of NSAIDs include gastritis, exacerbation of bronchospasm, platelet inhibition, nephrotoxicity, and water retention. Phenylbutazone

Table 15.7   Dosing Data for Acetaminophen (APAP) and NSAIDs

Drug	Usual Dose for Adults and Children >50 kg Body Weight	Usual Dose for Children and Adults <50 kg Body Weight
Acetaminophen and over-the-counter NSAIDs		
Acetaminophen III	650 mg q4h	10–15 mg/kg q4h
	975 mg q6h	15–20 mg/kg q4h (rectal)
Aspirin IV	650 mg q4h	10–15 mg/kg q4h
	975 mg q4h	15–20 mg/kg q4h (rectal)
Ibuprofen (Motrin, others)	400–600 mg q6h	10 mg/kg q6-8h
Prescription NSAIDs		
Carprofen (Rimadyl)	100 mg tid	
Choline magnesium trisalicylate VI (Trilisate)	1000–1500 mg tid	25 mg/kg tid
Choline salicylate (Arthropan) VI	870 mg q3-4h	
Diflunisal (Dolobid) VII	500 mg q12h	
Etodolac (Lodine)	200–400 mg q6-8h	
Fenoprofen calcium (Nalfon)	300–600 mg q6h	
Ketoprofen (Orudis)	25–60 mg q6-8h	
Ketorolac tromethamine VIII (Toradol)	10 mg q4-6h to a maximum of 40 mg/day	
Magnesium salicylate (Doan's, Magan, Mobidin, others)	650 mg q4h	
Meclofenamate sodium (Meclomen) VIIII	50–100 mg q6h	
Mefenamic acid (Ponstel)	250 mg q6h	
Naproxen (Naprosyn)	250–275 mg q6-8h	5 mg/kg q8h
Naproxen sodium (Anaprox)	275 mg q6-8h	

Taken from Reference 1.

may cause bone marrow toxicity. Naproxen use may result in pulmonary infiltrates, while use of ibuprofen, sulindac, and tolmetin may result in aseptic meningitis. Misoprostol, 200 mg bid effectively prevents NSAID-induced gastric ulcerations and is available in combination preparations. Extreme care should be taken to monitor renal function in patients on NSAIDs because of the risk of severe renal failure secondary to renal prostaglandin synthesis inhibition.

Tramadol is useful in controlling mild to moderate cancer pain. A 50-mg dose has the analgesic potency of 60 mg of codeine. It can be combined with acetaminophen in patients in whom the NSAIDs are contraindicated and in patients who wish not to use opioids.

Opiate Analgesics

Opiate analgesics are used in steps two and three of the WHO analgesic ladder (Dosing guidelines—Table 15.8). Codeine, dihydrocodeine, hydrocodone, oxycodone, and propoxyphene, in combination with acetaminophen, are used in the treatment of moderate pain. The usefulness of fixed combinations is often limited by the excessive amount of acetaminophen contained. Codeine must be converted to morphine to provide analgesia. Thus, inhibitors of facilitating enzyme systems, such as quinidine, cimetidine, or fluoxidine counteract its analgesic efficacy.

Persistent or severe pain should be medicated around-the-clock, with generous supplemental doses "as needed." Early aggressive treatment of side effects will permit upward titration to pain control and will prevent patient refusal of the drug. Opiates with no ceiling effect should be used for severe pain, and mixed agonist–antagonists should not be given at the same time with direct agonists so as to avoid opiate withdrawal syndrome. Administration of naloxone for opiate side effect reversal should be performed with small, titrated doses, to avoid reversal of analgesia. Opiates with potentially toxic active metabolites (such as propoxyphene and meperidine) should not be used if sustained opiate use is anticipated.[40]

Patient-Controlled Opiate Analgesia

Intravenous administration of opiates can provide rapid pain relief and, when used as patient-controlled analgesia (PCA), enhances the patient's sense of control. Along with the use of epidural opiates or opiate and local analgesic combinations, PCA is the preferred analgesic method for control of postoperative pain. Limitations in the intensive care unit may include the unconscious, heavily sedated, or confused patient. Physical limitations include patients with severe arthritis or other conditions that interfere with use of the PCA apparatus.

Potential complications include infiltration of the lines, infection, and the risk of excessive sedation if high doses of a continuous infusion are used. Additionally, total analgesic requirements show a large interpatient variability, which is partly age related. Morphine is the most commonly used agent, although meperidine hydrochloride (Demerol), fentanyl citrate (Sublimaze), sufentanil, hydromorphone, and others can also be used.

Initially, a loading dose may be appropriate if the patient has not been receiving other narcotics. Typically, 1–2 mg of MS (or equianalgesic) is administered every 15–30 minutes until pain relief is obtained. The PCA should then be adjusted to deliver the minimum effective analgesic concentration required to provide optimal analgesia with minimal side effects.[18,57] This can be easily achieved by appropriately setting the demand dose, lockout interval, and total hourly limit administered. Sample orders are shown in Table 15.9 and general guidelines for initial dosing are presented in Table 15.10. Otherwise, the amount of drug available for the patient should only be limited by the associated side effects. The PCA is intended to deliver a relatively constant analgesic dose range to patients in order to minimize wide fluctuations between underdosed pain and overdosed sedation and respiratory depression.

Table 15.8 Dose Equivalents for Opioid Analgesics in Opioid-Naive Adults and Children (≥50 kg Body Weight)

Drug	Approximate Equianalgesic Dose		Usual Starting Dose for Moderate to Severe Pain	
	Oral	Parenteral	Oral	Parenteral
Opioid agonist II				
Morphine III	30 mg q3-4h (repeat around-the-clockdosing) 60 mg q3-4h (single dose or intermittent dosing)	10 mg q3-4h	30 mg q3-4h	10 mg q3-4h
Morphine, controlled-release III, IV (MS Contin, Oramorph)	90–120 mg q12h	N/A	90–120 mg q12h	N/A
Hydromorphone III (Dilaudid)	7.5 mg q3-4h	mg q3-4h	6 mg q3-4h	1.5 mg q3-4h
Levorphanol (Levo-Duromoran)	4 mg q6-8h	2 mg q6-8h	4 mg q6-8h	2 mg q6-8h
Meperidine (Demerol)	300 mg q2-3h	100 mg q3h	N/R	100 mg q3h
Methadone (Dolophine, other)	20 mg q6-8h	10 mg q6-8h	20 mg q6-8h	10 mg q6-8h
Oxymorphone III (Numorphan)	N/A	1 mg q3-4h	N/A	1 mg q3-4h
Combination opioid/NSAID preparations				
Codeine (with aspirin or acetaminophen)	180–200 mg q3-4h	130 mg q3-4h	60 mg q3-4h	60 mg q2h (IM/SC)
Hydrocodone (in Lorcet, Lortab, Vicodin, others)	30 mg q3-4h	N/A	10 mg q3-4h	N/A

Taken from Reference 1.

460

Table 15.9   Patient-Controlled Analgesia (PCA) Basic Sample Orders

1. Disregard previous analgesic and sedative orders.

2. Intravenous fluids as ordered previously, or start IV D5/0.45 NS to keep open until PCA discontinued. If IV infiltrates and cannot be restarted, call MD.

3. PCA Orders:
   A. Agent used _____
   B. Concentration _____mg/ml
   C. PCA Dose _____mg
   D. Lockout interval _____minutes
   E. Continuous Basal rate _____mg/hr
   F. 4-hour limit _____mg

4. Keep 0.4 mg naloxone (Narcan) at bedside

5. Side effect medications:
   A. Droperidol 0.5 mg IV Push q4 hrs PRN Nausea
   B. Benadryl 25 mg IV or PO q4 hrs PRN pruritis
   C. If respiratory rate <8 or patient not arousable:
      1. Stop PCA STAT
      2. Administer naloxone 0.4 mg IVP STAT
      3. Notify MD STAT

Infusion of the ultrashort-acting opiate remifentanil is useful in the ICU setting to wean patients from long-acting opiates. This drug is easily titrated and termination of the effect occurs minutes after cessation of use. PCA can also be administered via subcutaneous infusion of hydromorphone and morphine, providing rapid pain relief in the absence of IV access.[30]

Epidural Opiates

Epidural opiates used in combination with local anesthetics tend to produce the best compromise between the quality of analgesia and the intensity of side effects in the control of postoperative pain.[20, 28] Lipid soluble drugs (opiates and local anesthetics) placed in the center of the segmental area targeted for pain control will produce excellent analgesia and minimal side effects. Properly trained nursing personnel and

Table 15.10   Initial Morphine Sulfate PCA Dosing Guidelines

	Age <50 years	Age 51–60 years	Age 61–70 years	Age <70 years
Bolus Dose (mg)	2	1.5	1	0.5
Basal Rate (mg/hr)	1–2	1–2	1	1
Lockout (min)	10	12	15	20
Total Dose limit (mg/4 hours)	30	20	15	10

good communication between the surgical and pain management team are essential to assure maximal benefits and minimal complications of this method. The most popular combinations are fentanyl 1–5 mcg/mL with bupivacaine 0.125%–0.25%. Sufentanil 0.2–0.5 mcg/mL and ropivacaine 0.1%–0.2% are reasonable alternatives.

For patients with poor pain control or for those experiencing intractable side effects, intrathecal and intracerebral administration may prove advantageous. Local anesthetics added to epidural or spinal opiates may dramatically improve the quality of analgesia.

The use of transdermal fentanyl provides an alternative delivery route for patients unable to tolerate oral drug delivery. The onset to peak plasma levels after placement of the initial patch or after increasing the dose is about 12 hours. The rectal route is a useful alternative when the oral or parenteral administration is not available. The onset of action is slow and this route is not widely accepted by patients.

Tolerance and physical dependence are expected with long-term opiate use and should not be regarded as "addiction." Abrupt discontinuation of opiates or administration of antagonists or agonist–antagonists will result in withdrawal, manifested by viral flu-like symptoms in mild cases. Severe pain, anxiety, chills, lacrimation, diaphoresis, nausea, abdominal cramps, and diarrhea may be seen in the more severe cases. The onset of withdrawal occurs from 6 to more than 24 hours after treatment discontinuation, depending on the agent's half-life. If discontinuation of opiates is required, a tapering schedule that reduces the amount of drug by about 10% per day minimizes withdrawal symptoms. Clonidine 0.1–0.2 mg/day transdermally will reduce the autonomic hyperactivity and anxiety associated with opioid withdrawal.

Prevention and treatment of opiate side effects is an often disregarded, important aspect of management. Nausea may be treated by a centrally acting antiemetic. Early administration of a bowel stimulant and a stool softener will usually insure one soft bowel movement every 1–2 days. Sedation typically resolves with time. It can be reduced with the use of methylphenidate, dextroamphetamine, and caffeine. Myoclonic spasms can be treated with a long-acting benzodiazepine, such as clonazepam. Changing to a different opiate may be necessary in some patients. Delirium may appear secondary to large doses of opiates or from other causes in the critically ill patient. If this occurs, decreasing the dose or changing to another potent opiate may be necessary.

Adjuvant Analgesic Drugs

The role of adjuvant therapy is to supplement opiate analgesia, treat specific types of pain, and control associated symptoms. Skeletal metastases, neuropathic pain syndromes, and visceral pain syndromes may respond well to co-analgesics. Commonly used drugs are antidepressants, anticonvulsants, corticosteroids, antiarrhythmics, alpha-1 antagonists, and alpha-2 agonists. Other types of drugs that can be used for special therapeutic reasons are the skeletal muscle relaxants, antihistamines, and antipsychotics. Substance P inhibitors and local anesthetics are used externally for the treatment of localized pain syndromes (Table 15.11).[16, 29, 38]

Table 15.11   Adjuvant Analgesic Drugs for Cancer Pain

Drug	Approximate Adult Daily Dose Range	Route of Administration	Type of Pain
Corticosteroids			
Dexamethasone II	16–96 mg	PO, IV	Pain associated with brain metastases and epidural spinal cord compression
Prednisone	40–100 mg	PO	
Anticonvulsants			
Carbamazepine III	200–1600 mg	PO	Neuropathic pain
Phenytoin IV	300–500 mg	PO	
Antidepressants			
Amitriptyline V	25–150 mg	PO	Neuropathic pain
Doxepin VI	25–150 mg	PO	
Imipramine VII	20–150 mg	PO	
Trazodone VIII	75–225 mg	PO	
Neuroleptics			
Methotrimeprazine VIII	40–80 mg	IM	Analgesia, sedation, antiemetic
Antihistamines			
Hydroxyzine VV	300–450 mg	IM	Adjuvant to opioids in postoperative and other types of pain; relief of complicating symptoms including anxiety, insomnia, nausea
Local anesthetics/antiarrhythmics			
Lidocaine VVI	5 mg/kg	IV/SC	Neuropathic pain
Mexiletine VVII	450–600 mg	PO	
Tocainide VVIII	20 mg/kg	PO	

Taken from Reference 1.

Antidepressants are useful for the treatment of neuropathic pain. They improve sleep as well as depression. However, anticholinergic, antihistaminic, antidopaminergic, and alpha-1 antagonist activity-related side effects may limit their therapeutic use. Also, pain relief may not be achieved for several weeks following initiation of therapy. Nortriptyline and desipramine are better tolerated than other tricyclic antidepressants. The initial dose should be low, followed by slow upward titration, limited by side effects.

Anticonvulsants are useful in the treatment of shooting, lancinating or shock-like pain, and enhance control of neuropathic pain when added to an antidepressant. A safer new agent in this class is gabapentin. Monitoring is required to avoid specific toxicities when other anticonvulsants are used. Antiarrhythmics are also effective in the treatment of neuropathic pain.

Corticosteroids are effective in pain associated with inflammation and may decrease pain due to CNS and spinal cord tumors. Alpha-1 antagonists and alpha-2 agonists are agents used in the treatment of sympathetically mediated pain. Blockade of alpha receptors located on the peripheral nerve terminals by the alpha-1 antagonists and inhibition of norepinephrine release from the postganglionic sympathetic terminals are considered to be their mechanisms of action.

Several drugs are used to secure comfort of patients undergoing palliative care. Subcutaneous midazolam infusion, titrated intravenous barbiturates and propofol, and oral, parenteral, and intrathecal ketamine have been used along with opiates with often dramatic improvement in patient comfort.[23, 30, 36, 52, 60, 71, 72, 74] Optimal use of co-analgesics often requires a pain specialist experienced in the treatment of the targeted conditions.

Nonpharmacological Measures

Nonpharmacological measures are important for maximizing both patient comfort and functional status. The use of physical therapy interventions such as heat, cold, electrical stimulation, massage, hands on mobilization, and stretching techniques and well as appropriate exercise programs may be very helpful in relieving pain such as mechanical low back pain or pain secondary to muscle spasm. Biofeedback and relaxation training, guided imagery conditioning, and cognitive restructuring may be helpful in decreasing pain and anxiety and in improving the patient's sense of self-control. Acupuncture has been used in the management of cancer pain, although outcome studies are inconclusive about its efficacy.

When pharmacological and other noninvasive means have proven insufficient in the management of a patient's pain, invasive management strategies may be appropriate. Palliative radiation therapy may be useful for the treatment of painful metastatic lesions. Neural blockade with local anesthetics and steroids can provide what is often temporary but significant relief of pain in localized areas.[22] Implanted epidural and intrathecal drug delivery systems may produce profound analgesia with minimal side effects in patients who experience insufficient pain relief or intolerable side effects from analgesics via other routes of administration. Neurolytic blockade and neurosurgical ablative procedures are usually steps of last choice.[5, 12, 22] These techniques bring with them the possibility of significant long-term side effects such as loss of motor of sensory function in the targeted area, while achieving the desired effect of pain relief is uncertain at best.

MONITORING OF PAIN MANAGEMENT QUALITY

The application of quality assessment and improvement methodologies is considered the most successful way to facilitate progress in the field of cancer pain relief. An interdisciplinary team effort is necessary to provide the required expertise and outcome analysis. Educational efforts should address the patients, their families, and also the caregivers. Active assessment of pain at all levels of care and efforts to assure continuity of care at all levels is imperative. Availability of pain specialists and allocation of funds for treatment, education and research are highly desirable.[1,2,9,10,32,51]

CONCLUSIONS

Optimal pain management remains an unrealized goal for many patients with gynecological tumors. However, the continued education of health-care providers and the increase in the number of physicians with specialty training in the management of pain provides the promise of significant progress toward this goal in the coming years. Global use of simple pharmacological methods and the addition of more complex interventions will allow the caregiver to minimize the patients pain and improve their functional capacity and quality of life.

REFERENCES

1. Jacox A, Carr DB, Payne R, et al. Management of Cancer Pain Guideline Panel. Management of Cancer Pain. Clinical Practice Guideline. AHCPR Pub. No. 94–0592. Rockville, MD: Agency for Health Care Policy and Research, Public Health Service, U.S. Department of Health and Human Services; 1994.
2. Acute Pain Management Guideline Panel. Acute Pain management: Operative or Medical Procedures and Trauma. Clinical Practice Guideline. AHCPR Pub. No. 92–0032. Rockville, MD: Agency for Health Care Policy and Research, Public Health Service, U.S. Department of Health and Human Services; 1992.
3. Ad Hoc Committee on Cancer Pain of the American Society of Clinical Oncology. Cancer pain assessment and treatment curriculum guidelines. J Clin Oncol 1992;10(12):1975–1982.
4. Adams F, Fernandez F, Andersson BS. Emergency pharmaco-therapy of delirium in the critically ill cancer patient. Psychosomatics 1986;27(1 suppl):33–38.
5. Amano K, Kawamura H, Tanikawa T, et al. Bilateral versus unilateral percutaneous high cervical cordotomy as a surgical method of pain relief. Acta Neurochir (Wien) 1991;52(suppl):143–145.
6. American Cancer Society. Cancer and the Poor: A Report to the Nation. American Cancer Society; Atlanta, GA, 1989.
7. American Cancer Society. Questions and Answers About Pain Control: A Guide for People with Cancer and Their Families. American Cancer Society and the National Cancer Institute; 1992. p 76.
8. American Cancer Society. Cancer Facts and Figures – 1994. Atlanta, GA: American Cancer Society Inc.; 1994. p 1.
9. American Pain Society. Committee on Quality Assurance Standards. Standards for monitoring quality of analgesic treatment of acute pain and cancer pain. Oncol Nurs Forum 1990;17: 952–954.
10. American Pain Society. Committee of quality assurance standards. American Pain Society quality assurance standards for relief of acute pain and cancer pain. In: Bond MR, Charlton JE, Woolf CJ, editors. Proceedings of the Sixth World Congress of Pain. New York, NY: Elsevier Science Publications; 1991. p 185–190.
11. American Pain Society. Principles of Analgesic use in the Treatment of Acute Pain and Chronic Cancer Pain: A Concise Guide to Medical Practice. Skokie, IL: American Pain Society; 1992.
12. Arbit E, Galicich JH, Burt M, et al. Modified open thoracic rhizotomy for treatment of intractable chest wall pain of malignant etiology. Ann Thorac Surg 1989;48(6):820–823.
13. Attard AR, Corlett MJ, Kidner NJ, et al. Safety of early pain relief for acute abdominal pain. Br Med J 1992;305: 554.

14. AU E, LOPRINZI CL, DHODAPKAR M, et al. Regular use of a verbal pain scale improves the understanding of oncology inpatient pain intensity (12 references). J Clin Oncol 1994;12(12):2751.

15. AVELLANOSA AM, WEST CR. Experience with transcutaneous electrical nerve stimulation for relief of intractable pain in cancer patients. J Med 1982;2(3):203–213.

16. BACH FW, JENSEN TS, KASTRUP J, et al. The effect of intravenous lidocaine on nociceptive processing in diabetic neuropathy. Pain 1990;40(1):29–34.

17. BARBOUR LA, McGUIRE DB, KIRCHHOFF KT. Nonanalgesic methods of pain control used by cancer outpatients. Oncol Nurs Forum 1986;13(6):56–60.

18. BAUMANN TJ, BATENHORST RL, GRAVES DA, et al. Patient-controlled analgesia in the terminally ill cancer patient. Drug Intell Clin Pharm 1986;20(4):297–301.

19. BECK SL. The therapeutic use of music for cancer-related pain. Oncol Nurs Forum 1991;18(8):1327–1337.

20. BEHAR M, MAGORA F, OLSHWANG D, et al. Epidural morphine in treatment of pain. Lancet 1979;1(8115):527–529.

21. BOLUND C. Suicide and cancer: II. Medical and care factors in suicide by cancer patients in Sweden 1973–76. J Paychosoc Oncol 1985;3: 17–30.

22. BONICA KK, BUCKLEY FP, MORICCA G, et al. Neurolytic blockade and hypophysectomy. In: BONICA JJ, editor. The Management of Pain. Vol. 1, 2nd ed. Philadelphia, PA: Lea and Febiger; 1990. p 1980–2039.

23. BOTTOMLEY DM, HANKS GW. Subcutaneous midazolam infusion in palliative care. J Pain Symptom Manage 1990;5: 259–261.

24. BREITBART W, HOLLAND JC. Psychiatric complications of cancer. In: BRAIN MC, CARBONE PP, editors. Current Therapy in Hematology-Oncology—3. Philadelphia, PA: BC Decker; 1988. p 268–274.

25. BREITBART W. Cancer pain and suicide. In: FOLEY K, BONICA JJ, VENTAFRIDDA V, editors. Advances in Pain Research and Therapy. Vol. 16. New York, NY: Raven Press; 1990. p 399–412.

26. BREITBART W. Suicide in cancer patients. Oncology 1987;1: 49–53.

27. BRENNAN SC, REDD WH, JACOBSEN PB, et al. Anxiety and panic during magnetic resonance scans. Lancet 1988;2(8609):512.

28. BROMAGE PR, CAMPORRESI EM, DURANT PA, NIELSEN CH. Rostral spread of epidural morphine. Anesthesiology 1982;56: 4341–4346.

29. BROSE WG, COUSINS MJ. Subcutaneous lidocaine for treatment of neuropathic cancer pain. Pain 1991;45(2):145–148.

30. BRUERA E, BRENNEIS C, MacDONALD RN. Continuous Sc infusion of narcotics for the treatment of cancer pain: an update. Cancer Treat Rep 1987;71(10):953–958.

31. BRUERA E, SCHOELLER T, MONTEJO G. Organic hallucinosis in patients receiving high doses of opiates for cancer pain. Pain 1992;48(3):397–399.

32. BRUNIER G, CARSON MG, HARRISON DE. What do nurses know and believe about patients with pain? Results of a hospital survey. J Pain Sympt Man 1995;10(6):436.

33. BURKBERG J, PENMAN D, HOLLAND JC. Depression in hospitalized cancer patients. Psychosom Med 1984;46(3):199–212.

34. BYRNE TN. Spinal cord compression from epidural metastases. N Engl J Med 1992;327(9):639–645.

35. CASSEL EJ. The nature of suffering and the goals of medicine. N Engl J Med 1982;306(11):639–645.

36. CHARAP AD. The knowledge, attitudes and experience of medical personnel treating pain in the terminally ill. Mt Sinai J Med 1978;45: 561.

37. CHERNY NI, PORTENOY RK. Cancer pain: principles of assessment and syndromes. In: WALL PD, MELZACK R, editors. Textbook of Pain. 3rd ed. Edinburgh: Churchill Livingstone; 1994. p 787.

38. CHINERY R, BEAUCHAMP RD, SHYR Y, et al. Antioxidants reduce cyclooxygenase-2 expression, prostaglandin production, and proliferation in colorectal cancer cells. Cancer Res 1998;58(11):2323–2327.

39. CHRISTENSEN O, CHRISTENSEN P, SONNENSCHEIN C, et al. Analgesic effect of intraarticular morphine: a controlled randomized and double-blind study. Acta Anaesth Scand 1996;40(7):842.

40. CLARK RF, WEI EM, ANDERSON PO. Meperidine: therapeutic use and toxicity. J Emerg Med 1995;13(6):797.

41. CLEELAND CS, GONIN R, HATFIELD AK, et al. Pain and its treatment in outpatients with metastatic cancer. New Engl J Med 1994;330: 592.
42. CLEELAND CS. The impact of pain on patients with cancer. Cancer 1984;54: 263–267.
43. CRYER B, FELDMAN M. Cyclooxygenase-1 and cyclooxygenase-2 selectivity of widely used nonsteroidal anti-inflammatory drugs. Am J Med 1998;104; 5: 413–421.
44. DAUT RL, CLEELAND CS. The prevalence and severity of pain in cancer. Cancer 1982;50: 1913–1918.
45. DEROGATIS LR, MARROW GR, FETTING J, et al. The prevalence of psychiatric disorders among cancer patients. JAMA 1983;249: 751–757.
46. EDWARDS WT. Optimizing opioid treatment of postoperative pain. J Pain Symptom Manage 1990;5: S24.
47. EISENBERG E, BERKEY CS, CARR DB, et al. Efficacy and safety of nonsteroidal antiinflamatory drugs for cancer pain: a meta-analysis. J Clin Oncol 1994;12(12):2756.
48. FOLEY KM. Pain syndromes in patients with cancer. In: BONICA JJ, WENTAFRIDDA V, editors. Advances in Pain Research and Therapy. Vol. 2. New York, NY: Raven Press; 1979. p 59.
49. FOLEY KM. The treatment of cancer pain. N Engl J Med 1985;313: 84–95.
50. FORSYTH PA, POSNER JB. Headaches in patients with brain tumors: a study of 111 patients. Neurology 1993;43(9):1678.
51. GONZALES GR, ELLIOTT KJ, PORTENOY RK, FOLEY KM. The impact of a comprehensive evaluation in the management of cancer pain. Pain 1991;47: 141.
52. GREENE WR, DAVIS WH. Titrated intravenous barbiturates in control of symptoms in patients with terminal cancer. South Med J 1991;84: 332–337.
53. GUPTA R, RAJA N. Chronic pain: pathophysiology and its therapeutic implications. Curr Rev Pain 1996;1: 1–9.
54. HAGEN NA, ELWOOD T, ERNST S. Cancer pain emergencies: a protocol for management. J Pain Sympt Man 1997;14(1):45.
55. HANKS GW, JUSTINS DM. Cancer pain: management. Lancet 1992;339: 1031–1036.
56. JANUSZ JM, YOUNG PA, RIDGEWAY JM. New cyclooxygenase-2/5 lipoxygenase inhibitors. 3. 7-*tert*-Butyl-2,3-dihydro-3,3-dimethylbenzofuran derivatives as gastrointestinal safe antiinflamatory and analgesic agents: variations at the 5 position. J Med Chem 1989;41(18):3515–3529.
57. LEHMAN KA. Patient-controlled analgesia for post-operative pain. In: MAX MM, PORTENOY RK, LASKA E, editors. Design of Analgesic Clinical Trials. New York, NY: Raven Press; 1991. p 481.
58. LEVIN D, CLEELAND CS, DAR R. Public attitudes toward cancer pain. Cancer 1985;56: 2337–2339.
59. MARKS RM, SACHAR EJ. Undertreatment of medical inpatients with narcotic analgesics. Ann Intern Med 1973;78: 173.
60. Moyle J. The use of propofol in palliative medicine. J Pain Symptom Manage 1995;10: 643–646.
61. NIV D, DEVOR M. Preemptive analgesia in the relief of postoperative pain. Curr Rev Pain 1996;1: 79–92.
62. PORTENOY RK, HAGEN NA. Breakthrough pain: definition, prevalence and characteristics. Pain 1990;41: 273.
63. PORTENOY RK, KORNBLITH AB, WONG G, et al. Pain in ovarian cancer: prevalence, characteristics, and associated symptoms. Cancer 1994;74: 907.
64. PORTENOY RK. Cancer pain: epidemiology and syndromes. Cancer 1989;63: 2298.
65. PORTENOY RK. Cancer pain: pathophysiology and syndromes. Lancet 1992;339; 1026–1031.
66. ROSEN SM. Procedural control of cancer pain. Semin Oncol 1994;21: 740–747.
67. SCHIRRMACHER V. Cancer metastasis: experimental approaches, theoretical concepts, and impacts for treatment strategies. Adv Cancer Res 1985;43: 1.
68. SCHUG SA, ZECH D, DORR U. Cancer pain management according to WHO analgesic guidelines. J Pain Symptom Manage 1990;5: 27–32.
69. SCHWARTZ PE. Cancer in pregnancy. In GUSBERG SB, editor. New York: Churchill Livingstone; 1988. p 725–754.
70. SUGARBAKER EV. Patterns of metastasis in human malignancies. Cancer Biol Rev 1981;2: 235.
71. TOBIAS JD, PHIPPS S, SMITH B, MULHERN RK. Oral ketamine premedication to alleviate the distress of invasive procedures in pediatric oncology patients. Pediatrics 1992;90(4):537.

72. TWYCROSS RG, FAIRFIELD S. Pain in far-advanced cancer. Pain 1982;14: 303.
73. VENTAFRIDDA V, CARACENI A, GAMBA A. Field-testing of the WHO guidelines for cancer pain relief: summary report of demonstration projects. In: FOLEY KM, BONICA JJ, VENTAFRIDDA V, editors. Proceedings of the Second International Congress of Cancer Pain. Advances in Pain Research and Therapy. Vol 16. New York, NY: Raven Press; 1990. p 451–464.
74. World Health Organization. Cancer Pain Relief and Palliative Care. Geneva: World Health Organization; 1990.
75. VESELIS RA. Intravenous narcotics in the ICU. Crit Care Clin 1990;6(2):305–313.

Chapter 16

Fertility Preservation in the Gynecologic Cancer Patient

Nicole Fleming, MD

INTRODUCTION

The American Society of Clinical Oncology has recently highlighted the lack of research on the reproductive concerns of cancer survivors.[1] Cancer treatment can negatively impact female fertility through surgical removal of all or part of the reproductive organs, administration of chemotherapy drugs that are toxic to the ovary, and radiation therapy which causes permanent ovarian failure and uterine damage in high doses.[2] In addition to the hormonal disruption and reproductive failure that may occur from treatment, female cancer survivors have also reported sexual morbidity, bowel and bladder changes, chronic menopausal symptoms, and emotional and relationship alterations.[3] With the recent advances in oncology, survival rates are increasing, and issues affecting long-term cancer survivors, such as fertility preservation, are becoming more widely recognized. Surgical, medical, and technological advances have enabled oncologists to provide fertility-sparing options for patients undergoing therapy. The options available to any particular cancer patient will depend on the age of the patient at the time of diagnosis and treatment, cancer type, severity, location, and type of treatment.[2]

RADIATION

The ovaries are radiation-sensitive organs with resulting progressive and irreversible damage at increasing dosages. The likelihood of permanent ovarian failure following radiation increases with advancing age. Individuals over the age of 40 years may experience permanent ovarian failure with exposure of as little as 500–600 cGy, while doses greater than 1500–2000 cGy are needed to produce permanent ovarian

Gynecologic Oncology: Evidence-Based Perioperative and Supportive Care, Second Edition.
Edited by Scott E. Lentz, Allison E. Axtell and Steven A. Vasilev.
© 2011 John Wiley & Sons, Inc. Published 2011 by John Wiley & Sons, Inc.

failure in women less than 40 years.[4] Patients who require high dose radiation therapy (4000–4500 cGy or more) to the whole pelvis, a standard treatment modality seen in many gynecologic cancers, should be counseled regarding the loss of reproductive capability.[5] The damaging effects of radiation are not only seen in the ovary, but direct exposure of pelvic radiation on the uterus can also produce long-term sequelae on pregnancy outcomes. Uterine radiation is associated with infertility, spontaneous pregnancy loss, and intrauterine growth restriction.[6] Direct effects on the uterus after abdominal radiation in young girls being treated for childhood cancers have included irreversible changes in uterine musculature and blood flow. Significantly decreased uterine volume, up to 40% of normal adult size, has been observed in this population, which is unresponsive to hormone therapy.[7] Doppler flow also decreased among patients who received radiation, suggesting damage to vasculature. Altogether these changes can lead to inadequate placentation and obstetrical complications. Spontaneous abortions occur at a rate of 38% compared to 12% in the general population, preterm labor 62% compared with 9%, and low birth weight infants 62% compared with 6%. There is no risk of teratogenicity if the radiation is not administered during the pregnancy.[8]

CHEMOTHERAPY

Chemotherapy affects rapidly dividing cells, and thus ovarian toxicity can occur through impairment of follicular maturation, depletion of primordial follicles, and ovarian stromal fibrosis.[9] Rates of amenorrhea vary based on the age of the patient and the duration and dose of chemotherapy delivered.[10] Alkylating agents, such as cyclophosphamide and ifosfamide, have been shown to have significant toxicity on developing oocytes and primordial follicles because they do not require cell proliferation for their cytotoxic action.[9] Other gonadotoxic chemotherapy agents include vinca alkaloids, antimetabolites, and platinum agents. In a study by Byrne et al., patients diagnosed with cancer and treated between ages 13 and 19 were four times more likely to undergo menopause between the ages of 21–25. There was significant increased relative risk of menopause during the early 20s after treatment with either radiotherapy alone (relative risk 3.7) or alkylating agents alone (relative risk 9.2). By age 31, 42% of these patients had reached menopause compared with 5% of controls[11] (**Level II-3**).

Reproductive function has been more specifically assessed in long-term ovarian germ cell tumor survivors after platinum-based chemotherapy. One hundred and thirty-two survivors from GOG (Gynecologic Oncology Group)-participating institutions were identified and matched to controls. Median survivor age at diagnosis was 24.3 years, with a median age at time of study entry of 35.5 years, giving an approximate 10-year follow-up. Of the survivors, 53.8% underwent fertility-sparing surgery, and 87% of fertile survivors were having menstrual function at the time of the study. Of the 71 patients who underwent fertility-sparing surgery and platinum-based chemotherapy, only two women (3%) had documented premature menopause. Twenty-four survivors had children after cancer treatment. Of these, the first pregnancy resulted in a live birth for 20 women (83%). Seven survivors (5.3%) reported having spontaneous abortions after cancer treatment[12] (**Level II-2**).

PRESERVATION OF OVARIAN FUNCTION DURING CHEMOTHERAPY

The impact of premature ovarian failure (POF) after chemotherapy and its associated infertility is of great importance to premenopausal women diagnosed with cancer. Fertility preservation options depend on the patient's age, type of treatment, diagnosis, whether she has a partner, the time available, and the potential that cancer involves or has metastasized to her ovaries.[13]

Embryo Cryopreservation

Embryo cryopreservation is considered an established fertility preservation method and has been routinely used for storing surplus embryos after *in vitro* fertilization (IVF) for infertility treatment. This approach typically requires approximately 2 weeks of ovarian stimulation with daily injections of follicle-stimulating hormone from the onset of menses. At the appropriate time, an injection of HCG is administered to start the ovulatory cascade, and the oocytes are collected by transvaginal needle aspiration. Oocytes are fertilized *in vitro* and cryopreserved after fertilization. Because stimulation must be started at the onset of menses and takes 2 weeks, a delay of 2–6 weeks in chemotherapy initiation may be required if the patient does not see a reproductive specialist early in her menstrual cycle. Live birth rates after embryo cryopreservation depend on the patient's age and the total number of embryos cryopreserved and may be lower than with fresh embryos.[14] The options of cryopreservation of embryos after IVF before chemotherapy are relevant to those who have a long-term partner, and may be unacceptable to single women. IVF might also not be relevant in patients who need urgent chemotherapy, or in diseases which could be aggravated by the increased pharmacologic levels of sex steroids.[15] This would also only be relevant in gynecologic malignancies whose type, stage, and grade of cancer could allow for fertility-sparing surgeries to be performed. For women with hormone-sensitive tumors, alternative hormonal stimulation approaches such as letrozole or tamoxifen have been developed to theoretically reduce the risk of estrogen exposure.[16] Recently, standard ovarian stimulation with coapplication of a progestin-releasing IUD has been reported to allow successful preservation of embryos in a patient with endometrial cancer[17] (**Level III**).

Oocyte Cryopreservation

Cryopreservation of unfertilized oocytes is another option for fertility preservation, especially for whom a partner is unavailable at the time of diagnosis. The oocytes are thawed later and fertilized *in vitro*. Ovarian stimulation and harvesting are similar to embryos.[14] Cryopreservation of unfertilized oocytes has been successful in rodents; however, research in human oocytes indicate that they are more prone to damage during cryopreservation than embryos. There have been approximately 120 deliveries with this approach, and the use of conventional slow-programmed cryopreservation and vitrification technologies may increase success rates[18] (**Level II-1**).

Ovarian Tissue Cryopreservation and Transplantation

One of the most promising options for fertility preservation prior to chemotherapy is ovarian tissue cryopreservation followed by transplantation of cryopreserved-thawed ovarian tissue. Ovarian transplantation can be to either orthotopic or heterotopic locations. Orthotopic transplantations consist of ovarian tissue grafts transplanted back to the ovary left *in situ*, ovarian fossa, or peritoneal sites, with most studies reporting recovery of ovarian function between 16 and 18 weeks (range 8–32 weeks)[19–24] (**Level III**). Heterotopic transplantation to other tissues such as subcutaneous, rectus abdominis, and breast tissue has also reported recovery of ovarian function between 12 and 18 weeks (range 8–26 weeks).[25–27] The world's first pregnancy and live birth with frozen-thawed ovarian tissue autotransplantation was reported by Donnez et al. (2004). The patient presented with stage IV Hodgkin's lymphoma and received multiagent chemotherapy and radiotherapy, and subsequently developed POF. Upon completion of treatment, her frozen-thawed ovarian cortical tissue was transplanted into a peritoneal window near the ovarian vessels and fimbria. The patient's follicle-stimulating hormone levels returned to normal at 9.5 months, and after 1 year of attempted natural conception, a successful spontaneous conception ending in a live birth was achieved.[19] Meirow et al. (2005) reported the first case of oocyte retrieval, IVF, and pregnancy in a 28-year-old non-Hodgkin's lymphoma patient, following orthotopic transplantation of cryopreserved-thawed ovarian tissue. The ovarian tissue was placed under the surface of the *in situ* ovary. The patient regained endocrine activity 9 months after transplantation, and a single mature oocyte was retrieved in the fourth IVF trial. Embryo transfer resulted in a normal pregnancy and delivery of a healthy baby.[21]

Ovarian Suppression

Ovarian suppression through gonadotropin-releasing hormone (GnRH) agonist or antagonist therapy, or with oral contraceptives (OC) during chemotherapy, is highly controversial as a method to maintain fertility. GnRH agonists act on the hypothalamic-pituitary axis to suppress ovarian function, protecting the germinal epithelium from the cytotoxic effects of chemotherapy. This hypothesis was first tested in 1981 by Glode et al., using a murine model which concluded that an antagonistic analog of GnRH appeared to protect male mice from the gonadal damage produced by cyclophosphamide.[28] However, human studies using GnRH agonists have been highly controversial. One of the largest studies to date evaluated 65 patients compared with retrospective controls showing a significant benefit in preserving menstrual function from ovarian suppression with GnRH analogs in women undergoing chemotherapy for Hodgkin's lymphoma. Two of 65 patients (3.1%) in the study group developed POF versus 17 of 46 patients (37%) in the control group ($p < 0.001$). Among the patients in the study group, 96.9% resumed cyclic ovarian function within 2 years and/or conceived versus 63% in the control group ($p < 0.001$). The relatively advanced ages (36 years old) of the two patients in the study group who developed POF may suggest that minimizing follicular loss may be efficient only in younger patients whose follicular reserve is above a certain limit[29] (**Level II-1**). Similarly, GnRH agonists appeared to prevent POF in premenopausal breast cancer patients being treated with chemotherapy[30] (**Level II-3**).

There have also been studies performed to determine whether suppression of ovarian function by OC would provide protection against ovarian cell death secondary to chemotherapy in young women. This was first looked at by Chapman and Sutcliffe in 1981 in six young women, aged 18–31 years, with Hodgkin's lymphoma treated with MVPP therapy (nitrogen mustard, vinblastine, procarbazine, and prednisone). Of the six women treated with OC during chemotherapy, five resumed normal menses at the end of MVPP, and one conceived[31] (**Level II-3**). However, Whitehead et al. (1983) found no protective effect from combination OC in patients receiving chemotherapy for Hodgkin's lymphoma. They studied 44 patients treated with MVPP, 9 of whom took OC during chemotherapy with median age 23 years. Seven of nine patients (77%) were either amenorrheic or oligomenorrheic after completion of treatment, and two (22%) resumed normal menses. These results were similar to the group not receiving OC, with 61% of patients amenorrheic or oligomenorrheic and 39% resuming normal menses[32] (**Level III**). Similarly, Elis et al. (2006) examined patients with non-Hodgkin's lymphoma, mean age 28 ± 7 years, who were treated with CHOP therapy (cyclophosphamide, adriamycin, vincristine, and prednisone). Twelve out of 36 women received either a GnRH analog or OC with chemotherapy. There were no significant differences between those patients receiving fertility-preserving measures versus the remainder concerning regular menstrual cycle recovery or pregnancies.[33] Due to the underpowered nature of these studies, no definitive conclusions can be reached. However, with recent data published by Behringer et al. (2005) showing statistically significant lower rates of amenorrhea in patients receiving OC and mostly BEACOPP therapy (bleomycin, etoposide, adriamycin, cyclophosphamide, procarbizine, and prednisone) (44.1% vs. 10.1%, $p < 0.0001$),[34] the role for OC for fertility preservation is uncertain and needs further investigation (**Level III**).

PRESERVATION OF OVARIAN FUNCTION DURING RADIATION

In a retrospective cohort multicenter study by the Childhood Cancer Survivor Study, factors associated with the development of acute ovarian failure were increased age at time of treatment, increased radiation doses (particularly >10 Gy), and exposure to alkylating agents (specifically procarbazine and cyclophosphamide)[35] (**Level II-3**).

In a separate cohort analyzed, women who received both an alkylating agent and abdominopelvic irradiation had a cumulative incidence of nonsurgical premature menopause of 30%[36] (**Level II-1**). Abdominopelvic radiotherapy as a part of the management of cancer clearly has deleterious effects on ovarian function. However, the modern age of computer-driven technology has permitted customization of radiation doses to conform to the tumor and spare normal tissues. It is important to recognize the tolerance doses of normal tissues with three-dimensional planning. The dose tolerance of the ovary is dependent on several factors including the volume irradiated, the total radiation dose, the fractionation schedule, and the patient's age at the time of treatment.[37] One of the early studies looking at the dose tolerance of the ovary was by the Children's Cancer Study Group. They assessed long-term female survivors of childhood acute lymphoblastic leukemia which showed a dose–response relationship of POF between 18 and 24 Gy for those patients receiving craniospinal irradiation[38] (**Level III**). More recently, Wallace et al. (2005) has calculated the effective sterilizing dose from birth to menopause. The effective sterilizing dose is the dose after which the primordial follicle population will decrease below 1000, or similarly, the dose that will induce immediate ovarian failure in 97.5% of the female population. The effective sterilizing dose for ovarian irradiation at birth is 20.3 Gy; at 10 years old, 18.4 Gy; at 20 years old, 16.5 Gy; and at 30 years old, 14.3 Gy[39] (**Level II-2**). The human oocyte is extremely radiosensitive with a low LD50 of approximately 2 Gy, or the dose of radiation required to destroy 50% of primordial follicles. Using such models can assist in predicting the age of ovarian failure after treatment with a known dose of radiotherapy.[40]

Modern improvements in radiation delivery allow the radiation oncologist to tailor highly conformal dose distributions to maximize target coverage and spare normal tissues. Radiation treatment planning systems now allow for meaningful assessment of the planned dose to the ovaries through dose–volume histograms.[37] Knowledge of the precise location of the ovaries during treatment is essential in determining ovarian dose during irradiation. Rigsby and Siegel (1994) found that the ovaries should be detectable on CT simulation for radiation planning in the majority of female patients older than 8 years old.[41] The position of the ovaries, however, can vary based on filling and emptying of the bladder. Nicholson et al. (2000) reported significant variation in the position of the ovaries was evident and around the pelvic inlet would have resulted in displacement of the ovaries into a region of high dose irradiation.[42] Instructing the patient on bladder filling and including a safety margin when delineating the ovary during radiation treatment planning may provide for better sparing of the ovaries. Alternatively, daily three-dimensional imaging may provide the framework to customize treatments to the appropriate anatomy immediately before treatment[37] (**Level III**).

Limiting the ovarian dose without compromising target coverage is the goal in preserving ovarian function. Transfixing the ovaries out of the radiation fields before therapy by a procedure called oophoropexy or ovarian transposition may allow for better sparing of the ovaries from radiation effects.[37] For primary pelvic malignancies, a lateral ovarian transposition technique is used; however, for cases of lymphoid irradiation, the ovaries are frequently moved medially behind the uterus away from the pelvic lymph node fields. Hadar et al. (1994) reported improved likelihood of shielding the ovaries during pelvic radiotherapy when a lateral ovarian transposition is performed as opposed to a medial transposition.[43] Thibaud et al. (1992) reported on 18 girls (median age 9.4 years) who underwent ovarian transposition before radiotherapy for various malignancies including Hodgkin's disease, Ewing's sarcoma, medulloblastoma, and gynecologic tumors. The ovaries were surgically transfixed just below the iliac crest (15 cases) or posterolateral to the uterus (3 cases). The calculated dose to the ovary was up to 9.5 Gy. At 8.6 ± 0.9 year follow-up after ovarian transposition, 16 of the 18 girls were menstruating.[44] Belinson et al. (1984) calculated that the scatter dose to transposed ovarian tissue when delivering 45 Gy in posterior-anterior pelvic fields was 15.8 Gy and using a four-field box technique (posterior-anterior, right and left laterals) 21.9 Gy[45] (**Level III**).

Historically, rates of cessation of ovarian function after transposition alone have been reported to be as high as 40%[45–48] (**Level III**). This suggests that surgery alone can cause enough insult to the ovary to cause POF by vascular compromise leading to atresia, loss of function, and fibrosis. Several early studies of ovarian transposition with radiation after radical hysterectomy for cervical cancer reported rates of ovarian preservation ranging between 50% and 70%.[49,50] More recently, Buekers et al. (2001) analyzed 102 women (median age 32.3 years) undergoing surgical management with ovarian retention for early stage cervical cancer. Eighty patients had one or both ovaries transposed at the time of exploration for radical hysterectomy or staging lymphadenectomy. For those patients undergoing pelvic radiation, unilateral oophorectomy, and contralateral ovarian transposition, ovarian survival was 4 months vs. 43 months ($p = 0.003$) in those who had both ovaries transposed. The mean age at menopause of those with unilateral oophorectomy was 34.2 years and all patients with concurrent unilateral oophorectomy lost ovarian function by 1 year after treatment. Forty-one percent of the patients undergoing radiotherapy with bilateral ovarian transposition had ovarian function after 1 year. The mean age at menopause for these patients was 36.6 years. Ninety-two percent of these patients reached menopause by age 46 years. This mean age at menopause was significantly different from the reported population mean of 51.3 years ($p < 0.0001$)[51] (**Level III**).

CERVICAL CANCER

The widespread use of cervical cancer screening has resulted in the overall younger age and earlier stage at diagnosis, and an increase in the number of younger women diagnosed who desire to preserve reproductive function. Early stage cervical cancer is treatable by either surgical therapy, consisting of radical hysterectomy, or radiation therapy. Neither form of therapy allows preservation of a functional utero-ovarian system for reproductive purposes. In the younger patient, surgical therapy is usually preferred in an attempt to preserve ovarian function and avoid potential long-term effects of definitive radiation therapy. Fertility issues will become more pronounced in the management of cervical cancer as more women have delayed childbearing.[52]

Squamous cell carcinoma *in situ* and FIGO (International Federation of Gynecologists and Obstetricians) stage IA1 invasive squamous cell cervical lesions (microscopic lesions with stromal invasion less than 3 mm in depth and less than 7 mm wide) can be managed by a cold knife cone biopsy. The margins of the cone biopsy need to be negative in stage IA1 lesions managed by cone biopsy as definitive therapy.[53] However, unlike squamous lesions, management of adenocarcinoma *in situ* (AIS) or microinvasive adenocarcinoma lesions is more complex. These lesions are usually multifocal and generally located high in the endocervical canal. Traditional management has been hysterectomy. However, some studies have analyzed more conservative treatment options for women desiring fertility preservation, with mixed results.[2] Early studies by Poynor et al. (1995) and McHale et al. (2001) found 47%–60% recurrence rates, respectively, for patients with either AIS or microinvasive adenocarcinoma managed conservatively. In addition, Poyner's study challenged the previously held belief that margin status was a helpful predictor of recurrence and treatment success, with 40% of patients with negative margins having a second surgical specimen containing AIS.[54,55] However, these studies have been criticized due to limited sample size. In contrast, a larger retrospective series was performed by Shin et al. (2000) of patients with AIS. Of 132 women treated with cone biopsy for AIS, 95 (72%) were managed conservatively after cold knife cone or loop electrical excisional procedure alone, and 37 (28%) underwent hysterectomy. Median age of diagnosis in the conservative management group was 29 years and 40 years in the hysterectomy groups ($p < 0.0001$). Of those who underwent hysterectomy, margin status was a more accurate predictor of residual disease. Thirteen (62%) of 21 patients with positive margins had residual disease in the hysterectomy specimen compared to 1 (6%) of 16 patients who had negative margins ($p < 0.0001$). Nine of 24 patients (38%) who underwent repeat cone biopsies for positive margins had residual AIS. Of those patients conservatively managed, nine women underwent repeat cone biopsies for abnormal follow-up, three of whom had cervical intraepithelial neoplasia. There were no recurrences of AIS or invasive adenocarcinoma.[56] Another retrospective multi-institutional study by Bull-Phelps et al. (2007) analyzed a total of 101 patients undergoing conization for AIS with median age 29 years. Cold knife conization had a higher efficacy at achieving negative margins (72% vs. 47%, $p = 0.036$) versus loop excision. Thirty-seven women underwent repeat conization during follow-up, with 21 being performed within 3 months due to positive or unevaluable margins. Of these 21 patients, 3 had residual AIS with positive margins, and 4 had residual AIS with negative margins. Thirty-five women had a total of 49 pregnancies during a mean follow-up of 51 months. No invasive cervical adenocarcinomas were observed during the study interval[57] (**Level III**). McHale had four patients with stage IA1 adenocarcinoma of the cervix treated with cone biopsy with negative margins. Three patients had successful subsequent pregnancies and there were no reported recurrences in all four patients.[55] Schorge et al. (2000) treated five patients with stage IA1 adenocarcinoma of the cervix with cold knife cone biopsy all with negative margins and no lymph-vascular space invasion. None of the patients developed recurrent disease in the limited follow-up period[58] (**Level III**). For young patients desiring to maintain reproductive capacity, AIS appears to be safely managed by cold knife conization and diligent surveillance. Microinvasive adenocarcinoma of the cervix has an excellent prognosis; however, conservative management with conization alone should be undertaken with caution until safety has been more extensively studied[59] (**Level III**).

In 1987, French surgeon Dargent developed a fertility-sparing surgical procedure for the treatment of FIGO stage IA2 to IB invasive squamous cell carcinoma or adenocarcinoma of the cervix. It was initially called a radical vaginal trachelectomy (RVT) but is now performed with a laparoscopic lymphadenectomy first, to evaluate for nodal metastases first on frozen section. The trachelectomy specimen is also sent for frozen section with a clear endocervical margin of 5–8 mm required for adequate treatment, and at least 1 cm of endocervix left for preservation of fertility. If adequate margins are achieved, a cerclage is then placed. Dargent covers the cerclage with vaginal epithelium to avoid ascending infections (Saling procedure). Cesarean section is necessary for delivery, and patency of the cervical os is digitally restored at the time of cesarean.[60] Early studies from a total of 224 women resulted in a 53% live birth rate, with 35% of births less than 34 weeks.[60–64] Sonoda et al. (2008) performed a retrospective review of 43 radical vaginal trachelectomies with laparoscopic lymphadenectomies at Memorial Sloan-Kettering Cancer Center. Median age was 31 years. FIGO stages for the group were IB1 (28), IA2 (7), and IA1 with lymphovascular invasion (8). Histologic type included squamous (24), adenocarcinoma (16), and adenosquamous (3). Two patients (5%) underwent complete hysterectomy due to extensive endocervical disease. Five patients (12%) underwent adjuvant chemoradiation for pathologic risk factors determined on final pathology. Eleven (79%) of 14 women who were trying to get pregnant were able to conceive. Four of these (36%) required assisted reproductive techniques to conceive. With a median follow-up of 21 months, one recurrence in a patient with IB1 adenocarcinoma of the cervix was reported. Postoperative complications included two patients requiring drainage of an infected lymphocyst by interventional radiology, one patient requiring hysterectomy due to vaginal bleeding 13 days posttrachelectomy, and one patient requiring temporary ureteral stents due to edema at the ureterovesical orifices.[52] Beiner et al. (2008) performed a case control analysis of 90 RVT patients matched to 90 radical hysterectomy patients with stage IA2 to IB cervical carcinomas. Median follow-up was 51 months and 58 months, respectively. Histology was matched with 49% of each group having adenocarcinoma and 43% squamous cell carcinoma of the cervix. All patients had negative pelvic lymph nodes. There were five (5.5%) recurrences diagnosed in the RVT group compared to one (1.1%) recurrence in the radical hysterectomy group. There were no recurrences in the remaining cervical stump or uterus, and four of five recurrences were outside the pelvis. The 5-year survival rates were 99% and 100%, respectively ($p = 0.55$)[65] (**Level II-2**). However, pregnancy rates were not assessed in this study. A recent review of the literature by Sonoda et al. (2008) totaling 548 patients revealed a 4% recurrence rate and 2.6% death rate after RVT alone.[52, 62, 63, 66–70] Pregnancy outcomes were also assessed in 435 patients after RVT. There were 204 conceptions leading a 23% first trimester loss rate, and a 10.3% second trimester loss rate. One hundred and sixteen (56.9%) patients successfully had a third trimester delivery with only eight (3.9%) patients delivering in the second trimester[52, 62, 67, 68, 70–72] (**Level III**). With favorable oncologic and obstetric outcomes reported in review of the literature, radical trachelectomy may provide young women an option for preserving their uterus for future childbearing while serving as an adequate treatment option for early stage cervical cancers.

ENDOMETRIAL CANCER

Endometrial cancer is primarily a disease of the postmenopausal woman, although 25% of the cases occur in premenopausal patients, with only 5% occurring in patients younger than 40 years of age.[5] Most cases occurring in younger women are due to hyperestrogenism related to obesity or chronic anovulation, and thus have well-differentiated histologies. Younger women who desire fertility preservation may want conservative over surgical management. Progestins have been routinely used to treat simple hyperplasia and complex hyperplasia without atypia in young women. Medroxyprogesterone acetate (Provera) 10 mg for 10–14 days each month or continuously for 3–6 months has regression rates reported in 98%–100% of patients. The OC pill has also been used. Depot medroxyprogesterone acetate (Depo-Provera) 150 mg intramuscularly every 3 months can also be given if compliance is an issue. Megestrol (Megace) 40 mg two to four times daily for 3–12 months has reported regression rates of 94%.[73]

The use of progestins in the treatment of endometrial adenocarcinoma has been supported in several retrospective studies and case reports[73–81] (**Level III**). Imai et al. (2001) treated 15 young women aged 24–38 years with grade 1 to 2 endometrial cancer with high dose medroxyprogesterone acetate (400–800mg) daily for 18–64 weeks. Median treatment length was 29 weeks. Endometrial sampling was performed every 4 weeks. Medroxyprogesterone acetate was maintained for 8–12 weeks after regression of the lesion by sampling. The patients were followed for a mean of 59 months from the start of progestin therapy. Seven of 12 patients with grade 1 lesions and one of the two with grade 2 lesions regressed (53%). Three of the initial responders and one additional patient on maintenance therapy (50%) recurred 19–28 weeks after discontinuation of treatment. Of the six patients attempting to conceive, two were successful, both requiring assisted reproductive technology.[80] Ramirez et al. (2004) reviewed the use of hormonal therapy in grade 1 endometrial adenocarcinoma in 81 patients. Sixty-two (76%) patients responded to treatment, with median time to response being 12 weeks (range 4–60 weeks). Fifteen (24%) patients who initially responded to treatment recurred. The median time to recurrence was 19 months (range 6–44 months). Ten (67%) patients with recurrence ultimately underwent total abdominal hysterectomy. Residual endometrial carcinoma was found in six patients (60%). Nineteen patients (23%) never responded. Twenty patients were able to become pregnant at least once after completing treatment. The median follow-up was 36 weeks (range 0 weeks to 30 years). No patients died of their disease.[81]

Because oral progestins have been associated with poor compliance and systemic side effects, the levonorgestrol-releasing intrauterine system (LNG-IUS) has been more recently used to treat endometrial hyperplasia or as an adjunct to oral progestin therapy for early endometrial cancer. There have been a few case reports with regression of stage I grade 1 endometrial cancer with LNG-IUS[82, 83] (**Level III**). Montz et al. (2002) reported treatment of 12 patients with presumed stage IA grade 1 endometrioid cancer. Histologic studies identified no residual carcinoma in 6 of 12 women at 3 months, 7 of 11 women at 6 months, 7 of 9 women at 9 months, and 6 of 8 women at 12 months. One patient with negative endometrial biopsies at 6 and 9 months had endometrioid carcinoma identified by dilation and curettage at 12 months. Further recurrence of endometrial cancer was not found in any of the 6 women who had complete regression at 12 months and continued the LNG-IUS for as long as 36 months. Three of the 12 patients had associated expulsion of the IUD between 6 and 9 months after placement[84] (**Level II-2**).

Altogether, progestin therapy can be considered in highly motivated and compliant patients with presumed stage I grade 1 endometrial cancers. A hysteroscopy and curettage should be performed pretreatment to assess the entire endometrial cavity.[2] Imaging and a CA 125 test should be performed to assess the ovaries, since a 16%–29% rate of ovarian metastasis or synchronous ovarian and endometrial cancers has been reported in young patients.[61] Endometrial sampling should be performed every 3–6 months or if the patient has any persistent bleeding on this regimen. Following treatment, the patient should attempt pregnancy.[2]

OVARIAN CANCER

Germ Cell Tumors

Malignant germ cell tumors account for <5% of all ovarian malignancies. However, most occur during adolescence and early adulthood, and decisions regarding management and fertility preservation become important. The current standard of treatment for all germ cell tumors is a unilateral salpingo-oophorectomy and staging consisting of an omentectomy, cytologic washings, peritoneal biopsies, and pelvic and para-aortic lymph node sampling. The contralateral ovary is not biopsied unless grossly involved with tumor due to risks of future infertility related to peritoneal adhesions or ovarian failure. Prompt initiation of appropriate chemotherapy is the critical factor for young patients with advanced malignant germ cell tumors, most notably the BEP (bleomycin, etoposide, and cisplatin) regimen. Gershenson et al. have reported effective treatment for these tumors with the BEP regimen with future fertility seemingly unaffected[85, 86] (**Level III**). Low et al. (2000) reviewed 74 patients undergoing conservative surgery for malignant ovarian germ cell tumors, retaining the uterus and contralateral ovary to preserve ovarian function, with or without chemotherapy. Mean age was 20.9 years (range 10–35 years). Majority of patients (75.7%) had stage I tumors, 4.1% stage II, 14.9% stage III, and 5.4% stage IV tumors. Adjuvant chemotherapy was administered to 47 patients (63.5%). Mean follow-up was 52.1 months. Survival for patients with stage I disease was 98.2% and for patients with advanced disease 94.4%. There were seven recurrences (99.5%) and two deaths (2.7%). During chemotherapy 61.7% of patients developed amenorrhea but 91.5% of patients resumed normal menstrual function on completion of chemotherapy. Fourteen live births were recorded in the chemotherapy group. Altogether, the surgical approach in young patients with malignant ovarian germ cell tumors confined to a single ovary should aim to preserve fertility. Advanced disease is not usually accompanied by contralateral ovarian disease and should not necessarily contraindicate conservative surgery[87] (**Level III**).

Tumors of Low Malignant Potential

Low malignant potential (LMP) tumors are epithelial ovarian tumors with histologic features of malignant tumors but without identifiable stromal invasion. They account for approximately 15% of all epithelial ovarian cancers, with more than 50% occurring in women under the age of 40.[88] Patients with LMP tumors have a 10-year survival rate of 95%. Unilateral salpingo-oophorectomy and staging is the standard treatment for younger women[89] (**Level III**). However, the risk of a new primary lesion or recurrence after conservative management ranges from 0% to 19%.[90–95] Rao et al. (2005) reviewed 38 (15%) of 249 women who underwent fertility-sparing surgery for ovarian LMP tumors. Median age was 26 years (range 15–39). Thirty-four (17%) of 196 stage I patients underwent fertility-sparing surgery versus 4 (98%) of 53 stage II to III patients. None of the 38 patients received adjuvant therapy. Six (16%) of 38 patients recurred with fertility-sparing surgery versus 1 (4%) when complete resection was performed[96] (**Level III**). This was similar to reports by Zanetta et al. (2001) who reported disease recurrence of 19% in women undergoing fertility-sparing surgery versus 5% with more radical surgery.[91] Because these tumors occur in young women, the role of ovarian cystectomy, rather than unilateral salpingo-oophorectomy, has also been reported in a small number of cases. Plante (2000) reported a recurrence rate after cystectomy for all stages which was similar to that after unilateral salpingo-oophorectomy, ranging from 12% to 15%.[61] However, Morice et al. (2001) found that the recurrence rate, treating all stages, after cystectomy was 36%. His analysis included 12 of 44 patients (27%) with stage II or III disease being treated conservatively with either cystectomy or unilateral salpingo-oophorectomy. Fourteen of 44 patients treated conservatively were able to achieve 17 pregnancies. Four achieved pregnancy after a repeat cystectomy for a tumor recurrence. He concluded that cystectomy be reserved for those with recurrent LMP tumor with previous history of contralateral unilateral salpingo-oophorectomy and a strong desire for fertility preservation.[97]

Invasive Epithelial Tumors

Although fertility-sparing surgery has been recommended for younger patients with nonepithelial ovarian tumors and LMP tumors, it has not been well defined in invasive epithelial ovarian cancers. A unilateral salpingo-oophorectomy and staging consisting of omentectomy, washings, multiple peritoneal biopsies, and pelvic and periaortic lymphadenectomy should be performed in patients desiring fertility preservation with stage I disease. Examination of the contralateral ovary is necessary with biopsies only performed for grossly visible abnormalities.[5] There have been a few studies looking at the safety and efficacy of conservative management in this patient population. Schilder and Thompson (2002) analyzed 52 patients with either stage IA (42 patients) or IC (10 patients) invasive epithelial ovarian cancer (grades 1 to 3) treated with unilateral adnexectomy and staging. Median follow-up was 68 months. Five patients developed a recurrence 8–78 months after initial surgery. Two patients with stage IA mucinous tumors recurred with metastatic disease 9 and 78 months after initial surgery and died of disease. The estimated 5-year and 10-year survival rates were 98% and 93%, respectively. Twenty-four patients attempted pregnancy and 17 (71%) conceived[98] (**Level III**). Park et al. (2008) reported a larger series of 62 patients with invasive epithelial ovarian cancer treated with fertility-sparing surgery. Thirty-six patients had stage IA disease, 2 had stage IB, 21 had stage IC, and one each had stages IIB, IIIA, and IIIC. Forty-one of 62 (66%) tumors had mucinous histology. Three patients underwent unilateral ovarian cystectomy, 10 unilateral oophorectomy, and 49 unilateral salpingo-oophorectomy. All patients had multiple peritoneal biopsies, washings, and at least a partial omentectomy. Only 18 patients underwent pelvic and/or para-aortic lymphadenectomy. Mean age was 26 years (range 13–40 years). Median follow-up was 56 months. Eleven patients had recurrence 6–58 months after initial surgery. For patients with stage IA, IB, IC, and above stage II disease, 5-year overall survival rates were 91%, 100%, 88%, and 33%, respectively ($p = 0.0014$). For patients with grades I, II, and III disease, the 5-year disease-free survival rates were 93%, 80%, and 15%, respectively ($p < 0.0001$), and the 5-year overall survival rates were 95%, 100%, and 42%, respectively ($p = 0.0002$). Even in patients with stage IA disease, grade III disease showed significantly poorer disease-free survival ($p < 0.001$) and overall survival ($p < 0.001$). Fifteen of 19 patients who attempted to conceive had successful pregnancies. Twelve of the 15 patients who became pregnant had received prior platinum-based chemotherapy. Their findings suggested that fertility-sparing surgery be considered safe even for stage IC epithelial cancers. However, fertility-sparing surgery should not be performed in patients with disease staged higher than IC or for grade III tumors[99] (**Level III**).

REFERENCES

1. LEE SJ, SCHOVER LR, PARTRIDGE AH. American Society of Clinical Oncology recommendations on fertility preservation. J Clin Oncol 2006;24:2917–2931.
2. SIMON B, LEE SJ, PARTRIDGE AH, et al. Preserving fertility after cancer. CA Cancer J Clin 2005;55:211–228.
3. SCHOVER L. Sexuality and Fertility After Cancer. New York: John Wiley and Sons, Inc.; 1997.
4. MEIROW D, NUGENT K. The effects of radiotherapy on female reproduction. Hum Reprod Update 2001;7:535–543.
5. HOSKINS WJ, PEREZ CA, YOUNG RC, et al. Principles and Practice of Gynecologic Oncology. 4th ed. Lippincott Williams & Wilkins; 2005.
6. WALLACE WH, THOMPSON AB. Preservation of fertility in children treated for cancer. Arch Dis Child 2003;88:493–496.
7. CRITCHLEY HO. Factors of importance for implantation and problems after treatment for childhood cancer. Med Pediatr Oncol 1999;33:9–14.

8. CRITCHLEY HO, BATH LE, WALLACE HB. Radiation damage to the uterus—review of the effects of treatment of childhood cancer. Hum Fertil 2002;5:61–66.

9. BLUMENFELD Z. Preservation of fertility and ovarian function and minimalization of chemotherapy associated gonadotoxicity and premature ovarian failure: the role of inhibin-A and -B as markers. Mol Cell Endocrinol 2002;187:93–105.

10. MEIROW D. Reproduction post-chemotherapy in young cancer patients. Mol Cell Endocrinol 2002;169:123–131.

11. BYRNE J, FEARS TR, GAIL MH, et al. Early menopause in long-term survivors of cancer during adolescence. Am J Obstet Gynecol 1992;166:788–793.

12. GERSHENSON DM, MILLER AM, CHAMPION VL, et al. Reproductive and sexual function after platinum-based chemotherapy in long-term ovarian germ cell tumor survivors: a Gynecologic Oncology Group study. J Clin Oncol 2007;25(19):2792–2797.

13. ROBERTS JE, OKTAY K. Fertility preservation: a comprehensive approach to the young woman with cancer. J Natl Cancer Inst Monogr 2005; 57–59.

14. LEE SJ, SCHOVER LR, PARTRIDGE AH, et al. American Society of Clinical Oncology recommendations on fertility preservation in cancer patients. J Clin Oncol 2006;24(18):2917–2930.

15. BLUMENFELD Z. How to preserve fertility in young women exposed to chemotherapy? The role of GnRH agonist cotreatment in addition to cryopreservation of embryo, oocytes, or ovaries. Oncologist 2007;12:1044–1054.

16. OKTAY K, BUYUK E, ROSENWAKS Z. Novel use of an aromatase inhibitor for fertility preservation via embryo cryopreservation in endometrial cancer: a case report. Fertil Steril 2003;80:144.

17. JURETZKA MM, O'HANLAN KA, KATZ SL, et al. Embryo cryopreservation after diagnosis of stage IIB endometrial cancer and subsequent pregnancy in gestational carrier. Fertil Steril 2005;83(4):1041.

18. OKTAY K, CIL AP, BANG H. Efficiency of oocyte cryopreservation: a meta-analysis. Fertil Steril 2006;86:70–80.

19. DONNEZ J, DOLMANS MM, DEMYLLE D, et al. Livebirth after orthotopic transplantation of cryopreserved ovarian tissue. Lancet 2004;364:1405–1410.

20. OKTAY K, KARLIKAYA G. Ovarian function after transplantation of frozen, banked autologous ovarian tissue. N Engl J Med 2000;342:1919.

21. MEIROW D, LEVRON J, ELDAR-GEVA T, et al. Ovarian tissue storing for fertility preservation in clinical practice: successful pregnancy, technology, and risk assessment. Fertil Steril 2005;84:S2.

22. RADFORD JA, LEIBERMAN BA, BRISON DR, et al. Lancet 2001;357:1172–1175.

23. SCHMIDT KL, ANDERSEN CY, LOFT A, et al. Follow-up of ovarian function post-chemotherapy following ovarian cryopreservation and transplantation. Hum Reprod 2005;20:3529–3546.

24. DONNEZ J, DOLMANS MM, DEMYLLE D, et al. Restoration of ovarian function after orthotopic (intraovarian and periovarian) transplantation of cryopreserved ovarian tissue in a woman treated by bone marrow transplantation for sickle cell anaemia: a case report. Hum Reprod 2006;21:183–188.

25. KIM SS, HWANG IT, LEE HC. Heterotopic autotransplantation of cryobanked human ovarian tissue as a strategy to restore ovarian function. Fertil Steril 2004;82:930–932.

26. CALLEGO J, SALVADOR C, MIRALLES A, et al. Long-term ovarian function evaluation after autografting by implantation with fresh and frozen-thawed human ovarian tissue. J Clin Endocrinol Metab 2001;86:4489–4494.

27. KIM SS, YANG HW, KANG HG, et al. Quantitative assessment of ischemic tissue damage in ovarian cortical tissue with or without antioxidant (ascorbic acid) treatment. Fertil Steril 2004;82:679–685.

28. GLODE LM, ROBINSON J, GOULD SF. Protection from cyclophosphamide induced testicular damage with an analogue of gonadotropin-releasing hormone. Lancet 1981;1:1132–1134.

29. BLUMENFELD Z, AVIVI I, ECKMAN A, et al. Gonadotropin-releasing hormone agonist decreases chemotherapy-induced gonadotoxicity and premature ovarian failure in young female patients with Hodgkin lymphoma. Fertil Steril 2008;89(1):166–173.

30. RECCHIA F, SAGGIO G, AMICONI G, et al. Gonadotropin-releasing hormone analogues added to adjuvant chemotherapy protect ovarian function and improve clinical outcomes in young women with early breast carcinoma. Cancer 2006;106:514–523.

References **483**

31. Chapman RM, Sutcliffe SB. Protection of ovarian function by oral contraceptives in women receiving chemotherapy for Hodgkin's disease. Blood 1981;58:849–851.
32. Whitehead E, Shalet SM, Bleckledge G, et al. The effect of combination chemotherapy on ovarian function in women treated for Hodgkin's disease. Cancer 1983;52:988–993.
33. Elis A, Tevet A, Yerushalmi R, et al. Fertility status among women treated for aggressive non-Hodgkin's lymphoma. Leuk Lymphoma 2006;47:623–627.
34. Behringer K, Breuer K, Reineke T, et al. Secondary amenorrhea after Hodgkin's lymphoma is influenced by age at treatment, stage of disease, chemotherapy regimen, and the use of oral contraceptives during therapy: a report from the German Hodgkin's Lymphoma Study Group. J Clin Oncol 2005;23:7555–7564.
35. Chemaitilly W, Mertens AC, Mitby P, et al. Acute ovarian failure in the childhood cancer survivor study. J Clin Endocrinol Metab 2006;91:1723–1728.
36. Sklar CA, Mertens AC, Mitby P, et al. Premature menopause in survivors of childhood cancer: a report from the childhood cancer survivor study. J Natl Cancer Inst 2006;98:890–896.
37. Stroud JS, Mutch D, Rader J, et al. Effects of cancer treatment on ovarian function. Fertil Steril (in press).
38. Hamre MR Robison LL, Nesbit ME, et al. Effects of radiation on ovarian function in long-term survivors of childhood acute lymphoblastic leukemia: a report from the Children's Cancer Study Group. J Clin Oncol 1987;5:1759–1765.
39. Wallace WH, Thomson AB, Saran F, et al. Predicting age of ovarian failure after radiation to a field that includes the ovaries. Int J Radiat Oncol Biol Phys 2005;62:738–744.
40. Wallace WH, Thomson AB, Kelsey TW. The radiosensitivity of the human oocyte. Hum Reprod 2003;18:117–121.
41. Rigsby CK, Siegel MJ. CT appearance of pediatric ovaries and uterus. J Comput Assist Tomogr 1994;18:72–76.
42. Nicholson R, Coucher J, Thornton A, et al. Effect of a full and empty bladder on radiation dose to the uterus, ovaries, and bladder from lumbar spine CT and X-ray examinations. Br J Radiol 2000;73:1290–1296.
43. Hadar H, Loven D, Herskovitz P, et al. An evaluation of lateral and medial transposition of the ovaries out of radiation fields. Cancer 1994;74:774–779.
44. Thibaud E, Ramirez M, Brauner R, et al. Preservation of ovarian function by ovarian transposition performed before pelvic irradiation during childhood. J Pediatr 1992;121:880–884.
45. Belinson JL, Doherty M, McDay JB. A new technique for ovarian transposition. Surg Gynecol Obstet 1984;159:157–160.
46. Hodel K, Rich WM, Austin P, et al. The role of ovarian transposition in conservation of ovarian function in radical hysterectomy followed by pelvic radiation. Gynecol Oncol 1982;13:195–202.
47. Husseinzadeh N, Nahhas WA, Velkly DE, et al. The preservation of ovarian function in young women undergoing pelvic radiation therapy. Gynecol Oncol 1984;18:373–379.
48. Husseinzadeh N, van Aken ML, Aron B. Ovarian transposition in young patients with invasive cervical cancer receiving radiation therapy. Int J Gynecol Cancer 1994;4:61–65.
49. Chambers SK, Chambers JT, Holm C, et al. Sequelae of lateral ovarian transposition in unirradiated cervical cancer patients. Gynecol Oncol 1990;39:155–159.
50. Feeney DD, Moore DH, Look KY, et al. The fate of the ovaries after radical hysterectomy and ovarian transposition. Gynecol Oncol 1995;56:3–7.
51. Buekers TE, Anderson B, Sorosky JI, et al. Ovarian function after surgical treatment for cervical cancer. Gynecol Oncol 2001;80:85–88.
52. Sonoda Y, Chi DS, Carter J, et al. Initial experience with Dargent's operation: the radical vaginal trachelectomy. Gynecol Oncol 2008;108:214–219.
53. Berek JS, Hacker NF. Practical Gynecologic Oncology. Philadelphia, PA: Lippincott Williams & Wilkins; 2000.
54. Poynor EA, Barakat RR, Hoskins WJ. Management and follow up of patients with adenocarcinoma in situ of the uterine cervix. Gynecol Oncol 1995;57:158–164.

484 Chapter 16 Fertility Preservation in the Gynecologic Cancer Patient

55. McHale M, Le TD, Burger RA et al. Fertility sparing treatment for in situ and early invasive adenocarcinoma of the cervix. Obstet Gynecol 2001;98:726–730.
56. Shin CH, Schorge JO, Lee KR, et al. Conservative management of adenocarcinoma in situ of the cervix. Gynecol Oncol 2000;79:6–10.
57. Bull-Phelps SL, Garner EI, Walsh CS, et al. Fertility-sparing surgery in 101 women with adenocarcinoma in situ of the cervix. Gynecol Oncol 2007;107:316–319.
58. Schorge JO, Lee KR, Sheets EE. Prospective management of stage IA1 cervical adenocarcinoma by conization alone to preserve fertility: a preliminary report. Gynecol Oncol 2000;78:217–220.
59. Shipman SD, Bristow RE. Adenocarcinoma in situ and early invasive adenocarcinoma of the uterine cervix. Curr Opin Oncol 2001;13:394–398.
60. Dargent D, Martin X, Sacchetoni A, et al. Laparoscopic vaginal radical trachelectomy. Cancer 2000;88:1877–1882.
61. Plante M. Fertility preservation in the management of gynecologic cancers. Curr Opin Oncol 2000;12:497–507.
62. Schlaerth JB, Spirtos NM, Schlaerth AC. Radical trachelectomy and pelvic lymphadenectomy with uterine preservation in the treatment of cervical cancer. Am J Obstet Gynecol 2003;188:29–34.
63. Covens A, Shaw P, Murphy J, et al. Is radical trachelectomy a safe alternative to radical hysterectomy for patients with stage IA-IB carcinoma of the cervix? Cancer 1999;86:2273–2279.
64. Roy M, Plante M. Pregnancies after radical vaginal trachelectomy for early-stage cervical cancer. Am J Obstet Gynecol 1998;179:1491–1496.
65. Beiner ME, Hauspy J, Rosen B, et al. Radical vaginal trachelectomy vs. radical hysterectomy for small early stage cervical cancer: a matched case-control study. Gynecol Oncol 2008;110:168–171.
66. Hertel H, Kohler C, Grund D, et al. Radical vaginal trachelectomy combined with laparoscopic pelvic lymphadenectomy: prospective multicenter study of 100 patients with early cervical cancer. Gynecol Oncol 2006;103:506–511.
67. Shepherd JH, Spencer C, Herod J, et al. Radical vaginal trachelectomy as a fertility-sparing procedure in women with early-stage cervical cancer-cumulative pregnancy rate in a series of 123 women. BJOG 2006;113:719–724.
68. Mathevet P, Laszlo de Kaszon E, Dargent D. Fertility preservation in early cervical cancer. Gynecol Obstet Fertil 2003;31:706–712.
69. Plante M, Renaud MC, Francois H, et al. Vaginal radical trachelectomy: an oncologically safe fertility-preserving surgery. An updated series of 72 cases and review of the literature. Gynecol Oncol 2004;94:614–623.
70. Burnett AF, Roman LD, O'Meara AT, et al. Radical vaginal trachelectomy and pelvic lymphadenectomy for preservation of fertility in early cervical carcinoma. Gynecol Oncol 2003;88:419–423.
71. Bernardini M, Barrett J, Seaward G, et al. Pregnancy outcomes in patients after radical trachelectomy. Am J Obstet Gynecol 2003;189:1378–1382.
72. Plante M, Renaud MC, Hoskins IA, et al. Vaginal radical trachelectomy: a valuable fertility-preserving option in the management of early-stage cervical cancer. A series of 50 pregnancies and review of the literature. Gynecol Oncol 2005;98:3–10.
73. Randall TC, Kurman RJ. Progestin treatment of atypical hyperplasia and well differentiated carcinoma of the endometrium in women under age 40. Obstet Gynecol 1997;90:434–440.
74. Bokhman JV, Chepick OF, Volkova AT, et al. Can primary endometrial carcinoma stage I be cured without surgery and radiation therapy? Gynecol Oncol 1985;20:139–155.
75. Sardi J, Anchezar Henry JP, Paniceres G, et al. Primary hormonal treatment for early endometrial carcinoma. Eur J Gynaecol Oncol 1998;19:565–568.
76. Kaku T, Yoshikawa H, Tsuda H, et al. Conservative therapy for adenocarcinoma and atypical endometrial hyperplasia of the endometrium in young women: central pathologic review and treatment outcome. Cancer Lett 2001;167:207–212.
77. Wang CB, Wang CJ, Huang HJ, et al. Fertility-preserving treatment in young patients with endometrial adenocarcinoma. Cancer 2002;94:2192–2198.

78. KIM YB, HOLSCHNEIDER CH, GHOSH K, et al. Progestin alone as primary treatment of endometrial carcinoma in premenopausal women. Report of seven cases and review of the literature. Cancer 1997;79:320–327.

79. GOTLIEB WH, BEINER ME, SHALMON B. Outcome of fertility-sparing treatment with progestins in young patients with endometrial cancer. Gynecol Oncol 2003;102:718–725.

80. IMAI M, JOBO T, SATO R, et al. Medroxyprogesterone acetate therapy for patients with adenocarcinoma of the endometrium who wish to preserve the uterus-usefulness and limitations. Eur J Gynaecol Oncol 2001;22:217–220.

81. RAMIREZ PT, FRUMOVITZ M, BODURKA DC, et al. Hormonal therapy for the management of grade 1 endometrial adenocarcinoma: a literature review. Gynecol Oncol 2004;95:133–138.

82. GIANNOPOULOS T, BUTLER-MANUEL S, TAILOR A. Levonorgestrol-releasing intrauterine system as a therapy for endometrial carcinoma. Gynecol Oncol 2004;95:762–764.

83. DHAR KK, NEEDHIRAJAN T, KOSLOWSKI M, et al. Is levonorgestrol intrauterine system effective for treatment of early endometrial cancer? Report of four cases and review of the literature. Gynecol Oncol 2005;97:924–927.

84. MONTZ FJ, BRISTOW RE, BOVICELLI A, et al. Intrauterine progesterone treatment of early endometrial cancer. Am J Obstet Gynecol 2002;186:651–657.

85. BREWER M, GERSHENSON DM, HERZOG CE, et al. Outcome and reproductive function after chemotherapy for ovarian dysgerminoma. J Clin Oncol 1999;17:2670–2675.

86. GERSHENSON DM, et al. Menstrual and reproductive function after treatment with combination chemotherapy for malignant ovarian germ cell tumors. J Clin Oncol 1988;6:270–275.

87. LOW JH, PERRIN LC, CRANDON AJ, et al. Conservative surgery to preserve ovarian function in patients with malignant ovarian germ cell tumors. Cancer 2000;89:391–398.

88. DISAIA PJ, CREASMAN WT. Clinical Gynecologic Oncology. 6th ed. St. Louis: Mosby-Year Book; 2002.

89. TRIMBLE CL, KOSARY C, TRIMBLE EL. Long-term survival and patterns of care in women with ovarian tumors of low malignant potential. Gynecol Oncol 2002;86:34–37.

90. CHAN JK, LIN YG, LOIZZI V, et al. Borderline ovarian tumors in reproductive-age women. Fertility-sparing surgery and outcome. J Reprod Med 2003;48:756–760.

91. ZANETTA G, ROTA S, CHIARI S, et al. Behavior of borderline tumors with particular interest to persistence, recurrence, and progression to invasive carcinoma: a prospective study. J Clin Oncol 2001;19:2658–2664.

92. MORRIS RT, GERSHENSON DM, SILVA EG, et al. Outcome and reproductive function after conservative surgery for borderline ovarian tumors. Obstet Gynecol 2000;95:541–547.

93. GOTLIEB WH, FLIKKER S, DAVIDSON B, et al. Borderline tumors of the ovary: fertility treatment, conservative management, and pregnancy outcome. Cancer 1998;82:141–146.

94. CAMATTE S, MORICE P, PAUTIER P, et al. Fertility results after conservative treatment of advanced stage serous borderline tumour of the ovary. BJOG 2002;109:376–380.

95. DONNEZ J, MUNSCHKE A, BERLIERE M, et al. Safety of conservative management and fertility outcome in women with borderline tumors of the ovary. Fertil Steril 2003;79:1216–1221.

96. RAO GG, SKINNER EN, GEHRIG PA, et al. Fertility-sparing surgery for ovarian low malignant potential tumors. Gynecol Oncol 2005;98:263–266.

97. MORICE P, CAMATTE S, HASSAN JE, et al. Clinical outcomes and fertility after conservative treatment of ovarian borderline tumors. Fertil Steril 2001;75:92–96.

98. SCHILDER J, THOMPSON A. Outcome of reproductive age women with stage IA or IC invasive epithelial ovarian cancer treated with fertility-sparing therapy. Gynecol Oncol 2002;87:1–7.

99. PARK JY, KIM DY, SUH DS, et al. Outcomes of fertility-sparing surgery for invasive epithelial ovarian cancer: oncologic safety and reproductive outcomes. Gynecol Oncol 2008;110:345–353.

Chapter 17

Perioperative Herbal and Supplement Use

Alexander Vasilev and Steven Vasilev, M.D.

The first written record of medicinal herb use dates back 5000 years from the Sumerians. Today chemicals derived from plants are found in approximately 25% of prescription drug formulations.[1] Surveys found enormous & widespread public enthusiasm for herbal medications in the presurgical population.[2,3] Many of these are recognized as being "dietary supplements," which the Food and Drug Administration (FDA) defines as any orally administered product that contains anything that acts to supplement an individual's diet.[4] These supplements include organ tissues, amino acids, enzymes, vitamins, minerals, metabolites, extracts, concentrates of substances, or herbs. In 2007, it was estimated that the dietary supplement market was worth $24–$25 billion, with herbal medication accounting for $5.8 billion.[5,6] The largest increase in medicinal herbal use was between 1990 and 1997 at 380%.[7] Recent reports suggest that there will be a continued double-digit growth of this industry due to trends aimed toward greater financing and globalization, better regulation, and an increased consumer-driven focus on health.

The popularity of herbal medication can be ascribed to the desire for individual control of health care, increased cultural exposure, high cost of traditional medicine, and ready availability to the general public.[8] In order to ascertain the relative efficacy of such alternative therapies, the National Institute of Health created the Office of Alternative Medicine in 1992.

Unfortunately, this billion-dollar industry is still relatively unregulated, which means that the safety of such supplements is not guaranteed. In 1994, the FDA enacted the Dietary Supplement Health and Education Act (DSHEA), which placed the sole responsibility of product safety and quality control on the manufacturer. As a result, these products are exempt from FDA safety and efficacy testing that is generally required for over-the-counter medications.[9] This means that manufacturers may sell any product without the consent of the FDA so long as the product has a disclaimer

Gynecologic Oncology: Evidence-Based Perioperative and Supportive Care, Second Edition. Edited by Scott E. Lentz, Allison E. Axtell and Steven A. Vasilev.

mentioning that the FDA has not approved its use and it does not claim to be effective for prevention or treatment of any disease.

Since its enactment, the DSHEA has raised numerous concerns regarding the risk of potential adulteration, lack of postmarketing reporting systems, scarcity of information regarding the interactions of herbs and other drugs, as well as standardization and quality of herbal products.[10, 11] Although many of these products are safe, there have been many reported cases of significant adverse effects.

It has been reported that approximately 70% of patients fail to inform their physicians of their herbal consumption for a myriad of reasons, which gives rise to risk for many potential perioperative complications.[12] These reasons may include fear that their physician is biased against herbal use, fear of reprisal for self-medication, as well as the belief that such products are safe because they are deemed "natural."[13] The failure to report alternative medications carries important implications for both adverse and beneficial effects when attempting to create and follow the best possible perioperative strategy.

In this chapter, the relationship between evidence-based and complementary and alternative medicine is examined. In addition, several substances most likely to be detrimental in the perioperative period are discussed, which include echinacea, ephedra, garlic, ginseng, ginkgo, kava, St. John's wort, and valerian root. The chapter concludes by addressing potentially beneficial substances such as arginine, chitosan, eicosapentaenoic acid, glutamine, ornithine ketoglutarate, and ribose. The aforementioned herbs and supplements are discussed alphabetically and their order does not reflect relative importance.

EVIDENCE-BASED AND COMPLEMENTARY AND ALTERNATIVE MEDICINE

Evidence-based medicine (EBM) is functionally a measuring stick with respect to the relative and specific efficacy of any given treatment plan. Specifically, this method uses rigorous clinical testing so that it can be concluded with relative certainty that a particular drug, acting alone, causes a specific effect. This facilitates optimal decision making in patient care. The growing popularity of complementary and alternative medicine (CAM), however, has led to widespread debate with respect to viability of relying solely on EBM to validate options. Research on many herbal and dietary supplements have concluded their relative association with beneficial or adverse reactions, yet, as the old saying goes, "correlation does not necessarily imply explicit causation." In other words, herbs and supplements generally interact synergistically with each other and with other elements in the body and, in these instances, EBM research is unable to conclude with certainty that the supplement was solely, or even partially, responsible for the observed clinical effect. It is here that it becomes apparent that scientific inquiry is much like a two-sided coin. One side begs the question "Does treatment X work?", which provides the general foundation for EBM. It is quite obvious that this is important in determining the correct treatment for each patient. The other side arises due to the inability of EBM to conclude that the supplement was the only factor responsible for the effect. It asks, "*How* does treatment X work?" It is apparent that there are a myriad of inherent difficulties with respect to conducting evidence-based CAM research, a few of which are discussed in the following text.[14]

The first challenge is that many CAM interventions involve the study of several simultaneous treatments, while EBM research usually focuses on one treatment at a time. In other words, conventional EBM research prefers to simplify complex treatments by studying individual reactions. By valuing this "simplistic" approach, traditional EBM may ignore the importance of synergistic reactions occurring within the body. CAM, on the other hand, attempts to account for the complexity of the human body. Rather than trying to oversimplify these complexities, which may inadvertently compromise research, it recognizes that some reactions arise solely from synergistic effects.

Second, it is hard to establish correlations between a certain CAM-based treatment and a patient's observed outcome, unless both are measured and defined precisely. For example, no two acupuncture sessions are exactly alike and each session only represents one out of an infinite amount of possible experiences. Here, labeling the treatment does not define the treatment itself. Thus, rather than ascribing a label to their treatments researchers should instead define the exact style or type of treatment implemented.

Third, biased studies or testing the wrong interactions may occur if there is insufficient preclinical knowledge or if wrong conclusions have been made with respect to a supplement's or herb's functional constituents. In other words, there is tension between the synergistic approach of studying the effect of the entire substance and the simplistic approach of studying the effect of each of the substance's constituents. Proponents of CAM argue that testing individual constituents may, in fact, weaken the observed clinically beneficial effects of the entire supplement or herb.

A fifth, somewhat subjective, challenge is that the use of blinded and randomized studies contradicts the fundamental philosophy of CAM, which places much value on patient preferences and self-empowerment. In other words, patients may relinquish their full range of preferences by agreeing to be a part of randomized or blinded trials. As a result, these studies may contradict the process of making totally informed decisions from the patient perspective.

Another challenge is that most CAM treatments are tailored to the individual, whereas EBM research relies on the standardization of a treatment's entire process. Standardizing these treatments takes away the patients ability to select from a variety of alternative treatments.

Seventh, all treatments, not just CAM, have both specific and nonspecific effects that are impossible to sort out. Specifically, it is sometimes impossible to ascribe the effects of a drug solely to its ingredients, while ignoring other reactions that may occur. This is illustrated with placebo studies, which may produce specific results not ascribed to the ingredients of the drug.

Finally, double-blind studies cannot be used to study the pharmacological activity of some CAM treatments. For example, hypnosis cannot possibly be studied in this fashion as it is obvious what treatment is being tested. As a result, it is apparent that the evidence provided by EBM research is not enough to make a decision. Patients instead make their choices based on comparisons of risk and benefit, cost, and personal values. When it comes to CAM-based research, two relatively new research methods are discussed: aptitude by treatment interaction research and practical clinical trials.

The aptitude by treatment interaction approach seeks to evaluate how certain results depend on the matching of specific treatments with the characteristics of the patient. As a result, researchers can examine whether treatments can be altered to maximize the results for each individual patient.[15, 16] One of the challenges of this approach is to avoid ascribing causal correlations between a particular treatment and the observed aptitude.

Although physicians try to effectively translate research evidence to respective clinical recommendations, it is nearly impossible to predict the decision-making process of patients. Usually, randomized controlled trials (RCTs) are done wherein most physicians are interested in comparison of risks, benefits and, in some cases, costs. However, this method ignores the fact that there is no universal "decision-making process" and many patients weigh costs or risks versus benefits differently. The use of practical clinical trials (PCTs) can address this because the hypothesis and experimental procedure are designed to explicitly address the decision-making process.[17] PCTs account for the intricate interactions in the treatment, such as the environment in which the therapy is administered and the effect it has on the general well-being of patients. Therefore, rather than following the RCT procedures that focus on which treatment is the "best," practical clinical trials instead focus on the optimal treatment, conditions, and procedure for each individual.

In summary, traditionally defined evidence-based research cannot account for the many complexities associated with application of CAM. In order to address the challenges associated with conducting evidence-based research on CAM, it has been suggested that physicians instead utilize aptitude by treatment interaction research and practical clinical trials. As such, it is somewhat artificial and often impossible to assign a traditional evidence level or grade to the data supporting herbal or supplement use. Nonetheless, one can glean enough information from the world's peer-reviewed literature to support some risk and benefit recommendations.

POTENTIALLY DETRIMENTAL PERIOPERATIVE SUBSTANCES

Echinacea

Currently three species of *Echinacea* are being used in marketed medicinal products. These include *Echinacea angustifolia, Echinacea pallida,* and *Echinacea purpurea.* Widely believed to be an immunostimulant, it is taken for the prophylaxis and treatment of many fungal, bacterial, and viral infections, especially those of the upper respiratory tract.[18] Unfortunately, the specific pharmacological activity has not been ascribed to a single compound. This is because echinacea's composition is relatively complex as many of its constituent chemicals differ in both effect and potency.

Studies show, however, that the alkylamides, various essential oils, and polyacetylenes existing in the lipophilic portion of echinacea are most likely responsible for the aforementioned effects.

Although echinacea is nontoxic and safe for some, its use has been correlated with allergic reactions that include, but are not limited to, anaphylaxis and hepatoxicity.[19] Therefore, patients with atopy, allergic rhinitis, asthma, and preexisting dysfunction of the liver should be especially cautious while taking echinacea. In addition, the pharmacokinetic activity of echinacea has not yet been extensively documented. Therefore, if there are any anticipated complications regarding blood flow to the liver or hepatic function in general, then it is recommended that patients discontinue their use of echinacea as far in advance as possible prior to surgery.

Many preclinical reports have shown that echinacea acts as an immunostimulant.[20–22] Therefore, consuming echinacea may decrease the effectiveness of certain immunosuppressive medications.[23] Thus, individuals undergoing surgical procedures that call for perioperative immunosuppression, such as organ transplantation, should be advised against its use. This is obviously not a consideration for gynecologic or gynecologic oncology–related procedures per se. Equally important, patients who are allergic to daisies, mums, marigolds, and ragweed may experience allergic reactions as a result of echinacea use.[23] Contrary to its short-term effects as an immunostimulant, using echinacea for a period longer than 8 weeks may potentially result in detrimental long-term effects that include immunosuppression and a theoretical increase in postsurgical complications that include opportunistic infections as well as poor wound healing.[24] In addition, this immunosuppressive effect may impact the course of their malignancy and treatment response in the long run.

Ephedra

Ephedra is a central Asian shrub that is more commonly known in Chinese medicine as *ma huang* and is reputed to be the world's oldest "medicine" having been discovered over 5000 years ago. Until 2004, when it was banned by the FDA, it was a common ingredient in not only energy-boosting products but also in products promoting weight loss. Although no longer available in products manufactured in the United States, it can still be obtained internationally. In addition, products that source raw materials from other countries could contain ephedra in unquantifiable amounts.

Ephedra has also been used in the treatment of conditions arising in the respiratory tract, including bronchitis and asthma. Its composition includes many alkaloids, such as ephedrine, norpseudoephedrine, norepinephrine, pseudoephedrine, and methylephedrine.[25]

Ephedra has been associated with complications such as palpitations, seizures, stroke, myocardial infarction, cardiovascular collapse from catecholamine depletion, hypertension, heart attack, and in some cases sudden death even in individuals that had no preexisting vascular or heart disease.[26, 27] While some recorded deaths were due to overdose, others died despite taking ephedra within the guidelines given by the manufacturer.[26] Because of its high potential for harm, ephedra is now recognized as one of the most dangerous herbal products, especially for perioperative patients.[28]

Individuals who use ephedra are at risk of dosage-dependent rises in both heart rate and blood pressure. The predominantly active constituent of ephedra is ephedrine, a noncatecholamine sympathomimetic agent. It exhibits $\alpha 1$, $\beta 1$, and $\beta 2$ activity due to its direct affect on the adrenergic receptors, which in turn cause the indirect release of endogenous norepinephrine.[29] As a result, these sympathomimetic effects have been responsible for more than 1070 undesirable events, which include fatalities due to complications of the central nervous and cardiovascular systems.[30]

It is common to use ephedrine for intraoperative hypotension and bradycardia. Therefore, unsupervised consumption of ephedra prior to surgery raises a myriad of concerns. For example, thrombotic stroke and myocardial infarction may be caused by related vasospasm and vasoconstriction of the cerebral and coronary arteries.[27] Cardiovascular function may also be affected by ephedra consumption as it may cause hypersensitivity myocarditis, which results in cardiomyopathy with infiltration of eosinophil and myocardial lymphocytes.[31] The risk of intraoperative ventricular arrhythmias is increased if individuals are anesthetized with halothane after ephedra consumption due to halothane sensitization of the myocardium, predisposing to an increased arrhythmia risk.[32] The long-term consumption of ephedra may also add to hemodynamic instability during the perioperative period via tachyphylaxis from endogenous catecholamine store depletion. Consequently, primary therapy of intraoperative bradycardia and hypotension may be better accomplished using direct-acting sympathomimetic agents. Furthermore, life-threatening coma, hypertension, and hyperpyrexia may be brought about by the simultaneous use of monoamine oxidase inhibitors and ephedra. Lastly, if used for prolonged periods, excessive ephedra consumption can be responsible for unusual cases of radiolucent kidney stones, which may impact perioperative symptoms and workup.[33,34]

Many studies have been conducted regarding the pharmacokinetic activity of ephedrine in humans.[35,36] It was found that nearly 70%–80% of the ephedrine compound remained unchanged as it was excreted in the urine. In addition, it was found to have a half-life lasting 5.2 hours. Based on this data and the known cardiovascular risks, it is recommended that the use of ephedra should be discontinued no later than 24 hours prior to surgery. Patients with heart conditions, neurological disorders, and hypertension in particular should especially avoid ephedra-containing or possible "ephedra-contaminated" supplements.

Garlic

Garlic has long been one of the most studied medicinal herbs. It may lower cholesterol and serum lipid levels as well as reduce thrombus formation and blood pressure.[37] As a result, garlic has the potential to change the risk associated with the development of atherosclerosis.[37] These beneficial effects can be ascribed to the compounds whose composition includes sulfur, specifically allicin and its metabolites. Equally important, commercially distributed garlic products may or may not be standardized to a specific allicin and allicin potency.

Among its adverse effects, garlic may cause a dose-dependent inhibition of platelet aggregation. The compound ajoene seems to cause irreversible effects that may increase the effect of other compounds that inhibit platelet aggregation, such as dipyridamole, forskolin, indomethacin, and prostacyclin.[38,39] While consistent documentation of such occurrences is unavailable, there are some interesting case reports. One of these discusses an elderly patient, who developed epidural hematomas that were attributed to excessive garlic use.[40] Specifically, the patient was reported to have ingested around 2000 mg of garlic on a daily basis for an unspecified period of time.[40] Aside from garlic's potential to cause prolonged bleeding, it may also lower blood pressure. Studies on laboratory animals have shown that allicin lowered blood pressure and caused a decline in both pulmonary and systemic vascular resistance.[41,42] Similar research on humans reveal that garlic has marginal antihypertensive effects.[43]

Pharmacokinetic research has revealed that garlic's constituent cycloallin is normally completely excreted via the urine after approximately 48 hours with peak plasma levels observed after 45 minutes to an hour after intravenous administration.[44] Based on this data, it is advised that patients discontinue their preoperative use of garlic at least 7 days in advance due to potential irreversible inhibition of platelet aggregation. This is particularly the case if other platelet inhibitors are given or if an increased risk of bleeding is anticipated.

Ginkgo

Derived from the *Ginkgo biloba* leaf, ginkgo has been used for the treatment of altitude sickness, vertigo, tinnitus, cognitive disorders, age-related macular degeneration, erectile dysfunction, and peripheral vascular disease. In addition, research implies individuals with multiinfarct dementia and Alzheimer disease may show signs of improved cognitive performance when taking ginkgo.[45,46] Among its constituents, flavonoids and terpenoids are responsible for the majority of ginkgo's pharmacological activity.

Ginkgo also seems to inhibit platelet-activating factor, act as an antioxidant, alter vasoregulation, and modulate neurotransmitter and receptor activity.[47–50] The inhibition of platelet-activating factor poses the greatest threat to patient health during the perioperative period because altered platelet function may occur. While a small number of patients undergoing clinical trials did not show bleeding complications, postoperative bleeding following laparoscopic cholecystectomy, spontaneous hyphema, and spontaneous intracranial bleeding have been attributed to ginko use.[51–56] In case reports, it was suspected to have contributed to a bilateral subdural hematoma in a 33-year-old woman who took 60 mg of ginkgo twice a day over a 2-year period, a frontal subdural hematoma in a 72-year-old woman who consumed 50 mg three times a day over a 6-month period, and a spontaneous hyphema in a 70-year-old man who consumed 40 mg of concentrated ginkgo extract two times a day in combination with 325 mg of aspirin over a 1-week period.[51,55]

When taken orally, terpenoids are very bioavailable and flavonoids are more bioavailable than originally believed. Flavonoid metabolism seems to involve glucuronidation, which increases water solubility whereby elimination is accelerated for most flavonoid subtypes.[57] However, pharmacokinetic studies have found that terpenoids have a relatively prolonged elimination half-life of up to 10 hours after oral administration.[58] Based on this data and the potential risk of bleeding, especially in perioperative patients, ginkgo use should be discontinued at least 2 days prior to surgery.

Ginseng

Asian and American ginseng are the most commonly described herbs with respect to their pharmacological effects. It is believed that this herb can restore homeostasis and alleviate body stress, which is why it is generally called an "adaptogen."[59] The constituents of ginseng believed to be responsible for its pharmacological activity are known as ginsenosides, which belong to the steroidal saponin compound group. However, commercially distributed ginseng products may or may not be standardized to specific ginsenoside concentration.

Ginseng's pharmacological activity is not yet completely understood due to the numerous heterogeneous and often conflicting effects of various ginsenosides.[60] Ginseng's ability to decrease postprandial blood glucose in patients with type 2 diabetes mellitus and those without diabetes suggests that it may be a possible therapeutic agent.[61] This effect, however, has the potential to cause unintentional hypoglycemia, especially in individuals who have fasted prior to surgery. Equally important, concern has grown regarding ginseng's adverse effects on coagulation pathways due to the ability of ginsenosides to cause the inhibition of platelet aggregation in vitro.[62–65] Laboratory tests on rats have shown that ginsenosides can prolong coagulation time, as measured by thrombin and activated partial thromboplastin (aPTT).[64] Although additional confirmation is required, prior research has implied that panaxynol (a compound in ginseng) may cause irreversible antiplatelet activity in humans.[65] Despite the potential inhibition of the coagulation cascade, one case report of ginseng consumption was associated with reduction in warfarin anticoagulation.[66]

Research on the pharmacokinetic activity of ginseng in laboratory rabbits has shown that the activity of the main ginsenoside subtypes has elimination half-lives that are widely varied, lasting 0.8–7.4 hours.[67] Although this data suggests that ginseng use should be discontinued 24 hours before surgery, the potential for ginseng to cause irreversible platelet inhibition suggests that patients should stop using ginseng about a week before surgery.

Kava

Kava, also known as kava kava, has become increasingly popular as both a sedative and anxiolytic. Clinical studies suggest that symptomatic treatment of anxiety may be possible through use of kava therapeutically.[68] Pharmacological activity has been ascribed to its constituent kavalactones.[69]

When drug–nutrient interaction studies were first initiated, kava was one of the first medicinal herbs anticipated to interact with anesthetics due to its psychomotor effects. In addition, the central nervous system's antiepileptic, neuroprotective, and local anesthetic properties may be affected by the kavalactones in a dose-dependent manner.[70,71] Kava also has the potential to function as a sedative-hypnotic by increasing the effect of γ-aminobutyric acid (GABA) inhibitory neurotransmission. Studies on laboratory animals have also shown that barbiturate-induced sleep is lengthened.[72] These results may also explain the case report of a patient in a semicomatose state that was associated with an interaction of alprazolam and kava.[73]

While kava can theoretically be abused, there is little information to confirm its long-term effects, which include addiction, tolerance, and acute withdrawal after its discontinued use. However, excessive kava use may lead to a condition known as *kava dermopathy*, which results in reversible scaly cutaneous eruptions.[74] As of 2002, kava has also been the subject of consumer safety warnings from the FDA as multiple cases of hepatotoxicity have been reported.[75]

Pharmacokinetic studies have shown that kavalactones have an elimination half-life of 9 hours and that peak plasma levels are generally reached 1.8 hours after oral administration.[69] Kavalactones as well as their metabolites are destroyed as they are passed through the digestive system and are excreted in feces and urine.[76] Based on this data as well as kava's potential to increase the sedative effects of anesthetics, it is recommended that patients discontinue kava consumption at least 24 hours before surgery.

St. John's Wort

St. John's wort is derived from *Hypericum perforatum*. Although it has shown success as a short-term solution for mild-to-moderate depression, clinical trial research has determined that it is not a viable treatment for major depression.[77,78] Studies suggest that the pharmacological activity of St. John's wort is ascribed to its constituents, hyperforin and hypericin.[79] Standardized and commercially distributed products usually contain a fixed 0.3% of hypericin.

St. John's wort consumption can result in a considerable increase of the metabolic pathways of many drugs that are concomitantly administered. This is an important consideration as many of these drugs are crucial during perioperative patient care. For example, the metabolic activity of cytochrome isoform P4503A4 is doubled.[80,81] Many studies have also observed the interactions between St. John's wort and numerous P4503A4 isoform substrates, such as cyclosporine, ethinyl estradiol, and indinavir sulfate.[82,83] In one case series, St. John's wort was correlated with an average decline of 49% of cyclosporine levels in the blood of organ transplant recipients.[84] There are many other P4503A4 substrates that are used throughout the perioperative period, such as serotonin receptor antagonists, calcium channel blockers, lidocaine, midazolam hydrochloride, and alfentanil. Aside from the P4503A4 isoform, there have also been reports that St. John's wort may also induce cytochrome isoform P4502C9, which includes the substrates warfarin and many nonsteroidal anti-inflammatory drugs. There have been at least seven instances reported where the anticoagulant effect warfarin was greatly reduced due to use of St. John's wort.[83] Equally important, if other enzyme inducers, such as other medicinal herbs, are used concomitantly, then the effects of St. John's wort enzyme induction may be more prominent. The pharmacokinetics of digoxin may also be affected by St. John's wort.[85]

Many effects of St. John's wort are due to the inhibition of neuron reuptake of dopamine, norepinephrine, and serotonin.[86, 87] The simultaneous consumption of St. John's wort with or without re-uptake inhibitors of serotonin may cause central serotonin syndrome.[88, 89] Research has also implied that one of constituent alkaloids in St. John's wort is a monoamine oxidase inhibitor (MAOI). While no contraindications exist involving the use of monoamine oxidase inhibitors (MAOI), with inhaled anesthetics, there are certain concerns as the combination of various narcotics and MAOIs may cause hypotension and has the potential to exaggerate the depressant effects of the narcotic in both the central nervous and respiratory systems.[90, 91] Therefore, if narcotic analgesia use is expected, then it is recommended that patients discontinue consumption of St. John's wort prior to surgery.

Steady-state and single-dose research data exists regarding the pharmacokintetic activity of hyperforin, pseudohypericin, and hypericin.[92, 93] When taken orally, it was found that hyperforin and hypericin, the active components of St. John's wort, had median elimination half-lives of 9 and 43.1 hours and had peak plasma levels after 3.5 and 6 hours, respectively. The consumption of St. John's wort poses certain perioperative risks due to its long half-life and its potential to change the metabolism of other drugs. Based on the aforementioned data, it is recommended that patients stop using St. John's wort at least 5 days before surgery. Furthermore, this consideration is particularly important for individuals who will receive postoperative anticoagulants as well as those awaiting organ transplants. In these cases, the patients should also be advised against the postoperative consumption of St. John's wort.

Valerian

Valerian is derived from the dried root of *Valeriana officinalis* and is commonly used as an anxiolytic or sedative. It is used to help treat insomnia and is a component of most medicinal sleep aids.[94] While many of its constituent components display synergistic interactions, research suggests that sesquiterpenes are responsible for the majority of the pharmacological activity seen in valerian. Commercially distributed products may be standardized to contain a fixed valerenic acid content.

Valerian induces hypnosis and sedation in a dose-dependent manner.[95] In addition, modulation of receptor function and GABA neurotransmission seem to mediate these particular effects.[96, 97] Studies on laboratory animals have also shown that valerenic acid (a valerian extract) increases the length of barbiturate-induced sleep.[98] This acid contributes to the sedative effects of valerian and causes the inhibition of γ-aminobutyric acid transaminase. There was also a case report of a valerian withdrawal that seemed to imitate an acute benzodiazepine withdrawal syndrome associated with postoperative cardiac complications and delirium. These withdrawal effects were calmed by the administration of benzodiazepine.[99] As a result, valerian should be expected to amplify the sedative properties of administered anesthetics and adjuvants, including midazolam, which function at the GABA receptor level.

Research on the pharmacokinetic activity of valerian indicates that it has an elimination half-life of about 1 hour with bimodal peak plasma levels observed after 1 and 5 hours.[100] Individuals should be cautioned against abruptly stopping valerian consumption due to the potential of physical dependence, which may mimic acute benzodiazepine withdrawal. In addition, it is advised that these individuals should gradually reduce their valerian use in the weeks prior to surgery to avoid the potential of such withdrawals. If tapering the dosage is not possible, then the patient should be advised to continue valerian consumption until the day prior to surgery. It has been shown that using benzodiazepines in the postoperative period helps to effectively treat symptoms of withdrawal if they were develop.[99]

POTENTIALLY BENEFICIAL PERIOPERATIVE SUBSTANCES

Arginine

L-arginine, more commonly known as arginine, is usually consumed orally and has been touted as an immunostimulant. Specifically, it is an amino acid that is necessary for protein synthesis and is found in red meat, fish, dairy, and poultry products.[101] L-arginine is often taken orally in combination with ribonucleic acid (RNA) and eicosapentaenoic acid (EPA) during either the pre- or postoperative period to shorten recovery time, reduce the risk of infection, and promote wound healing.[102–105] In addition, L-arginine has shown potential in the promotion of wound healing when applied topically. Intravenous administration of L-arginine has been reported to have numerous hemodynamic benefits with respect to heart failure, such as decreased average arterial pressure and heart rate and increased stroke volume and cardiac output.[106]

It is approved by the FDA and is considered safe when used orally or topically, although some adverse effects do exist.[107] Simultaneous use of L-arginine with herbs such as andrographis, cat's claw, and lycium may theoretically result in hypotensive complications. Patients with allergies or asthma should also use L-arginine with caution as allergic reactions, such as airway inflammation, may result because arginine has the potential to aggravate individual allergies.[108] In addition, blood pressure control may be affected by L-arginine during and after surgery, which is why it is advised that patients discontinue L-arginine use at least 2 weeks prior to elective surgery. Although additional evidence is required, topical postoperative administration is usually considered safe with a dose of 4 g of 12.5% L-arginine cream usually administered on the wound twice a day.[109]

Chitosan

Chitosan, a linear polysaccharide, has a number of potential uses in biomedical therapy. Specifically, the topical application of N-carboxybutyl chitosan has been shown to help promote tissue regeneration following plastic surgery.[110] Research has shown that the wound-healing and hemostatic activity exhibited by chitosan is likely due to the improvement of fibroblasts, polymorphonuclear leukocytes, and macrophages, which seems to be relatively independent of the classical coagulation cascade.[111,112] Its properties allow the more efficient clotting of blood than the traditional gauze dressing, which is why it has been approved for use in bandages in the United States.[113] In addition, chitosan has natural antibacterial and hypoallergenic properties, further supporting its usefulness in bandages.[114]

Although chitosan exhibits many beneficial properties, there are some possible adverse effects associated with its use. Specifically, chitosan is derived from shellfish, which makes its use particularly risky in patients with shellfish allergies.[115] There have also been reports that chitosan may potentiate warfarin's anticoagulant effects. However, it is generally safe when used topically. There is no typical dosage.[110,116–118]

EICOSAPENTAENOIC ACID

Eicosapentaenoic acid, also known as EPA, is effectively used as a dietary supplement in combination with L-arginine and RNA during the perioperative period and acts to promote wound healing, shorten recovery time, and reduce the risk of infection.[102,105,119,120] Although EPA does not greatly affect factors involved in the clotting process, it has been shown that it reduces platelet aggregation.[121] In addition, there is preliminary evidence suggesting that EPA also acts to reduce the activity of natural killer cells, which may reduce the likelihood of organ transplant and bone marrow rejection.[122] On the other hand, in the case of cancer therapy, this may be a counterproductive effect.

Although EPA is generally safe when administered intravenously or orally, there are harmful consequences, such as increased risk of bleeding and decreased blood coagulation, resulting from using doses in excess of 3 g a day.[123] Furthermore, patients who are pregnant or are allergic to aspirin should be advised against the use of EPA.[124] There are also other adverse reactions that may occur. Although patients generally tolerate oral consumption, some side effects may include diarrhea, nausea, epigastric discomfort, itching, nosebleed, skin rash, and joint, back, and muscle pain.[125] In addition, since reports indicate EPA present in fish oil may decrease natural killer cells, there is a potential increased risk of viral infection, cancer, and several detrimental immunologic effects.[122] Some patients who simultaneously use EPA with herbs such as garlic, ginkgo, and ginseng may be at an increased risk of bleeding.[121] Patients usually consume formulations with EPA and docosahexaenoic acid (DHA) in a wide range of doses. Typically, however, a dose of 5 g of fish oil is given that contains around 72–312 mg of DHA with 169–563 mg of EPA.

Glutamine

Glutamine, also known as GLN or glutamic acid, is the most abundant free amino acid in the body.[126] It has shown potential when given intravenously to help promote recovery following bone marrow transplant and abdominal surgery. About one-third of the nitrogen that mobilizes to repair wounds following surgery is from glutamine.[127] In addition, a decline in glutamine concentration during the postoperative period is associated with impaired function of monocytes and neutrophils, which raises the potential for infection.[128] Although not effective for all patients, reports suggest that oral administration of glutamine helps to decrease the length and severity of mucositis-related oral pain in patients undergoing bone marrow transplant.[129–132] While benefits are not experienced by all patients, intravenous use of glutamine-supplemented parenteral nutrition following abdominal and bone marrow transplant surgery results in lower microbial colonization rates, shorter hospital stay, increased hepatic function, lower rate of clinical infection, improved nitrogen balance, and increase lymphocyte recovery.[131,133–141]

Glutamine is considered safe when used intravenously and when taken orally in daily doses less than 40 g.[130,142–144] In addition, clinical studies have reported no significant adverse side effects in both orally and intravenously given glutamine.[138,144–146] Patients who should avoid using glutamine include those who are pregnant, allergic to monosodium glutamate, have mania, seizures, or severe liver disease.[147]

The recommended dosage for patients recovering from bone marrow transplant is 570 mg per day.[138] Patients recovering from other surgeries who are receiving parenteral nutrition have been given between 20 g and 300 mg a day of glutamine.[133,134] However, if glutamine dipeptide is given after surgery, then the daily dosage is usually 18–30 g of glutamine dipeptide in patients who weigh 60–70 kg. Higher doses are reserved for patients who have severe burns, multiple injuries, and immune deficiency.[148]

ORNITHINE KETOGLUTARATE

Ornithine ketoglutarate, commonly known as OKG, is commonly used to promote wound healing. Specifically, it seems to be effective at increasing the rate of wound healing in burn patients when administered orally.[149] In addition, OKG is intravenously used to prevent a decline in muscle-free glutamine concentrations, protein synthesis preservation following a stroke or total hip replacement, and after surgery to amplify the protein synthesis pathway of skeletal muscles. Although preclinical research suggests that OKG is an effective agent in the promotion of muscular protein synthesis, more evidence is needed before any significant claims are made with regards to its efficacy.[150,151]

Although it is generally considered safe when it is used intravenously, there is little reliable information with regards to the safety of oral administration.[150–153]

OKG continues to show potential as there are also no known adverse effects. The typical oral dosage given to burn victims is 30 g a day as an enteral bolus.[149] For other patients, a dosage of 350 mg a day is intravenously given to improve skeletal muscle protein synthesis in the postoperative period. The typical dosage used to preserve protein synthesis following hip replacement and to prevent a decline in free glutamine concentrations is 280 mg a day.[151]

Ribose

Ribose, also known as D-ribose, is used to increase athletic performance, boost muscle tissue energy, promote recovery of muscle function, and maintain or increase heart or muscle cell energy stores. For example, ribose is used after heart bypass surgery to promote the supply of energy to heart. Prior research suggests that immediate use of ribose during the postoperative period results in improved cardiac indices, although additional evidence is required to conclude this with certainty.[154] Recent research, however, corroborates with the aforementioned findings. Specifically, a controlled study was performed following heart bypass surgery in which one group received ribose and the other did not. Of the two groups, the individuals who received ribose experienced a cardiac index 30% higher than those who did not receive ribose supplementation.[155] It was suggested that ribose helps pump more blood to the heart simply by supplying more energy. The study also states that patients recovered within 3–4 weeks, with some out of the hospital in only a few days.[155] In addition to these benefits, some research implies that ribose may promote the preservation of hearts used for transplantation by helping to maintain ATP activity.[156]

Ribose use is generally considered safe when administered either intravenously or orally over a short-term period.[157–161] Unfortunately, there is insufficient information with regards to the long-term safety of ribose supplementation.

The general positive results noted were in patients undergoing cardiac surgery. Assumption of any benefits in other surgical patient populations is by extrapolation of plausible benefit only.

There are several adverse effects associated with ribose. Oral administration may cause decreased blood glucose, nausea, headache, diarrhea, gastrointestinal discomfort, decreased serum phosphate, increased levels of serum insulin, and hypoglycemia.[157,162–166] Therefore, caution should be used during the perioperative period as ribose has the potential to affect the control of blood glucose both pre- and postoperatively. Consequently, physicians should advise their patients to discontinue self-administered ribose use at least 2 weeks prior to elective surgery.

CONCLUSION

In conclusion we may say that CAM has many inherent risks and benefits. Because of their increasing popularity, it is important that physicians remember to ask their patients if they are using any alternative medicines, since the use of CAM may result in unforeseen health risks during the perioperative period. Equally important, physicians should also be aware that the use of such medications may be beneficial under alternative circumstances. Although subsequent research is required in many areas, alternative medicine has the potential to add a new range of possible treatment strategies for patients in the perioperative period.

REFERENCES

1. ERNST E. Herbal medicines: where is the evidence? BMJ 2000;321:395–396.
2. TSEN LC, SEGAL S, POTHIER M, et al. Alternative medicine use in presurgical patients. Anesthesiology 2000;93:148–151.
3. KAYE AD, CLARKE RC, SABAR R, et al. Herbal medications: current trends in anesthesiology practice – a hospital survey. J Clin Anesth 2000;12:468–471.
4. An FDA guide to dietary supplements. Available at: http://vm.cfsan.fda.gov/~dms/fdsupp.html. Accessed: February 6, 2003.
5. Herbal Health products, health facts for you. UW Health, University of Wisconsin Hospital, Madison. August 22, 2007. http://www.uwhealth.org/healthfacts/B_EXTRANET_HEALTH_INFORMATION-FlexMember-Show_Public_HFFY_1116944266659.html. Accessed: October 18, 2009.
6. THURSTON C. Dietary supplements: the latest trends & issues – nutraceuticals world. Nutraceuticals world – serving the dietary supplement, functional food and nutritional beverage industries. Available at: http://www.nutraceuticalsworld.com/articles/2008/04/dietary-supplements-the-latest-trends-issues. Accessed: October 18, 2009.
7. EISENBERG DM, DAVIS RB, ETTNER SL, et al. Trends in alternative medicine use in the united states, 1990–1997: results of a follow-up national survey. JAMA 1998;280:1569–1575.
8. SABAR R, KAYE AD, FROST EA. Perioperative considerations for the patient taking herbal medicines. Heart Dis 2001;3(2):87–96.
9. Dietary supplement health and education act of 1994. Available at: http://vm.cfsan.fda.gov/~dms/dietsupp.html. Accessed: February 6, 2003.
10. MARCUS DM, GROLLMAN AP. Botanical medicines—the need for new regulations. N Engl J Med 2002;347:2073–2076.
11. DE SMET PA. Herbal remedies. N Engl J Med 2002;347:2046–2056.
12. KAYE AD, CLARKE RC, SABAR R, et al. Herbal medicines: current trends in anesthesiology practice—a hospital survey. J Clin Anesth 2000;12:468–471.
13. ANG-LEE MK, MOSS J, YUAN CS. Herbal medicines and perioperative care. JAMA 2001;286:208–216.
14. CASPI O. Evidence-based medicine and clinical decision making. Integr Med 2006;7:43–56.
15. CASPI O, BELL IR. One size does not fit all: aptitude treatment interaction (ATI) as a conceptual framework for CAM outcome research: I. What is ATI research? J Altern Complement Med 2004;10:580–586.
16. CASPI O, BELL IR. One size does not fit all: aptitude treatment Interaction (ATI) as a conceptual framework for CAM outcome research: II. Research designs and their applications. J Altern Complement Med 2004;10:698–705.
17. TUNIS SR, STRYER DB, CLANCY CM. Practical clinical trials: increasing the value of clinical research for decision making in clinical and health policy. JAMA 2003;290:1624–1632.
18. MELCHART D, LINDE K, FISCHER P, et al. Echinacea for preventing and treating the common cold. Cochrane Database Syst Rev 2000; (2):CD000530.
19. MULLINS RJ. Echinacea-associated anaphylaxis. Med J Aust 1998;168:170–171.
20. PEPPING J. Echinacea. Am J Health Syst Pharm 1999;56:121–122.
21. SEE DM, BROUMAND N, SAHL L, et al. In vitro effects of echinacea and ginseng on natural killer and antibody-dependent cell cytotoxicity in healthy subjects and chronic fatigue syndrome or acquired immunodeficiency syndrome patients. Immunopharmacology 1997;35:229–235.

22. REHMEN J, DILLOW JM, CARTER SM, et al. Increased production of antigen-specfic immunoglobins G and M following in vivo treatment with the medicinal plants *Echinacea angustifolia* and *Hydrastis Canadensis*. Immunol Lett 1999;68:391–395.
23. Echinacea effectiveness, safety, and drug interactions on RxList. RxList: The Internet Drug Index. Available at: http://www.rxlist.com/echinacea/supplements.htm. Accessed: October 20, 2009.
24. BOULLATA JI, NACE AM. Safety issues with herbal medicine. Pharmacotherapy 2000;20:257–269.
25. GURLEY BJ, GARDNER SF, HUBBARD MA. Content versus label claims in ephedra-containing dietary supplements. Am J Helath Syst Pharm 2000;57:963–969.
26. SAMENUK D, LINK MS, HOMOUS MK, et al. Adverse cardiovascular events temporally associated with ma huang, an herbal source of ephedrine. Mayo Clin Proc 2002;77(1):12–16.
27. HALLER CA, BENOWITZ NL. Adverse cardiovascular and central nervous system events associated with dietary supplements containing ephedra alkaloids. N Engl J Med 2000;343:1833–1838.
28. MEYER TA, BAISDEN CE, ROBERSON CR, et al. Survey of preoperative patients' use of herbal products and other selected dietary supplements. Hosp Pharm 2002;37:1301–1306.
29. ANG-LEE M, MOSS J, CUN-SU Y. Herbal medicines and perioperative care. JAMA 2001;2:208–216.
30. NIGHTINGALE SL. From the Food and Drug Administration. JAMA 1997;278:15.
31. ZAACKS SM, KLEIN L, TAN CD, et al. Hypersensitivity myocarditis associated with ephedra use. J Toxicol Clin Toxicol 1999;37:485–489.
32. ROIZEN MK. Anesthetic implications of concurrent diseases. In: MILLER RD, editor. Anesthesia. 4th ed. New York, NY: Churchill Livingstone Inc; 1994. p 903–1014.
33. BLAU JJ. Ephedrine nephrolithiasis associated with chronic ephedrine abuse. J Urol 1998;160:825.
34. POWELL T, HSU FF, TURK J, et al. Ma-huang strikes again: ephedrine nephrolithiasis. Am J Kidney Dis 1998;32:153–159.
35. WHITE LM, GARDNER SF, GURLEY BJ, et al. Pharmacokinetics and cardiovascular effects of ma-huang (*Ephedra sinica*) in normotensive adults. J Clin Pharmacol 1997;37:116–122.
36. GURLEY BJ, GARDNER SF, WHITE LM, et al. Ephedrine pharmacokinetics after the ingestion of nutritional supplements containing *Ephedra sinica* (ma-huang). Ther Drug Monit 1998;20:439–445.
37. STEVINSON C, PITTLER MH, ERNST E. Garlic for treating hypercholesterolemia: a meta-analysis of randomized clinical trials. Ann Intern Med 2000;133:420–429.
38. SRIVASTAVA KC. Evidence for the mechanism by which garlic inhibits platelet aggregation. Prostaglandins Leukot Med 1986;22:313–321.
39. APITZ-CASTRO R, ESCALANTE J, VARGAS R, et al. Ajoene, the antiplatelet principle of garlic, synergistically potentiates the antiaggregatory action of prostacyclin, forskolin, indomethacin and dypiridamole on human platelets. Thromb Res 1986;42:303–311.
40. ROSE KD, CROISSANT PD, PARLIAMENT CF, et al. Spontaneous spinal epidural hematoma with associated platelet dysfunction from excessive garlic ingestion: a case report. Neurosurgery 1990: 26; 880–882.
41. KAYE AD, De WITT BJ, ANWAR M, et al. Analysis of responses of garlic derivatives in the pulmonary vascular bed of the rat. J App Physiol 2000;89:353–358.
42. ALI M, AL-QATTAN KK, AL-ENEZI F, et al. Effect of allicin from garlic powder on serum lipids and blood pressure in rats fed with a high cholesterol diet. Prostaglandins Leukot Essent Fatty Acids 2000;62:253–259.
43. SILAGY CA, NEIL HA. A meta-analysis of the effect of garlic on blood pressure. J Hypertens 1994;12:463–468.
44. ICHIKAWA M, MIZUNO I, YOSHIDA J, et al. Pharmacokinetics of cycloalliin, an organosulfur compound found in garlic and onion, in rats. Available at: http://cat.inist.fr/?aModele = afficheN&cpsidt = 18368283. *CAT. INIST*. Accessed: October 20, 2009.
45. Le BARS PL, KATZ MM, BERMAN N, et al. A placebo-controlled, double-blind, randomized trial of an extract of *Ginkgo biloba* for dementia: north american EGb study group. JAMA 1997;278:1327–1332.
46. OKEN BS, STORZBACH DM, KAYE JA. The efficacy of *Ginkgo biloba* on cognitive function in Alzheimer disease. Arch Neurol 1998;55:1409–1415.

47. JUNG F, MROWIETZ C, KIESEWETTER H, et al. Effect of *Ginkgo biloba* on fluidity of blood and peripheral microcirculation in volunteers. Arzneimittelforschung 1990;40:589–593.

48. MAITRA I, MARCOCCI L, DROY-LEFAIX MT, et al. Peroxyl radical scavenging activity of *Ginkgo biloba* extract EGb 761. Biochem Pharmacol 1995;49:1649–1655.

49. HOYER S, LANNERT H, NOLDNER M, et al. Damaged neuronal energy metabolism and behavior are improved by *Ginkgo biloba* extract (EGb 761). J Neural Transm 1999;106:1171–1188.

50. CHUNG KF, DENT G, MCCUSKER M, et al. Effect of a ginkgolide mixture (BN 52063) in antagonizing skin and platelet responses to platelet activating factor in man. Lancet 1987;1:248–251.

51. ROWIN J, LEWIS SL. Spontaneous bilateral subdural hematomas associated with chronic *Ginkgo biloba* ingestion. Neurology 1996;46:1775–1776.

52. VALE S. Subarachnoid hemorrhage associated with *Ginkgo biloba*. Lancet 1998;352:36.

53. GIBERT GJ. *Ginkgo biloba*. Neulogy 1997;48:1137.

54. MATTHEWS MK Jr. Association of *Ginkgo biloba* with intracerebral hemorrhage. Neurology 1998;50:1933–1934.

55. ROSENBLATT M, MINDEL J. Spontaneous hyphema associated with ingestion of *Ginkgo biloba* extract. N Engl J Med 1997;336:1108.

56. FESSENDEN JM, WITTENBORN W, CLARKE L. *Gingko biloba*: a case report of herbal medicine and bleeding postoperatively from a laparoscopic cholecystectomy. Am Surg 2001;67:33–35.

57. WATSON DG, OLIVEIRA EJ. Solid-phase extraction and gas chromatography—mass spectrometry determination of kaempferol and quercetin in human urine after consumption of *Ginkgo biloba* tablets. J Chrmatoger B Biomed Sci Appl 1999;723:203–210.

58. Ginkgo. In: MILLS S, BONE K, editors. Principles and Practice of Phytotherapy. New York, NY: Churchill Livingstone Inc; 2000. p 404–417.

59. BREKHAM II, DARDYMOV IV. New substances of plant origin which increase nonspecific resistance. Annu Rev Pharmacol 1969;9:419–430.

60. ATTELE AS, WU JA, YUAN CS. Ginseng pharmacology: multiple constituents and multiple actions. Biochem Pharmacol 1999;58:1685–1693.

61. VUKSAN V, SIEVENPIPER JL, KOO VY, et al. American ginseng (*Panax quinquefolius L*) reduces post-prandial glycemia in nondiabetic subjects and subjects with type 2 diabetes mellitus. Arch Interm Med 2000;160:1009–1013.

62. KIMURA Y, OKUDA H, ARICHI S. Effects of various ginseng saponins on 5-hydroxytryptamine release and aggregation in human platelets. J Pharm Pharmacol 1988;40:838–843.

63. KUO SC, TENG CM, LEE JC, et al. Antiplatelet components in *Panax ginseng*. PLanta Med 1990;56:164–167.

64. PARK HJ, LEE JH, SONG YB, et al. Effects of dietary supplementation of lipophilic fraction from *Panax ginseng* on cGMP and cAMP in rat platelets and on blood coagulation. Biol Pharm Bull 1996;19:1434–1439.

65. TENG CM, KUO SC, KO FN, et al. Antipletelet actions of panaxynol and ginsenosides isolated from ginseng. Biochem Biophys Acta 1989;990:315–320.

66. JANETZKY K, MORREALE AP. Probable interaction between warfarin and ginseng. Am J Health Syst Pharm 1997;54:692–693.

67. CHEN SE, SAWCHUK RJ, STABA EJ. American ginseng: III, pharmacokinetics of ginsenosides in the rabbit. Eur J Drug Metab Pharmacokinet 1980;5:161–168.

68. PITTLER MH, ERNST E. Efficacy of kava extract for treating anxiety: systematic review and meta-anaylsis. J Clin Psychopharmacol 2000;20:84–89.

69. PEPPING J. Kava: p*iper methysticum*. Am J Health Syst Pharm 1999;56:957–958, 960.

70. MEYER HJ. Pharmacology of kava. 1. Psychopharmacol Bull 1967;4:10–11.

71. BACKHAUSS C, KRIELSTEIN J. Extract of kava (*Piper. methysticum*) and its methysticin constituents protect brain tissue against ischemic damage in rodents. Eur J Pharmacol 1992;215:265–269.

72. JAMIESON DD, DUFFIELD PH, CHENG D, et al. Comparison of the central nervous system activity of the aqueous and lipid extract of kava (*Piper methysticum)*. Arch Int Pharmacodyn Ther 1989;301:66–80.

73. ALMEIDA JC, GRIMSLEY EW. Coma from the health food store: interaction between kava and alprazolam. Ann Intern Med 1996;125:940–941.

74. NORTON SA, RUZE P. Kava dermopathy. J Am Acad Dermatol 1994;31:89–97.

75. FDA Consumer Advisory. Kava-containing dietary supplements may be associated with severe liver injury. Available at: http://www.cfsan.fda.gov/~dms/addskava.html. Accessed: February 10, 2003.

76. RASMUSSEN AK, SCHELINE RR, SOLHEIM E, et al. Metabolism of some kava pyrones in the rat. Xenobiotica 1979;9:1–16.

77. GASTER B, HOLROYD J. St John's wort for depression: a systematic review. Arch Intern Med 2000;160:152–156.

78. SHELTON RC, KELLER MB, GELENBERG A, et al. Effectiveness of St John's wort in major depression. JAMA 2001;285:1978–1986.

79. MULLER WE, SINGER A, WONNEMANN M, et al. Hyperforin represents the neurotransmitter reuptake inhibiting constituent of hypericum extract. Pharmacopsychiatry 1998;31(suppl 1):16–21.

80. OBACH RS. Inhibition of human cytochrome P450 enzymes by constituents of St. John's wort, an herbal preparation used in the treatment of depression. J Pharmacol Exp Ther 2000;294:88–95.

81. ERNST E. Second thoughts about safety of St. John's wort. Lancet. 1999;354:2014–2016.

82. PISCITELLI SC, BURSTEIN AH, CHAITT D, et al. Indinavir concentrations and St. John's wort. Lancet 2000;355:547–548.

83. YUE QY, BERGQUIST C, GERDEN B. Safety of St. John's wort. Lancet 2000;355:576–577.

84. BREIDENBACH T, HOFFMANN MW, BECKER T, et al. Drug interaction of St. John's wort with cyclosporine. Lancet 2000;355:1912.

85. JOHNE A, BROCKMOLLER J, BAUER S, et al. Pharmacokinetic interaction of digoxin with an herbal extract from St. John's wort. (*Hypericum perforatum*). Clin Pharmacol Ther 1999;66:338–345.

86. NEARY JT, BU Y. Hypericum LI 160 inhibits uptake of serotonin and norepinephrine in astrocytes. Brain Res 1999;816:358–363.

87. FRANKLIN M, CHI J, MCGAVIN C, et al. Neuroendocrine evidence for dopaminergic actions of hypericum extract (LI 160) in healthy volunteers. Biol Psychiatry 1999;46:581–584.

88. LANTZ MS, BUCHALTER E, GIAMBANCO V. St. John's wort and antidepressant drug interactions in the elderly. J Geriatr Psychiatry Neurol 1999;12:7–10.

89. BROWN TM. Acute St. John's wort toxicity. Am J Emerg Med 2000;18:231–232.

90. STACK CG, ROGERS P, LINTER SP. Monoamine oxidase inhibitors and anaesthesia. A review. Br J Anaesth 1988;60:222–227.

91. FERRILL MJ, MURAKAMI KE; Drugdex editorial staff. *Isocarboxazid (Drug Evaluation)*. In: HUTCHISON TA, SHAHAN DR, editors. Drugdex System. Greenwood Village, CO: Micromedex; 2001.

92. KERB R, BROCKMOLLER J, STAFFELDT B, et al. Single-dose and steady-state pharmacokinetics of hypericin and pseudohypericin. Antimicrob Agents Chemother 1996;40:2087–2093.

93. BIBER A, FISCHER H, ROMER A, et al. Oral biovailability of hyperforin from hypericum extracts in rats and human volunteers. Pharmacopsychiatry 1998;31(suppl 1):36–43.

94. HOUGHTON PJ. The scientific basis for the reputed activity of valerian. J Pharm Pharmacol 1999;51:505–512.

95. HENDRIKS H, BOS R, ALLERSMA DP, et al. Pharmacological screening of valerenal and some other components of essential oil of *valeriana officinalis*. Planta Med 1981;42:62–68.

96. ORTIZ JG, NIEVES-NATAL J, CHAVEZ P. Effects of *Valeriana officinalis* extracts on [^{3}H] flunitrazepam binding, synaptosomal [^{3}H] GABA uptake, and hippcampal [^{3}H] GABA release. Neurochem Res 1999;24:1373–1378.

97. SANTOS MS, FERREIRA F, CUNHA AP, et al. Synaptosomal GABA release as influenced by valerian root extract- involvement of the GABA carrier. Arch Int Pharmacodyn Ther 1994;327:220–231.

98. LEUSCHNER J, MULLER J, RUDMANN M. Characterization of the central nervous depressant activity of a commercially available valerian root extract. Arzneimittelforschung 1993;43:638–641.

99. GARGES HP, VARIA I, DORAISWAMY PM. Cardiac complications and delirium associated with valerian root withdrawal. JAMA 1998;280:1566–1567.

100. ANDERSON GD, ELMER ED, TEMPLETON IE, et al. Pharmacokinetics of valerenic acid after administration of valerian in healthy subjects. International Bibliographic Information on Dietary

Supplement, September 19, 2005. Available at: http://grande.nal.usda.gov/ibids/index.php?mode2 = detail&origin = ibids_references&therow = 786227. Accessed: October 20, 2009.
101. TENEBAUM A, FISMAN EZ, MOTRO M. L-arginine: rediscovery in progress. Cardiology 1998;90: 153–155.
102. DALY JM, LIEBERMAN MD, GOLDFINE J, et al. Enteral nutrition with supplemental arginine, RNA, and omega-3 fatty acids in patients after operation: immunologic, metabolic and clinical outcome. Surgery 1992;112:56–67.
103. SENKAL M, KEMEN M, HOMANN HH, et al. Modulation of postoperative immune response by enteral nutrition with a diet enriched with arginine, RNA, and omega-3 fatty acids in patients with upper gastrointestinal cancer. Eur J Surg 1995;161:115–122.
104. KEMEN M, SENKAL M, HOMANN HH, et al. Early postoperative enteral nutrition with arginine-omega-3 fatty acids and ribonucleic acid-supplemented diet vs placebo in cancer patients: an immunologic evaluation of impact. Crit Care Med 1995;23:652–659.
105. TEPASKE R, VELTHUIS H, Oudemans-van STRAATEN HM, et al. Effect of preoperative oral immune-enhancing nutritional supplement on patients at high risk of infection after cardiac surgery: a randomised placebo-controlled trial. Lancet 2001;358:696–701.
106. BOCCHI EA, VILELLA DE MORAES AV, ESTEVES-FILHO A, et al. L-arginine reduces heart rate and improves hemodynamics in severe congestive heart failure. Clin Cardiol 2000;23:205–210.
107. MCKEVOY GK, editor. AHFS Drug Information. Bethesda, MD: American Society of Health-System Pharmacists; 1998.
108. TAKANO H, LIM HB, MIYABARA Y, et al. Oral administration of L-arginine potentiates allergen-induced airway inflammation and expression of interleukin-5 in mice. J Pharmacol Exp Ther 1998;286:767–771.
109. FOSSEL ET. Improvement of temperature and flow in feet of subjects with diabetes with use of a transdermal preparation of L-arginine: a pilot study. Diabetes Care 2004;27:284–285.
110. BIAGINI G, BERTANI A, MUZZARELLI R, et al. Wound management with N-carboxybutyl chitosan. Biomaterials 1991;12:281–286.
111. RAO SB, SHARMA CP. Use of chitosan as a biomaterial: studies on its safety and hemostatic potential. J Biomed Mater Res 1997;34:21–28.
112. UENO H, MORI T, FUJINAGA T. Topical formulations and wound healing applications of chitosan. Adv Drug Deliv Rev 2001;52:105–115.
113. PUSATERI AE, MCCARTHY SJ, GREGORY KW, et al. Effect of a chitosan-based hemostatic dressing on blood loss and survival in a model of severe venous hemorrhage and hepatic injury in swine. Journal of Trauma 2003;4(1):177–182.
114. MCCUE K. "New Bandage Uses Biopolymer." American Chemical Society. Available at: http://www.chemistry.org. Created: March 3, 2003. Accessed: October 16, 2009.
115. GUERCIOLINI R, RADU-RADULESCU L, BOLDRIN M, et al. Comparative evaluation of fecal fat excretion induced by orlistat and chitosan. Obes Res 2001;9:364–367.
116. MUZZARELLI R, BIAGINI G, PUGNALONI A, et al. Reconstruction of parodontal tissue with chitosan. Biomaterials 1989;10:598–603.
117. MUZZARELLI RA, BIAGINI G, BELLARDINI M, et al. Osteoconduction exerted by methylpyrrolidinone chitosan used in dental surgery. Biomaterials 1993;14:39–43.
118. MUZZARELLI R, TARSI R, FILLIPPINI O, et al. Antimicrobial properties of N-carboxybutyl chitosan. Antimicrob Agents Chemother 1990;34:2019–2023.
119. SENKAL M, KEMEN M, HOMANN HH, et al. Modulation of postoperative immune response by enteral nutrition with a diet enriched with arginine, RNA, and omega-3 fatty acids in patients with upper gastrointestinal cancer. Eur J Surg 1995;161:115–122.
120. KEMEN M, SENKAL M, HOMANN HH, et al. Early postoperative enteral nutrition with arginine-omega-3 fatty acids and ribonucleic acid-supplemented diet vs placebo in cancer patients: an immunologic evaluation of impact. Crit Care Med 1995;23:652–659.
121. TERANO T, HIRAI A, HAMAZAKI T, et al. Effect of oral administration of highly purified eicosapentaenoic acid on platelet function, blood viscosity and red cell deformability in healthy human subjects. Atherosclerosis 1983;46:321–331.

122. THIES F, NEBE-VON-CARON G, POWELL JR, et al. Dietary supplementation with eicosapentaenoic acid, but not with other long-chain n-3 or n-6 polyunsaturated fatty acids, decreases natural killer cell activity in healthy subjects aged >55 y. Am J Clin Nutr 2001;73:539–548.

123. FDA. Center for Food Safety and Applied Nutrition. Letter regarding dietary supplement health claim for omega-3 fatty acids and coronary heart disease. Available at: http://vm.cfsan.fda.gov/~dms/ds-ltr11.html. Accessed: October 15, 2009.

124. EPA (eicosapentaenoic acid) effectiveness, safety, and drug interactions on RxList. RxList: The Internet Drug Index. Available at: http://www.rxlist.com/epa_eicosapentaenoic_acid/supplements.htm. Accessed: October 20, 2009.

125. YOKOYAMA M, ORIGASA H, MATSUZAKI M, et al. Effects of eicosapentaenoic acid on major coronary events in hypercholesterolaemic patients (JELIS): a randomised open-label, blinded endpoint analysis. Lancet 2007;369:1090–1098.

126. MEDINA MA. Glutamine and cancer. J Nutr 2001;131:2539S–2542S.

127. WILMORE DW. The effect of glutamine supplementation in patients following elective surgery and accidental injury. J Nutr 2001;131:2543S–2549S.

128. FURUKAWA S, SAITO H, INOUE T, et al. Supplemental glutamine augments phagocytosis and reactive oxygen intermediate production by neutrophils and monocytes from postoperative patients in vitro. Nutrition 2000;16:323–329.

129. ANDERSON PM, RAMSAY NK, SHU XO, et al. Effect of low-dose oral glutamine on painful stomatitis during bone marrow transplantation. Bone Marrow Transplant 1998;22:339–344.

130. COCKERHAM MB, WEINBERGER BB, LERCHIE SB. Oral glutamine for the prevention of oral mucositis associated with high-dose paclitaxel and melphalan for autologous bone marrow transplantation. Ann Pharmacother 2000;34:300–303.

131. SCHLOERB PR, SKIKNE BS. Oral and parenteral glutamine in bone marrow transplantation: a randomized, double-blind study. J Parenter Enteral Nutr 1999;23:117–122.

132. COGHLIN DICKSON TM, WONG RM, NEGRIN RS, et al. Effect of oral glutamine supplementation during bone marrow transplantation. J Parenter Enteral Nutr 2000;24:61–66.

133. MORLION BJ, STEHLE P, WACHTLER P, et al. Total parenteral nutrition with glutamine dipeptide after major abdominal surgery: a randomized, double-blind, controlled study. Ann Surg 1998;227:302–308.

134. POWELL-TUCK J, JAMIESON CP, BETTANY GE, et al. A double blind, randomised, controlled trial of glutamine supplementation in parenteral nutrition. Gut 1999;45:82–88.

135. VAN DER HULST RR, VAN KREEL BK, VON MEYENFELDT MF, et al. Glutamine and the preservation of gut integrity. Lancet 1993;341:1363–1365.

136. JIAN ZM, CAO JD, ZHU XG, et al. The impact of alanyl-glutamine on clinical safety, nitrogen balance, intestinal permeability, and clinical outcome in postoperative patients: a randomized, double-blind, controlled study of 120 patients. J Parenter Enteral Nutr 1999;23:S62–S66.

137. MERTES N, SCHULZKI C, GOETERS C, et al. Cost containment through L-alanyl-L-glutamine supplemented total parenteral nutrition after major abdominal surgery: a prospective randomized double-blind controlled study. Clin Nutr 2000;19:395–401.

138. ZIEGLER TR, YOUNG LS, BENFELL K, et al. Clinical and metabolic efficacy of glutamine-supplemented parenteral nutrition after bone marrow transplantation. A randomized, double-blind, controlled study. Ann Intern Med 1992;116:821–828.

139. BROWN SA, GORINGE A, FEGAN C, et al. Parenteral glutamine protects hepatic function during bone marrow transplantation. Bone Marrow Transplant 1998;22:281–284.

140. ZIEGLER TR, BYE RL, PERSINGER RL, et al. Effects of glutamine supplementation on circulating lymphocytes after bone marrow transplantation: a pilot study. Am J Med Sci 1998;315:4–10.

141. WILMORE DW, SCHLOERB PR, ZIEGLER TR. Glutamine in the support of patients following bone marrow transplantation. Curr Opin Clin Nutr Metab Care 1999;2:323–327.

142. NOYER CM, SIMON D, BORCZUK A, et al. A double-blind placebo-controlled pilot study of glutamine therapy for abnormal intestinal permeability in patients with AIDS. Am J Gastroenterol 1998;93:972–975.

143. Den HOND E, HIELE M, PEETERS M, et al. Effect of long-term oral glutamine supplements on small intestinal permeability in patients with Crohn's disease. J Parenter Enteral Nutr 1999;23:7–11.

144. GARLICK PJ. Assessment of the safety of glutamine and other amino acids. J Nutr 2001;131:2556S–2561S.

145. JEBB SA, OSBORNE RJ, MAUGHAN TS, et al. 5-fluorouracil and folinic acid-induced mucositis: no effect of oral glutamine supplementation. Br J Cancer 1994;70:732–735.

146. RUBIO IT, CAO Y, HUTCHINS LF, et al. Effect of glutamine on methotrexate efficacy and toxicity. Ann Surg 1998;227:772–778.

147. Glutamine effectiveness, safety, and drug interactions. RxList: The Internet Drug Index. Available at: http://www.rxlist.com/glutamine/supplements.htm. Accessed: October 20, 2009.

148. FURST P. New developments in glutamine delivery. J Nutr 2001;131:2562S–2568S.

149. DE BANDT JP, COUDRAY-LUCAS C, LIORET N, et al. A randomized controlled trial of the influence of the mode of enteral ornithine alpha-ketoglutarate administration in burn patients. J Nutr 1998;128:563–569.

150. WERNERMAN J, HAMMARQVIST F, VON DER DECKEN A, et al. Ornithine-alpha-ketoglutarate improves skeletal muscle protein synthesis as assessed by ribosome analysis and nitrogen use after surgery. Ann Surg 1987;206:674–678.

151. BLOMQVIST BI, HAMMARQVIST F, VON DER DECKEN A, et al. Glutamine and alpha-ketoglutarate prevent the decrease in muscle free glutamine concentration and influence protein synthesis after total hip replacement. Metabolism 1995;44:1215–1222.

152. MOUKARZEL AA, GOULET O, SALAS JS, et al. Growth retardation in children receiving long-term total parenteral nutrition: effects of ornithine alpha-ketoglutarate. Am J Clin Nutr 1994;60:408–413.

153. WERNERMAN J, HAMMARKVIST F, ALI MR, et al. Glutamine and ornithine-alpha-ketoglutarate but not branched-chain amino acids reduce the loss of muscle glutamine after surgical trauma. Metabolism 1989;38:63–66.

154. PERKOWSKI D, WAGNER S, MARCUS A, et al. Ribose enhances ventricular function following off pump coronary artery bypass surgery. J Altern Complement Med 2005;11:745.

155. PERKOWSKI D, WAGNER S, St. Cyr J. D-ribose and 'off' pump coronary artery bypass revascularization aids cardiac indices following acute myocardial infarction; presented at the 13th World Congress on Heart Disease, July 2007.

156. MULLER C, ZIMMER HG, GROSS M, et al. Effect of ribose on cardiac adenine nucleotides in a donor model for heart transplantation. Eur J Med Res 1998;3:554–558.

157. GROSS M, REITER S, ZOLLNER N. Metabolism of D-ribose administered continuously to healthy persons and to patients with myoadenylate deaminase deficiency. Klin Wochenschr 1989;67:1205–1213.

158. ZOLLNER N, REITER S, GROSS M, et al. Myoadenylate deaminase deficiency: successful symptomatic therapy by high dose oral administration of ribose. Klin Wochenschr 1986;64:1281–1290.

159. WAGNER DR, GRESSER U, ZOLLNER N. Effects of oral ribose on muscle metabolism during bicycle ergometer in AMPD-deficient patients. Ann Nutr Metab 1991;35:297–302.

160. FALK DJ, HEELAN KA, THYFAULT JP, et al. Effects of effervescent creatine, ribose, and glutamine supplementation on muscular strength, muscular endurance, and body composition. Strength Cond Res 2003;17:810–816.

161. KREIDER RB, MELTON C, GREENWOOD M, et al. Effects of oral D-ribose supplementation on anaerobic capacity and selected metabolic markers in healthy males. Int J Sport Nutr Exerc Metab 2003;13:76–86.

162. BURKE ER. D-Ribose What You Need To Know. Garden City Park, NY: Avery Publishing Group; 1999. p. 1–43.

163. PLIML W, VON ARNIM T, STALEIN A, et al. Effects of ribose on excercise-induced ischaemia in stable coronary artery disease. Lancet 1992;340:507–510.

164. SEGAL S, FOLEY J. The metabolism of D-ribose in man. J Clin Invest 1958;37:719–735.

165. PERLMUTTER NS, WILSON RA, ANGELLO DA, et al. Ribose facilitates thallium-201 redistribution in patients with coronary artery disease. J Nucl Med 1991;32:193–200.

166. HEGEWALD MG, PALAC RT, ANGELLO DA, et al. Ribose infusion accelerates thallium redistribution with early imaging compared with late 24-hour imaging without ribose. J Am Coll Cardiol 1991;18:1671–1681.

Chapter 18

End-of-Life Decision Making

Scott E. Lentz

"Life is a chronic condition that uniformly results in death."

—Penn State University College of Medicine

Medicare estimates that it spends one third of an individual's cancer costs in the final year of life, and 78% of that spending in a patient's final month. One recent study found that in the final month of life admission to the ICU as well as hospital admissions have increased, while prolonged admissions (more than 14 days) in the final month of life have remained unchanged.[1] At the same time, evidence shows that quality of life is better and overall costs are 35% lower in patients who have had end-of-life discussions.[2] With health-care dollars becoming more and more scarce, physicians and other health-care practitioners must carefully consider the value of interventions near the end of life. A large percentage of cancer patients will ultimately succumb to their disease, and many of those patients will require numerous hospital admissions, medication changes, and/or surgical procedures as the natural history of their cancer plays out. This chapter seeks to explore the common events associated with death and dying, with special attention paid to the quality of evidence related to interventions aimed at managing these common conditions.

In a descriptive analysis of the final year of life in ovarian cancer patients, Von Gruenigan found a significant difference in the number of hospital-based deaths among terminally ill patients who were on chemotherapy (but no chemotherapy-related deaths) as well as a significant increase in the number of hospitalizations in the final 3 months of life. Remarkably, only a small percentage of their patients (23%) had adequate documentation of "do not resuscitate" orders. While not intended to be an advisor on the best management of dying patients with ovarian cancer, it is one of the few publications that outlines the natural course in gynecologic cancer patients[3] **Level III**.

The interconnected nature of many of the most common situations becomes apparent as a patient progresses toward death. While the topics here are presented

Gynecologic Oncology: Evidence-Based Perioperative and Supportive Care, Second Edition. Edited by Scott E. Lentz, Allison E. Axtell and Steven A. Vasilev.
© 2011 John Wiley & Sons, Inc. Published 2011 by John Wiley & Sons, Inc.

individually, it is clear that many of the items outlined are intrinsically associated. The distinctions made here are clearly arbitrary ones and every attempt has been made to clarify the particular evidence-based item that a specific reference is directed toward.

PAIN CONTROL

Adequate pain control has become a bellwether for quality care and management. The World Health Organization opened the door on effective pain management in a 1986 monograph entitled *Cancer Pain Relief*.[4] In response to the understanding that medical trainees had little formal training in pain evaluation and control, the "cancer pain ladder" laid the basic groundwork for a productive discourse on best practices in pain control. The significance of the pain problem over the past 20 years has evolved into the acknowledgement that "pain is the 5th vital sign." The vast number of publications concerning pain control are a testament to the level of interest that this subject has garnered.

Pain management can become one of the most challenging aspects of cancer care, particularly because inadequate pain control can spiral into an ever larger morass of clinical symptoms, psychiatric hurdles, and subsequent interventions. Alternatively, adequate pain control can aid the clinician by allowing the patient to constructively participate in her care plan and maximize the quality of life of both the patient and her family.

While the "silver bullet" of cancer pain control remains an elusive goal, a better understanding of the active process of stimulus and response has led to a more comprehensive approach to management. Pain is believed to occur on three separate levels: peripheral, spinal, and supraspinal. Pain can be alleviated at any or all of the three levels, and various combinations of methods have been put forward as optimal management strategies. One of the more recent theories in the pain process is that pain is an active process rather than a passive one and results in fundamental changes in the nervous system. Labeled neuronal plasticity, this theory explains the exaggerated sensitivity, chronic inflammation, and neuropathic pain that commonly results in significant debilitation in cancer patients.[5]

A complete discussion of pain assessment and management is outside the scope of this chapter. The majority of pain management literature centers on assessment instruments that require the patient to participate in quantifying their level of pain as well as the degree of effect produced by an intervention. This is commonly not possible in terminally ill patients, as their medical status precludes adequate participation in assessments. When clinicians attempt to determine the degree of a patient's pain using indirect measures (such as behavioral cues), undertreatment is a real and frequent result.[6] Attempts have been made to correct the deficiency, and two separate assessment tools are available for patients who cannot assist in evaluating their pain.

It is no surprise that the intensive care setting has been the source of a large body of literature for evaluating patient's who cannot participate in assessing subjective symptoms. The development of standardized scoring systems provides a mechanism for objectifying the severity of symptoms, including pain management. In ventilator-dependent patients, the Behavioral Pain Scale was developed for this purpose.[7] It is reliable between different raters, is internally consistent, and is discriminant.[8, 9] Another simple instrument for determining pain level in adults who cannot self-report is the Pain Assessment Behavior Scale. This method is internally consistent and reliable between interpreters and demonstrates a high correlation of pain presence and intensity when tested with able patients.[10]

INTESTINAL OBSTRUCTION

Gastrointestinal dysfunction is one of the more common causes for hospitalization among cancer patients, best demonstrated in the advanced ovarian cancer patient. Intestinal problems can result from any number of sources in the cancer patient, from causes such as direct or ancillary medication effect, posttreatment scarring, central nervous system metastasis, or overt tumor growth in the gastrointestinal tract. The literature in managing terminal intestinal obstruction (TIO) is critically flawed by the inconsistent definition of a successful intervention. Some researchers have traditionally used survival postintervention, but this is counterintuitive in a population of patients where prolonging survival may not be a primary goal. Other researchers have examined rates of discharge or the ability to tolerate oral intake, but these are misleading as they do not directly comment on the effect of a single intervention. Work should proceed to evaluate these interventions based on patient (and family) perceived outcomes as the primary measure. To date, no such publications exist.

The term malignant bowel obstruction (MBO) has been used in various ways covering a spectrum of intestinal problems. The only commonality in each of the cases is that the obstruction is caused by the intra-abdominal growth of tumor. Surgeons who routinely care for these patients can understand that the limitless number of possible recurrence patterns can each result in obstruction, but no two malignant obstructions are the same. Solitary abdominal masses causing strangulation of an isolated segment of intestine are far simpler to resolve than widespread carcinomatosis that has obliterated the mesenteric root. Studies that evaluate MBO need to differentiate between these categories of obstruction, as favorable outcomes in the former situation are far more likely than in the latter. In an attempt to standardize nomenclature such that evidence-based conclusions in MBO patients could be accomplished, a palliative care consensus conference in 2007 clarified the definition of MBO (Table 18.1).

Table 18.1   Definition of Malignant Bowel Obstruction

1. Clinical evidence of bowel obstruction
2. Bowel obstruction beyond the ligament of Treitz
3. Intra-abdominal primary cancer with incurable disease
4. Non-intra-abdominal primary cancer with clear intraperitoneal spread

Excerpted from Reference 11.

The clinical presentation of MBO is notable in that it is distinctly different than other causes of bowel obstruction. These cases generally show a long, slow, progressive development rather than the abrupt onset more typical of a complete small bowel obstruction. As their time course is different, they allow for deliberate evaluation and therapeutic planning. Clinical judgment can become clouded when the insidious history of an MBO is not carefully identified, and this can lead to errors in management of a terminally ill patient. This is not to suggest that surgical emergencies do not occur in MBO patients, rather that the clinical situation demands careful consideration and discussion among the patient, family, surgeon, and oncologist to ensure that the clinical decision making meets the needs of the dying patient. The clinical manifestations common to MBO are variable and often nonspecific. Most commonly, the clinical situation is one that evolves over a long period of time, when significant changes in the clinical examination are commonplace and continual reassessment is needed to determine the best course of action.

As a general rule, the development of MBO suggests an overall survival of less than 1 year and in most cases less than 6 months. Summarized in detail in Table 18.2, the survival rates and operative morbidity among a large number of retrospective case series in gynecologic cancer patients show remarkable consistency **Level II-3**. Operative complication rates are disproportionately high, median survival is abysmally low, and the benefit to these operations is questionable. While Level I data in this phenomenon is unlikely for ethical reasons, the uniformity among the differing publications is noteworthy.

Table 18.2 Case Reports in Malignant Bowel Obstruction

Author	Tumor Site	Number of Patients	Operative Complications %	Median Survival (Months)
Lund et al.	Ovary	25	32	2
Tunca et al.	Ovary	127	NR	7
Piver et al.	Ovary	60	7	2.5
Krebs, et al.	Ovary	98	12	3.1
Clarke-Pearson et al.	Ovary	49	49	4.5
Beattie et al.	Ovary	11	9	7
Soo et al.	Gynecologic	64	15.5	2.5
Pictus et al.	Ovary	60	31	2.5
Van Oojen et al.	Ovary	20	90	1.0
Jong et al.	Ovary	53	42	3.0
Sun et al.	Ovary	57	39	3.0
Redman et al.	Ovary	26	42	2.5
Butler	Various	25	50	2.5
Chan et al.	Various	10	80	2
Woolfson et al.	Various	32	48	7

Adapted from Reference 12.

While the diagnosis of a bowel obstruction is a clinical one, the role of radiologic evaluation must be addressed. Locating an obstruction is an important part of choosing appropriate therapy in any obstruction picture but is more important in the terminal patient who may choose to decline certain interventions (such as laparotomy). Both CT and MRI have been evaluated in their ability to diagnose MBO. The inclusion of CT information altered the management of 21% of cases in one study, confirming the central role that imaging can play in treating these cases.[13] Sensitivity (93%–95%), specificity (100%), and accuracy (94%–96%) for CT and MRI are similar in reported literature,[14, 15] but one head-to-head comparison of the two modalities in the same institution found a marked improvement with the MRI technique.[14] In all trials examining efficacy CT or MRI, the experience of the radiologist is a determining factor in the utility of one modality or another.

The idea of symptom control in MBO patients provides the widest degree of variability. About 42%–80% of patients are reported to have symptom resolution as a result of surgery for MBO, but the inconsistency of the definition of resolution makes comparison impossible. For example, survival for a proscribed period of time as a resolution measure does not address whether obstructive symptoms are managed, and with no validated measuring tools to assess obstructive symptoms, an evaluation of symptom relief is too subjective to draw conclusions. Reobstruction rates are reported on the order of 10%–50%, but time to obstruction is not routinely reported and makes the relationship to surgical intervention suspect. It is unfortunate that the data quality in this subject is so poor, as the morbidity and mortality in these operations is likely one of the driving forces to avoid such procedures. Reported rates of 30-day mortality are in the range of 5%–32%, generally exceeding the usually accepted mortality in elective procedures.

One of the poorly addressed issues of MBO in the terminal patient is whether there is a population for whom surgery should NOT be chosen. This is different from those in whom surgery is contraindicated, the patients in question here are those who could tolerate surgery in all probability but who would derive so little benefit that the risks of the procedure outweigh any benefit of intervention. The inability of CT to accurately identify small volume disease is a clinical conundrum well known in gynecologic oncology. CT accuracy has been documented to be poor (<20%) in cases where the cancer is <0.5 cm, particularly in ovarian and colorectal cancers.[16–18] In these patients, failure rates with surgical interventions are high, and even in highly selected patients, morbidity and mortality remain very high.[19]

A United Kingdom report of the National Confidential Enquiry into Perioperative Deaths[20] stated that surgeons are performing too many "inappropriate and aggressive" operations on patients who are frail or terminally ill. This report was notable in that it highlighted a frequent problem in terminally ill patients and raises the question of when an operation should be avoided. The question is not easily answered, and led to a 1999 review of the published literature to that point which dealt with terminal obstruction in cancer patients. The vast majority of the literature available to the authors was confined to ovarian cancer patients, and the most telling finding was that all of the publications were of the lowest quality **Level III**. No statistical comparison was possible because of the low methodological quality of the studies, and the authors were left to a descriptive analysis only. The results are difficult to synthesize, but do provide a basis to begin further study.

The decision to operate on a terminally ill patient is never an easy one. The patient with a bowel obstruction can present a unique clinical dilemma, as it may be very difficult to help patients understand why a surgical option may not be appropriate. The literature concerning laparotomy in MBO is largely dedicated to those patients early in their disease course, the decision to perform laparotomy is centered around factors concerning the patient, the disease and the procedure. There is no comprehensive score sheet that can accurately tabulate the likely outcome after considering all of these factors; however, evidence of the lowest quality does stipulate that risk factors in any one of the areas should be sufficient to temper the rush to surgery. In ovarian cancer patients, mortality as high as 44% has been predicted when two adverse features are present[21] **Level III**. Prognostic clinical indicators have been culled from the literature and summarized expertly by Ripamonte[12] in a series of publications (Table 18.3).

Age was identified as a prognostic variable in survival of ovarian cancer patients (with or without cachexia),[21,22] a separate colon cancer study showed an increase in

Table 18.3   Prognostic Features Suggesting Poor Outcome from Surgery for Malignant Bowel Obstruction

---

Absolute contraindications
Intestinal motility problems due to diffuse intraperitoneal carcinomatosis
Ascites requiring frequent paracentesis
Diffuse palpable intra-abdominal masses and liver involvement
A recent laparotomy that demonstrated that further corrective surgery was not possible
Previous abdominal surgery that showed diffuse metastatic cancer
Involvement of proximal stomach

Relative contraindications
Widespread tumor
Patients older than 65 years and in association with cachexia
Low serum albumin level and low serum prealbumin level
Previous radiotherapy of the abdomen or pelvis
Distant metastases, pleural effusion, or pulmonary metastases
Elevated blood urea nitrogen levels, elevated alkaline phosphatase levels, advanced tumor
    stage, short diagnosis to obstruction interval
Poor performance status
Extra-abdominal metastases producing symptoms that are difficult to control (e.g., dyspnea)

Other poor prognostic signs
Obstruction secondary to cancer
Patients with nutritional deficits
Multiple partial bowel obstruction with prolonged passage time on radiograph examination

---

Adapted from Reference 12.

odds ratio of dying of 1.85 for each decade from 65 to 85 years.[23] This same trial also showed an increase in odds of dying of 3.3 when ASA class increased from 1 to 2. Malnutrition is a well-known negative prognostic factor in surgical patients, and is a hallmark of terminally ill patients. In MBO patients with malnutrition, there is a threefold increase in the likelihood of death following laparotomy.[24, 25] A very small retrospective review in patients with ovarian carcinomas found that successful palliation (defined as ability to tolerate some form of oral intake for 60 postoperative days) occurred in only 30% of their cases and 40% of the surgical cases experienced some form of postoperative mortality[26] **Level III**.

Procedure-related factors are also paramount in the terminally ill patient, as the surgical maxim to provide maximum benefit with minimal risk is easily evident. Emergent surgery in an MBO patient is clearly associated with increased morbidity and mortality[23], but no studies have been performed in the terminally ill as a specific group. This may be a reflection of the need for careful planning in this circumstance. Disease-related factors such as tumor biology and disease spread are generally not a consideration in the palliative setting, and these issues carry less impact in decision making as compared to the initial presentation of malignancy.

Octreotide

Palliation of obstruction in the inoperable patient has been dramatically improved with the addition of corticosteroids and octreotide to the armamentarium. The Cochrane database found only a trend toward improvement in MBO patients using 6–16 mg dexamethasone **Level II-1**; octreotide is better supported in the literature. In three randomized small trials, octreotide resulted in more rapid removal of nasogastric suction, better control of gastric secretions, and improved nausea control.[27–29]

In addition to managing nausea, the role of octreotide deserves to be expanded in the management of obstructed patients. Supportive care literature shows that octreotide does not alter the lumen of the obstructed bowel above the level of obstruction and does not result in permanent pathologic change above the obstructed bowel. Concerns of poor anastomotic healing in bowel exposed to octreotide were also allayed in this study, where successful anastomosis was performed with ease.[30] Furthermore, octreotide reduces gastric secretions when used in conjunction with percutaneous gastrotomy procedures. Octreotide deserves to be considered earlier in the management of the patient with MBO.

Stent Placement

Endoscopic transluminal stent placement is a relatively new addition to the range of options for MBO. The procedure allows for resolution of obstruction without a formal laparotomy and under conscious sedation. A self-expanding stent (either metal or plastic) is inserted under fluoroscopic or endoscopic guidance. Three separate reviews comparing stent placement to traditional laparotomy confirm that the procedure is successful in the majority of patients and has few complications.[31-33] The appropriate candidates are rare and limited to isolated obstructions in the left colon. Colonic stents in other locations (transverse or splenic flexure) are prone to failure due to redundant colon. Rectal stenting is also problematic as the stent has a tendency to migrate outward after placement. A retrospective series of colonic stenting in obstructed ovarian cancer patients showed that successful stent placement was possible in 77% of their cases, but 56% of their cases required some additional form of surgical intervention (23% because a stent could not be placed and a further 33% in cases where the stent was initially successful)[34] **Level III**. Unfortunately, no assessment of the improvement of quality of life was performed in these cases.

The final palliation in obstructed patients is percutaneous decompression. Known as the venting gastrotomy, this intervention acts a "pressure-release valve" to limit gastric distension and minimize nausea and vomiting. This is generally limited to patients who are not responsive to medical management of nausea and who are not candidates for other surgical procedures. There are no randomized trials in venting gastrotomy, some researchers advocate that response to nasogastric decompression can be used to predict the effectiveness of gastrotomy **Level III**.

The idea of symptom control in MBO patients provides the widest degree of variability, and 42%–80% of patients are reported to have symptom resolution as a result of surgery for MBO, but the inconsistency of the definition of resolution makes comparison impossible. For example, survival for a proscribed period of time as a resolution measure does not address whether obstructive symptoms are managed, and with no validated measuring tools to assess obstructive symptoms, an evaluation of symptom relief is too subjective to draw conclusions. Reobstruction rates are reported on the order of 10%–50%, but time to obstruction is not routinely reported and makes the relationship to surgical intervention suspect. It is unfortunate that the data quality in this subject is so poor, as the morbidity and mortality in these operations is likely one of the driving forces to avoid such procedures. Reported rates of 30-day mortality are in the range of 5%–32%, generally exceeding the usually accepted mortality in elective procedures.

NUTRITIONAL MANAGEMENT

As GI function declines, nutritional support becomes a common concern. Frequently, this feature is the initial signal to family and friends that there has been a change in the status of the patient's disease. Temporal wasting, loss of fat stores, and generalized cachexia are all classically taught as signs of advanced cancer. Management of these issues is less well taught in medical school and patients are increasingly turning to outside sources for support and advice. This is not without consequence as some interventions advocated by alternative sources are potentially harmful, but others have proven effectiveness. Traditional nutritional support measures have been confined to pharmacologic appetite stimulation, enteral nutrition, and parenteral nutrition. Each is considered in detail here. The impact of cancer cachexia is important in that several sources have independently confirmed that "anorexia and weight loss are validated predictors of early death" in advanced cancer patients.[35]

Terminal malignancy of any sort ultimately evolves into anorexia. As the disease process moves forward, patients lose the stimulus to maintain adequate nutritional intake, and this proceeds to outright wasting and malnutrition. Many cancers present with anorexia as an initial symptom, but frequently effective anticancer therapy resolves this anorexia and patients return to their pretreatment weight. However, once a cancer diagnosis reaches the terminal stage, anorexia is nearly impossible to avoid.

Sources of anorexia are both intrinsic and extrinsic. The mechanisms involved in tumor-related anorexia are still poorly understood but are likely related to a complex interaction among tumor cytokine factors. Extrinsic effects producing anorexia are more easily explained and are largely related to mechanical effects by the tumor on the gastrointestinal tract. The previous discussion of intestinal obstruction outlines the evidence related to procedures on the GI tract for symptom resolution. Other non-surgical interventions are also potentially helpful in mitigating anorexia in terminally ill patients.

Pharmacologic Support

Pharmacologic support of nutrition is largely limited to megestrol acetate. The original reference for this intervention comes from an incidental finding in breast cancer patients from a 1987 publication using variable doses of the medication. Since that time, megestrol has become a standard in resolving cancer-related cachexia and has also found use in other wasting syndromes, notably in the AIDS population. Despite the large body of literature in support of the use of megestrol for weight gain, there is still dispute about the exact mechanism of appetite stimulation. A large body of Level I data supports the practice of megestrol use, led by a very large placebo-controlled trial that found that 800 mg/day resulted in improved appetite in 70% of the patients studied as well as a weight gain of at least 15 pounds in 16% of the study population.[36] The same trial contains an important caveat though—in the placebo group, a full 44% reported improved appetite, a fact that should not detract from the statistical significance of the results, but highlight the dramatic placebo effect in this symptom.

Despite the positive effect of megestrol on weight gain, this may not translate into improved survival. If the sign of weight loss in cancer patients portends early demise, the logical connection would be that reversing that trend should improve survival. In a randomized, placebo-controlled trial in lung cancer patients, no difference was found when megestrol versus placebo was added to standard chemotherapy[37] **Level I**. Furthermore, global quality of life is not improved with the addition of megestrol. Despite the clear improvement in appetite, this does not extrapolate to other areas of the debilitated patient.

Other agents have been tested against megestrol in head-to-head fashion, without much success. The most commonly reported alternates to the progestational agent are eicosapentaenoic acid nutritional supplements or the marijuana derivative, dronabinol. In both cases, direct randomized comparisons failed to show benefit above that of the megestrol[38,39] **Level I**. Corticosteroids have been shown to perform equivalent to megestrol, and may be associated with better global quality of life improvements. This concept is less well studied and must also be weighed against the detrimental effects of prolonged corticosteroid use.

Parenteral Nutrition

Total parenteral nutrition (TPN) is an item that is generally disdained in patients with advanced solid tumors. This is reflected in a consensus opinion statement from the American College of Physicians, which is based upon randomized clinical trials that fail to demonstrate clinical benefit when TPN is used for these patients.[40] TPN is shown to increase costs and may be associated with an increased likelihood of tumor progression and death. Weight gain on TPN is the result of water weight and fat deposition, but no increase in lean body mass. The contribution of lean body mass to overall well-being should not be underestimated. As an example, in the HIV population, loss of more than 40% of lean body mass is a direct predictor of survival[41] **Level I**. All information on tumor progression on TPN is limited to animal models only. No randomized trials in humans with solid tumors have analyzed the behavior of tumors related to hyperalimentation alone. Despite these facts, the use of TPN in terminally ill patients continues.

One poorly studied, but frequently cited use for TPN is the effect of improved quality of life. Many times this takes the form of improving one's health to allow further treatment—usually in the form of chemotherapy. This was specifically evaluated in ovarian cancer patients with what was termed a Terminal Intestinal Obstruction (TIO). Patients with TIO were categorized as such if they were declared inoperable and had an irreversible obstruction that precluded any form of enteral feeding. TPN usage in this trial was at the discretion of the treating physician as was the case for chemotherapy administration as well. Despite the inherent bias in the study design, the results are notable for the finding that the median survival appeared to be increased in the TPN group, but once the confounding effect of chemotherapy was resolved, overall survival was statistically shorter in the TPN group[42] **Level II-3**. Unfortunately, no cost or quality of life assessment was included in this limited report.

ELECTROLYTE CHANGES

Nutritional derangement ultimately leads to electrolyte abnormality. Commonly, these are the root source of many hospital admissions, and the direct effects of malignancy can also lead to catastrophic electrolyte derangements.

Hypercalcemia deserves a particular mention as one of the electrolytes commonly associated with cancer. Two common situations result in hypercalcemia: either a paraneoplastic syndrome or a direct lytic effect from bony metastases. Hypercalcemia is often associated with breast cancers and small cell lung cancers, but is not unusual in gynecologic malignancies, including those at the end of life.

The mechanism of tumor-induced hypercalcemia (TIH) is based on a dysregulation between osteoblast and osteoclast activity. Additionally, renal reabsorption of calcium is increased through a direct effect of parathyroid hormone–related protein (PTHrP).[43,44] Unlike hyperparathyroidism, the effects of PTHrP lead to an increased ratio of deoxypyridinoline and osteocalcin, causing an "uncoupling" of bone formation and resorption. This effect is established by the observation that collagen cross link excretion increases in patients with TIH.[45]

Hypercalcemic patients rapidly dehydrate as excreted calcium brings water along with it and this exacerbates the clinical dilemma. Paradoxically, furosemide therapy has been advocated as an initial step in the management of hypercalcemia. Remarkably, the evidence for this intervention is scant and publications on the topic are both outdated and of poor quality **Level III**. A comprehensive review of the subject clarifies that furosemide therapy is both counterintuitive and probably incorrect.[46]

Bisphosphonate therapy should probably be considered the treatment of choice for TIH. A large body of randomized-controlled trials comparing all of the clinically available agents were able to normalize calcium levels in 70%–90% of patients with minimal side effects **Level I**. The most commonly used agents are clodronate and pamidronate, but the newer agents ibandronate and zoldronate have also been tested in this condition. In the palliative setting, clodronate may be the most useful, as it can be given as a subcutaneous injection. A once daily, 1500-mg dose was found to be effective at normalizing 80% of hypercalcemic patients (**Level II-1**), but this has not been specifically tested in the palliative setting.[47] Pamidronate has a larger body of literature and is associated with normocalcemia in up to 90% of cases. In a randomized head-to-head comparison, a single infusion of 90 mg given intravenously over 2–24 hours produced normocalcemia for a period of 4 weeks compared to 2 weeks using clodronate[48] **Level II-2**. Limited quality evidence exists for ibadronate, and the optimal dose is not yet known. Phase 2 data with this agent show comparable effectiveness with pamidronate, but there have been no direct comparisons. The advantage in ibadronate seems to be the tolerability of prolonged administration, but further studies are required. Zoledronate holds promise because very low doses (1–2 mg) and very short treatments (30 minutes) seem to be effective in TIH. Further data is also necessary in this compound, as only phase 1 data is available in small numbers of patients[49] **Level III**.

NAUSEA AND VOMITING

Nausea and vomiting are probably the most feared cancer-related symptoms, both during therapy and at the end of life. Nausea and vomiting may be better tolerated during treatment as patients can conceptualize a future where the symptoms will disappear once therapy is concluded. However, at the end of life this same hopefulness is not present, and the despair brought with nausea and vomiting is magnified by hopelessness. This is further exacerbated by the truth that commonly nausea (and vomiting) may be unavoidable side effects of other symptomatic efforts—most notably pain control. Whether nausea is a mechanical process from gastric overdistension or is a central phenomenon controlled at the brainstem, the ultimate product causes anxiety for patients and family members and leads to frequent contacts with caregivers. This may occur through the hospice care services, or may escalate as far as inpatient admission in order to resolve the problem.

Management of nausea and vomiting in the dying patient often involves a consideration of many other causes, and a careful determination of which interventions are suitable for discontinuation versus those that are not. A common example is the nauseating effect of pain medications. If other causes have been excluded, and the source of nausea is narcotic related, patients and caregivers are forced to consider whether cessation of narcotics to resolve nausea is worth the potential increase in unmanaged pain. If substitute medications can limit nausea while providing effective pain control, these interventions are the best initial first management step.

As elaborated in the NCCN guidelines, initial pharmacologic management of nausea includes metoclopramide for gastroparesis, with or without the addition of dopamine receptor antagonists. Benzodiazepines can help those in whom anxiety exacerbates the nausea, but alone, these drugs have no antiemetic effect. Changes in the route of administration may also improve effectiveness, particularly in those who are unable to tolerate oral intake. For persistent nausea and vomiting, the addition of corticosteroids or continuous infusion of antiemetics can alleviate suffering. Finally, if all else fails, palliative sedation or other nonpharmacologic interventions may be helpful.

As regards nonpharmacologic management of nausea and vomiting, acupuncture has seen the largest recent increase in interest. This intervention has not yet been tested in the terminally ill, but studies in cancer patients undergoing chemotherapy have shown promise. A Chinese trial compared acupuncture with vitamin B6 against acupuncture alone or vitamin B6 alone. The study found that the combination group had significantly fewer emesis episodes than either of the other groups[50] **Level II-2**.

Other acupuncture literature predates the routine use of anticipatory antiemetics with prolonged half-lives, and the largest comprehensive analysis suggested that the beneficial effects of acupressure were of unclear clinical merit.[51] This was based on the fact that the most robust analysis was on an admittedly small number of patients (only 139 in three trials) and that the chosen acupuncture points were arbitrary and in some cases incomplete. This feature highlights the largest criticism of acupuncture, namely that the treatment is technician dependent. The highest quality study on the subject of acupuncture in chemotherapy-related nausea was performed in the pediatric oncology population. A multicenter crossover study in patients receiving highly emetogenic treatments did show a significantly lower need for rescue medication as well as fewer treatment-induced vomiting episodes among patients who were receiving acupuncture[52] **Level II-1**. In addition to its design, this trial is notable for the fact that acupuncturists were allowed to tailor therapy to the individual. This trial is limited by the lack of a placebo arm (sham acupuncture) as well as a limited number of participants. Even so the conclusions suggest that there is a role for acupuncture in managing nausea and vomiting and the benefit may be extended to the terminally ill, particularly when other interventions are fruitless.

CONSTIPATION

Different from obstruction, the constipated patient is no less uncomfortable. Interventions are notably less invasive, but often require a larger amount of "tinkering" before adequate bowel function is achieved. Again, these symptoms are commonly an unintended side effect of another therapy and are best managed in a proactive manner rather than a reactive one. Constipation is universally recognized as a common side effect of many medications given in cancer care, and most palliative and supportive care physicians recommend the routine administration of cathartic measures when ordering any form of narcotics in the terminally ill patient. Recommendations for the optimum laxative regimen are based largely on clinical opinion and are lacking experimental supportive evidence.

A comprehensive review by the Cochrane Database in 2008[53] found only three trials in palliative care patients that met their rather broad inclusion criteria. In reviewing the literature, specifically included were palliative care patients (but not required to have cancer) and specifically excluded were any trials that included healthy volunteers. This resulted in a very small sample size of patients (163), which did not allow for data pooling. Five laxative agents were utilized among the three trials: senna, lactulose, danthron combined with poloxamer, Misrakasneham, and magnesium hydroxide combined with liquid paraffin. In head-to-head comparisons of the five agents, there were no statistically significant differences between the agents to make one more potent than another. The relationship to opioid use was examined in two of the trials evaluated, and while a statistical difference was not found, a trend toward improved response to laxatives in the nonopioid patients as opposed to those using strong opioids was seen. Notably, when patient preference was reported in constipation trials, taste was the primary determinant of preference rather than stool frequency. In an area where there seems to be little high quality evidence, perhaps the motivating force for choosing laxatives should be patient preference.

In cancer patients who require laxatives, no differences have been found between lactulose and senna. The pair used in combination is more effective than either agent alone in patients who can tolerate both. Bulk-forming laxatives (fiber or methylcellulose) should be carefully considered in terminally ill patients. If these agents are used in the absence of adequate water supplies, constipation will worsen rather than improve. In the terminally ill patient who is not capable of supplying sufficient water, these agents should be avoided. The popularity of lactulose in the palliative setting is well documented, but the excessive side effects (flatulence, bloating, and abdominal pain) have caused others to consider alternatives.[54] A "laxative ladder" conceptually similar to the analgesic ladder from the WHO had been proposed but lacks any published evidence of its usefulness **Level III**.

A final comment on the concept of opioid rotation. This management strategy was introduced in the early 1990s for the management of opioid-induced constipation. The theory in this method is that by alternating opioids in patients who are chronically dependent on such pain medications, clinicians can limit the degree of constipation. Rotations that have been promoted in the literature are based on replacing an opioid with a nonsteroidal agent (e.g., morphine and tramadol), choosing altered routes of administration (oral morphine vs. transdermal fentanyl), or by alternating agonist only narcotics with agonist/antagonist agents (morphine vs. methadone). Clinical evidence for this behavior is scant. There are no randomized clinical trials to support this sort of action, but low quality data does indicate that opioid rotation can reduce the level of opioid side effects[55] **Level III.**

ASCITES

Gynecologic oncology is well acquainted with the dilemma of tumor-related ascites, but terminal ascites represents quite a different dilemma than ascites as a presenting symptom. Aggressive anticancer therapy commonly resolves ascites in the initial setting, but once cancers have become resistant to cytotoxic therapy or once patients are too infirm to tolerate the side effects of chemotherapy, treatment options become severely limited. Patients commonly fixate on the benefit of percutaneous drainage and may be unaware that without an effective strategy to manage the underlying cause of the ascites, needle drainage is a temporary solution for a permanent problem. Repetitive drainage also leads to loculation of the fluid making continued drainage efforts more difficult and less effective. The ultimate outcome is that repeated drainage attempts can become very painful for patients, leading to frustration for the patient and the clinician as well as possible infectious seeding and procedural complication.

The pathophysiology of malignant ascites separates it from other causes of ascites with respect to management and outcomes. Originally, malignant ascites was considered to be a mechanical phenomenon, the result of lymphatic channel blockages and subsequent lymphangitic edema. This concept has been amended to include other nonobstructive processes, predominantly immunomodulators. A comprehensive discussion of the pathophysiology of malignant ascites is outside the scope of this book, but animal studies have found that cell-free malignant ascites can cause an increase in edema most likely related to an increase in capillary permeability.

Standard therapeutic options for malignant ascites remain diuretic therapy and paracentesis. As most terminally ill patients will have therapy-resistant tumors or may be too deconditioned to tolerate further anticancer therapy, treatments directed at the source of ascites are generally not available to the terminal patient. Diuretic therapy is generally resisted in newly diagnosed ovarian cancer patients, but may be beneficial when ascites is the result of portal hypertension from liver metastases. Despite the limitations described above, periodic paracentesis remains the most effective method of management, but reaccumulation is the rule and the question of needless interventions in a dying patient becomes a legitimate concern.

Alternates to paracentesis are the percutaneous drainage systems. Numerous publications have reviewed the various options, ranging from pigtail catheter drainage to the placement of long-term shunting therapies. In 2005, the FDA approved the use of the PleurX™ pleural catheter for use in drainage of malignant ascites. In all of the methods for percutaneous drainage, the primary complicating factor is the potential for migration of bacteria along the catheter and into the peritoneal cavity. Shunt therapy aims to resolve the infectious risks, but this comes at the cost of more severe complications such as permanent occlusion, pulmonary edema, venous thrombosis, and DIC. The TIPS procedure has high quality data[56] (**Level I**) supporting its use in reducing portal hypertension and improving sodium excretion, but this data is confined to patients whose ascites is the result of portal venous congestion. Since portal hypertension is felt to be the cause of ascites in only 15% of cancer patients, the role of this procedure in malignant ascites is questionable.

Novel therapies are in process, but the evidence to support them remains poor. A number of trials have evaluated intraperitoneal immunotherapy with either interferon alfa-2b or tumor necrosis factor alpha (TNF-α). Interferon was associated with a 36% complete response rate (defined as the inability to withdraw fluid during paracentesis) and a 9% partial response rate (**Level III**) in ovarian cancer patients.[57] A second small study in patients with malignant ascites (including 10 ovarian cancer patients) confirmed TNF-α as effective in 22 out of 29 patients[58] **Level III**. A larger case control trial used intraperitoneal infusion of the streptococcal antigen OK-432 and found a 56% response rate as well as a significant increase in overall survival (10.2 vs. 3.1 months)[59] **Level II-2**. All of these have been tested only in the primary setting and no information exists in their use on dying patients.

Both VEGF and matrix metalloprotinases have been targeted in an attempt to limit ascites, but neither has sufficient evidence to suggest use in any clinical setting. Anti-VEGF is yet to be tested in human subjects despite promising effect in cell culture and animal models.[60] A single trial using the metalloproteinase inhibitor batimastat in humans also showed promise, but animal models demonstrated a contradictory effect, which requires further analysis.[61]

The role of VEGF in ascites has been further highlighted by the rapid adoption of bevacizumab into clinical practice. First reported in a safety/efficacy trail in refractory malignant ascites, bevacizumab has been found to be effective in advanced ovarian cancer patients. The mechanism is not completely understood at this time, but appears to relate to the increased serum VEGF levels found in patients with malignancy. Serum VEGF is highest in patients with chemoresistant, progressive disease and ascites production is felt to be the result of the increased vascular permeability produced by VEGF. Bevacizumab has been tested in both intravenous administration as well as intraperitoneal routes, with promising results. Responses range from 1 to 4 months in heavily pretreated patients, all reporting marked clinical response and the ability to abandon repetitious paracenteses while using bevacizumab. The side effect profile remains mild, with no reported major side effects in the palliative use of this agent[62–64] (**Level II-3**).

RESPIRATORY FUNCTION

It is those patients who are unfortunate enough to contend with respiratory compromise at the end of life who provide the most compelling and heartbreaking dilemmas. Pulmonary metastases that lead to altered gas exchange at the alveolar level ultimately progress to overt tachypnea and a clinical picture reminiscent of COPD. As the brainstem respiratory centers are driven by serum concentrations of O_2 and CO_2, efforts to alleviate symptoms are commonly short lived. Most researchers agree that terminal intubation is both uncomfortable and potentially harmful, and patients generally view mechanical ventilation as an unacceptable intrusion in the final time. Control of respiratory symptoms is usually focused on "outwitting" the symptoms.

Patients commonly report that the sensation of a fan moving air across the face will provide a sense of security. While a common house fan cannot produce air flow sufficient to improve air entry, there is a secondary effect produced by cooling the face in the area served by the second and third branches of the trigeminal nerve.[65] Randomized-controlled trials have demonstrated the benefit of passive flow of oxygen or air by an unknown mechanism.[66,67,108] Highest quality data on the effect of this simple intervention are forthcoming as a fully powered randomized-controlled trial is presently underway.[68]

A newer therapeutic option in cancer patients may be the idea of noninvasive ventilation (NIV). The process is similar to the more well-known BIPAP, but has recently been extended to the end-stage cancer patients with solid tumors in a small trial in Italy. There was no difference found in the mortality rates when patients were randomly assigned between NIV and standard passive oxygenation, but there were marked differences in quality of life in the patients in the NIV group. One of the notable effects was a reduction in morphine use in the NIV group, which allowed for better communication between patients and caregivers[69] **Level III**. While the evidence is limited in this intervention, it does represent an active attempt to manage respiratory debilitation while limiting painful and high risk interventions.

Pharmacological Management

Opioids

Evidence is widely available and of the highest quality (**Level I**) that opioids are effective in alleviating breathlessness. In a large meta-analysis of randomized, double blind, placebo-controlled trials (18 studies included), opioid use provided improved symptom control over placebo regardless of the mode of delivery. In a secondary analysis, the mode of delivery was also evaluated and found that there was a statistical difference favoring parenteral administration over nebulized opioids.[70] Oral administration can offer a similar effect, as demonstrated in a randomized-controlled trial in opioid naive patients. Using a visual analog scale measurement, a 20-mg sustained-release morphine formulation provided a 5%–10% improvement in dyspnea as well as improved sleep in all patients studied[71] **Level II-1**. Dosing schedules are inconsistent among available published literature and the optimal schedule had not been determined. Fears of excess mortality as a result of chronic narcotic use, which limit widespread utilization of this intervention, have never been demonstrated in any published studies.

Benzodiazepines

Empirical use of benzodiazepines is widespread, primarily to alleviate anxiety associated with breathlessness rather than the symptom itself. Existing evidence does not support this maneuver, as there are no randomized-controlled trials to document its effectiveness. One trial did examine the combination of midazolam and morphine and found an improvement in control of cancer dyspnea. This finding is limited by the quality of the trial, especially as no placebo control arm was employed[72] **Level III**.

Unconventional Therapies

Several novel approaches have been considered for use in patients with terminal breathlessness. One such option is heliox. Heliox has been used as a bridging maneuver for some time in patients with airway obstruction, but because of its cost has not been considered for the terminally ill. By replacing the nitrogen in inspired air with helium, the helium:oxygen mixture is able to reduce the work of breathing and improve alveolar ventilation by reducing airway turbulence. A small trial in lung cancer patients (**Level II-2**) found that oxygen saturation and exercise capacity was improved by the use of heliox compared to oxygen-enriched air.[73] An alternate option may prove to be inhaled furosemide. When inhaled in mist form, frusemide can act to limit bronchoconstrictive stimuli and prevent cough. This intervention is both cost effective and easily managed, making it an attractive option. No controlled trials have been performed in the terminally ill, but limited Level III data are intriguing.[74–76]

FATIGUE

The medical term *fatigue* is not only a symptom, but can also be a syndrome as well as a disease on its own. Fatigue has been estimated in 60%–90% of cancer patients while on treatment, and there is no discernable difference between the fatigue seen in patients on chemotherapy and those receiving radiation therapy. There are no pharmacologic methods to manage fatigue and the contribution of anemia to fatigue is overestimated by both patients and the media. Recent studies in this field have outlined the limited effect that management of anemia has on improving fatigue scores, and notably, the effects of exercise and activity have been shown to be the most beneficial. Perhaps most distressing is a lack of understanding that patients and clinicians show for the duration required to resolve fatigue.

Evaluating Fatigue

Assessment of fatigue has been a primary barrier to completing research designed to alleviate this symptom. Of the myriad of quality-of-life assessment tools that have arisen in the past 15 years, several have included questions that address fatigue; but the assessment of fatigue is not the primary target of these questionnaires. The most widely used tool is the Functional Assessment of Cancer Therapy (FACT).[77] The advantage of this tool is that it has been validated across several countries and ethnic groups, and the FACT assessment is commonly included in the quality-of-life arm of most cooperative group trials.

The limitation in FACT assessment is that the tool is not specific for fatigue, and this has led to attempts to create instruments that are specific to fatigue and to the many dimensions of its burden. To date, there are no tools that have been prospectively validated across a multitude of cultures, but the Multidimensional Fatigue Index (MFI) is a promising start. This index has the advantages of being easily administered, requires minimal patient input, is easily interpreted and scored, and is readily translated for cross-cultural applicability. Despite the reproducible nature of this instrument in several populations, it has not yet garnered full international acceptance.[78]

Patterns of fatigue are notable in that they do not always demonstrate the same resilience that other physical processes do following treatment. High quality fatigue assessment examines the subdimensions of fatigue. There is little agreement of how many different subdimensions constitute a complete fatigue assessment but as an example, items such as general fatigue, reduced motivation, reduced activity, mental fatigue, and physical fatigue can be individually assessed. There have been no fatigue assessments specific to gynecologic oncology, but a comprehensive assessment in Hodgkin's lymphoma patients showed a remarkable pattern.[79] While a portion of patients will return to normal levels of functioning after therapy, there are other groups who *never* regain full functionality even after improving once treatment stops; the most concerning group shows that functionality remains low after treatment and actually decreases over time, despite the fact that the patients are cancer free **Level II-2**.

Treatment

Treatment of fatigue remains an elusive goal. The most comprehensive assessment of interventions designed to correct fatigue was performed by the U.S. Agency for Healthcare Research and Quality. Their report evaluated all randomized clinical trials in patients with cancer-related fatigue, and perhaps the most telling finding was that there were only 10 evaluated trials. None of the included trials were performed in gynecologic cancer patients, and the commentary on this report cited several flaws in the included studies. The most widely publicized aspect of the AHRQ report is the 2001 report, which confirmed that erythropoietin alpha used for cancer-related anemia resulted in a statistically significant correlation between hemoglobin level and overall quality of life. In the AHRQ report, this is the only pharmacologic intervention study, the remaining nine studies examined nonpharmacologic methods, which showed promising outcomes for actions such as psychotherapy, relaxation therapy, support groups, and exercise therapy.[80]

Table 18.4   Bleeding Control Measures in the Advanced Cancer Patient

Topical measures	Procedural measures
Nonadherent dressings	Radiotherapy
Hemostatic dressings	Surgery
Absorbable gelatin	Vessel ligation
Microfibrillar collagen	Tissue resection
Absorbable collagen	Endoscopy
Oxidized cellulose	Interventional radiology
Fibrin sealants	Transcutaneous embolization
Alginates	Transcutaneous balloon
Hemostatic agents	**Systemic measures**
Epinephrine	Vitamin K
Acetone	Vasopressin
Thrombin/	Somatostatin analogues
thromboplastin	Antifibrinolytic agents
Topical cocaine	Tranexamic acid
Prostaglandin E2/F2	Aminocaproic acid
Silver nitrate	Aprotinin
Formalin	Blood products
Aluminum	Platelets
astringents	Fresh frozen plasma
Sucralfate	Coagulation factors

BLEEDING

Bleeding is a symptom that may be more frequently found in gynecologic cancer patients than in other malignancies. Not only a direct cause of anemia, bleeding is a very distressing sign for patients, is a clinical conundrum for physicians, and may eventually be the proximate cause of death. Agents to control hemorrhage can be classified into either local or systemic approaches (Table 18.4).

PACKED RED BLOOD CELLS

Locoregional Therapy

The interventions discussed here are directed at identifiable bleeding; occult bleeding does not generate the same degree of anxiety among patients. The choice of the level of intervention must first consider the overall patient condition and outlook. Many of the methods to control bleeding require hospitalization or outpatient procedures, something that may be inappropriate or unfeasible in a terminally ill patient. Furthermore, the administration of sedative agents in order to complete an invasive procedure may result in an alteration of sensorium that the patient or her family dislike. This section merely outlines the basic interventions available, clinical judgment must dictate the most appropriate for a specific patient.

Evidence to support one intervention over another is lacking. Most literature on this subject is in the form of case reports **Level III**. Among the locally applied hemostatic agents, there are no reports of superiority of one agent over another and the best option is generally guided by patient-specific factors. Radiotherapy for hemostatic control is well known to the gynecologic oncologist, but there is disagreement over the most appropriate dosing schedule. Radiotherapy will control up to 80% of acute bleeding,[92–95] but this option may not available in the end-of-life setting, as many gynecologic cancer patients will have received irradiation as a primary treatment modality. Patients who recur within the previously irradiated field pose a special challenge as their treatment options become limited.

Endoscopic control of hemorrhage has become more effective as the instrumentation for operative endoscopy has improved. Again, the specific methods of endoscopic hemostasis are largely confined to case reports and small series, but the evidence for direct hemostasis is superior to balloon tamponade[96] **Level III**. Hemostatic agents can include ethanol, hyperosmotic saline, gelatin solutions, as well as electrocautery, thermocautery, or laser cautery.

Interventional radiology has also evolved to provide a crucial component of hemorrhage control. These procedures are generally limited to situations where acute bleeding is confined to areas with a clearly defined arterial supply and where major organs are not involved. The procedures generally require some form of arterial cannulation with fluoroscopic guidance of a flexible catheter. Again, case reports (Level III) dominate the literature where hemorrhage is concerned, and there are no reported series demonstrating interventional radiology as superior to other methods of local control.

Systemic Therapy

Systemic agents to control bleeding are generally directed at restoring the normal clotting cascade, inhibiting clot resolution, or causing small vessel spasm to affect clot formation. Vitamin K is essential for the extrinsic pathway of clot formation and has been shown to effectively reverse excessive anticoagulation. Vitamin K is available in parenteral, subcutaneous and oral formulations, and there is conflicting evidence on the best route of administration. In a trial comparing the various methods of administration, intravenous use resulted in the most rapid resolution of anticoagulation, but was also the most likely to overcorrect[97] **Level II-1**. In a separate trial, subcutaneous administration was felt to be the optimal route of administration as all patients given subcutaneous vitamin K were able to achieve normal INR within 72 hours of drug administration[98] **Level II-1**.

Vasopressin and somatostatin analogues (octreotide acetate) have been advocated in the control of gastrointestinal bleeding. These agents both work via the splanchnic circulation but using different mechanisms. Vasopressin causes direct arteriolar constriction in the splanchnic circulation and can be administered both intravenously or intra-arterially. In oncologic use, about 50% of patients with upper gastrointestinal malignancy were able to achieve bleeding control with vasopressin continuous infusion using 0.1–0.4 mg[99] **Level II-1**. Side effects are consistent with vascular constriction, most significant in the myocardial, cerebrovascular, or mesenteric circulation. Octreotide acts via splanchnic vasodilation resulting in lowered vessel pressures and decreased portal venous flow. This medication must be titrated to achieve maximal effectiveness and may require additional time (as compared to vasopressin) to resolve hemorrhage. No reports exist regarding the use of octreotide in cancer patients with the exception of prophylactic use in postoperative pancreatic cancer resections. There are no reports of use of octreotide use as hemorrhage control in the terminally ill.

The final category of systemic agents consist of the fibrinolysis inhibitors. These agents are synthetic products that block plasminogen binding and result in decreased fibrin clot lysis. These agents are well described in the nononcologic setting, and are used frequently following dental extractions and in gastrointestinal hemorrhage.[100] In cancer patients, the role of these agents is as yet unclear. Data in support[101–107] is limited to Level III and no controlled studies are forthcoming.

DECISION MAKING

End-of-life decision making can produce the most compelling and dramatic moments in a patient's life. Hospice and palliative care have made it a priority to educate physicians and caregivers that consideration should be given to end-of-life decision making early and often in the disease of a terminally ill patient. As most clinicians will attest, this discussion is more easily done in the artificial environment of a professional gathering rather than in the setting of direct patient care. Patient's lives are sloppy, and they are commonly unprepared to discuss difficult subjects such as death at a time when they want to be focused on treatments and living. Furthermore, routine office visits generally do not lend themselves to long compelling discussions that involve philosophy and theology.

Patients commonly designate a primary decision maker, either by direct identification or by evolution as the disease process proceeds. In cases where patients are unable or unwilling to choose a proxy for health-care decisions, the state will designate one for them. Laws designating the health-care proxy vary according to governmental body, and this too can lead to conflict among families. Conventional legal boundaries defining a proxy may be no better than a stranger in making critical decisions in an age when families are separated by thousands of miles, contain half-siblings, and include step-families. Surrogate decision making is governed by a series of landmark legal decisions that are by no means comprehensive or exhaustive. Table 18.5 outlines the basic framework that decision making falls under, specific details differ by state, and are generally vague by design.

This specific issue was examined in detail in a composite analysis of published literature on proxy decision making. The analysis is revealing in that only 16 publications were available that provided empirical data concerning decision making. The outcomes were even more compelling. Not only were patient-designated decision makers (68% accurate) no better than those chosen by state law (69% accurate), there was also no improvement in surrogate accuracy when patients had discussed their treatment preferences with their surrogates. This same study did confirm that

Table 18.5   Landmark Legal Principles in End-of-Life Ethics

- Competent patients have a right to determine how their bodies can be used
- Informed consent is required prior to therapeutic interventions
- Competent patients have a right to refuse interventions
- In the absence of competence, surrogates may act on the best interests of patients
- Surrogates have the authority to refuse any and all interventions on behalf of patients
- In the absence of known patient wishes, decision making can proceed using a best interest standard if the burden of an intervention outweighs its benefit
- Individual states have the authority to set the level of evidence required to determine the prior wishes of an incompetent patient

Adapted from Reference 81.

patient surrogates were more accurate than physicians in making patient choices, thus affirming the role of the surrogate in substituted judgment[82] (**Level II-2**).

Much of the current literature on end-of-life care has come from the ICU literature, a clinical setting where death and dying are both common and frequently dramatic. One of the more recent paradigm changes coming from the ICU literature is the idea of family-centered care. Patient autonomy has been one of the basic fundamentals of medicine in the United States, but autonomy requires that the patient be capable of participating in discussion and decision making with a clear sensorium. Terminally ill patients are little different than critical care patients in this regard, many are limited in their cognitive capability due to effects from the disease itself (brain metastases, endotracheal intubation), or from side effects of treatment to palliate symptoms (narcotics, sedatives). To resolve this potential impasse, the model of family-centered care places the patients at the center of a web of relationships between themselves, traditional family, and extended support. In this way, a comprehensive model of care emerges that can lead to more effective management and outcome.[83, 84]

The most difficult decision concerning end-of-life decisions is one that requires either the withdrawal or withholding of care. The current U.S. opinion concerning this causes significant contention and vehement disagreement within the medical community, but is fortunately consistent throughout the legal system. There are three principles that address directly to terminal care:

1. Withholding and withdrawing life support are equivalent.
2. There is an important distinction between killing and allowing to die.
3. The doctrine of "double effect" provides an ethical rationale for providing relief of pain and other symptoms with sedatives even when this may have the foreseen (but not intended) consequence of hastening death.[85–88]

The specifics of these three principles are outlined nicely in a 2008 publication in the critical care literature.[81] The specifics lay the foundation for compassionate care of the terminally ill without fear of retribution or legal harassment. What the authors do codify is that clear and concise documentation of the intentions of the treating physician is the primary factor in determining whether or not care falls within the boundaries of propriety. It may be that these principles are not needed, and recent publications argue that terminal sedation and analgesia does not hasten death,[89–91] but their statement does allow for open discussion of very sensitive topics.

EVIDENCE SUMMARY

The following points have been discussed in this chapter and are arranged here in order of quality for summary purposes:

Level I
- Addition of megestrol acetate to chemotherapy to prevent weight loss does not result in improved overall survival in lung cancer patients.
- Megestrol acetate is as effective as eicosapentaenoic acid nutritional supplements or dronabinol at increasing weight gain.
- Loss of >40% of lean body mass is a direct predictor of survival.
- Bisphosphonates are the treatment of choice in tumor-induced hypercalcemia.
- TIPS is highly effective at reducing portal hypertension and improving sodium excretion in patients with portal venous congestion.
- Opioids are effective and compassionate at alleviating breathlessness in terminally ill patients.

Level II-1
- Octreotide acetate resulted in more rapid removal of nasogastric suction and improved nausea control compared to corticosteroids.
- Acupuncture can reduce the number of treatment-related episodes and the need for rescue antiemetic medication among chemotherapy patients.
- Sustained-release morphine improves dyspnea and sleep in terminally ill cancer patients.
- Intravenous vitamin K is the most effective agent for correcting anticoagulation. Subcutaneous vitamin K can achieve normal INR within 72 hours in patients with upper GI malignancy—50% of patients are successful at resolving hemorrhage with vasopressin infusions.

Level II-2
- Pamidronate provides for more prolonged control of hypercalcemia compared to clodronate.
- Acupuncture combined with vitamin B6 is superior to either acupuncture alone or vitamin B6 alone in managing chemotherapy-induced nausea and vomiting.
- Heliox can reduce the work of breathing in ventilated patients.
- Despite being cancer free, a population of patients never regain their former energy level, and in fact, the fatigue may worsen with time.
- Patient surrogates are more accurate than physicians in making patient choices.

Level II-3
- Overall survival in terminally obstructed cancer patients is shortened by the addition of TPN to end-of-life treatments.

Level III
- Less than 25% of terminally ill ovarian cancer patients have adequate documentation of DNR orders at the time of their terminal admission.
- Patients with terminal bowel obstructions tolerate surgery poorly.
- Operative mortality approaches 44% when two negative predictors are present in malignant bowel obstructions.
- Only 30% of patients who receive surgery for MBO achieve success (defined as the ability to tolerate oral intake).
- Colonic stent placement is successful in 77% of obstructed ovarian cancer patients, and 56% of patients will require additional surgical intervention.
- Nasogastric suction can serve as a test for the effectiveness of percutaneous gastrostomy in terminally ill patients.
- Furosemide therapy should not be considered in the treatment of cancer-related hypercalcemia.
- Opioid rotation and laxative escalation to manage constipation lack high quality data.
- Immunotherapy holds promise as effective at managing recalcitrant ascites.
- Non-invasive ventilation can improve communication between patients and caregivers when terminal respiratory compromise is present. Combining midazolam with morphine may further improve dyspnea hemostatic agents to control bleeding in terminally ill patients are more effective than balloon tamponade.

REFERENCES

1. EARLE CC, NEVILLE BA, LANDRUM MB, et al. Trends in the aggressiveness of cancer care near the end of life. J Clin Oncol 2004;22(2):315–321.
2. ZHANG B, WRIGHT AA, HUSKAMP HA, et al. Health care costs in the last week of life: associations with end-of-life conversations. Arch Intern Med 2009;169(5):480–488.
3. VON GRUENIGEN V, FRASURE H, REIDY AM, et al. Clinical disease course during the last year in ovarian cancer. Gynecol Oncol 2003;90:619–624.
4. JADAD AR, BROWMAN GP. The WHO analgesic ladder for cancer pain management. Stepping up the quality of its evaluation. JAMA 1995;274(23):1870–1873.
5. WOOLF CJ, SALTER MW. Neuronal plasticity; increasing the gain in pain. Science 2000;288:1765–1769.
6. HALL P, SCHRODER C, WEAVER L. The last 48 hours of life in long-term care: a focused chart audit. J Am Geriatr Soc 2002;50:501–506.
7. PAYEN JF, BRU O, BOSSON JL, et al. Assessing pain in critically ill sedated patients by using a behavioral pain scale. Crit Care Med 2001;29:2258–2263.
8. AISSAOUI Y, ZEGGWAGH AA, ZEKRAOUI A, et al. Validation of a behavioral pain scale in critically ill, sedated, and mechanically ventilated patients. Anesth Analg 2005;101:1470–1476.
9. YOUNG J, SIFFLEET J, NIKOLETTI S, et al. Use of a Behavioural Pain Scale to assess pain in ventilated, unconscious and/or sedated patients. Intensive Crit Care Nurs 2006;22:32–39.

10. CAMPBELL ML, RENAUD E, VANNI L. Psychometric testing of a Pain Assessment Behavior Scale. Paper presented at: Midwest Nursing Research Society, Cincinnati, OH, March 2005.
11. HEYLER L and EASSON AM. Surgical approaches to malignant bowel obstruction. J Sup Oncol 2008;6(3):105–113.
12. RIPAMONTE C and BRUERA E. Palliative management of malignant bowel obstruction. Int J Gynecol Cancer 12:135–143.
13. TAOREL PG, FABRE JM, PRADEL JA, et al. Value of CT in the diagnosis and management of patients with suspected acute small bowel obstruction. Am J Roentgenol 1995;165:1187–1192.
14. BEALL D, FORTMAN B, LAWLER B, et al. Imaging bowel obstruction: a comparison between fast magnetic resonance imaging and helical computed tomography. Clin Radiol 2002;57: 719–724.
15. SURI S, GUPTA S, SUDHAKER P, et al. Comparative evaluation of plain films, ultrasound and CT in the diagnosis of intestinal obstruction. Acta Radiol 1999;40:422–428.
16. PECTASIDES D, KAYIANNI H, FACOU A, et al. Correlation of abdominal computed tomography scanning and second-look operation finding in ovarian cancer patients. Am J Clin Oncol 1991;14:457–462.
17. DE BREE E, KOOPS W, KROGER R, et al. Peritoneal carcinomatosis from colorectal or appendiceal origin: correlation of preoperative CT with intraoperative findings and evaluation of interobserver agreement. J Surg Oncol 2004;86:64–73.
18. JACQUEST P, JELINEK J, STEVES M, et al. Evaluation of computed tomography in patients with peritoneal carcinomatosis. Cancer 1993;72:1631–1636.
19. HELYER LK, LAW CH, BUTLER M, et al. Surgery as a bridge to palliative chemotherapy in patients with malignant bowel obstruction from colorectal cancer. Ann Surg Oncol 2007;14:1264–1271.
20. Report of the National Confidential Enquiry into Perioperative Deaths 1996/1997. NCEPOD.
21. KREBS H, GOPELRUD D. Surgical management of bowel obstruction in advanced ovarian carcinoma. Obstet Gynecol 1983;61:327–330.
22. FERNANDES J, SEYMOUR R, SUISSA S. Bowel obstruction inpatients with ovarian cancer: a search for prognostic factors. Am J Obstet Gynecol 1988;158:244–249.
23. TEKKIS P, KINSMAN R, THOMPSOM M, et al. The Association of Coloproctology of Great Britain and Ireland study of large bowel obstruction caused by colorectal cancer. Ann Surg 2004;240: 76–81.
24. BAINES MJ. ABC of palliative care: nausea, vomiting, and intestinal obstruction. BMJ 1997;315: 1148–1150.
25. PARKER MC, BAINES MJ. Intestinal obstruction in patients with advanced malignant disease. Br J Surg 1996;83:1–2.
26. POTHURI B, MEYER L, GERARDI M, et al. Reoperation for palliation of recurrent malignant bowel obstruction in ovarian carcinoma, Gynecol Oncol 2004;95:193–195.
27. MERCADANTE S, RIPAMONTI C, CASUCCIO A, et al. Comparison of octreotide and hyoscine butylbromide in controlling gastrointestinal symptoms due to malignant inoperable bowel obstruction. Support Care Cancer 2000;8:188–191.
28. RIPAMONTI C, MERCADANTE S, GROFF L, et al. Role of octreotide, scopolamine butylbromide and hydration in symptom control of patients with inoperable bowel obstruction and nasogastric tubes: a prospective randomized trial. J Pain Symptom Manage 2000;19:23–34.
29. MYSTAKIDOU K, TSLIKA E, KALAIDOPOULOU O, et al. Comparison of octreotide administration vs conservative treatment in the management of inoperable bowel obstruction in patients with far advanced cancer: a randomized double blind, controlled clinical trial. Anticancer Res 2002;22:1187–1192.
30. MERCADANTE S, AVOLA G, MADDALONI S, et al. Octreotide prevents the pathological alterations of bowel obstruction in cancer patients. Support Care Cancer 1996;4:393–394.
31. BHARDWAJ R, PARKER M. Palliative therapy of colorectal carcinoma: stent or surgery? Colorectal Dis 2003;5:518–521.
32. TILNEY H, LOVEGROVE R, PURKAYASTHA S, et al. Comparison of colonic stenting and open surgery for malignant large bowel obstruction. Surg Endosc 2007;21:225–233.

33. KHOT UP, LANG AW, MURALI K, et al. Systematic review of the efficacy and safety of colorectal stents. Br J Surg 2002;89:1096–1102.

34. CACERES A, ZHOU Q, IASONOS A, et al. Colorectal stents for palliation of large-bowel obstructions in recurrent gynecologic cancer: An updated series. Gynecol Oncol 2008;108:482–485.

35. MATEENA F, JATOIB A. Megestrol acetate for the palliation of anorexia in advanced, incurable cancer patients. Clin Nutr 2006;25:711–715.

36. LOPRINZI CL, ELLISON NM, SCHAID DJ, et al. Controlled trial of megestrol acetate for the treatment of cancer anorexia and cachexia. J Natl Cancer Inst 1990;82:1127–1132.

37. ROWLAND KM, LOPRINZI CL, SHAW EG, et al. Randomized double-blind placebo-controlled trial of cisplatin and etoposide plus megestrol acetate/placebo in extensive-stage small cell lung cancer: a North Central Cancer Treatment Group study. J Clin Oncol 1996;14:135–141.

38. JATOI A, ROWLAND K, LOPRINZI CL, et al.; North Central Cancer Treatment Group. An eicosapentaenoic acid supplement versus megestrol acetate versus both for patients with cancer-associated wasting: a North Central Cancer Treatment Group and National Cancer Institute of Canada collaborative effort. J Clin Oncol 2004;22:2469–2476.

39. JATOI A, WINDSCHITL HE, LOPRINZI CL, et al. Dronabinol versus megestrol acetate versus combination therapy for cancer-associated anorexia: a North Central Cancer Treatment Group study. J Clin Oncol 2002;20:567–573.

40. American College of Physicians-Position Paper. Parenteral nutrition in patients receiving cancer chemotherapy. Ann Int Med 1989;110(9):734–736.

41. KOTLER DP, TIERNEY AR, WANG J, et al. Magnitude of body cell mass depletion and the timing of death from wasting in AIDS. Am J Clin Nutr 1989;50:444–447.

42. BRARD L, WEITZEN S, STRUBEL-LAGAN SL, et al. The effect of total parenteral nutrition on the survival of terminally ill ovarian cancer patients. Gynecol Oncol 2006;103:176–180.

43. GRILL V, HO P, BODY JJ, et al. Parathyroid hormone-related protein: elevated levels in both humoral hypercalcemia of malignancy and hypercalcemia complicating metastatic breast cancer. J Clin Endocrinol Metab 1991;73:1309–1315.

44. GRILL V, RANKIN W, MARTIN TJ. Humoral hypercalcemia of malignancy: the discovery of PTHrP. In: BODY JJ, editor. Tumor Bone Diseases and Osteoporosis in Cancer Patients: Pathophysiology, Diagnosis and Therapy. New York, NY: Marcel Dekker; 2000. p 21–40.

45. BODY JJ, DELMAS PD. Urinary pyridinium crosslinks as markers of bone resorption in tumor-associated hypercalcemia. J Clin Endocrinol Metab 1992;74:471–475.

46. LEGRAND S, LESKUSKI D, ZAMA I. Narrative review: furosemide for hypercalcemia: an unproven yet common practice. Ann Intern Med 2008;149:259–263.

47. O'ROURKE NP, MCCLOSKEY EV, VASIKARAN S, et al. Effective treatment of malignant hypercalcaemia with a single intravenous infusion of clodronate. Br J Cancer 1993;67:560–563.

48. PUROHIT OP, RADSTONE CR, ANTHONY C, et al. A randomised double-blind comparison of intravenous pamidronate and clodronate in the hypercalcaemia of malignancy. Br J Cancer 1995;72:1289–1293.

49. BODY JJ, LORTHOLARY A, ROMIEU G, et al. A dose-finding study of zoledronate in hypercalcemic cancer patients. J Bone Miner Res 1999;14:1557–1561.

50. YOU Q, YU H, WU D, et al. Vitamin B6 points PC6 injection during acupuncture can relieve nausea and vomiting in patients with ovarian cancer. Int J Gynecol Can 2009;19(4):567–571.

51. EZZO J, VICKERS A, RICHARDSON MA, et al. Acupuncture-point stimulation for chemotherapy-induced nausea and vomiting. J Clin Oncol 2005;23:7188–7198.

52. GOTTSCHLING S, REINDL TK, MEYER S, et al. Acupuncture to alleviate chemotherapy-induced nausea and vomiting in pediatric oncology—a randomized multicenter crossover pilot trial. Klin Padiatr 2008;220:365–370.

53. MILES CL, FELLOWES D, GOODMAN ML, et al. Laxatives for the management of constipation in palliative care patients. Cochrane Database Syst Rev 2006;4:CD003448. DOI: 10.1002/14651858. CD003448.pub2.

54. KLASCHIK E, NAUCK F, OSTGATHE C. Constipation—modern laxative therapy. Support Care Cancer 2003;11:679–685.

55. QUIGLEY C. Opioid switiching to improve pain relief and drug tolerability. Cochrane Database Syst Rev 2004;3:CD004847.

56. SAAB S, NIETO JM, LY D, et al. TIPS versus paracentesis for cirrhotic patients with refractory ascites. Cochrane Database Syst Rev 2006;18(4):CD004889.

57. BEREK JS, HACKER NF, LICHTENSTEIN A, et al. Intraperitoneal recombinant alpha 2 interferon for salvage immunotherapy in persistent epithelial ovarian cancer. Cancer Treat Rev 1985;12(suppl B):23–32.

58. RATH U, KAUFMANN M, SCHMID H, et al. Effect of intraperitoneal recombinant human tumour necrosis factor alpha on malignant ascites. Eur J Cancer 1991;27:121–125.

59. KATANO M, TORISU M. New approach to management of malignant ascites with a streptococcal preparation, OK-432, II: intraperitoneal inflammatory cell-mediated tumor cell destruction. Surgery 1983;93:365–373.

60. BEATTIE GJ, SMYTH JF. Phase I study of intraperitoneal metalloproteinase inhibitor BB94 in patients with malignant ascites. Clin Cancer Res 1998;4:1899–1902.

61. LOW JA, JOHNSON MD, BONE EA, et al. The matrix metalloproteinase inhibitor batimastat (BB-94) retards human breast cancer solid tumor growth but not ascites formation in nude mice. Clin Cancer Res 1996;2:1207–1214.

62. NUMNUM TM, ROCCONI RP, WHITWORTH J, et al. The use of bevacizumab to palliate symptomatic ascites in patients with refractory ovarian carcinoma. Gynecol Oncol 2006;102:425–428.

63. HAMILTON CA, MAXWEL GL, CHERNOFSKY M, et al. Intraperitoneal bevacizumab for the palliation of malignant ascites in refractory ovarian cancer. Gynecol Oncol 2008;111(3):530–532.

64. EL-SHAMI K, ELSAID A, EL-KERM Y. Open-label safety and efficacy pilot trial of intraperitoneal bevacizumab as palliative treatment in refractory malignant ascites. J Clin Oncol 2007; 25(18S).

65. SCHWARTZSTEIN RM, et al. Cold facial stimulation reduces breathlessness induced in normal subjects. Am Rev Respir Dis 1987;136:58–61.

66. BOOTH S, et al. The use of oxygen in the palliation of breathlessness. A report of the Expert Working Group of the Scientific Committee of the Association of Palliative Medicine. Respir Med 2004;98:66–77.

67. BRUERA E, SCHOELLER T, MACEACHERN T. Symptomatic benefit of supplemental oxygen in hypoxemic patients with terminal cancer: the use of the N of 1 randomized controlled trial. J Pain Symptom Manage 1992;7:365–368.

68. BOOTH S, MOOSAVI SH, HIGGINSON IJ. The etiology and management of intractable breathlessness in patients with advanced cancer: a systematic review of pharmacological therapy. Nat Clin Prac Oncol 2008;5(2):90–100.

69. NAVA S, ESQUINAS A, FERRER M, et al. Multicenter, randomized study of the use of non-invasive ventilation (NIV) vs. oxygen therapy (O_2) in reducing respiratory distress in end-stage cancer patients. American Thoracic Society's International Conference Proceedings, 2008.

70. JENNINGS AL, DAVIES AN, HIGGINS JP, et al. A systematic review of the use of opioids in the management of dyspnoea. Thorax 2002;57:939–944.

71. ABERNETHY A, CURROW DC, FRITH P, et al. Randomised, double blind, placebo controlled crossover trial of sustained release morphine for the management of refractory dyspnoea. BMJ 2003;327:523–528.

72. NAVIGANTE AH, CERCHEITTI LC, CASTRO MA, et al. Midazolam as adjunct therapy to morphine in the alleviation of severe dyspnea perception in patients with advanced cancer. J Pain Symptom Manage 2006;31:38–47.

73. AHMEDZAI SH, LAUDE E, ROBERTSON A, et al. A double blind, randomised, controlled phase II trial of Heliox28 gas mixture in lung cancer patients with dyspnoea on exertion. Br J Cancer 2004;90:366–371.

74. KOHARA H, UEOKA H, AOE K, et al. The effect of nebulized furosemide in terminally ill cancer patients with dyspnoea. J Pain Symptom Manage 2003;26:962–967.

75. SHIMOYAMA N, SHIMOYAMA M. Nebulized furosemide as a novel treatment for dyspnea in terminal cancer patients. J Pain Symptom Manage 2002;23:73–76.

76. STONE P, KUROKAWA A, TOOKMAN A, et al. Nebulized frusemide for dyspnoea. Palliat Med 1994;8:258.

77. CELLA DF, TULSKY DS, GRAY G, et al. The functional assessment of cancer therapy scale: development and validation of the general measure. J Clin Oncol 1993;11:570–579.

78. SMETS EM, GARSSEN B, BONKE B, et al. The multidimensional fatigue inventory (MFI) psychmoetric qualities of an instrument to assess fatigue. J Psychosom Res 1995;39:315–325.

79. FLETCHNER H, RUEFFER JU, HENRY-AMAR M, et al. Quality of life assessment in Hodgkins Disease: a new comprehensive approach. Ann Oncol 1998;9(suppl 5):S147–S154.

80. CARR D, GOUDAS L, LAWRENCE D, et al. Management of cancer symptoms: pain, depression, and fatigue. Evidence Report/Technology Assessment No. 61. AHRQ Publication No. 02-E032. Rockville, MD: Agency for Healthcare Research and Quality; 2002.

81. TRUOG RD, CAMPBELL ML, CURTIS JR, et al. Recommendations for end-of-life care in the intensive care unit: a consensus statement by the American Academy of Critical Care Medicine. Crit Care Med 2008;36(3):953–963.

82. SHALOWITZ DI, GARRETT-MAYER E, DAVID WENDLER D. The accuracy of surrogate decision makers. Arch Intern Med 2006;166:493–497.

83. Institute of Medicine. Committee on Care at the End of Life: Approaching Death. Washington, DC: National Academy Press; 1997.

84. National Consensus Project for Quality Palliative Care. Clinical Practice Guidelines for Quality Palliative Care. Pittsburgh, PA: National Consensus Project; 2004.

85. QUILL TE, DRESSER R, BROCK DW. The rule of double effect—A critique of its role in end-of-life decision making. N Engl J Med 1997;337:1768–1771.

86. LO B, RUBENFELD G. Palliative sedation in dying patients: "We turn to it when everything else hasn't worked." JAMA 2005;294:1810–1816.

87. QUILL TE. The ambiguity of clinical intentions. N Engl J Med 1993;329:1039–1040.

88. SULMASY DP. Commentary: double effect—intention is the solution, not the problem. J Law Med Ethics 2000;28:26–29.

89. SYKES N, THORNS A. Sedative use in the last week of life and the implications for end-of life decision making. Arch Intern Med 2003;163:341–344.

90. SYKES N, THORNS A. The use of opioids and sedatives at the end of life. Lancet Oncol 2003;4:312–318.

91. CHAN JD, TREECE PD, ENGELBERG RA, et al. Narcotic and benzodiazepine use after withdrawal of life support: association with time to death? Chest 2004;126:286–293.

92. BRUNDAGE MD, BEZJAK A, DIXON P, et al. The role of palliative thoracic radiotherapy in non-small cell lung cancer. Can J Oncol 1996;6(suppl 1):25–32.

93. Medical Research Council Lung Cancer Working Party. A Medical Research Council (MRC) randomised trial of palliative radiotherapy with two fractions or a single fraction in patients with inoperable non-small-cell lung cancer (NSCLC) and poor performance status. Br J Cancer 1992;65:934–941.

94. HOSKIN PJ. Radiotherapy in symptom management. In: DOYLE D, HANKS GWC, MACDONALD N, editors.Oxford Textbook of Palliative Medicine 2nd ed. New York: Oxford University Press; 1998: 278–280.

95. LANGENDIJK JA, TEN VELDE GP, AARONSON NK, et al. Quality of life after palliative radiotherapy in non-small cell lung cancer: a prospective study. Int J Radiat Oncol Biol Phys 2000;47: 149–155.

96. BURNETT DA, RIKKERS LF. Nonoperative emergency treatment of variceal hemorrhage. Surg Clin North Am 1990;70:291–306.

97. WHITLING AM, BUSSEY HI, LYONS RM. Comparing different routes and doses of phytonadione for reversing excessive anticoagulation. Arch Intern Med 1998;158:2136–2140.

98. NEE R, DOPPENSCHMIDT D, DONOVAN DJ, et al. Intravenous versus subcutaneous vitamin K1 in reversing excessive oral anticoagulation. Am J Cardiol 1999;83:286–288, A6–A7.

99. ALLUM WH, BREARLEY S, WHEATLEY KE, et al. Acute haemorrhage from gastric malignancy. Br J Surg 1990;77:19–20.

100. PEREIRA J, PHAN T. Management of bleeding in patients with advanced cancer. Oncologist 2004;9:561–570.
101. DEAN A, TUFFIN P. Fibrinolytic inhibitors for cancer-associated bleeding problems. J Pain Symptom Manage 1997;13:20–24.
102. DE BOER WA, KOOLEN MGJ, ROOS CM, et al. Tranexamic acid treatment of haemothorax in two patients with malignant mesothelioma. Chest 1991;100:847–848.
103. KAUFMAN B, WISE A. Antifibrinolytic therapy for haemoptysis related to bronchial carcinoma. Postgrad Med J 1993;69:80–81.
104. COOPER DL, SANDLER AB, WILSON LD, et al. Disseminated intravascular coagulation and excessive fibrinolysis in a patient with metastatic prostate cancer: response to epsilon aminocaproic acid. Cancer 1992;70:656–658.
105. SHPILBERG O, BLUMENTHAL R, SOFER O, et al. A controlled trial of tranexamic acid therapy for the reduction of bleeding during treatment of acute myeloid leukemia. Leuk Lymphoma 1995;19:141–144.
106. AVVISATI G, BULLER HR, TEN CATE JW, et al. Tranexamic acid for control of haemorrhage in acute promyelocytic leukaemia. Lancet 1989;2:122–124.
107. HASHIMOTO S, KOIKE T, TATEWAKI W, et al. Fatal thromboembolism in acute promyelocytic leukemia during all-trans retinoic acid therapy combined with antifibrinolytic therapy for prophylaxis of hemorrhage. Leukemia 1994;8:1113–1115.
108. COMROE JH. Some theories on the mechanism of dyspnea in breathlessness. In: CAMPBELL E, HOWELL JBL, editors. Proceedings of an International Symposium Held on 7 and 8 April 1965 under the Auspices of the University of Manchester. London: Blackwell Scientific; 1966.

Index